Immunopharmacology

AF794183

Comprehensive Immunology

Series Editors: ROBERT A. GOOD and STACEY B. DAY
Sloan-Kettering Institute for Cancer Research
New York, New York

---

1 Immunology and Aging
Edited by TAKASHI MAKINODAN and EDMOND YUNIS

2 Biological Amplification Systems in Immunology
Edited by NOORBIBI K. DAY and ROBERT A. GOOD

3 Immunopharmacology
Edited by JOHN W. HADDEN, RONALD G. COFFEY, and FEDERICO SPREAFICO

4 The Immunopathology of Lymphoreticular Neoplasms
Edited by J. J. TWOMEY and ROBERT A. GOOD

Immunopharmacology

Edited by
JOHN W. HADDEN and RONALD G. COFFEY
Sloan-Kettering Institute for Cancer Research
New York, New York

and
FEDERICO SPREAFICO
"Mario Negri" Institute for Pharmacological Research
Milan, Italy

Springer Science+Business Media, LLC

Library of Congress Cataloging in Publication Data

Main entry under title:

Immunopharmacology.

(Comprehensive immunology; 3)
Includes index.
1. Immune response–Regulation. 2. Immunotherapy. 2. Cyclic nucleotides. I. Hadden, John W. II. Coffey, Ronald G. III. Spreafico, Federico. IV. Series. [DNLM: 1. Immunology. 2. Pharmacology. 3. Immunochemistry. 4. Endocrinology. W1 Co4523 v. 3/QW504 I366]
QR186.I47 615.7 77-23915

ISBN 978-1-4615-7251-0 ISBN 978-1-4615-7249-7 (eBook)
DOI 10.1007/978-1-4615-7249-7

© Springer Science+Business Media New York 1977
Originally published by 1977 Plenum Publishing Corporation
Softcover reprint of the hardcover 1st edition 1977

All rights reserved

No part of this book may be reproduced, stored in a retrieval system, or transmitted, in any form or by any means, electronic, mechanical, photocopying, microfilming, recording, or otherwise, without written permission from the Publisher

Contributors

Alessandro Anaclerio Laboratory of Tumor Chemotherapy and Immunology, Istituto di Ricerche Farmacologiche "Mario Negri", Milan, Italy

K. Frank Austen Departments of Medicine, Harvard Medical School and the Robert B. Brigham Hospital, Boston, Massachusetts

Henry R. Bourne Division of Clinical Pharmacology, Departments of Medicine, Pharmacology, and the Cardiovascular Research Institute, University of California, San Francisco, California

Vincent P. Butler, Jr. Department of Medicine, Columbia University College of Physicians and Surgeons, New York, New York

Charles B. Carpenter Immunology Laboratory, Renal Division, Department of Medicine, Peter Bent Brigham Hospital and Harvard Medical School, Boston, Massachusetts

Ronald G. Coffey Laboratory of Immunopharmacology, Memorial Sloan-Kettering Cancer Center, New York, New York

Philip Coffino Division of Clinical Pharmacology, Departments of Medicine and Microbiology, University of California, San Francisco, California

Philip Davies Merck Institute for Therapeutic Research, Rahway, New Jersey

Lilian Delmonte Memorial Sloan-Kettering Cancer Center, New York, New York

Arthur Englard Laboratory of Immunopharmacology, Memorial Sloan-Kettering Cancer Center, New York, New York

James R. Gavin, III Department of Internal Medicine, Barnes Hospital, Washington University School of Medicine, St. Louis, Missouri

Elizabeth Gillespie Division of Clinical Immunology, The Johns Hopkins University School of Medicine at The Good Samaritan Hospital, Baltimore, Maryland

Edward J. Goetzl Departments of Medicine, Harvard Medical School and the Robert B. Brigham Hospital, Boston, Massachusetts

John W. Hadden Laboratory of Immunopharmacology, Memorial Sloan-Kettering Cancer Center, New York, New York

Louis J. Ignarro Department of Pharmacology, Tulane University School of Medicine, New Orleans, Louisiana

Paul A. Insel Division of Clinical Pharmacology, Departments of Medicine, Pharmacology, and the Cardiovascular Research Institute, University of California, San Francisco, California

Frederick A. Kuehl, Jr. Merck Institute for Therapeutic Research, Rahway, New Jersey

Kenneth L. Melmon Division of Clinical Pharmacology, Departments of Medicine, Pharmacology, and the Cardiovascular Research Institute, University of California, San Francisco, California

Elliott Middleton, Jr. Allergy Laboratories, Buffalo General Hospital, State University of New York at Buffalo, Buffalo, New York

Herbert F. Oettgen Memorial Sloan-Kettering Cancer Center, New York, New York

Robert J. Perper Merck Institute for Therapeutic Research, Rahway, New Jersey

Edgar Pick Department of Human Microbiology, Tel Aviv University Sackler School of Medicine, Tel Aviv, Israel

Tak C. Poon Division of Clinical Pharmacology, Departments of Medicine, Pharmacology, and the Cardiovascular Research Institute, University of California, San Francisco, California

G. M. Shearer Immunology Branch, National Cancer Institute, National Institutes of Health, Bethesda, Maryland

Jocelyn Spragg Departments of Medicine, Harvard Medical School and the Robert B. Brigham Hospital, Boston, Massachusetts

Federico Spreafico Laboratory of Tumor Chemotherapy and Immunology, Istituto di Ricerche Farmacologiche "Mario Negri", Milan, Italy

Terry B. Strom Immunology Laboratory, Renal Division, Department of Medicine, Peter Bent Brigham Hospital and Harvard Medical School, Boston, Massachusetts

James Watson Department of Medical Microbiology, College of Medicine, University of California, Irvine, California

Yacob Weinstein Division of Clinical Pharmacology, Departments of Medicine, Pharmacology, and the Cardiovascular Research Institute, University of California, San Francisco, California; present address: Department of Hormone Research, Weizmann Institute of Science, Rehovot, Israel

Introduction

Immunopharmacology: A New Discipline of Immense Potential

Among the looming triumphs of the biologic revolution is the rapidly developing understanding of the mechanisms of bodily defense. In the short span of 35 years, knowledge of immunologic machinery has progressed from crudest description to major understanding in cellular and molecular terms. Antibodies, immunoglobulins, and the complement system have been almost completely defined in detailed molecular terms. Organs, like thymus, spleen and lymph nodes—so long enigmatic black boxes—are beginning to be understood not only in cellular terms but in molecular, physiologic, and endocrinologic terms.

With this surging new information about the immune system comes the possibility of developing a pharmacology which can modulate and control immunologic functions. Immunopharmacology most broadly conceived must address (1) control of development and function of the cellular components of the immunologic apparatus; (2) facilitation and suppression of function of the immunologically competent cells of the several subclasses, like T helpers, suppressors, and effectors, and B effectors and suppressors; (3) manipulation and repair of the major biologic amplification systems, e.g., the complement system and kinin-kallikrein system, and (4) utilization, modulation, and inhibition of the galaxy of molecules generated by T lymphocytes, the lymphokines. This new pharmacology must deal with the fundamental effector mechanisms of immunity, namely inflammation, phagocytosis, vascular reactivity, and blood coagulation. Furthermore, immunopharmacology must address and manipulate cell–cell communication and interaction, so vital to control of the immunological apparatus.

This volume represents a major effort by leaders from outstanding laboratories who are feverishly working to develop the field of immunopharmacology. The editors have brought together much that is extant in this rapidly developing science. From the studies and perspectives collected in this volume one can recognize that a vigorous new discipline is taking shape.

Evidence that thymic hormones can drive stem cells through a succession of differentiative steps by selective gene action to the several classes and subclasses of functional T cells is already at hand (Komuro and Boyse, 1973; G. Goldstein *et al.*,

1977; Incefy and Good, 1976; Storrie *et al.*, 1976). As an example, both mouse and human precursors can be differentiated by thymopoietin (G. Goldstein *et al.*, 1977; Schlesinger and Goldstein, 1975) by processes which involve several steps, each of which utilizes RNA and protein synthesis, which seem to be separated by quantal proliferations (Touraine *et al.*, 1977). Hormones that can exercise powerful influences on lymphoid cellular development are rapidly becoming well defined molecules. They carry names like thymopoietin (Schlesinger and Goldstein, 1975), thymosin α_1 (A. L. Goldstein *et al.*, 1977), and Facteur serique thymique (Bach *et al.*, 1977). Some of these molecules are relatively simple peptides which have been fully defined and which contain very short amino acid sequences (active sites) of extraordinary biologic activity. These short sequences and a variety of congeners that will be generated by enterprising chemists will become drugs for this new immunopharmacology. The immunopharmacologic development, I am sure, will present vistas of immense potential. I feel certain we will soon be speaking of an immunopharmacology that can control development and involution of the immunologic systems. It is difficult to predict how far this will go, but one can conceive of consequences that are immense. Control and manipulation of the development of antibody-producting cells has also begun, and the recent studies of Hämmerling *et al.*, (1976) employing the peptide molecule ubiquitin (Schlesinger *et al.*, 1975) to develop precursors to antibody-producing cells are encouraging. Similar progress in cellular and molecular terms can be seen in the studies of specific and nonspecific helper cells and suppressor molecules (Gershon, 1974; Tada, 1975; Kapp *et al.*, 1977; Waldmann *et al.*, 1974; Siegel *et al.*, 1976; Shou *et al.*, 1976; Schwartz *et al.*, 1977). The possibilities of using chemically defined adjuvants that can generate selectively helper T cells for IgG production while inducing suppressor T cells for IgE production promises at long last "immunization against allergy or unwanted immunity" as a product of the new immunopharmacology (Kishimoto and Ishizaka, 1975; Kishimoto *et al.*, 1976). Even defined sequences of the Fc portion of the IgE molecule already elucidated could represent exciting immunopharmaceuticals of great potential (Hamburger, 1975).

As impressive as they are, these extraordinary achievements may pale before pharmacological developments which are coming from molecular analysis of those powerful agents called lymphokines. Among these are some of the most active molecules known. Studies of the cellular and molecular control of lymphokine generation and release, for example, the molecular and cellular basis of their action on macrophages, are developing rapidly. Inquiry into and understanding of the language by which these fascinating molecules "talk" to the granular leukocytes, macrophages, and platelets represents a major challenge. It seems clear from several communications in this volume that substantial progress has been made in this important segment of the new discipline of immunopharmacology.

Furthermore, ingenious model systems have been developed to study in broad perspective as well as in fine detail the processes of immunopotentiation, immunomodulation, and immunostimulation. Better understanding of the controls that underlie activation to involvement in inflammation of platelets, macrophages, mast cells, and eosinophils, and stimulation of these cells to deliver or secrete their cellular production is developing rapidly. This surge too promises to provide real bases for a powerful pharmacology and, ultimately, for drug development.

Progress toward understanding of the molecular basis of cell–cell interactions and communication, the role of the cell membrane in cell interactions and communication, the details of hormonal influences on the physical state and chemistry of the membranes, the nature of the surface-to-nuclear signals generated by membrane perturbations that lead to either proliferation or differentiation and secretion, perhaps more than any of the developments in this field, proceeds so rapidly it is difficult to project its trajectory. Can the Yin-Yang concept of Goldberg *et al.*, (1974) concerning the cyclic nucleotides be harnessed to control cellular behavior? Will study of the prostaglandins really have a big payoff in cellular control? These are important questions to be answered by this research.

We can be certain that these fundamental pharmacological analyses will ultimately yield new and powerful means of prediction, manipulation, and control of the vital immunological apparatus. There is little question, from studying the chapters of this volume and the immense literature they reflect, that the field of immunopharmacology has a good start and extraordinary growth potential. It holds great promise for control of those vital immunological processes, which, in the aggregate, ensure our individuality. We can all look forward with excitement to the further development of this important new discipline.

Robert A. Good

References

Bach, J. F., Dardenne, M., and Pleau, J.-M., 1977, *Nature* **266**:55–56.

Gershon, R. K., 1974, in: *Contemporary Topics in Immunobiology,* Vol. 3 (M. D. Cooper and N. L. Warner, eds.), pp. 1–40, Plenum, New York.

Goldberg, N. D., Haddox, M. K., Dunham, E., Lopez, C., and Hadden, J. W., 1974, in: *Control of Proliferation in Animal Cells* (B. Clarkson and R. Baserga, eds.), pp. 609–626, Cold Spring Harbor Press, Cold Spring Harbor.

Goldstein, A. L., Low, T. L. K., McAdoo, M., McClure, J., Thurman, G. B., Rossio, J., Lai, C.-Y., Chang, D., Wang, S.-S., Harvey, C., Ramel, A. H., and Meienhofer, J., 1977, *Proc. Natl. Acad. Sci. U.S.A.* **74**:725–729.

Goldstein, G., Scheid, M., Boyse, E. A., Brand, A., and Gilmour, D. G., 1977, *Cold Spring Harbor Symp. Quant. Biol.* **41**:5–8.

Hamburger, R. N., 1975, *Science* **189**:389–390.

Hämmerling, U., Chin, A. F., and Abbott, J., 1976, *Proc. Natl. Acad. Sci. U.S.A.* **73**:2008–2012.

Incefy, G. S., and Good, R. A., 1976, in: *Immune Reactivity of Lymphocytes: Development, Expression and Control* (M. Feldman and A. Globerson, eds.), pp. 41–50, Plenum, New York.

Kapp, J. A., Cantor, H., Pierce, C. W., and Benacerraf, B., 1977, *Fed. Proc.* **36**:1224 (abstr.).

Kishimoto, T., and Ishizaka, K., 1975, *J. Immunol.* **114**:1177–1184.

Kishimoto, T., Hirai, Y., Suemura, M., and Yamamura, Y., 1976, *J. Immunol.* **117**:396–404.

Komuro, K., and Boyse, E. A., 1973, *J. Exp. Med.* **138**:479–482.

Schlesinger, D. H., and Goldstein, G., 1975, *Cell* **5**:361–365.

Schlesinger, D. H., Goldstein, G., and Niall, H. D., 1975, *Biochemistry* **14**:2214–2218.

Schwartz, S. A., Choi, Y. S., Shou, L., and Good, R. A., 1977, *J. Clin. Invest.* **59**:1176–1187.
Shou, L., Schwartz, S. A., and Good, R. A., 1976, *J. Exp. Med.* **143**:1100–1110.
Siegal, F. P., Siegal, M., and Good, R. A., 1976, *J. Clin. Invest.* **58**:109–122.
Storrie, B., Goldstein, G., Boyse, E. A., and Hämmerling, U., 1976, *J. Immunol.* **116**:1358–1362.
Tada, T., 1975, in: *Proceedings of the Ninth Leukocyte Culture Conference* (A Rosenthal, ed.), p. 771, Academic Press, New York.
Touraine, J. L., Hadden, J. W., and Good, R. A., 1977, *Proc. Natl. Acad. Sci. U.S.A.* (in press).
Waldmann, T. A., Durm, M., Broder, S., Blackman, M., Blaese, R. M., and Strober, W., 1974, *Lancet* 2:609–613.

Contents

Chapter 1

Cyclic Nucleotides in Lymphocyte Proliferation and Differentiation 1

John W. Hadden

1. Introduction 1
2. Cyclic Nucleotide Biochemistry 2
3. Hormonal and Pharmacological Modulation of Lymphocyte Proliferation 4
4. Cyclic Nucleotides in the Early Events of Mitogenic Action 9
5. Calcium in the Early Events of Mitogenic Action 12
6. Other Components of Mitogenic Action 13
7. Lymphocyte Nuclear Activation and Cyclic Nucleotides 15
8. Cyclic GMP and Calcium as the Intracellular Mitogen Signal 18
9. Hormone Induction of Thymocyte Differentiation 20
10. Cyclic Nucleotides in Thymocyte Differentiation 22

References 25

Chapter 2

Involvement of Cyclic Nucleotides as Intracellular Mediators in the Induction of Antibody Synthesis 29

James Watson

1. Introduction 29
2. Induction and Paralysis 30
3. Effect of Cyclic Nucleotides on the Induction of Antibody Synthesis 32
4. Mitogen-Induced B-Lymphocyte Proliferation: Immunologic Effects 34
5. Cyclic Nucleotides and B-Lymphocyte Proliferation and Differentiation 37

References 43

Chapter 3
Regulation of Alloimmunity by Cyclic Nucleotides 47
Terry B. Strom and Charles B. Carpenter

1. Introduction 47
2. Cyclic Nucleotides 47
3. Pharmacological Abrogation of Target-Cell Lysis Mediated by Cytotoxic T Lymphocytes 48
4. Pharmacological Augmentation of Target-Cell Lysis Mediated by Cytotoxic T Lymphocytes 50
5. Pharmacological Abrogation of K-Cell-Mediated Lysis of Antibody-Coated Target Cells (Antibody-Dependent Lymphocyte-Mediated Cytotoxicity 52
6. Pharmacological Augmentation of K-Cell-Mediated Lysis by Cyclic GMP 52
7. Modulation of Graft-vs.-Host Proliferation by Cyclic Nucleotides 52
8. Modulation of Mixed Lymphocyte Culture Proliferation by Cyclic Nucleotides 53
9. Discussion 54
References 58

Chapter 4
Regulation of Polymorphonuclear Leukocyte, Macrophage, and Platelet Function 61
Louis J. Ignarro

1. Introduction 61
2. Polymorphonuclear Leukocytes (Neutrophils) 62
3. Mononuclear Phagocytes (Macrophages) 71
4. Platelets 74
5. Summary and Conclusions 81
References 83

Chapter 5
Molecular Aspects of Macrophage Activation and Proliferation 87
John W. Hadden and Arthur Englard

1. Introduction 87
2. Macrophage Activation *in Vivo* 87
3. Macrophage Activation *in Vitro* 91
4. Mechanism of Action of Macrophage Mitogenic Factor 95
5. Lysosomal Enzyme Induction in the Mediation of Macrophage Activation 95
6. Other Mechanisms of Macrophage Activation 97
7. Summary 97
References 98

Chapter 6
Pharmacological Control of Mediator Release from Leukocytes 101
Elizabeth Gillespie

1. Introduction 101
2. General Properties of Histamine Release 101
3. Mechanism of Action of Antigen 107
4. The Phenomenon of Desensitization 108
5. Release of Mediators Other Than Histamine 108
6. Summary 110
References 110

Chapter 7
Generation, Function, and Disposition of Chemical Mediators of the Mast Cell in Immediate Hypersensitivity 113
Edward J. Goetzl and K. Frank Austen

1. Introduction 113
2. Generation and Release of Chemical Mediators 114
3. Characteristics of the Chemical Mediators 115
4. Modulation of Mediators of Immediate Hypersensitivity 120
5. Summary 122
References 123

Chapter 8
Plasma Factors: The Hageman-Factor-Dependent Pathways and the Complement Sequence 125
Jocelyn Spragg and K. Frank Austen

1. Introduction 125
2. Hageman-Factor-Dependent Pathways 125
3. Complement 133
4. Interactions with Other Mediator Systems 138
5. Pharmacological Modulation 138
References 139

Chapter 9
Prostaglandins in the Regulation of Immune and Inflammatory Responses 145
Frederick A. Kuehl, Jr.

1. Introduction 145
2. Biological Function of the Prostaglandins 147
3. Inflammatory and Immunologic Diseases 149
4. Summary and Speculation 157
References 159

Chapter 10

Lymphokines: Physiologic Control and Pharmacological Modulation of Their Production and Action **163**

Edgar Pick

1. Introduction: What Are Lymphokines? 163
2. Macrophage Migration-Inhibitory Factor (MIF) 165
3. Macrophage Activation 178
4. Evidence for a Role of MIF *in Vivo* 179
5. Physiologic Control of MIF 181
6. Pharmacological Modulation of MIF 182
7. Physiologic Control and Pharmacological Modulation of Other Lymphokines 187
8. *In Vivo* Realities—Role of Lymphokines in Immunity and Nonimmunologic Processes 195

References 197

Chapter 11

Mechanism of Action of Antiallergic Drugs and Relationship of Cyclic Nucleotides to Allergy **203**

Ronald G. Coffey and Elliott Middleton, Jr.

1. Introduction 203
2. Cyclic Nucleotide Metabolism and Actions 204
3. Pathophysiology of Asthma 207
4. Drugs Used in Treatment of Asthma 212
5. Summary and Speculation 219

References 221

Chapter 12

Modulation of the Expression of the Immune Response by Antiinflammatory Drugs **227**

Robert J. Perper and Philip Davies

1. Introduction 227
2. Effect of Antiinflammatory Agents on Lymphocytes and the Immune Response 228
3. Neutrophils 233
4. Macrophages 234
5. Conclusions 240

References 241

Chapter 13
Immunosuppressive Agents 245
Federico Spreafico and Alessandro Anaclerio

1. Introduction and General Remarks 245
2. Steroids 249
3. Azathioprine and 6-Mercaptopurine 254
4. Cyclophosphamide 257
5. Other Chemical Immunodepressants and the Problem of Selective Immunosuppression 264
6. Nonspecific Biological Immunodepressants 267
7. Perspective for Immunologic Control 272
References 274

Chapter 14
Mechanisms of Immunopotentiation 279
John W. Hadden, Lilian Delmonte, and Herbert F. Oettgen

1. Introduction 279
2. Biological Substances 280
3. Chemical Immunopotentiators 292
4. Products of the Immune System 299
5. Conclusions 304
References 305

Chapter 15
Immunoassay of Drugs and the Biological Use of Antidrug Antibodies 315
Vincent P. Butler, Jr.

1. Introduction 315
2. Production of Antidrug Antibodies 316
3. Characterization of Antidrug Antibodies 317
4. Use of Antibodies in Immunoassays 321
5. Biological Properties of Antibodies to Drugs and to Other Compounds of Pharmacological Importance 326
References 328

Chapter 16
Receptors for Low-Molecular-Weight Hormones on Lymphocytes 331
Kenneth L. Melmon, Yacob Weinstein, Tak C. Poon, Henry R. Bourne, G. M. Shearer, Philip Coffino, and Paul A. Insel

1. Introduction 331

2. Determination of the 'Physiologic' Importance of Leukocyte Receptors 332
3. Somatic Genetic Analysis of Cyclic AMP Action as a Means of Assessing Receptor Function 334
4. Separation of Cells on the Basis of a Physiologic Function 339
5. Conclusions 353
References 354

Chapter 17

Polypeptide Hormone Receptors on Lymphoid Cells: Application to the Study of Receptor Alterations and Radioreceptor Assay of Polypeptide Hormones 357

James R. Gavin, III

1. Introduction 357
2. Existence of Insulin Receptors on Circulating Cells 360
3. Characteristics of the Insulin Receptor on Lymphoid Cells 369
4. Effects of Insulin on Lymphoid Cells 370
5. Existence of Human Growth Hormone (hGH) Receptors on Lymphoid Cells 373
6. Existence of Calcitonin Receptors on Human Lymphoid Cells 375
7. Radioreceptor Assay of Polypeptide Hormones Using Lymphoid Cell Receptors 376
8. Further Applications of Polypeptide Hormone Receptors on Lymphoid Cells 381
9. Conclusions 384
References 384

Chapter 18

Assays for Cyclic Nucleotides Including Clinical Applications 389

Ronald G. Coffey

1. Introduction 389
2. Extraction, Purification, and Measurement of Cyclic Nucleotides 390
3. Clinical Applications 401
References 407

Index 413

1

Cyclic Nucleotides in Lymphocyte Proliferation and Differentiation

JOHN W. HADDEN

1. Introduction

The last fifteen years have seen a marked increase in the experimental evidence supporting the central roles played by cyclic nucleotides in the regulation of diverse processes in cells and tissues of organisms throughout the plant and animal kingdom. Beginning with the observations of Sutherland and Rall (1960) that indicated that cyclic 3′,5′-adenosine monophosphate (cAMP) mediates the intracellular action of epinephrine and glucagon to induce glycogenolysis in liver, the concept of the cAMP "second messenger" system has been generalized to virtually every cell of the mammalian organism, and the system has been linked to the induction and regulation of central cellular processes in these cells. In general, cAMP participates in those processes that involve the promotion of preprogrammed events consistent with the differentiated phenotype, i.e., the dominant functions for which that cell type is developed—for the liver, glucose production from glycogen stores; for the adrenal gland, steroid production; for fat tissue, lipolysis; and so on.

Since 1970, another candidate for a second messenger system has emerged: cyclic 3′,5′-guanosine monophosphate (cGMP). cGMP would appear to be as ubiquitously distributed in nature as cAMP, and the biological events to which it has been linked appear, in general, to oppose in function those linked to cAMP. The apparent contrasting roles of the two cyclic nucleotides, the only two consistently found in nature, was recently cast in a dualism hypothesis of biological regulation (Goldberg *et al.*, 1974). While admittedly tentative in its presentation, this hypothesis, in offering a balanced view of cellular regulation, has provided useful guidelines for experimental approaches.

JOHN W. HADDEN • Laboratory of Immunopharmacology, Memorial Sloan-Kettering Cancer Center, New York, New York 10021.

The initial concepts of the cyclic nucleotides as intracellular messengers derived principally from studies of how hormones or hormonelike agents that act at the cell surface induce a particular biological event through the intracellular production of the cyclic nucleotide. The cyclic nucleotide initiates the biological event inside the cell by activating one or another intracellular biochemical process. Since these first concepts were developed, it has become apparent that the cyclic nucleotides are involved in mediating a number of environmental influences and factors, in addition to hormones. Such diverse influences include temperature, pH, contact, nutrient availability, growth-promoting substances, growth inhibitors, differentiation-inducing factors, and a number of nonhormone factors involved in inflammation, intercellular communication, and environmental recognition. Indeed, the cyclic nucleotides have taken a central role in the emergence of a broad field of interdisciplinary interest in the cell surface as the translator of diverse environmental cues into intracellular instructions involved in events ranging from the regulation of cellular homeostasis to that of cellular proliferation and maturation. The emergence of the cell surface as a dominant issue in cellular regulation has introduced the concept of a balanced interaction between the cellular environment as translated by the cell surface and genetic determinants housed in the nucleus. This interactive concept has provided considerable impetus to the study of cyclic nucleotides in the regulation of nuclear processes related to the initiation and modification of genetic transcription. In no field has this concept of the regulatory roles played by cyclic nucleotides had more impact than in immunology. This chapter will attempt to deal with the development of cyclic nucleotide pharmacology as it pertains specifically to the proliferation and differentiation of lymphocytes related to the thymus, i.e., the thymus-derived T lymphocyte and its precursor, the prothymocyte.

2. Cyclic Nucleotide Biochemistry

As preface to the subject of this chapter, a review of certain aspects of cyclic nucleotide biochemistry appears relevant. cAMP and cGMP are both present in lymphocytes, and their levels depend on the source of the cells. In general, cAMP levels are detected at 1–60 pmol/mg protein and, with our techniques, approximate 11, 27, and 8 pmol/mg protein for lymphocytes from spleen, peripheral blood, and thymus, respectively. Similar values were reported by M. Bach (1975). cGMP levels for lymphoid tissues have varied considerably in literature reports, from 0.02 to 2 pmol/mg protein; with our methods, they average 0.5, 0.3, and 0.2 pmol/mg protein for spleen, peripheral blood, and thymus, respectively. These levels must be considered in light of the sample size and the methods used for cell purification for the extraction and purification techniques, and for cyclic nucleotide assay. Such considerations are important in evaluating the varying levels reported in the literature for these different lymphocyte populations. Based on measurements of comparable sample size (10^6 lymphocytes/ml), cAMP levels in lymphoid cells average 10- to 100-fold greater than those of cGMP.

The cyclic nucleotides are produced from their corresponding 5′-triphosphates, ATP and GTP, by specific cyclic nucleotide cyclases termed *adenylate cyclase* and *guanylate cyclase*, respectively. These enzymes differ in their optimum cation requirements—magnesium for adenylate cyclase and calcium and manganese for guanylate cyclase. They also differ in their degree of plasma membrane association.

The greater part of adenylate cyclase (approximately 90%) appears to be associated with the plasma membrane, while the remainder may be soluble. Recent experiments suggest that a small portion may be associated with the nuclear membrane and be activated differently from the plasma membrane cyclase (Parker *et al.*, 1974). Direct activators of adenylate cyclase in lymphocytes include β-adrenergic catecholamines such as isoproterenol and epinephrine, prostaglandin E_1 (PGE_1), and sodium fluoride. Guanylate cyclase, in contrast, appears to be mainly soluble and approximately 70% cytoplasmic (Deviller *et al.*, 1975), and the membrane-associated enzyme may be more easily solubilized than adenylate cyclase on disruption of cells. Like its activity in other tissues (Schultz *et al.*, 1975), guanylate cyclase activity of lymphoid cells is dependent on calcium (Katagiri *et al.*, 1976). No direct stimulant of guanylate cyclase of lymphocytes has been reported; however, indirect stimulation was observed with phytohemagglutinin (PHA) (Deviller *et al.*, 1975) and concanavalin A (Con A) (Katagiri *et al.*, 1976). The cyclic nucleotides are catabolized by the appropriate cyclic nucleotide phosphodiesterases to their respective 5′-monophosphates. The cAMP phosphodiesterase of lymphocytes is stimulated by imidazole (MacManus and Whitfield, 1971) and cGMP and inhibited by caffeine (Whitfield *et al.*, 1971). Although the cGMP phosphodiesterase was not examined directly, it is thought to be inhibited by imidazole (Hadden *et al.*, 1975a,b). In addition, a number of agents alter cyclic nucleotide levels in lymphocytes, but have not been specifically studied as to their biochemical actions.

The intracellular actions of the cyclic nucleotides in lymphocytes have received inadequate attention to date. The general assumption is that the action of cAMP in lymphocytes, as in other tissues, is mediated by activation of a protein kinase that, when liberated from its regulatory subunit, to which cAMP binds, phosphorylates various protein substrates and leads to their enzymatic activation. cAMP-dependent protein kinases have been isolated from lymphocytes, and have been demonstrated to phosphorylate protein substrates common to those phosphorylated by protein kinases from other tissues (Farago *et al.*, 1973; E. M. Johnson *et al.*, 1975b). Induced increases in cAMP yield glycogenolysis in lymphocytes (Hadden *et al.*, 1971a,c), a process that in liver has been established to result from protein-kinase-mediated phosphorylation and activation of phosphorylase, which catalyzes glycogen breakdown. Also, in experiments with intact lymphocytes, cAMP has been related to phosphorylation of nonnuclear proteins (Wedner and Parker, 1975). These observations indicate that the action of cAMP in lymphocytes is linked to protein kinase activation and the phosphorylation of protein substrates. A number of observations indicate that cAMP may modulate processes that do not involve a protein kinase. These processes include the inhibition of phosphorylation of nuclear proteins (E. M. Johnson and Hadden, 1975), the inhibition of glucose and potassium transport (Hadden *et al.*, 1971b; Coffey *et al.*, 1975a), the enhancement of RNA synthesis (Cross and Ord, 1971; Hirschhorn *et al.*, 1970; Webb *et al.*, 1973a) and of gluconeogenesis (Hadden *et al.*, 1971a), and the inhibition of phosphoribosyl pyrophosphate (PRPP) synthetase activity (Chambers *et al.*, 1974). A variety of potential actions of cAMP may be possible, and the conservative hypothesis that cAMP-dependent protein kinase represents the only mechanism appears to be unnecessarily restrictive. Much investigation is warranted, particularly in the area of direct demonstration of enzymatic pathways influenced by cAMP in lymphocytes.

The actions of cGMP in lymphocytes are similarly assumed to involve a cGMP-dependent protein kinase analogous (but opposite) in function to the cAMP enzyme. cGMP in lymphocytes has been indirectly linked to the phosphorylation of nonhistone acidic nuclear proteins (E. M. Johnson and Hadden, 1975), thus suggesting such a mechanism; however, no publication concerning a cGMP-dependent protein kinase in lymphocytes has appeared to date. Other processes indirectly linked to cGMP in lymphocytes that may or may not involve this phosphorylation mechanism include glycogen accumulation (Hadden *et al.*, 1971c) and increased RNA and protein synthesis (Hadden *et al.*, 1975b; L. Johnson and Hadden, 1975). At least two direct actions of cGMP on enzymes have been observed that do not appear to depend on a phosphorylation mechanism: cGMP stimulation of PRPP synthetase (Chambers *et al.*, 1974) and RNA polymerase (L. Johnson and Hadden, unpublished observations). Without a comparable body of experimental evidence as exists for cAMP on which to evaluate the action of cGMP in lymphocytes, it appears premature to suggest that the action of cGMP is restricted to any particular single mode.

With this introduction to the biochemistry of cyclic nucleotide generation, action, and catabolism in lymphocytes, we will now deal with their history and current status as they relate to lymphocyte proliferation and differentiation. It is relevant to point out before this discussion, however, that this area is not without its controversial aspects. In an effort to ensure fair representation of what might be considered opposing views of the data accumulated to date, the reader is referred to other recent reviews (Parker *et al.*, 1974; MacManus *et al.*, 1975). Within the perspective of this chapter, certain controversial aspects will be noted.

3. Hormonal and Pharmacological Modulation of Lymphocyte Proliferation

The mature circulating lymphocyte is a resting cell (restricted "G_1") the biology of which includes, among other responses, clonal proliferation on exposure to antigen. Clonal proliferation provides an expansion process by which a few antigen-sensitive cells can generate a multitude of responding cells. *In vivo,* this expansion process is characterized by the transformation of small lymphocytes into large lymphocytes with abundant pyroninophilic cytoplasm and large euchromatic nuclei with prominent nucleoli. The culture of human lymphocytes *in vitro* and their study following stimulation to proliferate and transform by plant lectins such as PHA has enjoyed a growing experimental following since the early 1960s (see Ling and Kay, 1975), and as the corresponding growth in cAMP-related studies in the other cell types developed in the late 1960s, it became natural to question the role played by cAMP in lymphocyte proliferation in these circumstances. The first experiments concerning the role of cyclic nucleotides in lymphocyte proliferation dwelt on an analysis of the effects of cyclic nucleotides and agents that increased cellular cyclic nucleotide levels when they were added to cultures of human peripheral blood lymphocytes.

3.1. Agents That Increase Cyclic AMP

The initial experiments of May *et al.* (1970), Hirschhorn *et al.* (1970) and Hadden *et al.* (1970) indicated that isoproterenol, an activator of adenylate cyclase, cAMP, and theophylline, an inhibitor of cAMP phosphodiesterase, when added concomitantly with the mitogen PHA, inhibited lymphocyte proliferation (as measured by tritiated thymidine incorporation). A minor effect of cAMP and theophylline, that of increasing background thymidine incorporation in lymphocytes not stimulated by PHA, was noted by Hirschhorn *et al.* (1970) and others (Rigby and Ryan, 1970; Webb *et al.*, 1973a). While it became apparent that cAMP and its dibutyryl derivative could augment PHA-induced proliferation under certain circumstances dependent on such factors as concentration of the nucleotide and the absence of serum (Gallo and Whang-Peng, 1971; McCrery and Rigby, 1972; Webb *et al.*, 1973b), many laboratories (L. D. Johnson and Abell, 1970; Rigby and Ryan, 1970; Smith *et al.* 1971; Webb *et al.*, 1973b) confirmed the initial observation that agents that increase cAMP levels inhibit mitogen-induced lymphocyte proliferation.

These initial experiments were designed with the assumption that the addition of these agents did indeed result in an accumulation of lymphocyte levels of cAMP. The initial measurements of lymphocyte adenylate cyclase and cellular cAMP levels by Smith *et al.* (1971), Makman (1971), and Novogrodsky and Katchalski (1970) indicated that agents such as isoproterenol and prostaglandin PGE_1 stimulated adenylate cyclase directly and induced accumulation of cAMP in lymphocytes, and that this accumulation was augmented in the presence of a phosphodiesterase inhibitor such as theophylline. It was not until Webb *et al.* (1973b) measured lymphocyte cAMP levels under the influence of exogeneously added cAMP that it became apparent that extracellular cAMP and even cGMP could lower intracellular cAMP levels. In retrospect, it has become clear that under experimental circumstances most closely approximating the physiologic, agents that increase cAMP in lymphocytes are not mitogenic and are inhibitory to a variety of mitogenic stimuli (for further reviews of this topic, see Abell and Monahan, 1973; Hadden *et al.*, 1975b; Ling and Kay, 1975).

The circumstances under which this statement holds true refer quite specifically to the early events associated with the induction of proliferation by the mitogen. It should be noted that preincubation of lymphocytes with an agent such as isoproterenol or cAMP followed by the removal of the agent may enhance the proliferative response to a mitogen added subsequently (L. D. Johnson and Abell, 1970), and that addition of the agent more than 6 hr following the mitogen may have no effect (Smith *et al.*, 1971), or if in association with the late phases of the cell cycle, may augment proliferation (MacManus and Whitfield, 1969; Hadden *et al.*, 1970).

This antiproliferative role of cAMP demonstrated in lymphocytes conforms to that observed in a variety of cellular systems in which the initiation of proliferation has been studied (see Pastan *et al.*, 1975), and is consistent with the hypothesized role of cAMP in the maintenance of the differentiated, nonproliferative state. A natural question arises: if, as is the case in most tissues, cAMP is involved with the initiation of preprogrammed cellular events consistent with the differentiated nonproliferative state, what then are these events for the lymphocytes? While the answer to this question has not been obtained, certain insights that are reviewed later in this chapter indicate that cAMP is involved in the process of lymphocyte differentiation.

It is important to note that the biology of the lymphocyte is intimately related to proliferation, and it is the process of antigen-induced clonal proliferation that is thought to be the major mechanism for generating an immune response. The lymphocyte then appears to be an exception to most other tissues in that its dominant response appears to be antagonized rather than promoted by cAMP. As is attested to by other chapters in this volume, it appears that cAMP participates as a negative regulator of the functions of virtually every cell involved in the expression of immune response, including the B lymphocyte, macrophage, polymorphonuclear and basophilic leukocyte, mast cell, and platelet.

3.2. Agents That Act on ATPase: α-Adrenergics and Insulin

With the knowledge that cAMP acts to antagonize the induction of lymphocyte proliferation, it became important to analyze the action and mechanism of action of hormone and hormonelike agents that do not act via cAMP and that might augment lymphocyte proliferation. In 1970, we observed that in addition to the antiproliferative effect exhibited by catecholamines acting through a β-adrenergic receptor mechanism, there existed a proliferation-augmenting action resulting from an α-adrenergic mechanism (Hadden *et al.,* 1970). Investigations oriented toward probing the mechanism of this action led to the observations that α-adrenergic stimulation augments glucose uptake and utilization, glycogen accumulation, and potassium transport in lymphocytes (Hadden *et al.,* 1971a–c; Coffey *et al.,* 1975a), and to the observation that norepinephrine acts through an α-adrenergic mechanism to directly stimulate adenosine triphosphatases (ATPases) of isolated lymphocyte plasma membranes (Coffey *et al.,* 1975a). These ATPases represent a variety of membrane enzymes based on function and cation dependence, and are generally considered to consist of at least three separate systems, a Mg^{2+}-, Na^{+}-, and K^{+}-dependent enzyme involved in the efflux of Na^{+} and influx of K^{+}; a Ca^{2+}-dependent enzyme involved in active Ca^{2+} efflux; and a Mg^{2+}-dependent enzyme involved in Mg^{2+} influx (and perhaps glucose transport). While effects of cAMP to indirectly inhibit these enzymes and their functions have been observed, the relationship of the cyclic nucleotides to these transport-linked enzymes remains unclear at this time. The action of norepinephrine has been linked to cGMP in vas deferens (Schultz *et al.,* 1975) and in platelets (see Chapter 4); to date, however, this link has not been reported in lymphocytes, nor has a direct link of cGMP to membrane ATPases been established.

Another agent shown to act on lymphocytes is insulin. Insulin has been shown to augment glucose uptake and potassium and α-aminoisobutyrate transport in lymphocytes (Hadden *et al.,* 1972a; Goldfine *et al.,* 1972) and to augment lymphocyte proliferation in response to PHA and allogeneic stimulation (Weber, 1970; Pallavincini and Nichols, 1975), as well as "T"-lymphocyte cytotoxicity (Strom *et al.,* 1975a). Despite apparently clear-cut biological effects of insulin on lymphocyte functions, a controversy has developed over whether peripheral blood lymphocytes, prior to stimulation by phytomitogens such as PHA and Con A, have measurable insulin receptors (Gavin *et al.,* 1972a; Krug *et al.,* 1972). It would appear that the controversy rests on observations with lymphocytes prepared by different means. It has been demonstrated that lymphocyte insulin receptors are easily solubilized during cell preparation (Gavin *et al.,* 1972b), and that lymphocytes purified by nylon columns lack receptors (Krug *et al.,* 1972; Olefsky and Reaven, 1974). These observations do not preclude a small subpopulation that bears receptors or even the involvement of a nonlymphocyte mononuclear population, as has been suggested (Schwartz *et al.*, 1975). It appears feasible that the alterations of biological response of lymphocytes attributed to insulin might result from insulin action on nonlymphocytes such as macrophages to produce factors such as lymphocyte-activating factor (LAF), which in turn acts on lymphocytes (Gery *et al.*, 1972); however, that lymphoblasts of both the T and the B type have receptors for insulin (or an insulinlike substance) appears to be strong evidence for assuming that nondividing lymphocytes have insulin receptors but their detection is obscured either by certain methods of preparation of lymphocytes or by the ease of their shedding from the cell surface. (See Chapters 2 and 17 for further discussion of insulin effects and receptors.)

The mechanism of insulin action in augmenting lymphocyte functions has not been fully clarified. As has been observed in other tissues, actions of insulin in decreasing cAMP levels or in inhibiting its accumulation by other agents through inhibition of adenylate cyclase or stimulation of cAMP phosphodiesterase or both have not been studied critically in lymphocytes. In association with its ability to stimulate glucose and potassium uptake in density-gradient-prepared lymphocytes and in cell-line lymphoblasts, insulin directly stimulates a number of ATPases in isolated lymphoblast plasma membrane fractions (Hadden *et al.*, 1972a). Insulin action has been linked to cGMP accumulation (Goldberg *et al.*, 1974) in fibroblasts, an observation confirmed in fibroblasts (Jimenez de Asua *et al.*, 1975) and fat and liver (Illiano *et al.*, 1973). Our own unpublished observations (Hadden and Goldberg) indicate that insulin increases cGMP 2- to 3-fold in density-gradient-prepared lymphocytes. The action of insulin in augmenting lymphocyte functions may result from insulin actions on ATPase either in conjunction with or dissociated from its action to increase cellular cGMP levels. One important point concerning insulin action in relation to the biology of the immune response is that unlike the catecholamines and acetylcholine, for which a modulatory role can be easily developed in relation to the functions and activities of the autonomic nervous system, the action of insulin on lymphocytes may well be a tonic one that contributes to the integrity of the system and the effect of which is clearly discerned only *in vivo* in relation to the insulin-deficient state. Certainly, impairments of immunologic functions are implied by the greater susceptibility of the diabetic person to infection.

3.3. Agents That Increase Cyclic GMP

With the developing information implicating the sympathetic limb of the autonomic nervous system in the modulation of lymphocyte function, it seemed relevant to examine the possibility that the parasympathetic counterpart of this nervous system might also be involved. The relevance of this notion was provided by the observation of George *et al.* (1970) that the action of acetylcholine (ACh) is linked to cGMP. The action of ACh in the heart is opposite to that of the β-adrenergic catecholamines, i.e., depressed vs. augmented rate and force of contraction. While β-adrenergic stimulation has been linked by others to cAMP, Dr. Goldberg's group found that ACh increased cGMP and lowered cAMP levels in the heart. This observation constituted the first to suggest that cGMP represents another second messenger system.

In collaboration with Dr. Goldberg, we examined the possibility that ACh and therefore cGMP might be involved in the regulation of the function of lymphocytes.

We observed that ACh increased cGMP levels in lymphocytes and produced a modest augmentation of thymidine incorporation in PHA-stimulated lymphocytes (Goldberg *et al.*, 1973; Hadden *et al.*, 1974, 1975b). While not mitogenic itself in lymphocytes, ACh augmented RNA and protein synthesis in both PHA-stimulated and unstimulated lymphocytes. This action of ACh involves an atropine-sensitive muscarinic receptor mechanism, which implies that such effects *in vivo* would occur as a result of parasympathetic influences mediated by the vagus nerve.

This cholinergic action to augment proliferation of lymphocytes was confirmed by Strom *et al.* (1975b), and independently demonstrated to be involved in the augmentation of T-lymphocyte cytotoxicity (Strom *et al.*, 1972). Correspondingly, cholinergic stimulation augments antigen-induced lymphokine production (Hadden *et al.*, 1974).

We have been unable to show that ACh exerts any positive influence on the flux of calcium or the transport of nutrients in lymphocytes (Hadden *et al.*, 1975b), further suggesting that the action of ACh, unlike the actions of norepinephrine and insulin, is discretely linked to cGMP and does not involve transport-related mechanisms.

Pharmacological efforts to increase cGMP in lymphocytes through inhibition of cGMP phosphodiesterase and by exogenous addition of cGMP or its 8-bromo derivative to lymphocytes have offered further indication that cGMP is involved in the positive regulation of proliferation. Imidazole, a presumed cGMP phosphodiesterase inhibitor in lymphocytes, augments human lymphocyte proliferation induced by PHA, and augments both the background and PHA-induced proliferation of mouse splenic and thymic lymphocytes; it does so in close relationship with its ability to increase cGMP levels in the mouse cells (Hadden *et al.*, 1975a). While imidazole lowers cAMP in these cells, no correlation with proliferation exists. The actions of imidazole (10^{-7} M) in modifying both proliferation and cyclic nucleotide levels of lymphocytes are consistent with known effects of imidazole (10^{-3} M) on the cyclic nucleotide phosphodiesterases; these low-concentration effects cannot be interpreted to be mediated by phosphodiesterase, however, until appropriate measurements are performed.

Added cGMP or its derivatives are not mitogenic for human peripheral blood lymphocytes and do not augment PHA-induced proliferation (Hadden *et al.*, 1975b). In contrast, mouse spleen cells are augmented in their proliferation, and so significantly as to suggest that cGMP is directly stimulatory (Weinstein *et al.*, 1975). Diamantstein and Ulmer (1975b) suggested that cGMP does not act directly, but induces a factor from macrophages that mediates this proliferation-promoting action on lymphocytes. This factor is likely to be the LAF referred to earlier. On the basis of a number of observations to be developed in the next section, one would not expect cGMP to be directly mitogenic, since hormones acting through cGMP are not mitogenic. These observations do serve to underscore the notion that agents that act to increase cellular levels or turnover of cGMP augment proliferation induced by mitogenic agents.

The foregoing discussion on the influence of hormonal and pharmacological manipulations of cyclic nucleotide levels and lymphocyte proliferation was derived completely from *in vitro* studies. *In vivo* studies are needed to demonstrate the predicted modification of immunologic response that would result from such manipulations *in vivo* (i.e., overactivity or ablation of the sympathetic or parasympathetic limbs of the autonomic nervous system or overactivity or lack of pancreatic function). Not studied, either *in vitro* or *in vivo,* are the many other possible hormones that can be envisioned to influence the function of lymphocytes and other cells involved in the expression of immune response. Likely candidates appear to be pituitary growth hormone and thyroid hormone, since the integrity of both glands appears to be essential for the normal expression of immunity. Also likely are such hormones as the sex hormones, glucagon, prolactin, bradykinin, oxytocin, and parathormone, which have been demonstrated to modify the proliferation of thymocyte precursors (MacManus *et al.,* 1975; Morgan *et al.,* 1975). Perhaps more speculative is the possibility of a variety of hormonelike substances from the macrophage (e.g., LAF) and from the thymus that may act to modify T-lymphocyte proliferation through mediation of the cyclic nucleotides. It is evident from the foregoing presentation that the lymphocyte is a cell in which important questions concerning the influence and interactions of hormones and their mechanisms of action have been fruitfully studied. These studies have provided the basis for approaching the questions of how mitogens and other growth-inducing factors act to initiate cell division.

4. Cyclic Nucleotides in the Early Events of Mitogenic Action

The discovery that a number of mitogenic agents such as PHA and Con A could induce populations of resting thymus-derived lymphocytes to undergo blast transformation and to divide have provided the basis for in-depth experimental analyses of the early biochemical events of lymphocyte activation. The results of studies in this area have had considerable impact on the interdisciplinary efforts to understand the regulation of cellular proliferation (see Clarkson and Baserga, 1974).

Before the advent of cyclic-nucleotide-related research in this area, it was apparent that within minutes of stimulation of the lymphocyte by mitogenic agents such as PHA, a variety of cellular and nuclear processes are activated, and that within hours, RNA and protein synthesis increase, followed ultimately by DNA synthesis and cellular replication within 24 hr.

Several observations indicate that lymphocyte-triggering represents a discrete process in time and suggest that if the early events were understood, they might define how lymphocytes, in particular, and perhaps cells, in general, are triggered to divide. Studies on the interaction of PHA with lymphocytes indicated that:

1. PHA binds to lymphocytes within 30 min (Kay, 1971).
2. PHA could be applied to lymphocytes for short periods and the unbound PHA removed without significant reduction in proliferation measured 72 hr later (Soren, 1973).
3. Pharmacological agents introduced for short periods (1 hr) concomitant with PHA could modify the proliferative response measured at 72 hr (Hadden *et al.,* 1970).
4. PHA bound to Sepharose beads, and therefore not able to enter the cell, could initiate lymphocyte proliferation (Greaves and Bauminger, 1972).

These observations offered support for the hypothesis that PHA finds its final action at the cell membrane and there initiates events that ultimately yielded clonal proliferation.

4.1. Cyclic AMP

Smith *et al.* (1971) observed that PHA induced small increases in lymphocyte levels of cAMP within minutes of addition. Despite the otherwise contradictory evidence that nonmitogenic agents that induce similar increases in cAMP levels inhibit the induction of proliferation, this observation led to the hypothesis that cAMP is involved in the initiation of lymphocyte proliferation (see Parker *et al.*, 1974, for a review).

The initial observation of Smith *et al.* (1971) was apparently confirmed by the finding that PHA could activate adenylate cyclase of lymphoid cells (Winchurch *et al.*, 1971). A controversy ensued, however, when two laboratories employing a more highly purified PHA (PHA-P vs. PHA-M) could not demonstrate increases in levels of cAMP or of adenylate cyclase activity in lymphoid cells (Novogrodsky and Katchalski, 1970; Makman, 1971). Subsequently, it was confirmed that at optimal mitogenic concentrations, PHA-M did produce small increases in lymphocyte levels of cAMP, but that purified PHA-MR69 and Con A, at concentrations equally mitogenic, did not (Hadden *et al.*, 1972b). We suggested that the greater agglutinating potential of the impure PHA preparations was responsible for the cAMP increase. Since that suggestion was made, reports have continued to appear on both sides of the controversy (Krishnaraj and Talwar, 1973; DeRubertis *et al.*, 1974; Lyle and Parker, 1974; Webb *et al.*, 1975), even though more highly purified mitogenic substances were employed.

Rather than to recapitulate the technical differences of cell preparation and incubation and cyclic nucleotide assay procedures employed by those participating in this controversy, it seems relevant to conclude that mitogen-induced cAMP increases can occur and to discern under what biological conditions such increases are observed and analyze them within the perspective of correlated events that might or might not be related to the mitogenic signal.

It appeared to us that if PHA and Con A could increase cAMP levels in lymphocytes and if cAMP were antiproliferative, then perhaps mitogens lose their mitogenic action at high concentrations as a result of the generation of a countersignal related to cAMP.

A simple experimental approach to confirming this suggestion was provided by the work of Edelman and co-workers (Gunther *et al.*, 1973; Edelman, 1974). These workers purified and determined the structure of Con A and found that in its native form, it existed as a tetramer. They further found that succinylation of native Con A yields dimers with different biological activity. Importantly, succinylated Con A, in contrast to native Con A, does not exhibit a loss of proliferation-inducing capacity at high concentrations. We reasoned that these two forms of Con A might provide the tools to clarify the role of cAMP in mitogen action.

We (Hadden *et al.*, 1976) confirmed that succinylated Con A does not demonstrate a loss of mitogenic potential at concentrations up to 10 times the optimal mitogenic concentration for native Con A. The two preparations of Con A are equally mitogenic at 50 μg/ml under the culture conditions employed. In analyzing the effects of the two forms of Con A on lymphocyte levels of cAMP, we observed that native Con A produces negligible increases in cAMP levels at 25 μg/ml, but a progressive increase in cAMP levels at concentrations ranging up to 250 μg/ml. The concentration-dependent increase in cAMP induced by native Con A was inversely related to the degree of proliferation measured; i.e., the greater the concentration of Con A, the greater the cAMP increase and the less the proliferation. In contrast, succinylated Con A, over a concentration range of 25–250 μg/ml, produced no significant increase in cAMP. On the basis of these experiments, we suggested that supraoptimal concentrations of Con A inhibit proliferation as a result of an action to increase cAMP.

The foregoing observations appear to us to be ample evidence on which to conclude that cAMP acts in the lymphocyte, as in other models for the study of cellular proliferation, as an antiproliferative influence when the levels are increased in temporal association with the action of a mitogen. It is noteworthy that in the collected studies of the effects of PHA and Con A on lymphocyte cAMP levels, no consistent decreases in cAMP levels have been observed. This point is relevant to note, since in experiments with mitogenic agents in confluent (growth-inhibited) cells, these agents frequently produce a decrease in cAMP levels, and this decrease has been interpreted as an active signal in the induction of proliferation (see Pastan *et al.*, 1975).

4.2. Cyclic GMP

The search for a positive signal generated at the plasma membrane by mitogenic agents led us to investigate the possible role of cGMP in mitogen action. We observed that PHA-M, PHA-MR69, and Con A all produced early and significant increases in human peripheral blood lymphocyte levels of cGMP (Hadden *et al.*, 1972b). The increases were observable within 2 min, and the peak responses occurred at 20 min following mitogen addition. We found similar increases in confluent 3T3 fibroblasts induced to divide with insulin, serum, and phorbol myristate acetate (Goldberg *et al.*, 1974; Estensen *et al.*, 1974). These observations were confirmed by a number of laboratories with mitogen-stimulated lymphocytes (Heidrick, 1975; Schumm *et al.*, 1974; Webb *et al.*, 1975; Watson, 1975; Whitfield *et al.*, 1975; Katagiri *et al.*, 1976; Haddox *et al.*, 1976), fibroblasts (Armelin *et al.*, 1974; Seifert and Rudland, 1974; Rudland *et al.*, 1974; Jimenez de Asua, 1975; Moens *et al.*, 1975), uterus (Kuehl *et al.*, 1974), epidermal cells (Voorhees *et al.*, 1974), and salivary gland (Durham *et al.*, 1974). In virtually all these systems, the cGMP increases represent rapid and early increases of varying magnitude (from 2- to 70-fold), which return to or near control levels within 30 min.

Under the conditions in which the high-dose effects of Con A were studied in comparison to succinylated Con A (Hadden *et al.*, 1976), we observed that succinylated Con A produces comparable increases in cGMP over a concentration range from 25 to 250 μg/ml; however, native Con A from 50 to 250 μg/ml produces a concentration-dependent blunting of the increases in cGMP, suggesting that the progressive increases in cAMP observed under the latter conditions may have produced the blunted cGMP response. In general, the magnitude of cGMP increases induced by various concentrations of the two forms of Con A correlated with the degree of proliferation observed.

On the basis of our original observation (Hadden *et al.*, 1972b), we suggested that this increase in cGMP might represent an active signal for the induction of proliferation. It appears that in virtually every system that has been studied by laboratory workers with demonstrated ability to measure tissue levels of cGMP, increases have been observed in mitogen-stimulated cells. A few notable exceptions (Wedner *et al.*, 1975; Miller *et al.*, 1975; Burleson and Sage, 1976) are discussed in detail in Chapter 18.

5. Calcium in the Early Events of Mitogenic Action

Considerable general importance has been ascribed to calcium in the control of cellular activity (see Berridge, 1975), and the actions of lectin mitogens in stimulating lymphocytes have been extensively examined in this regard. Calcium is required to activate lymphocytes, particularly during the early times of the initiation process. The addition of EDTA or a chelator that is more selective for calcium, EGTA, inhibits the induction of proliferation by PHA (Alford, 1970; Whitney and Sutherland, 1973). This effect can be reversed with the addition of excess calcium and to a much lesser degree, magnesium. The dependency of mitogen action on the presence of calcium does not result from a requirement for calcium in receptor-binding, but rather from actions of the mitogen in influencing the interaction of extracellular calcium with the cell. Within the first 2 min (Freedman *et al.*, 1975), and certainly within the first 10 min (Hadden, unpublished observations), mitogens induce transient increases in cell-associated calcium (measured by ^{45}Ca uptake). The transient and reversible nature of these increases suggests that the calcium is briefly membrane-associated and does not actually enter the cell. Mitogens have an action that is apparent early—at 0 min using a technique involving at least a 10-min lag for washing (Whitney and Sutherland, 1972), or at 10 min using a filter technique (Hadden *et al.*, 1975b)—to induce an irreversible and progressive uptake of calcium by lymphocytes. This uptake measured at 1 hr has been correlated with proliferogenic potential of various lectins (Parker, 1974), and when inhibited with hydrocortisone or cAMP, it has been correlated with the degree of suppression of proliferation (Hadden *et al.*, 1975b; Freedman *et al.*, 1975). While no direct evidence has been presented to indicate that such uptake actually represents entry into the cell, the subsequent modification of a number of intracellular processes thought to be related to calcium certainly implies such an entry.

The understanding of the significance of this mitogen-induced calcium influx into lymphocytes was further advanced recently by experiments using a divalent cation ionophore (A23187, Lilly). This ionophore, which is known to activate a number of processes in various cells, was found to induce lymphocyte proliferation in a calcium-dependent manner (Maino *et al.*, 1974; Luckasen *et al.*, 1974). The ionophore was shown to induce calcium influx into lymphocytes in a manner comparable to its induction by lectin mitogens (Freedman *et al.*, 1975; Hadden, unpublished observations), thus suggesting that calcium influx alone may be the initial step in mitogenic action.

Of critical interest is the relationship that calcium influx may have to cGMP accumulation and turnover in lymphocytes, particularly since guanylate cyclase appears to be regulated by calcium (Katagiri *et al.*, 1976), and mitogens have not been demonstrated to directly activate guanylate cyclase of lymphocytes (Deviller *et al.*, 1975; Katagiri *et al.*, 1976). Lectin-mitogen-induced increases in cGMP appear to be dependent, in great part, on extracellular calcium (Whitfield *et al.*, 1975; Coffey *et al.*, 1975b). In addition, we observed that the calcium ionophore A23187 induces increases in lymphocyte levels of cGMP, and that it does so in a calcium-, but not magnesium-, dependent manner (Coffey *et al.*, 1975b). Further, inhibition of calcium uptake by hydrocortisone results in a corresponding reduction of cGMP accumulation in lymphocytes (Hadden and Goldberg, unpublished observations). These observations indicate that the presence of calcium and perhaps its influx are intimately linked with cGMP generation.

Certain observations suggest, however, that the influx of calcium may not be responsible for guanylate cyclase activation. These observations are that (1) mitogen-induced increases in cGMP levels in lymphocytes precede observable calcium influx and (2) cholingergic agents increase cGMP in lymphocytes without observable calcium influx (Hadden *et al.*, 1975b). The nature of the relationship between calcium and cGMP generation therefore remains to be clarified. It may well be that cholinergic or mitogenic activation of membrane-bound guanylate cyclase requires calcium as a cofactor, and that the influx of calcium occurs as an independent event induced by mitogenic but not by cholinergic stimulation.

6. Other Components of Mitogenic Action

We will present a brief discussion of other cell-surface-related events that have been attributed to mitogenic action; the reader is referred to Resch (1976) for a further discussion of these issues. These events may or may not relate to cGMP generation and calcium influx. In evaluating this body of information, a conservative hypothesis will be employed; i.e., if an action of a mitogen is not generally shared by other mitogens, then presumably that action is not essential for the induction of proliferation. This hypothesis assumes that lymphocytes are triggered to divide by only a single constellation of actions. While this approach is restrictive, it will allow the definition of, on one hand, the critical constellation and, on the other, the exceptions to the rule.

Among the early events associated with the binding of mitogenic lectins at the cell surface are certain phenomena related to the aggregation of receptors, and the formation of receptor patches and caps and their eventual removal from the cell surface. These events have been extensively examined in the laboratory of Dr. Gerald Edelman and were recently reviewed (Edelman, 1974). One interpretation of these findings is that because the succinylated form of Con A is equivalently mitogenic to native Con A and does not induce receptor cross-linking sufficient to allow or to induce gross patch formation and a colchicine-sensitive freezing of the membrane, these events are unrelated to mitogenic action. As suggested by these workers (Wang *et al.*, 1975) and supported by our cAMP observations (Hadden *et al.*, 1976), these events would appear to be related to actions of the mitogen that are antagonistic to the induction of proliferation. This interpretation implies that microtubular function *per se* is not directly related to the early events of mitogenic action. Following binding of the mitogen to cell-surface receptors, a variety of membrane changes have been observed to occur within 30 min. Changes related to phospholipid metabolism include increased incorporation of phosphate into phosphatidyl inositol and synthesis of phosphatidic acid (Fisher and Mueller, 1971), increased incorporation of fatty acid moieties into lecithin (Ferber *et al.*, 1974), and calcium-dependent activation of acyltransferase (Ferber and Resch, 1973; Ferber *et al.*, 1974). While the significance of these changes is not currently clear, it has been suggested that they are consistent with alterations that would relate to a more fluid and perhaps then more permeable membrane structure (Ferber *et al.*, 1974; Resch, 1976). Support for this suggestion using a variety of membrane probes to detect changes in membrane viscosity has been conflicting as to when they develop (Barnet *et al.*, 1974; Inbar and Shinitsky, 1975), making it difficult to assess the significance of this proposed membrane alteration at this time. On the basis of a variety of observations in other cell systems employed to study the induction of cellular proliferation, this proposal remains attractive to explain certain receptor-mobility and enzyme-activation phenomena and deserves rigorous experimental evaluation.

Among the changes observed in phospholipid metabolism, the preferential incorporation of arachidonic acid into lecithin and its subsequent liberation by phospholipase A (Resch *et al.*, 1971; Resch and Ferber, 1975) has interesting implications in terms of the possible role played by prostaglandins (PGs) in lymphocyte proliferation. Arachidonic acid represents the substrate for synthesis of PGs of both the E and F series, and it is generally recognized that the availability of arachidonic acid as substrate for prostaglandin synthesis represents the rate-limiting step in PG synthesis (see Chapter 9). The possibility exists that mitogens act to increase the level of arachidonic acid, which induces PG synthesis. That this synthesis is part of the triggering process for division appears unlikely, since if mitogens induce PG synthesis in lymphocytes, it does not occur early (Ferraris and DeRubertis, 1974), if it occurs at all (Jahng, 1975), and prevention of that synthesis with indomethacin, a PG synthetase inhibitor, does not block mitogen-induced proliferation and under certain circumstances may even augment it (Muscoplat *et al.*, unpublished observations). On the other hand, lymphocyte mitogens such as PHA and Con A do act on macrophages (Hadden *et al.*, unpublished observations), and macrophages represent a source of PGs (Bray *et al.*, 1975). It appears possible that the observations related to mitogen-induced PG synthesis may refer not to lymphocytes but to monocytes or macrophages that are also present in the mononuclear cell preparations. One explanation is that mitogen-induced macrophage PG synthesis and secretion may represent a feedback or suppressor influence on lymphocyte proliferation. This speculation is supported by the observations that PGE_1 inhibits lymphocyte proliferation (Smith *et al.*, 1971) and that under certain circumstances, the presence of macrophages inhibits the response of lymphocytes to mitogens (Folch and Waksman, 1973), an inhibition that is reversed by the removal of glass-adherent cells or the introduction of the PG synthesis inhibitor indomethacin (Muscoplat *et al.*, unpublished observations). While the role of PGs in lymphocyte proliferation, and in both helper and suppressor function for that matter, remains unclear, the observations of Yamamoto and Webb (1975) and Webb and Osheroff (1976) on the role of PGs in immune response *in vivo* indicates that considerably more work in this area is warranted.

In addition to changes in phospholipid metabolism, a number of membrane transport functions are altered in the lymphocyte early following mitogenic stimulation. These alterations include the increased transport of nutrients such as glucose (Peters and Hausen, 1971; Estensen *et al.*, 1974), choline, uridine, and leucine (Peters and Hausen, 1971), and α-aminoisobutyric acid (Vanden Berg and Betel, 1973). While an increase in the uptake of a large number of metabolites occurs, or can be envisioned to occur, within hours of the initiation of cellular proliferation, these early alterations in transport probably reflect direct changes in membrane function, and may relate to any or all of the following: alterations in membrane fluidity, membrane ATPase activities, and shifts in cations, particularly sodium.

Of the mechanisms that are possibly related to these alterations in transport, only the membrane ATPases have been studied to any extent. These membrane enzymes are involved in the transport of ions such as sodium, potassium, calcium, and magnesium, and perhaps nutrients such as sugars, amino acids, and nucleosides. Of these enzymes, only the Na^{+}–K^{+} transport enzyme has been extensively studied in lymphocytes. It has been observed that virtually immediately following addition of mitogen to lymphocytes, active, ouabain-sensitive K^{+} transport is increased (Quastel and Kaplan, 1970). The enzyme itself was shown to be activated when isolated from intact mitogen-stimulated lymphocytes, and Con A directly activates the enzyme in broken cell preparations (Novogrodsky, 1972). The significance of the activation of this enzyme system during mitogen stimulation in terms of alterations in cellular levels of Na^{+}, K^{+}, or ATP^{+}, of modified transmembrane potential, or of altered transport remains to be clarified; however, the general significance of K^{+} and ATP in particular in the regulation of cellular processes would indicate that a clearer understanding of these systems is needed.

With respect to these various changes in phospholipid transport and membrane ATPase activities, relatively little can be said about cyclic nucleotide involvement. It is generally considered that neither cyclic nucleotide is directly involved in these mechanisms. Evidence in the lymphocyte was presented to indicate that isoproterenol, an agent that increases levels of cAMP, antagonizes the transport of both glucose and potassium and does so in part through an indirect effect of cAMP in inhibiting the Na^{+}–K^{+} transport ATPase (Hadden *et al.*, 1972a; Coffey *et al.*, 1975a). In contrast, ACh, which increases cGMP levels in lymphocytes, does not increase transport of uridine, leucine, glucose, or K^{+} (Hadden *et al.*, 1975b, and unpublished observations). Thus, there may be inhibition of transport by cAMP in the absence of stimulation by cGMP. No other evidence directly links cGMP or calcium to these transports and their enzymatic processes; we therefore conclude that like the actions of insulin and norepinephrine (α-adrenergic), those of the mitogens on these processes represent independent, non-cyclic-nucleotide-related manifestations of their action at the cell surface. The ultimate role of these enzymes in the initiation of cellular proliferation remains to be determined.

7. Lymphocyte Nuclear Activation and Cyclic Nucleotides

Of the many processes considered to be involved in initiating cellular proliferation, those that occur in the nucleus early appear to be the most important. Several experiments have examined these early nuclear changes following the addition of either PHA or Con A to intact lymphocytes, and a number of processes have been observed to be modified within the first hour following stimulation. Those that occur within the first 15 min include the acetylation of histones, particularly the arginine-rich fraction (Pogo *et al.*, 1966), the phosphorylation of a number of acidic, nonhistone nuclear proteins (Kleinsmith *et al.*, 1966; E. M. Johnson *et al.*, 1974), an increase in RNA polymerase I activity (Pogo, 1972), and the synthesis of RNA (Pogo *et al.*, 1966), particularly ribosomal RNA (Cooper, 1970). While the interrelationship of these events has not been definitively established, a prevalent assumption is that the acetylation of histones and the phosphorylation of acidic proteins serve to unmask specific transcription sites on the DNA, and promote the initiation of RNA synthesis. The "primed" DNA is therefore available for any RNA polymerase I of nucleolar location (perhaps independently activated) to initiate ribosomal RNA synthesis.

While cyclic nucleotides have been observed to influence RNA synthesis in a number of systems, a direct effect of a cyclic nucleotide on a transcriptive enzyme was only recently described (L. Johnson and Hadden, 1975). In eukaryotic organisms, it has been hypothesized that many if not all biological effects of cyclic nucleotides are mediated by activation of specific cyclic-nucleotide-dependent protein kinases and the resultant phosphorylation of specific substrates. On the basis of observations of *Escherichia coli*, in which the cyclic nucleotides affect transcription by altering, with phosphorylation, the affinity of a receptor protein for the lac operon and thereby regulating the initiation of synthesis by RNA polymerase, it is likely that in mammalian cells, cyclic nucleotides may influence transcription indirectly through a mechanism involving protein receptor intermediates. These cyclic nucleotide receptor proteins may interact directly with transcriptive enzymes, or they may modify the activity of these enzymes through a mechanism involving the modification of proteins regulatory to the DNA. The latter mechanism would appear to be the most likely to involve a protein-kinase-dependent process insofar as histones represent known substrates for both cAMP- and cGMP-dependent protein kinases (Donnelly *et al.*, 1973), and the nonhistone acidic nuclear proteins are phosphorylated by a mechanism linked to cyclic nucleotides (E. M. Johnson and Hadden, 1975).

In experiments involving mitogen stimulation of intact lymphocytes, it was observed that within minutes, there occurs an increase in the synthesis of specific cytoplasmic proteins that enter the nucleus and bind to the chromatin (E. M. Johnson *et al.*, 1974). The concept that this nuclear protein flux and chromatin binding may serve a function related to the control of cell proliferation is reinforced by the observation that similar proteins bind to chromatin during the early G_1 and early S phases of the HeLa cell cycle (Karn *et al.*, 1974). In both lymphocytes and HeLa cells, increased nuclear flux has been associated with increased phosphorylation of the proteins involved. These results suggest that phosphorylation may serve either to regulate the nuclear entry of these specific proteins or to increase their ability to stimulate transcription (Teng *et al.*, 1971). Con A stimulates the phosphorylation of a number of these acidic DNA-binding proteins, and most specifically a species of approximately 52,000 molecular weight (E. M. Johnson *et al.*, 1974). This phosphorylation may represent a cyclic-nucleotide-mediated event, since ACh, carbachol, imidazole, and cGMP itself will qualitatively reproduce these changes (E. M. Johnson and Hadden, 1975; Hadden *et al.*, 1975b). The stimulation by these agents is of less magnitude and shorter duration; however, the profiles of phosphorylation of specific proteins separated on SDS–polyacrylamide gels are directly parallel. To the converse, cAMP and agents that increase its levels in lymphocytes inhibit the phosphorylation of this particular and other acidic nuclear proteins. This observation not only reinforces the notion that mitogen action within the nucleus may be mediated by cGMP, but also serves to indicate that the cholinergic modulation of RNA synthesis referred to earlier may be regulated through this mechanism. This latter indication is important in suggesting that because the action of ACh, in contrast to that of the mitogen, appears to be unrelated to calcium influx into lymphocytes, this process of acidic nuclear protein phosphorylation may involve cGMP in a manner independent of changes in calcium concentration.

To date, the question as to whether cyclic nucleotides are involved in the processes of histone acetylation in the mitogen-stimulated lymphocyte has not been examined. In addition, the observation that cAMP may be involved in the phosphorylation of histones has not been developed in the lymphocyte (Langan, 1968). The process of overall RNA synthesis has been probed with experiments using the extracellular addition of cAMP to intact lymphocytes. In these experiments, a small increase of RNA synthesis was observed with the addition of dibutyryl cAMP. However, considering that hydrocortisone—which increases lymphocyte cAMP levels—produced no such effect, and that dibutyryl cAMP may actually lower rather than increase intracellular cAMP levels (Webb *et al.*, 1973b), this effect of dibutyryl cAMP of increasing RNA synthesis needs to be further clarified and confirmed before it can be interpreted. While experiments with nuclei or nuclear fractions isolated from lymphocytes stimulated by cyclic nucleotides or related agents lend support to the notion that the nuclear effects produced by mitogens are mediated by cGMP and antagonized by cAMP, this support is at best correlative and indirect.

The most convincing support and the clearest insight have been generated by studying nuclei from nonstimulated lymphocytes using cGMP and calcium as probes and attempting to reproduce in the isolated nucleus those early events known to occur in the nucleus of the intact, mitogen-stimulated lymphocyte. The approach was prompted by the hypothesis that cGMP might represent a membrane-to-nucleus signal mechanism that mediates the mitogen's intracellular action (Hadden *et al.*, 1972b). We began these experiments following the studies of Osawa *et al.* (1957), who had demonstrated that lymphocyte nuclei, when isolated under isotonic conditions, behave (unlike those of other cells) as intact subcellular entities capable of respiring and regenerating ATP, but unable to take up triphosphates from the incubation media. For this reason, we incubated nuclei in medium containing [^{3}H]uridine as the precursor and measured its incorporation into acid-insoluble, RNase-sensitive nuclear constituents. Although this method is fraught with problems of reproducibility and "viability" of nuclei, it yielded evidence that cGMP in low concentrations (10^{-11}–10^{-9} M) stimulated nuclear RNA synthesis. This effect of cGMP was dependent on the presence of calcium in the incubation medium, and was greatly diminished or not observed at higher concentrations of cGMP (Hadden *et al.*, 1973; Goldberg *et al.*, 1974).

These studies prompted further experiments to analyze RNA synthesis more directly and in a way that would militate against extranuclear effects of the cyclic nucleotide in modifying the RNA synthesis. Applying the RNA polymerase assays as described by Pogo (1972) to lymphocyte nuclei prepared with detergents, we were initially unsuccessful. We subsequently found that if the lymphocyte nuclei were prepared under hypotonic conditions in the absence of detergents, we could obtain a nuclear preparation responsive to cGMP as measured by the incorporation of triphosphate precursors into acid-insoluble RNA. Employing definitions of RNA polymerases I, II, and III activity based on cation requirement and inhibitor sensitivity (Wolff *et al.*, 1967), we examined the effects of cGMP, in the presence and absence of calcium, on RNA polymerase activity in these nuclei. We (Hadden *et al.*, 1975b; L. Johnson and Hadden, 1975) observed that in the absence of calcium, cGMP had small effects in increasing RNA polymerase I activity, and that calcium potentiated this action and itself had small effects in stimulating such activity. cGMP produced optimal stimulation at concentrations ranging from 10^{-11} to 10^{-8} M, depending on the concentration of nuclei in the incubation medium. At concentrations at or above 10^{-7} M, cGMP reduced RNA synthesis to control (absence of both cGMP and calcium) levels. The magnitude of cGMP stimulation of RNA polymerase I corresponded to that observed in the nucleus of the intact lymphocyte stimulated with PHA. Nuclei from lymphocytes prestimulated with PHA for 2 hr had an increased RNA polymerase I activity that was less sensitive to cGMP stimulation. Ten times the concentration of cGMP was required to observe effects equivalent to those in the unstimulated nucleus under comparable conditions. In unstimulated nuclei, cGMP and calcium inhibited RNA polymerase II activity, as occurs intitially in the nuclei of intact lymphocytes stimulated with PHA. Correspondingly, nuclei from lymphocytes prestimulated with PHA show an elevation in RNA polymerase II activity at 2 hr that is insensitive to inhibition by cGMP and calcium. These observations serve to demonstrate that cGMP at levels achieved in mitogen-stimulated lymphocytes is capable of reproducing in the isolated nucleus precisely those changes in RNA polymerase I and II activity that occur in the intact mitogen-stimulated lymphocyte.

These effects of cGMP required the concomitant presence of calcium. In experiments with nuclei exposed to a minimal detergent treatment in which no effects of either cGMP or calcium alone were observed, the combination stimulated, thus implying an obligate copresence of the two compounds. These studies provide experimental support for the hypothesis that cGMP and calcium are copartners in a membrane-to-nucleus mitogen signal sequence leading to nuclear events involved in the initiation of cell division (Hadden *et al.*, 1975b; L. Johnson and Hadden, 1975).

Our recent studies indicate that in protein fractions isolated from lymphocyte nuclei, there exist both specific chromatin receptor proteins (both histone and nonhistone acidic nuclear proteins) that bind either cAMP or cGMP specifically (Allfrey *et al.*, 1976), and that chromatographically separated RNA polymerase I also binds cGMP and is activated in a calcium-independent manner (L. Johnson and Hadden, in preparation). One protein obtained from the basic nuclear fraction binds cGMP in a concentration-dependent fashion parallel to the response of RNA polymerase I, and when bound by cGMP, shows increased affinity for native DNA (E. M. Johnson *et al.*, 1975a). These observations serve to indicate that cGMP has actions in the lymphocyte nucleus that can be related to the presence of specific cyclic-nucleotide-binding proteins.

8. Cyclic GMP and Calcium as the Intracellular Mitogen Signal

The significance of the relationship of cGMP increases observed in mitogen-stimulated lymphocytes to the subsequent proliferation must be considered in the following perspective:

1. Can Sutherland's criteria be applied to demonstrate that the increase in cGMP mediates the intracellular action of the mitogen?

2. What actions does cGMP have in the lymphocyte that relate to initiation of proliferation?
3. Are the other early alterations that occur in lymphocytes stimulated by mitogenic agents related to other aspects of the mitogen's action or to the cellular changes in cGMP or calcium or both?

The answer to the first question is complicated by the fact that cGMP does not lend itself to exactly the same criteria that apply to cAMP, and that a mitogen cannot be envisioned to obey the simple formula applied to hormones. Nevertheless, a strong case can be made for cGMP and calcium as the principal components of the intracellular mitogen signal. The evidence as applied to PHA is as follows:

> Mitogenic agents induce increases of cGMP in lymphocytes that exceed in magnitude those induced by nonmitogenic cholinergic agents (Hadden *et al.*, 1975b). The increases begin virtually immediately, and therefore precede the biological response (Hadden *et al.*, 1972b). The mitogen-induced increases in cGMP and the proliferative response are potentiated by a cGMP phosphodiesterase inhibitor, imidazole (Hadden *et al.*, 1975a). The mitogen does not stimulate guanylate cyclase activity directly, but does induce early increases following stimulation of intact lymphocytes (Deviller *et al.*, 1975). Mitogenic stimulation, but not nonmitogenic cholinergic stimulation, induces calcium influx in lymphocytes (Allwood *et al.*, 1971; Whitney and Sutherland, 1972; Hadden *et al.*, 1975b). Extracellular calcium is necessary to the mitogen-induced increases in cellular levels of cGMP (Whitfield *et al.*, 1975; Coffey *et al.*, 1975b) and also for proliferation (Alford, 1970; Allwood *et al.*, 1971; Whitney and Sutherland, 1972). Calcium influx induced by a calcium ionophore (A23187, Lilly) both induces proliferation in lymphocytes (Maino *et al.*, 1974) and increases cGMP levels (Hadden *et al.*, 1975b). Finally, cGMP and calcium together can reproduce in the isolated lymphocyte nucleus those changes in RNA synthesis and RNA polymerase activity that occur in the nucleus of the intact lymphocyte stimulated by the mitogen (Hadden *et al.*, 1973; Goldberg *et al.*, 1974; L. Johnson and Hadden, 1975).

This evidence suggests that both calcium and cGMP are involved in the intracellular action of the mitogen, and that this action is differentiated, at least in the lymphocyte, from that of a hormonal, cholinergic agent in that the hormone's action involves cGMP in the absence of observable calcium influx.

An important point raised by the foregoing discussion concerns the relationship between calcium action at the cell surface and the generation of cGMP. Two hypotheses seem relevant: (1) The mitogen induces increases in membrane-bound or intracellular calcium that lead directly or indirectly to the activation of guanylate cyclase and the generation of cGMP. (2) The mitogen induces a concomitant activation of calcium influx and guanylate cyclase, and the two events, although independent, are interactive. The available information is insufficient to resolve the question of which of these two hypotheses is correct.

It is clear from the foregoing presentation that more critical experimentation concerning the interactions of membrane-bound calcium and guanylate cyclase are needed to resolve the issue. Since the guanylate cyclase activated by the mitogen in intact lymphocytes is in a soluble form, one must assume either that it is rendered soluble and thereby activated by the mitogen, at the cell surface, or that an intermediate step involving calcium or another enzymatic process or both is involved. The resolution of this issue appears to be of critical importance in establishing the essential components of mitogenic action in the lymphocyte.

While a large variety of processes occur early during the initiation of lymphocyte proliferation, and many of them may be regulated by cyclic nucleotides, much experimental work is required to distinguish those processes that are regulatory ones directly controlled by cyclic nucleotides and lead directly to the replication process.

9. Hormone Induction of Thymocyte Differentiation

The endocrine nature of the thymus was first envisioned when the role of the thymus gland in cell-mediated immunity was discovered; it was subsequently shown that it was possible to restore the immunocompetence of neonatally thymectomized mice by grafting a thymus within a millipore chamber that allowed the passage of macromolecules but not of cells (Osaba and Miller, 1964; Stutman *et al.*, 1970). The experiments of Klein *et al.* (1965) and Trainin and Small (1970) indicated that a cell-free bovine thymic fraction was capable of restoring cellular immune function in neonatally thymectomized mice, as measured by graft-vs.-host (GVH) reaction and skin graft rejection.

Several groups of investigators have analyzed the active moieties of these cell-free extracts, and have reported activity in thymus fractions with molecular weights ranging from 1000 to 12,500 (see White, 1975). Of those factors that influence the activity of T-cell precursors, three derived from thymus and one derived from serum have emerged. Table 1 represents a summary of these factors, their approximate molecular weights, and some of their biological effects on T-cell precursors *in vitro* and *in vivo*.

This tabulation is admittedly inadequate to describe the breadth of efforts in this field; however, it serves to make several critical points: A number of factors have been described that have apparently similar biological action yet distinct biochemical characteristics. While contamination of crude preparations with nonspecific substances that stimulate adenylate cyclase, such as ubiquitin (G. Goldstein *et al.*, 1975), remains a possibility to explain differences in activities, a central feature emerges: thymopoietin, thymosin, thymic humoral factor, and thymic factor all share the capacity to induce T-cell differentiation antigens *in vitro* and *in vivo*, and all appear to reconstitute cell-mediated immune response *in vivo* in mice without a thymus (nude or thymectomized, irradiated, anti-theta-treated, bone-marrow-reconstituted).

According to current information, the following represents an outline of the ontogeny of the T lymphocyte: The thymocyte develops within the thymus as a result of the differentiation of a precursor derived from hematopoietic populations of the spleen and bone marrow of mice. The initial steps of this process involve the appearance on this cell of markers characteristic of the intrathymic lymphocyte (e.g., *TL, Thy, Ly*); after a period of delay, functions such as mitogen and mixed leukocyte culture (MLC) responsiveness appear.

It has been found that thymocyte precursors in mouse spleen (concentrated by discontinuous albumin gradient centrifugation) can be stimulated *in vitro* by thymopoietin or thymosin to demonstrate within 2 hr the appearance of cell-surface markers previously defined as thymus differentiation antigen markers. These markers include *Thy-1* (θ), *TL*, *Ly-1,2,3,5*, G_{IX}, and *MSLA* (Komuro and Boyse, 1973; Scheid *et al.*, 1973, 1975). The display of these markers involves the expression of six or more discrete genes, and the induction of their display by thymopoietin involves new mRNA synthesis consistent with their first appearance, rather than a redisplay (Storrie *et al.*, 1976).

TABLE 1. Summary of Factors That Influence the Activity of T-Cell Precursors

			In vitro inductive action		*In vivo* inductive action			
Factor	Molecular weight	Source	T-cell markers	Mitogen responsiveness	MLC or GVH activity	Markers	CMI[a]	Purity
Thymopoietin (G. Goldstein *et al.*, 1975)	5,700	Thymus	+	+	?	+	+	Completely purified and sequenced
Thymosin (Hooper *et al.*, 1975)	12,500	Thymus	+	+	+	+	+	Partially purified
Thymic humoral factor (Trainin *et al.*, 1975)	3,000	Thymus	+	+	+	+	+	Partially purified
Thymic factor (J. F. Bach *et al.*, 1975)	1,000	Serum	+	?	?	+	+	Partially purified

[a]Increased cell-mediated immunity in nude or neonatally thymectomized mice.

While the action of thymopoietin has been intensively studied in splenic precursors, using the Komuro–Boyse assay, it can be conceived that the principal action is in fact occurring in precursor cells on arrival at the thymic cortex. These cells represent an actively cycling population that undergoes a suppression of proliferation in association with migration into the thymic medulla. This migration is associated with the subsequent acquisition of the functions of allogeneic responsiveness (i.e., MLC and GVH responsiveness) and mitogen responsiveness. These functions are thought to represent distinct subsets. The analysis of thymic hormone action in relation to the changes in proliferative activity that these cells undergo as they mature includes the following: Thymosin has been shown to increase thymidine incorporation in lymphoid cells in short-term (4-hr) culture (A. L. Goldstein *et al.*, 1966), and thymopoietin preserves splenic proliferative potential and enhances responsiveness to Con A following a preexposure of 24 hr (Basch and Goldstein, 1975a,b). We (Sunshine *et al.*, 1977, submitted) observed that thymopoietin increases the proliferative responses to MLC and Con A stimulation in mature thymocytes and lymph node cells. Trainin and associates noted that their thymic humoral factor (THF) decreases thymidine incorporation early (at 1 hr) in splenic cells of neonatally thymectomized mice; that in thymocytes, it prevents mitogen responsiveness, if continuously present; but that it augments mitogen responsiveness of both following a preexposure, then removal (Rotter and Trainin, 1975; Kook and Trainin, 1975). Basch and Goldstein (1975a,b) observed that their thymic factor increases splenic cell responsiveness to Con A. Touraine *et al.* (1975) reported that thymosin induces Con A and MLC responsiveness in human thymocytes following preexposure and removal. Barker and Moore (1977) observed that when thymocytes are treated *in vitro* with thymosin and reinjected, their distribution to spleen and lymph nodes and their responses to mitogenic stimulation are increased.

These observations may appear discordant in indicating that certain factors under certain conditions inhibit proliferation if present at the time of mitogen addition, while other factors under similar conditions promote proliferation when present at the time of mitogen addition. An integrated view of these apparently disparate observations might be that thymic hormone(s) may be antiproliferative at one stage of the development, i.e., the prothymocyte stage, and pro-proliferative at a later stage, i.e., the mature thymocyte. Another possibility is that contamination of thymic hormone preparations with ubiquitin, a known activator of adenylate cyclase through a β-adrenergic receptor mechanism, may be introducing anomalous increases in cAMP irrespective of the stage of thymocyte development, and that the action of the thymic hormone is thus being obscured. In either case, from the viewpoint of cyclic nucleotide mediation, a complex action of the thymic hormone(s) is implied.

10. Cyclic Nucleotides in Thymocyte Differentiation

Considerable pharmacological evidence exists to indicate that the action of thymic hormone(s) in inducing differentiation is mediated by cyclic nucleotides. On the basis of the lead provided by J. F. Bach *et al.* (1973) indicating that their thymic factor could be mimicked by extracellular cAMP, Scheid *et al.* (1973) presented a convincing array of evidence to indicate that a number of agents known to increase cAMP will mimic the action of thymosin and thymopoietin in the Komuro–Boyse induction assay system. These agents include polyA:polyU, endotoxin, PGE_1, and isoproterenol. In addition, agents that increase cGMP in lymphocytes, e.g., insulin, α-adrenergics, and imidazole, all antagonize the initial induction event. These pharmacological observations indicate that cAMP plays a role in the induction and that cGMP is antagonistic to that induction.

Direct evidence that cAMP mediates thymic hormone action has been somewhat inconsistent. Kook and Trainin (1974, 1975) and Trainin *et al.* (1975) presented evidence that their THF increases cAMP levels in unfractionated mouse thymocytes. Similarly, Astaldi *et al.* (1976) observed a thymus-dependent serum factor that increases cAMP in thymic lymphocytes. Using thymopoietin, we have not been able to confirm these observations in albumin gradient fractionated spleen cells or unfractionated thymocytes (Sunshine *et al.*, 1977, submitted). Similarly, thymosin and thymic factors have not been shown to increase cAMP levels in inducible cells (M. Bach and A. Goldstein, personal communication). The discrepancies among these experimental observations require further clarification using enriched precursor cells; however, they do not exclude the possibility that thymic hormone(s) increases cAMP levels in prothymocytes.

Kook and Trainin (1974, 1975) demonstrated that their THF factor increases adenylate cyclase activity of intact cells preincubated for 5–60 min with the factor. In experiments using an extremely sensitive modification of the adenylate cyclase assay, we have been unable to reproduce these observations with thymopoietin in enriched spleen cells. In addition, we have been unable to show direct effects of thymopoietin on adenylate cyclase activity of plasma membrane preparations of inducible cells. The difference here may result from ubiquitin contamination of the THF preparation. These studies are convincing to us in indicating that thymopoietin, in contrast to such nonspecific inducers as isoproterenol and PGE_1, does not directly stimulate adenylate cyclase. Whether adenylate cyclase activity increases in cells induced to differentiate remains to be clarified.

Some evidence also exists to indicate that PG synthesis may be involved in the action of at least one factor. M. A. Bach (1974) presented evidence that the effects of THF on induction are blocked by the PG synthesis inhibitor indomethacin. We observed that indomethacin (10^{-5} M) does not block the action of thymopoietin (Hadden, unpublished observations). These observations suggest that Bach's factor may act initially to stimulate PG synthesis, and that the PG is responsible for cAMP accumulation through stimulation of adenylate cyclase, or perhaps inhibition of cAMP phosphodiesterase.

Our observations that thymopoietin promotes Con-A-induced proliferation in mature thymocytes separated on albumin gradients when it was present at the same time as Con A suggested to us that cGMP might be involved in an action of thymopoietin on already differentiated thymocytes. Our preliminary measurements of cGMP levels in thymocytes and T-cell-rich spleen fractions stimulated by thymopoietin support this suggestion. In addition, thymosin was observed to enhance proliferation and other functions of postthymic T cells (Barker and Moore, 1977), actions that are quite consistent with a cGMP-mediated action of thymic hormone(s). While much work is required to clarify the action of these various thymic substances and to determine whether they are distinct or subcomponents of each other, a similarity of actions and mechanism of action appears to us to be common to them all (excepting ubiquitin, of course). An operational view of mechanism of action we would like to propose is that thymic hormone(s) induces prothymocyte differentiation in association with an initial antiproliferative action linked to cAMP and also enhances mature thymocyte proliferation through mediation of cGMP. This view implies that during ontogeny, the thymus-derived lymphocyte maintains sensitivity to a single hormone or class of hormones, yet the mechanism of the hormone's action shifts from cAMP to cGMP mediation. Such an evolution of mechanism of responsiveness is attractive in comparison with the combined differentiation and growth-promoting influences of other "poietin"-type substances such as nerve growth factor, colony stimulating factor, and erythropoietin.

One inadequacy of this view involves the lack of understanding of events involved in intrathymic evolution of the prothymocyte to the mature T lymphocyte. The immature cortical lymphocyte is thought to be a cell with a high rate of proliferation, while the more mature medullary lymphocyte has a low rate of proliferation. One must hypothesize proliferation-regulating mechanisms between these two stages. While such mechanisms have not been examined in relation to the action of thymic hormone(s), the collected works of MacManus *et al.* (1975) suggest that a variety of hormones may be involved. Using a model system involving the analysis of the flow of a population of thymus cortical cells into mitosis during a 6-hr incubation, these investigators developed a complex view of what appears to be intracycle (i.e., G_1–S boundary) regulation of thymocyte proliferation. One analysis of these collected data (Morgan *et al.,* 1975) indicates that dependent on the presence of calcium, a number of hormonal agents including parathormone, ACh, histamine, and insulin promote the flow of these cells into mitosis. This action appears to be mediated by cGMP and is antagonized by agents that increase cAMP, by magnesium, and by estradiol. In contrast, and dependent on the presence of magnesium, a number of hormonal agents including epinephrine, PGE_1, glucagon, and dopamine promote the flow of these cells into mitosis. This action appears to be mediated by cAMP and is antagonized by calcium and by testosterone. These observations suggest that two quite opposing mechanisms are involved in mediating the same event in these cells, i.e., the promotion of the flow of cells into mitosis from a midcycle position. The existence of such regulation *in vivo* implies either of two possibilities: (1) the existence of two independent thymocyte subsets with contrasting modulation or (2) a single population with a bidirectional modulation involving two distinct mechanisms. The experimental evidence mitigates the first possibility. The second seems more likely, and is supported by a similar set of observations in marrow precursor cells (Byron, 1973). One hypothesis that serves to integrate these observations with the foregoing ones would be that there is in the G_1–S boundary of differentiating cells an intracycle regulatory mechanism that determines which of two possible daughter cells (i.e., lymphocyte subsets) is produced. Which cyclic nucleotide is involved would then determine which subset results. The possible testing of such a hypothesis is now available using the Whitfield–MacManus assay and the analysis of distinctive cell-surface antigens of the *Ly* series, or of functions such as T helper vs. suppressor, or of mitogen vs. MLC response following differential cyclic nucleotide/cation manipulation. The clarification of this mechanism in relation to that of the variety of thymic hormones appears important in terms of determining the role of thymic hormones and their mechanisms in achieving thymocyte differentiation into T-cell subsets responsible for helper or suppressor functions, cytotoxicity, and allogeneic, mitogen, and antigen responsiveness.

Abell, C. W., and Monahan, T. M., 1973, *J. Cell. Biol.* **59**:549–558.

Alford, R. H., 1970, *J. Immunol.* **104**:698–703.

Allfrey, V. G., Inoue, A., Karn, J., Johnson, E. M., Good, R. A., and Hadden, J. W., 1976, in: *The Structure and Function of Chromatin, Ciba Found. Symp.* **28**:199–228.

Allwood, G., Asherson, G. L., Davey, M. J., and Goodford, P. J., 1971, *Immunology* **21**:509–515.

Armelin, H. A., Nishakawa, K., and Sato, G. H., 1974, in: *Cold Spring Harbor Symp.: Control of Proliferation in Animal Cells* (B. Clarkson and R. Baserga, eds.), pp. 97–104, Cold Spring Harbor Press, Cold Spring Harbor, New York.

Astaldi, A., Astaldi, G. C. B., Schellekens, P., and Eijsvoogel, V. P., 1976, *Nature (London)* **260**:713–715.

Bach, J. F., Dardenne, M., and Bach, M., 1973, *Transplant. Proc.* **5**:99–104.

Bach, J. F., Dardenne, M., Pleau, J. M., and Bach, M., 1975, *Ann. N. Y. Acad. Sci.* **249**:186–210.

Bach, M. A., 1974, *C. R. Acad. Sci. Paris* **278**:3023–3025.

Bach, M., 1975, *J. Clin. Invest.* **55**:1074–1081.

Barker, A., and Moore, V. S., 1977, in: *Progress in Cancer Research and Therapy II* (M. Chirigos, ed.), pp. 289–303, Raven Press, New York.

Barnet, R. E., Scott, R. E., Furcht, L. T., and Kersey, J. H., 1974, *Nature (London)* **249**:465, 466.

Basch, R. S., and Goldstein, G., 1975a, *Ann. N. Y. Acad. Sci.* **249**:290–299.

Basch, R. S., and Goldstein, G., 1975b, *Cell Immunol.* **20**:218–228.

Berridge, M. J., 1975, *Adv. Cyclic Nucleotide Res.* **6**:1–97.

Bray, M. A., Gordon, D., and Morley, J., 1975, *Nature (London)* **257**:227, 228.

Burleson, D. G., and Sage, H. J., 1976, *J. Immunol.* **116**:696–703.

Byron, J. W., 1973, *Nature (London) New Biol.* **241**:152–154.

Chambers, D. A., David, W. M., Jr., and Weinstein, Y., 1974, *Cell* **3**:375–380.

Clarkson, B., and Baserga, R., 1974, *Control of Proliferation in Animal Cells,* Cold Spring Harbor Press, Cold Spring Harbor, New York.

Coffey, R. J., Hadden, E. M., and Hadden, J. W., 1975a, *Endocr. Res. Commum.* **12**:179–198.

Coffey, R. J., Hadden, E. M., and Hadden, J. W., 1975b, *Fed. Proc. Fed. Am. Soc. Exp. Biol.* **34**:1029.

Cooper, H. L., 1970, in: *Proceedings of the Fifth Leukocyte Culture Conference* (J. Harris, ed.), pp. 15–32, Academic Press, New York.

Cross, M. E., and Ord, M. G., 1971, *Biochem. J.* **124**:241–248.

DeRubertis, F. R., Zenser, T. V., Alder, W. H., and Hudson, T., 1974, *J. Immunol.* **113**:151–161.

Deviller, Y., Chille, Y., and Betuel, M., 1975, *Enzyme* **19**:300–319.

Diamantstein, T., and Ulmer, A., 1975a, *Immunol. Commun.* **4**:51–62.

Diamantstein, T., and Ulmer, A., 1975b, *Nature (London)* **256**:418, 419.

Donnelly, T. E., Kuo, J. F., Reyes, P. L., Liu, Y. P., and Greengard, P., 1973, *J. Biol. Chem.* **248**:190–198.

Durham, J. P., Baserga, R., and Butcher, F. R., 1974, *Biochem. Biophys. Acta* **327**:196–217.

Edelman, G. M., 1974, in: *Control of Proliferation in Animal Cells,* (B. Clarkson and R. Baserga, eds.), pp. 357–378, Cold Spring Harbor Press, Cold Spring Harbor, New York.

Estensen, R. D., Hadden, J. W., Hadden, E. M., Touraine, J. L., Haddox, M. K., and Goldberg, N. D., 1974, in: *Control of Proliferation in Animal Cells* (B. Clarkson and R. Baserga, eds.), pp. 627–634, Cold Spring Harbor Press, Cold Spring Harbor, New York.

Farago, A., Antoni, F., Takats, A., and Fabian, F., 1973, *Biochem. Biophys. Acta* **297**:517–526.

Ferber, E., and Resch, K., 1973, *Biochem. Biophys. Acta* **296**:335–349.

Ferber, E., Reilly, C. E., dePasquale, G., and Resch, K., 1974, in: *Lymphocyte Recognition and Effector Mechanism* (K. Lindhal-Kissling and D. Osoba, eds.), pp. 529–534, Academic Press, New York.

Ferraris, V. A., and DeRubertis, P. D., 1974, *J. Clin. Invest.* **54**:378–386.

Fisher, D. B., and Mueller, G. C., 1971, *Biochem. Biophys. Acta* **248**:434–448.

Folch, H., and Waksman, B. H., 1973, *Cell. Immunol.* **9**:12–24.

Freedman, M. H., Raff, M. C., and Gomperts, B., 1975, *Nature (London)* **255**:378–382.

Gallo, R. C., and Whang-Peng, J., 1971, *J. Natl. Cancer Inst.* **47**:91–94.

Gavin, J. R., Roth, J., Jen, P., and Freychet, P., 1972a, *Proc. Natl. Acad. Sci. U.S.A.* **69**:747–751.

Gavin, J. R., Buell, D. N., and Roth, J., 1972b, *Science* **178**:168–169.

George, W. J., Polson, J. B., O'Toole, A. G., and Goldberg, N. D., 1970, *Proc. Natl. Acad. Sci. U.S.A.* **66**:398–403.

Gery, I., Gershon, R. K., and Waksman, B. H., 1972, *J. Exp. Med.* **136**:128–130.

Goldberg, N., Haddox, M., Hartle, D., and Hadden, J., 1973, in: *Proceedings of the Fifth International Congress of Pharmacology,* Vol. 5, pp. 146–169, S. Karger, Basel.

Goldberg, N. D., Haddox, M. K., Dunham, E., Lopez, C., and Hadden, J., 1974, in: *Control of Proliferation in Animal Cells* (B. Clarkson and R. Baserga, eds.), pp. 609–626, Cold Spring Harbor Press, Cold Spring Harbor, New York.

Goldberg, N. D., Haddox, M. R., and O'Dea, R. F., 1975, in: *Advances in Cyclic Nucleotide Research* (G. I. Drummon, P. Greengard, and G. A. Robinson, eds.), Vol. 5, pp. 307–338, Raven Press, New York.

Goldfine, I. O., Gardner, J. D., and Neville, D. M., Jr., 1972, *J. Biol. Chem.* **21**:6919–6926.

Goldstein, A. L., Slater, F. D., and White, A., 1966, *Proc. Natl. Acad. Sci. U.S.A.* **56**:1010–1017.

Goldstein, G., Scheid, M., Hammerling, U., Boyse, E. A., Schlesinger, D. H., and Niall, H. D., 1975, *Proc. Natl. Acad. Sci. U.S.A.* **72**:11–15.

Greaves, M. F., and Bauminger, S., 1972, *Nature (London) New Biol.* **235**:67–69.

Gunther, G. R., Wang, J. L., Yahara, I., Cunningham, B. A., and Edelman, G. M., 1973, *Proc. Natl. Acad. Sci. U.S.A.* **70**:1012–1016.

Hadden, J. W., Hadden, E. M., and Middleton, E., 1970, *J. Cell Immunol.* **1**:583–595.

Hadden, J. W., Hadden, E. M., and Good, R. A., 1971a, *Biochem. Biophys. Acta* **237**:339–347.

Hadden, J. W., Hadden, E. M., and Good, R. A., 1971b, *Exp. Cell Res.* **68**:217–219.

Hadden, J. W., Hadden, E. M., Middleton, E., Jr., and Good, R. A., 1971c, *Int. Arch. Allergy Appl. Immunol.* **40**:526–539.

Hadden, J. W., Hadden, E. M., Wilson, E. E., Good, R. A., and Coffey, R. G., 1972a, *Nature (London) New Biol.* **234**:174–176.

Hadden, J. W., Hadden, E. M., Haddox, M. K., and Goldberg, N. D., 1972b, *Proc. Natl. Acad. Sci. U.S.A.* **69**:3024–3027.

Hadden, J. W., Hadden, E. M., Meetz, G., Good, R. A., Haddox, M. K., and Goldberg, N. D., 1973, *Fed. Proc. Fed. Am. Soc. Exp. Biol.* **32**:1022.

Hadden, J. W., Hadden, E. M., and Goldberg, N. D., 1974, in: *Cyclic AMP Cell Growth and the Immune Response* (W. Braun, L. M. Lichtenstein, and C. W. Parker, eds.), pp. 237–246, Springer-Verlag, New York.

Hadden, J. W., Hadden, E. M., Coffey, R. G., Corrales-Lopez, E., and Sunshine, G., 1975a, *Cell. Immunol.* **20**:98–103.

Hadden, J. W., Johnson, E. M., Hadden, E. M., Coffey, R. G., and Johnson, L. D., 1975b, in: *Immune Recognition* (A. S. Rosenthal, ed.), pp. 359–390, Academic Press, New York.

Hadden, J. W., Hadden, E. M., Sadlik, J. R., and Coffey, R. J., 1976, *Proc. Natl. Acad. Sci. U.S.A.* **73**:1717–1721.

Haddox, M. K., Furcht, L. T., Stephenson, J. H., Moser, M. E., and Goldberg, N. D., 1976, *Fed. Proc. Fed. Am. Soc. Exp. Biol.* **35**:295.

Heidrick, M. L., 1975, *J. Cell Biol.* **59**:139a.

Hirschhorn, R., Grossman, J., and Weissman, G., 1970, *Proc. Soc. Exp. Biol. Med.* **133**:1361–1363.

Hooper, J. A., McDaniel, M. C., Thurman, G. B., Cohen, G. H., Schulof, R. S., and Goldstein, A. L., 1975, *Ann. N. Y. Acad. Sci.* **249**:125–144.

Illiano, G., Tell, G. P. E., Siegal, M. I., and Cuatrecasas, P., 1973, *Proc. Natl. Acad. Sci. U.S.A.* **70**:2443–2447.

Inbar, M., and Shinitsky, M., 1975, *Eur. J. Immunol.* **5**:170–175.

Jahng, H. N., 1975, *Fed. Proc. Fed. Am. Soc. Exp. Biol.* **34**:1030.

Jimenez de Asua, L., Clingan, D., and Rudland, P. S., 1975, *Proc. Natl. Acad. Sci. U.S.A.* **72**:2724–2728.

Johnson, E. M., and Hadden, J. W., 1975, *Science* **187**:1198–1200.

Johnson, E. M., Karn, J., and Allfrey, V. G., 1974, *J. Biol. Chem.* **249**:4990–4999.

Johnson, E. M., Inoue, A., Crouse, L., Allfrey, V. G., and Hadden, J. W., 1975a, *Biochem. Biophys. Res. Commun.* **65**:714–720.

Johnson, E. M., Hadden, J. W., Inoue, A., and Allfrey, V. G., 1975b, *Biochemistry* **14**:3873–3884.

Johnson, L. D., and Abell, C. W., 1970, *Cancer Res.* **30**:2718–2723.

Johnson, L., and Hadden, J. W., 1975, *Biochem. Biophys. Res. Commun.* **65**:714–721.

Karn, J., Johnson, E. M., Vidali, G., and Allfrey, V. G., 1974, *J. Biol. Chem.* **249**:667–677.
Katagiri, T., Terao, T., and Osawa, T., 1976, *J. Biochem.* **79**:849–852.
Kay, J. W., 1971, in: *Proceedings of the Fourth Annual Leukocyte Culture Conference* (O. Ross mcIntyre, ed.), pp. 21–35, Appleton-Century-Crofts, New York.
Klein, J. J., Goldstein, A. L., and White, A., 1965, *Proc. Natl. Acad. Sci. U.S.A.* **53**:812–817.
Kleinsmith, L. J., Allfrey, V. G., and Mirsky, A. E., 1966, *Science* **154**:780, 781.
Komuro, K., and Boyse, E. A., 1973, *J. Exp. Med.* **138**:479–482.
Kook, A. I., and Trainin, N., 1974, *J. Exp. Med.* **139**:193–207.
Kook, A. I., and Trainin, N., 1975, *J. Immunol.* **114**:151–157.
Krishnaraj, R., and Talwar, G. P., 1973, *J. Immunol.* **111**:1010–1017.
Krug, V., Krug, F., and Cuatrecasas, P., 1972, *Proc. Natl. Acad. Sci. U.S.A.* **69**:2604–2608.
Kuehl, F. A., Ham, E. A., Zanetti, M. E., Sanford, C. H., Nicol, S. E., and Goldberg, N. D., 1974, *Proc. Natl. Acad. Sci. U.S.A.* **71**:1866–1871.
Langan, T. A., 1968, *Science* **162**:579–581.
Ling, H. R., and Kay, J. E., 1975, *Lymphocyte Stimulation,* American Elsevier, New York.
Luckasen, J. R., White, J. G., and Kersey, J. H., 1974, *Proc. Natl. Acad. Sci. U.S.A.* **71**:5088–5090.
Lyle, L. R., and Parker, C. W., 1974, *Biochemistry* **13**:5415–5420.
MacManus, J. P., and Whitfield, J. F., 1969, *Exp. Cell Res.* **58**:188–191.
MacManus, J. P., and Whitfield, J. F., 1971, *Exp. Cell Res.* **69**:281–288.
MacManus, J. P., Whitfield, J. F., Boynton, A. L., and Rixon, B. H., 1975, in: *Advances in Cyclic Nucleotide Research* (G. I. Drummon, P. Greengard and G. A. Robinson, eds.), Vol. 5, pp. 719–734, Raven Press, New York.
Maino, V. C., Green, M. N., and Crumpton, M. J., 1974, *Nature (London)* **25**:324–327.
Makman, M. K., 1971, *Proc. Natl. Acad. Sci. U.S.A.* **68**:885–889.
May, C. D., Lyman, M., and Alberto, R., 1970, *J. Allergy* **46**:21–28.
McCrery, S. E., and Rigby, P. G., 1972, *Proc. Soc. Exp. Biol. Med.* **140**:1456–1459.
Miller, Z., Lovelace, E., Gallo, M., and Pastan, I., 1975, *Nature (London)* **257**:1213–1215.
Moens, W., Vokawe, A., and Kram, R., 1975, *Proc. Natl. Acad. Sci. U.S.A.* **72**:1063–1067.
Morgan, J. I., Hall, A. K., and Perris, A. D., 1975, *Biochem. Biophys. Res. Commun.* **66**:188–194.
Novogrodsky, A., 1972, *Biochem. Biophys. Acta* **266**:343–349.
Novogrodsky, A., and Katchalski, E., 1970, *Biochem. Biophys. Acta* **215**:291–296.
Olefsky, J., and Reaven, G. M., 1974, *J. Clin. Endocrinol. Metab.* **38**:554–560.
Osaba, D., and Miller, J. A., 1964, *J. Exp. Med.* **119**:177–194.
Osawa, S., Allfrey, V. G., and Mirsky, A. E., 1957, *J. Gen. Physiol.* **40**:491–513.
Pallavincini, M. G., and Nichols, W. K., 1975, *Fed. Proc. Fed. Am. Soc. Exp. Biol.* **34**:760.
Parker, C. W., 1974, *Biochem. Biophys. Res. Commun.* **61**:1180–1186.
Parker, C. W., Sullivan, T. J., and Wedner, H. J., 1974, in: *Advances in Cyclic Nucleotide Research* (P. Greengard and G. A. Robinson, eds.), Vol. 4, pp. 1–80, Raven Press, New York.
Pastan, I. H., Johnson, G. S., and Anderson, W. B., 1975, *Annu. Rev. Biochem.* **44**:491–522.
Peters, J. M., and Hausen, P., 1971, *Eur. J. Biochem.* **19**:502–508.
Pogo, B. G. T., 1972, *J. Cell Biol.* **53**:635–641.
Pogo, B. G. T., Allfrey, V. G., and Mirsky, A. E., 1966, *Proc. Natl. Acad. Sci. U.S.A.* **55**:805–812.
Quastel, M. R., and Kaplan, J. G., 1970, *Exp. Cell Res.* **63**:230–233.
Resch, K., 1976, in: *Receptors and Recognition* (P. Cuatrecasas and M. F. Greaves, eds.), pp. 61–117, Chapman & Hall, London.
Resch, K., and Ferber, E., 1975, in: *Immune Recognition* (A. S. Rosenthall, ed.), pp. 281–312, Academic Press, New York.
Resch, K., Ferber, E., Ooenthall, J., and Fisher, H., 1971, *Eur. J. Immunol.* **1**:162–165.
Rigby, P. G., and Ryan, C. W., 1970, *Rev. Eur. Etudes Clin. Biol.* **15**:774–777.
Rotter, V., and Trainin, N., 1975, *Cell. Immunol.* **16**:413–421.
Rudland, P. S., Gospardowicz, D., and Seifert, W. E., 1974, *Nature (London)* **250**:741–744.
Scheid, M. D., Hoffman, M. K., Komuro, K., Hammerling, U., Abbott, J., Boyse, E. A., Cohen, G. H., Hooper, J. A., Schulof, R. S., and Goldstein, A. L., 1973, *J. Exp. Med.* **138**:1027–1032.
Scheid, M. P., Goldstein, G., Hammerling, U., and Boyse, E. A., 1975, *Ann. N. Y. Acad. Sci.* **249**:531–540.
Schultz, G., Hardman, J. G., Schultz, K., Davis, J. W., and Sutherland, E. W., 1973, *Proc. Natl. Acad. Sci. U.S.A.* **12**:3889–3893.

Schultz, G., Schultz, K., and Hardman, J. G., 1975, *Metabolism* **24**:429–437.
Schumm, D. E., Morris, H. P., and Webb, T. E., 1974, *Eur. J. Cancer* **10**:107–113.
Schwartz, R. H., Bianco, A. R., Handwerger, B. S., and Kahn, C. R., 1975, *Proc. Natl. Acad. Sci. U.S.A.* **72**:474–478.
Seifert, W. E., and Rudland, P. S., 1974, *Nature (London)* **248**:138–140.
Smith, J. W., Steiner, A. L., and Parker, C. W., 1971, *J. Clin. Invest.* **50**:442–449.
Soren, L., 1973, *Exp. Cell. Res.* **78**:201–208.
Storrie, B., Goldstein, G., Boyse, E. A., and Hammerling, U., 1976, *J. Immunol.* **115**:1358–1362.
Strom, T. B., Deisseroth, A., Morganroth, J., Carpenter, C. B., and Merrill, J. P., 1972, *Proc. Natl. Acad. Sci. U.S.A.* **69**:2995–2999.
Strom, T. B., Bear, R. A., and Carpenter, C. B., 1975a, *Science* **187**:1206–1208.
Strom, T. B., Hirsh, M. S., Black, P. H., Carpenter, C. B., Phillips, S. M., and Merrik, J. B., 1975b, *Transplant. Proc.* **7**:305–307.
Stutman, O., Yunis, E., and Good, R. A., 1970, *J. Exp. Med.* **132**:583–612.
Sunshine, G., Scheid, M., Coffey, R. G., Goldstein, G., and Hadden, J. W., 1977, submitted to *Nature*.
Sutherland, E. W., and Rall, T. W., 1960, *Pharmacol. Rev.* **12**:265–299.
Teng, C. S., Teng, C. T., and Allfrey, V. G., 1971, *J. Biol. Chem.* **246**:3597–3609.
Touraine, J. L., Touraine, F., Incefy, G. S., Goldstein, A. L., and Good, R. A., 1975, in: *Biological Activity of Thymic Hormones* (D. W. vanBekkum, ed.), PPBI Kook YGR Publications, Rotterdam.
Trainin, N., and Small, M., 1970, *J. Exp. Med.* **132**:885–897.
Trainin, N., Kook, A. I., Umiel, T., and Albala, M., 1975, *Ann. N. Y. Acad. Sci.* **294**:349–361.
Vanden Berg, K. J., and Betel, I., 1973, *FEBS Lett.* **29**:1498–1500.
Voorhees, J., Stawiski, M., Duell, M., Haddox, M., and Goldberg, N. D., 1974, in: *Control of Proliferation in Animal Cells* (B. Clarkson and R. Baserga, eds.), pp. 653–648, Cold Spring Harbor Press, Cold Spring Harbor, New York.
Wang, J. L., McClain, D. A., and Edelman, G. M., 1975, *Proc. Natl. Acad. Sci. U.S.A.* **72**:1917–1921.
Watson, J., 1975, *J. Exp. Med.* **141**:97–111.
Webb, D. R., and Osheroff, P. L., 1976, *Proc. Natl. Acad. Sci. U.S.A.* **73**:1300–1314.
Webb, D. R., Stites, O. P., and Fudenberg, H. H., 1973a, *Immunol. Commun.* **2**:353–360.
Webb, D. R., Stites, D. P., Perlman, J. D., Loong, D., and Fudenberg, H. H., 1973b, *Biochem. Biophys. Res. Commun.* **53**:1002–1008.
Webb, D. R., Belohradsky, B., Hanes, D., Stites, D. O., Perlman, J. D., and Fudenberg, H. H., 1975, *Clin. Immunol. Immunopathol.* **4**:226–240.
Weber, W. T., 1970, *Clin. Exp. Immunol.* **6**:919–940.
Wedner, H. J., and Parker, C. W., 1975, *Biochem. Biophys. Res. Commun.* **62**:808–815.
Wedner, H. J., Dankner, R., and Parker, C. W., 1975, *J. Immunol.* **115**:81–1687.
Weinstein, Y., Segal, S., and Melmon, K. L., 1975, *J. Immunol.* **115**:112–117.
White, A., 1975, *Ann. N. Y. Acad. Sci.* **249**:523–532.
Whitfield, J. F., MacManus, F., Franks, D. J., Gillan, D. J., and Youadale, T., 1971, *Proc. Soc. Exp. Biol. Med.* **137**:453–457.
Whitfield, J. F., MacManus, J. P., Boynton, A. L., Gillan, D. J., and Isaacs, R. J., 1975, *J. Cell. Physiol.* **84**:445–458.
Whitney, R. B., and Sutherland, R. M., 1972, *J. Cell. Physiol.* **82**:9–20.
Winchurch, R., Ishizuka, M., Webb, D., and Braun, W., 1971, *J. Immunol.* **106**:1399–1400.
Wolff, J. S., III, Langstaff, J. A., Weinberg, G., and Abell, C. W., 1967, *Biochem. Biophys. Res. Commun.* **26**:336–371.
Yamamoto, I., and Webb, D. R., 1975, *Proc. Natl. Acad. Sci. U.S.A.* **72**:2320–2324.

2

Involvement of Cyclic Nucleotides as Intracellular Mediators in the Induction of Antibody Synthesis

JAMES WATSON

1. Introduction

Antibody forming cells are produced in the terminal stage of a specialized differentiation sequence. As hematopoietic stem cells develop along the pathway to antibody-forming cells, they become committed to an increasingly limited fate. The changes that occur in the phenotypic characteristics of these differentiating cells must result from temporal variations in responsiveness to new external stimuli and the expression of new genetic information.

The immediate precursors of antibody-forming cells in the developmental sequence are the antigen-sensitive lymphocytes derived from bone marrow (B cells). These B cells are found in the various peripheral lymphoid organs in a growth-arrested state, and have already differentiated to a state in which they are committed to the production of unique immunoglobulin (Ig) which is found on the surface membrane as an antigen-binding receptor. Antigen-sensitive cells are thus committed to the expression of antibody, but they respond to interactions with antigen *either* by differentiation to antibody-forming cells (induction) *or* by inactivation in that they are no longer inducible (paralysis). The paralytic pathway is important for the maintenance of a state of tolerance to self antigens. The interaction of antigen with Ig receptors on the antigen-sensitive cells is involved as an external stimulus for both the inductive and the paralytic pathway. In this chapter, I

JAMES WATSON • Department of Medical Microbiology, College of Medicine, University of California, Irvine, California 92717.

will consider how antigen is involved in the initiation of these opposing pathways in B cells, and the involvement of intracellular cyclic nucleotides in regulating the expression of the inductive and paralytic pathways.

2. Induction and Paralysis

The interaction of specific antigen with antigen-sensitive B cells is required for the induction of antibody synthesis. From the initial observations by Miller (1961) showing the necessity for thymus-derived (T) cells in the induction of antibody responses to the subsequent experiments analyzing the role of T cells in activating B cells, the question has continually arisen whether the recognition of antigenic determinants by specific Ig receptors on B cells is all that is required as the inductive stimulus. The finding that animals depleted of T cells respond well to some antigens but poorly to others has led to the division of antibody responses into T-cell-independent and T-cell-dependent. Thus, a variety of antigens, including polymeric agents such as bacterial lipopolysaccharides and flagella, pneumococcal carbohydrate and other polysaccharides, polyvinylpyrrolidone (Davies *et al.*, 1970; B. Andersson and Blomgren, 1971; Nossal and Ada, 1971), dinitrophenylated ficoll (Paul *et al.*, 1974), and numerous synthetic polypeptides (Mitchell *et al.*, 1972), have been termed *thymus-independent antigens,* while erythrocyte antigens, serum proteins, and other hapten–protein conjugates have been termed *thymus-dependent antigens* (Mitchison, 1971). Several general statements can be made concerning this division: First, the antigens that elicit comparable antibody (IgM) responses in intact and T-cell-deficient mice are generally polymeric molecules. Second, most IgG antibody responses are highly T-cell-dependent, whereas many IgM responses are not.

The question that must be asked is whether the existence of T-cell-independent and T-cell-dependent antigens reflects (1) different mechanisms for inducing the maturation of any given antigen-sensitive B cell to an antibody-forming cell, (2) a relative difference in the manner in which various antigens utilize the same induction mechanism for antibody synthesis, or (3) the existence of two classes of antigen-sensitive B cells, i.e., those that respond only to T-cell-independent antigens and those that respond only to T-cell-dependent antigens.

Any consideration of T-cell-independent antigens must also concern the nature of the mechanism that activates the paralytic pathway in B cells (Bretscher and Cohn, 1970). Evidence for the existence of a direct inactivation pathway in B cells is obtained from experiments that show that haptens coupled to immunogenic carriers elicit hapten-specific immune responses, whereas haptens on nonimmunogenic carriers induce hapten-specific unresponsiveness (Weigle, 1965; Katz *et al.*, 1971a,b 1974; Golan and Borel, 1971; Hamilton and Miller, 1973a,b). Carrier moieties are nonimmunogenic because their interactions with T cells have somehow been limited. In several cases, adoptive transfer experiments have been performed and have revealed that B cells have been directly inactivated, or paralyzed. Since haptens on nonimmunogenic carriers interact with B cells, but apparently not with T cells, the interaction between haptenic determinants and Ig receptors on the surface of B cells initiates the intracellular events that lead to inactivation. A number of haptens on nonimmunogenic carriers have been shown to elicit hapten-specific immune responses when another signal acting on B cells is simultaneously provided, by the use of either allogeneic lymphocytes (Katz *et al.*, 1971a) or bacterial lipopolysaccharide (LPS) (Chiller and Weigle, 1973; Schmidtke and Dixon, 1972), implying that the T-cell signal diverts those cells binding hapten from a paralytic to an inductive pathway. Three general statements can be made concerning the nature of the inductive and paralytic stimuli: (1) The interaction of antigenic determinants with Ig receptors on B cells, in the absence of T-cell help, tends to lead to the inactivation of B cells. (2) The interaction of antigenic determinants with Ig receptors on B cells, in the presence of T-cell help, leads to the induction of antibody synthesis. (3) T-cell-independent and T-cell-dependent antigens are operational terms. The terms may reflect differences in the apparent T-cell help that is required to activate B cells; the terms *do not* necessarily mean that these antigens activate B cells via different inductive mechanisms. It appears unlikely that T-cell-independent antigens activate B cells to either an inductive or a paralytic pathway *solely* on the basis of pattern or density presentation of determinants to surface Ig receptors.

2.1 Intracellular Mediators of B-Cell Expression

The inductive and paralytic pathways in B cells appear to be regulated by antigenic and T-cell interactions, presumably at their surface membranes. For those agents that act at the surface of the cell, an intracellular mediator is required to convey the signal from the exterior to the interior of the cell. While antigen is known to bind to surface Ig receptors on B cells, the chemical nature of the T-cell signal or its cellular site of action remains unknown.

For antigen or the T-cell signal to interact with the B cell to initiate the inductive or paralytic pathway, it is clear that these agents by themselves, or synergistically, must activate a complex set of metabolic reactions. While it is not possible to define these reactions, it is feasible to question how these changes are initiated. That it is feasible was recognized by Hershko *et al.* (1971), who termed the coordinated biochemical components of any regulatory program a *pleiotypic* response. This term can be applied to the expression of antigen-sensitive cells. The pleiotypic responses, or pathways expressed by these cells, are a function of limited genetic information they can express as a consequence of prior differentiation events. In B cells, the inductive pathway may be considered a positive pleiotypic response, whereas the paralytic pathway may be considered a negative pleiotypic response (Watson, 1975b).

I will consider here the evidence that indicates that cyclic AMP (cAMP) and cyclic GMP (cGMP) may be involved as the intracellular mediators of the antigenic and T-cell signals in B cells. Thus, agents that interact with B cells and selectively affect the metabolism of cAMP and cGMP may initiate either a positive or a negative pleiotypic response in these cells. Four groups of agents may be used to examine B-cell expression in this way: (1) exogenously added cAMP or cGMP; (2) agents such as adrenergic or cholinergic agonists that interact with receptors on lymphoid cells and selectively increase intracellular cyclic nucleotide levels; (3) phosphodiesterase activators or inhibitors, which also lead to an increase or decrease in intracellular cyclic nucleotide levels; (4) lymphocyte mitogens (Watson *et al.*, 1973a–c; Watson, 1974).

In considering the effects of these various agents on cyclic nucleotide metabolism in lymphoid cells, it is apparent that the changes observed may be specific for select subpopulations of cells. For example, agents that appear to be mitogenic for antigen-sensitive B cells also act as a differentiation stimulus for subpopulations of lymphocytes that precede the antigen-sensitive cell stage. Whereas cGMP appears to be involved in the mitogenic stimulus, cAMP may be involved in the differentiation stimulus. The inference from these observations is that intracellular cyclic nucleotide levels affect the expression of lymphocytes in various ways that depend on their stage of differentiation. Understanding how the same intracellular mediators acquire the ability to affect the expression of different sets of genetic information during development may be fundamental to all differentiation processes.

3. Effect of Cyclic Nucleotides on the Induction of Antibody Synthesis

3.1. Stimulatory Effects of Cyclic AMP and Cyclic GMP

It was originally shown by Ishizuka *et al.* (1970, 1971) that immune responses to erythrocyte antigens *in vivo* could be enhanced by double-stranded poly A:U. This action of poly A:U was potentiated by the phosphodiesterase inhibitor theophylline (Braun and Ishizuka, 1971a,b). Although poly A:U has little effect on intracellular cAMP levels (Winchurch *et al.*, 1971), it was suggested that it acts synergistically with antigen to increase intracellular cAMP levels. Higher levels of poly A:U inhibited immune responses to sheep red blood cells (SRBC) (Ishizuka *et al.*, 1970, 1971). It was suggested that the interaction of antigen with Ig receptors on B cells stimulated the synthesis of cAMP, and that this increase was the activation signal for induction.

There are several reports that the intravenous injection of SRBC results in a 2- to 3-fold increase in splenic cAMP levels (Plescia *et al.*, 1975; Yamamoto and Webb, 1975). This change occurred in response to heterologous erythrocytes, but not to autologous erythrocytes or nonimmunogenic carbon particles. Also, poly A:U enhanced the response when given with SRBC when the cAMP level was rising, and was immunosuppressive if given when the cAMP level was decreasing. It is extremely unlikely that the 2- to 4-fold enhancement of cAMP levels is due specifically to antigen-stimulated B cells, since these cells contribute less than 0.01% of the spleen cell population.

There are two major difficulties in studying the effect of cyclic nucleotides on the induction of immune responses. The first is that the small number of specific antigen-binding cells in any given lymphoid population and the difficulties associated with their purification impose restrictions on how biochemical events can be studied in cells following the addition of antigen to cultures. To study the involvement of cyclic nucleotides in the activation of B cells by antigen, we can add cyclic nucleotides or cyclic-nucleotide-elevating agents to cultures with antigen and examine the effects on the appearance of specific antibody-forming cells, but the responding cells are a minority of the population. The second difficulty concerns the many types present in lymphoid cell cultures. In view of the effects cyclic nucleotides exert on secretory processes (Bourne *et al.*, 1974), it may be difficult to distinguish between a direct effect of a cyclic nucleotide on a B cell and an indirect effect of an agent secreted by another cell type.

The addition of dibutyryl cAMP, or agents known to stimulate increases in the intracellular levels of cAMP, inhibits the induction of primary immune responses to erythrocyte antigens in spleen cultures (Watson *et al.*, 1973c; Watson, 1974).

Dibutyryl cAMP and monobutyryl cAMP, but not 5′-AMP, inhibit the induction of immune responses in the range of 10^{-4}–10^{-3} M, indicating that it is cAMP and not one of its various metabolites that is responsible for the inhibition. At extracellular concentrations between 10^{-4} M and 10^{-6} M, cAMP and its butyrated derivatives have an enhancing effect on the induction of *in vitro* immune responses (Watson *et al.*, 1973c; Teh and Paetkau, 1976a,b; Bösing-Schneider, 1975) similar to the *in vivo* enhancements of immune responses observed (Ishizuka *et al.*, 1970; Braun and Ishizuka, 1971a,b). In contrast, similar concentrations (10^{-3}–10^{-6} M) of cGMP or agents that stimulate increases in intracellular cGMP in lymphoid cells have little effect on the induction of immune responses in mouse spleen cultures (Watson *et al.*, 1973c; Watson, 1974, 1975a). There are numerous reports that poly A:U as well as a number of cAMP-elevating agents enhance specific immune responses *in vitro* and *in vivo* (Winchurch *et al.*, 1971; Jaroslow and Ortiz-Ortiz, 1972; Mozes *et al.*, 1974).

The addition of cGMP or its butyrated derivatives to T-cell-depleted cultures has two effects on the induction of primary immune responses to SRBC. In the absence of SRBC, small background immune responses are observed. In the presence of SRBC, there is a definite synergistic effect, resulting in stimulations of immune responses above the background responses. In many experiments, these stimulations have consistently been in the range of 5-fold. cAMP or cAMP-elevating agents show no stimulation of immune responses in T-cell-depleted cultures (Watson *et al.*, 1973c; Watson, 1974).

3.2. Inactivation of B Cells by Cyclic AMP

The treatment of mouse spleen cultures for short periods (<12 hr) with concentrations of dibutyryl cAMP (10^{-3} M) or isoproterenol (10^{-4} M) that normally inhibit the induction of immune responses generally stimulates subsequent immune responses to erythrocyte antigens (Watson, 1974; Teh and Paetkau, 1976a,b). However, treatment for longer periods inhibits immune responses. Since at least three cell types are required for the induction of immune responses, the cAMP could be affecting any one of the three types to inhibit immune responses. The specific effect of cAMP on the activity of B cells was studied by incubating nude spleen cells for various times with cAMP-elevating agents, washing the cultures, and challenging with erythrocyte antigens and fresh, nontreated accessory cell types (Watson *et al.*, 1973c). Between 12 and 20 hr after the addition of the cAMP-elevating agents to cultures, the activity of B cells begins to decrease. By about 30 hr, the ability of B cells to respond to antigen has been lost. Since the maturation to antibody-forming cells requires cell proliferation, and cAMP is known to inhibit proliferation in a variety of normal and malignant cells, it is not surprising that these agents inhibit the induction of antibody synthesis. The problem here is whether to regard the inactivation of precursor cells by cAMP as merely a nonspecific toxic effect, or as a consequence of a specific cAMP-induced biochemical pathway, i.e., a pleiotypic effect. There are a number of indirect reasons that favor inactivation via a specialized cell pathway. While high concentrations of cAMP inhibit the growth of other mammalian cell types, the inhibitory effects tend to be reversible for considerable periods. These high concentrations of cAMP also cause the expression of differentiated functions characteristic of specialized cells (Scheid *et al.*, 1973;

Hämmerling *et al.*, 1975) (see Section 5.2). Also, tumors derived from T lymphocytes have been found that are rapidly killed by raising intracellular levels of cAMP, not merely growth-arrested as are other mammalian cells (Daniel *et al.*, 1973). Inactivation of B cells by cAMP is partially or completely prevented by the simultaneous presence of cGMP (Watson *et al.*, 1973c). This preventive effect may not be expected if the inactivation process is due to a general toxic effect. It is unlikely that cGMP is merely competing with cAMP for uptake into cells to reduce the effective intracellular concentration of cAMP in these experiments, since carbachol, the cholinergic agonist, partially reverses the inactivating effects of both cAMP and isoproterenol, the β-adrenergic agonist (Watson, 1974). The intracellular levels of cAMP are not affected by carbachol and possibly not by cGMP in these reversal experiments; thus, the reversal effects indicate that it is not the absolute level of intracellular cAMP that leads to the inactivation, but rather the intracellular ratio of cAMP to cGMP.

The enhancement of *in vitro* immune responses by dibutyryl cAMP was also reported not to be a direct B-cell effect, but to inhibit the function of a suppressor cell type that normally lowers immune responsiveness (Teh and Paetkau, 1976a,b).

4. Mitogen-Induced B-Lymphocyte Proliferation: Immunologic Effects

4.1. Lymphocyte Mitogens

The difficulty in analyzing the biochemical response of a B cell to the antigenic or T-cell stimulus lies in the small number of cells in any given lymphocyte population that respond to a specific antigen. Instead of adding cyclic-nucleotide-enhancing agents and examining their effects on the induction of antigen-specific immune responses, an alternative approach is to find agents that nonspecifically induce most B cells to mature to antibody-forming cells and examine the biochemical action of such agents.

A large number of agents have now been shown to exert mitogenic activity on B cells. These agents include bacterial LPSs, a purified protein derivative (PPD) from tuberculin (J. Andersson *et al.*, 1972; Sultzer and Nilsson, 1972; Coutinho *et al.*, 1974; Gronowicz *et al.*, 1974), numerous polymerized proteins, polysaccharides, polyanions, and polyribonucleotides (Coutinho *et al.*, 1974; Diamantstein *et al.*, 1974; Gronowicz *et al.*, 1974; Scher *et al.*, 1973; Strong *et al.*, 1974), an activated complement component (Dukor and Hartmann, 1973), a water-soluble extract of *Nocardia opaca* (Bona *et al.*, 1974), and cGMP (Watson, 1974, 1975a; Weinstein *et al.*, 1974, 1975). In contrast to the dual requirement for antigen and T helper cells in the induction of antibody synthesis, nonspecific B-cell mitogens appear to directly stimulate cells to division. When the responding B cells also mature to antibody-forming cells, a polyclonal response is observed. Since these B-cell mitogens mimic the action of antigen and T cells in the inductive stimulus, they provide valuable tools for dissecting the inductive pathway.

4.2. Bacterial Lipopolysaccharide as a Probe of T Helper Cell Function

Of all the B-cell mitogens studied, bacterial LPS has been used the most to modulate B cell expression. The LPS isolated from gram-negative bacteria acts as a specific mitogen for B lymphocytes from mice (J. Andersson *et al.*, 1972) and as a highl, immunogenic antigen (Rudbach, 1974). LPS can be viewed as a composite of two distinct functional moieties: (1) the *O*-polysaccharide, which has been characterized as the major antigen (Luderitz *et al.,* 1971) and which is linked via a trisaccharide of 2-keto-3-deoxyoctanoic acid (KDO) to (2) the Lipid A structure, which is responsible for the mitogenic activity of LPS (Chiller *et al.,* 1973). LPS has been shown to possess a number of immunologic activities in mice that relate to the inductive or the paralytic pathway:

1. LPS stimulates polyclonal B cell activation (Coutinho and Möller, 1973). This process is antigen-independent, and results in the maturation of many B cells to antibody-forming cells.
2. LPS may replace T helper cells in the induction of antigen-dependent immune responses. LPS stimulates immune responses to heterologous erythrocyte antigens in T-cell-depleted spleen cultures (Watson *et al.,* 1973a) and stimulates immune responses to determinants that, because of their size or structure, are nonimmunogenic (Schmidtke and Dixon, 1972; Watson *et al.,* 1973b; Trenkner, 1974). In contrast to the polyclonal activation of B cells, this response is an antigen-dependent process that demonstrates *synergy* between LPS and antigen. It is evident that whether a polyclonal or a synergistic response is induced by LPS depends on the concentration of LPS used in spleen cultures. Low concentrations of LPS in the presence of antigen show synergy, whereas high concentrations of LPS suppress these synergistic responses with antigen, but show enhanced antigen-independent or polyclonal responses.
3. LPS interferes with the induction of tolerance to human γ-globulin (HGG) (Golub and Weigle, 1967) and to bovine γ-globulin (Claman, 1963).

These diverse immunologic activities of LPS have been related to a common mechanism utilizing the C3H/HeJ strain of mouse, the spleen cells of which, as originally described by Sultzer and Nilsson (1972), do not support a mitogenic response to LPS, whereas spleen cultures prepared from related C3H strains (C3H/St, C3H/DiSn, C3HeB/FeJ) all support mitogenic responses similar to those reported from other strains of mice (Watson and Riblet, 1974). Other B-cell mitogens, the PPD from tuberculin, dextran sulfate, polyinosinic acid (Poly I), and trypsin all stimulate mitogenic responses in C3H/HeJ spleen cultures comparable in magnitude to the mitogenic responses elicited by these mitogens using other C3H strains of mice. Thus, C3H/HeJ mice are selectively unresponsive to B-cell mitogens, indicating that the mode of action of LPS differs in at least one step from that of PPD, dextran sulfate, Poly I, and trypsin (Watson and Riblet, 1974, 1975).

Genetic back-cross experiments revealed that the loss of mitogenic responsiveness in C3H/HeJ mice is due to a single gene defect, and cell-mixing experiments indicated that this gene is expressed on B cells (Watson and Riblet, 1974, 1975). The gene that limits LPS-induced immunologic activities in C3H/HeJ mice may affect a cell-surface "receptor" for LPS on B lymphocytes. The interaction of Lipid A with this "receptor" site on B lymphocytes in other strains of mice may result in the initiation of intracellular events that lead to DNA synthesis and cell division. Radioactive LPS was shown to bind equally well to C3H/HeJ and C3HeB/FeJ spleen cells (Watson and Riblet, 1975). Therefore, if the gene defect in C3H/HeJ mice does control the expression of LPS "receptors," it does so without quantitatively reducing the capacity of the receptors to bind LPS in the C3H/HeJ cells.

4.3 Lipopolysaccharide and the Inductive Pathway

The expression of B cells is normally governed physiologically by interactions at *two* different sites, presumably on their surface membranes. The first site is where antigen binds to Ig receptors; the second site is where a stimulus from T helper cells is received. The finding that the interaction of LPS with B cells is all that is required to stimulate these cells to mature to antibody-forming cells (polyclonal response) gave rise to the question whether antigens and T cells, on the one hand, and nonspecific mitogens, on the other, initiate the same intracellular responses in B cells (Coutinho and Möller, 1973; Cohn, 1972; Watson, 1975b).

Genetic experiments with C3H/HeJ mice indicated that the interaction of LPS with B cells is *all* that is required to stimulate cell division and polyclonal expression. Therefore, the expression of cell division and antibody synthesis appears to be *coordinately linked*. This apparent linking suggests that the physiologic inductive stimuli delivered to B cells via interactions with antigen and T helper cells merely complement each other to form a similar mitogenic stimulus (Watson and Riblet, 1974, 1975; Watson *et al.*, 1975).

It has been considered that the interaction of antigenic determinants with surface Ig receptors on B cells is sufficient to stimulate B cells to divide, but that a T-cell stimulus is then required to allow these dividing cells to mature to antibody-forming cells (Dutton, 1974; Hunig *et al.*, 1974); i.e., cell division and maturation to antibody-forming cells are *not* coordinately linked. The experiments that led to this suggestion involved immune responses to erythrocyte antigens in spleen cultures prepared from nude mice. Such cultures contain T cells; therefore, it is difficult to rule out the presence of a few T helper cells, which, with antigen, stimulate B cells to DNA synthesis. There may not be sufficient T helper cells to provide the constant stimulation for B cells necessary for continued division, so that some form of T-cell-replacing activity is required after 48 hr to allow cells to divide further (Dutton, 1974; Hunig *et al.*, 1974). It appears unlikely that antigenic determinants provide a mitogenic stimulus to B cells, and that T helper cells provide a differentiation signal to the dividing cells as suggested (Dutton, 1974; Hunig *et al.*, 1974); rather, cell proliferation and antibody synthesis are coordinately linked if one accepts the interpretation that the mitogen experiments using LPS show that cell division and maturation are coordinately expressed in antigen-sensitive B cells.

4.4 Lipopolysaccharide and the Paralytic Pathway

LPS also has the capacity to modulate the induction of a specific state of tolerance or paralysis in mice to the thymus-dependent antigen human IgG (HGG) into a specific state of immunity to HGG (Chiller and Weigle, 1973). Mice treated with LPS shortly after the injection of a paralytic dose of deaggregated HGG (DHGG) not only fail to become tolerant to HGG, but also demonstrate a delayed primary response to HGG, and, as well, respond anamnestically to a subsequent immunogenic challenge of aggregated HGG (AHGG) (Chiller *et al.*, 1974a,b). The immune response to HGG that is seen as the result of dual treatment of mice with DHGG and LPS appears to occur despite the normal induction of tolerance in both HGG-specific thymocytes and peripheral T cells (Louis *et al.*, 1973; Chiller *et al.*, 1974a,b). That it is suggests that LPS not only prevents the initiation of the paralytic pathway in B cells, but also overcomes the normal requirement for HGG-specific T helper cells in the inductive pathway. In contrast, LPS fails to inhibit paralysis to HGG in C3H/HeJ mice. The lack of an effect of LPS in the C3H/HeJ is not due to an inability of this strain to respond to the antigen HGG, since this strain responds as well as other strains to an immunogenic challenge with AHGG (Chiller *et al.*, 1974a,b). A back-cross experiment was performed to determine whether the gene that limits mitogenic responses to LPS in C3H/HeJ mice is involved in the interference of paralysis to DHGG by LPS. A total of 24 mice were individually tested by immunizing with DHGG and LPS, followed 3 weeks later by a challenge with AHGG. Of these 24 mice, 15 supported both high *in vivo* immunogenic and *in vitro* mitogenic responses to LPS, as well as immune responses to AHGG, indicating that LPS had inhibited paralysis to DHGG. In contrast, the remaining 9 mice supported only low mitogenic and immune responses to LPS, and also failed to respond to AHGG, indicating that LPS had no effect on paralysis to HGG in these mice (Skidmore *et al.*, 1975; Watson *et al.*, 1975).

The coordinate expression of these two immunologic effects of LPS in these back-cross mice suggests not only that the cellular site of action of LPS is confined to B lymphocytes, but also that its subcellular mode of action in the paralytic pathway may result from the delivery of a signal to antigen-specific B cells that is a stimulus for mitogenesis. The role of a mitogenic signal would be to divert B cells from the paralytic pathway initiated by the interaction of DHGG with Ig receptors clonally expressed on specific B cells to the inductive pathway, as a consequence of the interaction of the Lipid A moiety of LPS with an LPS "receptor" nonclonally expressed on all B cells.

The mitogenic activity of LPS therefore provides a probe not only for analyzing how a B cell may distinguish between *inductive* and *paralytic* stimuli, but also for examining the biochemical events that are involved in the expression of these pathways.

5. Cyclic Nucleotides and B-Lymphocyte Proliferation and Differentiation

5.1. Cyclic GMP as a Proliferation Signal

It was originally reported by Hadden *et al.* (1972) that the addition of the T-cell mitogens concanavalin A (Con A) and phytohemagglutinin (PHA) to lymphocyte populations stimulated rapid but transient 5- to 50-fold increases in intracellular levels of cGMP. Purified PHA and Con A had no effect on cAMP levels. However, although stimulation of cGMP levels through the activation of cholinergic receptors did not produce mitogenic responses in these cells, both the mitogenic and the cholinergic stimulation of lymphocytes are associated with early changes in the rate of RNA and protein synthesis (Hadden *et al.*, 1974).

The addition of mitogenic concentrations of LPS to mouse spleen cultures stimulates rapid but transient increases in the intracellular levels of cGMP with little concomitant change in cAMP levels (Watson, 1974, 1975a). At high LPS concentrations, a small increase in cAMP levels can be observed (Watson, 1974). The increases in cGMP levels are generally in the range of 3-fold, reach a maximum by

15 min, and then decrease to a level that is approximately similar to the levels observed in nonstimulated cultures.

The addition of either cGMP itself or its butyrated derivatives to lymphoid cell cultures, or to mouse spleen cultures depleted of T cells, stimulates DNA synthesis. The magnitude of the stimulation varies, and is undoubtedly related to the stability of cGMP in serum-free or supplemented media (Watson, 1974, 1975a; Weinstein *et al.,* 1974, 1975; Diamantstein and Ulmer, 1975). Maximum stimulation of DNA synthesis is generally seen between 24 hr and 48 hr after addition of cGMP to cultures, when more than 10% of the spleen cells show significant activity by autoradiography (Watson, 1975). 5′-GMP has also been shown to exert smaller stimulatory effects on DNA synthesis in mouse spleen cultures, and these effects may be related to the general enhancing effects that purines exert on mammalian cell cultures (Schor and Rozengurt, 1971). However, while LPS and cGMP both stimulate DNA synthesis in mouse spleen cultures, it has also been shown that agents that raise intracellular levels of cGMP in lymphoid cells are not necessarily mitogenic. Agents such as carbamylcholine chloride, which interact with cholinergic receptors to stimulate guanylate cyclase activity, do not have significant effects on DNA synthetic responses (Watson, 1974, 1975a,b). There are similarities and differences between the effects of LPS and cGMP on mouse lymphoid cells. Both stimulate DNA synthesis in murine B cells, but not in T cells. However, cGMP does not stimulate the same striking polyclonal effects as does LPS.

An increasing body of data from other mammalian systems indicates that rapid increases in intracellular cGMP levels are produced by the interaction of mitogens with cell-surface membranes. The stimulation of cGMP synthesis by Con A was reported in rat thymocyte cultures (Whitfield *et al.,* 1974), in which it was also shown that the increases in intracellular cGMP synthesis are optimal in medium containing low concentrations of calcium. Mouse fibroblast cells can be growth-arrested in the G_0 phase of the cell cycle by serum deprivation in culture. The addition of cGMP or its butyrated derivatives to such quiescent cells stimulates DNA synthesis, which is first detected some 12–16 hr later, followed by cell division (Seifert and Rudland, 1974). The addition of serum to fibroblasts growth-arrested by serum deprivation also results in rapid, transient increases in intracellular levels of cGMP. The addition of a purified fibroblast growth factor (FGF) to quiescent mouse fibroblast cells also stimulates intracellular cGMP synthesis, DNA synthesis, and cell division (Rudland *et al.,* 1974a). Phorbol myristate acetate (PMA) stimulates cultures of confluent mouse fibroblasts to DNA synthesis and cell division (Estensen *et al.,* 1974). PMA causes an increase of intracellular cGMP concentrations greater than 20-fold after 45 sec. By 1 or 2 min, these levels have returned to around normal. PMA is also mitogenic for human lymphoid cells.

Levamisole, an immunopotentiator, was compared with its parent molecule, imidazole, in its effects on lymphocyte proliferation and cyclic nucleotide levels. Both levamisole and imidazole augment PHA-induced proliferation of human peripheral blood lymphocytes, mouse thymocytes, and T-cell-enriched splenocytes. Both agents increase cGMP levels of T-cell-enriched mouse spleen cells with a dose–response curve that closely parallels their effects on proliferation. Both agents lower cAMP levels in these cells. The data are consistent with the interpretation that the potentiation of PHA responses induced by levamisole may result from increases in levels of lymphocyte cGMP levels (Hadden *et al.,* 1975).

In contrast to the reported changes in intracellular cGMP levels in cells following mitogen stimulation, there are reports that cAMP levels also change (Parker *et al.*, 1971; Smith *et al.*, 1971; Webb *et al.*, 1973; Krishnaraj and Talwar, 1973). In general, the addition of high concentrations of cAMP or cAMP-elevating agents to mouse spleen cultures has marked inhibitory effects on mitogen-induced events. The addition of high concentrations of dibutyryl cAMP or isoproterenol, a β-adrenergic agonist, inhibits the induction of DNA synthesis by LPS (Watson, 1974), as well as by PPD, dextran sulfate, and polyribonucleotides. Similar inhibitory effects of cAMP on the activity of the T-cell mitogens Con A and PHA have been widely observed (see Chapter 1). Agents that elevate cAMP levels in mammalian cells growing in culture are well known to inhibit cell growth (Burger *et al.*, 1972; Pastan and Perlman, 1971; Smets, 1972; Sheppard, 1972). In contrast to the inhibitory effects of cAMP, high concentrations of cGMP or cGMP-elevating agents have little effect on the mitogenic activity of mitogens (Watson, 1974, 1975a,b).

If cGMP is specifically involved as an intracellular mediator of B-cell mitogen action, the question arises as to how these various mitogens activate guanylate cyclases, the enzymes that synthesize cGMP. There are two general ways in which this activation may be achieved: (1) The mitogen may bind to a receptor or membrane component that is linked *directly* to the intracellular enzymes. (2) The binding of the mitogen to the surface membrane may initiate a series of changes that lead *indirectly* to the activation of intracellular guanylate cyclases.

In the absence of extracellular calcium, intracellular cGMP levels decrease, and cells do not respond to a wide variety of cGMP-elevating agents (Schultz *et al.*, 1973). The removal of calcium from the medium inhibits the mitogenic effects of PHA (Alford, 1970; Whitney and Sutherland, 1973), and prevents the stimulation of guanylate cyclase by Con A (Whitfield *et al.*, 1974). These inhibitions can all be reversed by the addition of calcium to the medium. An ionophore specific for divalent cations, the *Streptomyces* antibiotic A23187, initiates events similar to those caused by PHA in pig lymphocytes (Maino *et al.*, 1974). A23187 forms a lipid-soluble complex with a divalent cation and enables it to diffuse across membranes. The ionophore stimulates DNA synthesis in pig lymphocytes but not murine lymphocytes, and requires calcium in the culture medium for mitogenic activity, implying that its mitogenic effects may be due to the transport of calcium across the membrane (Maino *et al.*, 1974). PHA was shown to stimulate calcium uptake in human blood lymphocytes (Allwood *et al.*, 1971). These various findings suggest that in B cells, the means by which mitogens activate guanylate cyclase may also be via changes in cation transport across surface membranes. It has been reported, however, that Con A induces increased radioactive calcium uptake in the mouse T lymphocytes, but not B lymphocytes, within 45 sec of the addition of Con A (Freedman *et al.*, 1975). This effect is short-lived and is inhibited by high concentrations of dibutyryl cAMP, but enhanced by dibutyryl cGMP. B-cell mitogens such as LPS apparently did not cause measurable increases in radioactive calcium uptake (Freedman *et al.*, 1975). As with the mitogenic effects of extracellular cGMP on B cells but not on T cells, this finding may reflect subtle differences in the activation of B and T cells.

Calcium has many effects on proliferative processes. When rat thymocytes are placed in a complex synthetic medium without calcium, the movement of cells from the G_1 to the S phase is arrested (Whitfield *et al.*, 1973). The addition of cAMP, agents that increase intracellular levels of cAMP, or calcium allows cells arrested in the late G_1 phase to enter the S phase. B cells are growth-arrested in early G_1 and do not respond to cAMP as do rat thymocytes growth-arrested in late G_1 in the calcium-free medium. B cells are activated by agents that elevate intracellular cGMP levels, but not by agents that elevate intracellular cAMP levels, whereas rat thymocytes are activated by both types of agents. Low concentrations of cAMP or cGMP replace calcium and cause blocked thymocytes in calcium-free medium to initiate DNA synthesis as effectively as raising the calcium levels (MacManus and Whitfield, 1969; Whitfield *et al.*, 1971, 1973, 1974). A large number of agents have been shown to induce blocked rat thymocytes in low-calcium medium, but not in calcium-free medium, to DNA synthesis and cell division. Such agents appear to share in common the ability to increase calcium uptake into cells (MacManus *et al.*, 1975), and they may also be cGMP-elevating agents. Thus, the ability of cAMP and cGMP to act as proliferative signals to cells may depend very much on what stage of the cell cycle a cell is in at the time of cyclic nucleotide treatment.

Since B-cell mitogens may stimulate rapid, transient increases in the levels of cGMP, and the initiation of DNA synthetic activity is not observed until some 12–14 hr later, the question arises as to how a transient change in cGMP can be a signal for an event that is not detected until a number of hours later. Agents that raise cGMP levels in B cells are *not* necessarily mitogenic; thus, cells must respond to more than a mere change in cGMP levels (Watson, 1974, 1975a,b). There is evidence that the cell responds not to the absolute level of cGMP, but to the intracellular ratio of cAMP to cGMP. The experiments that support this view are of two general types: First, a survey of many nondividing and dividing cell cultures has shown that while the intracellular levels of cAMP and cGMP vary from one cell type to another, there is *always* a striking difference between the ratio of cAMP to cGMP in nondividing and the ratio in dividing cells. This ratio is always high in nondividing cells and much lower in dividing cells (Rudland *et al.*, 1974b; Watson, 1975a,b). The transient elevation of intracellular levels of cGMP following LPS stimulation may not be as important as the prolonged decrease in the ratio of cAMP to cGMP as a mitogenic signal to cells. The second type of experiments that implicate this ratio as important in signal delivery are those that show that the addition of cAMP-elevating agents to spleen cultures inhibits the mitogenic effects of LPS. Since the absolute level of cGMP is considered to be unchanged by the addition of these agents, the ratio of cAMP to cGMP is expected to increase (Watson, 1974).

5.2. Cyclic AMP as a Differentiation Signal in B Lymphocytes

B cells are known to pass through several differentiation steps in their ontogeny, and there exist a number of surface markers unique to B cells that appear during development and may be used as surface markers for different phases. When bone marrow and spleen cells of mice are fractionated by density-gradient procedures, a small fraction of Ig-bearing cells can be induced to express the *Ia* alloantigen (Hämmerling *et al.*, 1975). Induction can be effected by various catecholamines, prostaglandin PGE_1, cAMP, LPS, and Lipid A. This process is similar to the prothymocyte induction that results in the expression of the thymocyte phenotype as characterized by the *TL*, *Thy-1*, and *Ly* alloantigens (Scheid *et al.*, 1973).

In both these systems, it appears that agents that elevate cAMP levels in the progenitor B or T cells are responsible for inducing new surface markers on cells. This observation is particularly interesting with respect to the mode of action of LPS. In murine spleen cultures, LPS is a cGMP-elevating agent. That it is suggests that the cyclic-nucleotide-enhancing activity of LPS is selective for different cell types. Specifically, less mature B cells (Ia^- cells) may respond to LPS by elevations in cAMP levels, and more mature B cells (Ia^+ cells) may respond by changes in cGMP levels. Three different explanations may be proposed for this phenomenon:

1. The LPS-receptor sites utilized for the mitogenic response in Ia^+ cells and for the maturation step in Ia^- cells are different.
2. The LPS-receptor sites are the same. As a B cell matures from an Ia^- cell to an Ig^+ cell, however, the intracellular enzyme systems associated with the LPS-receptor sites may undergo a change such that adenylate cyclase is activated in the less mature cell and guanylate cyclase in the more mature cell. This interchange of adenylate and guanylate cyclases associated with a receptor may occur frequently in developing biological systems. For example, in the rat atrium, an interchange of adenylate and guanylate cyclases has been proposed for the transformation of β- to α-adrenergic responses (Amer and Byrne, 1975).
3. LPS activates adenylate cyclase activity in all cells. In antigen-sensitive B cells, however, increases in cAMP levels lead to an enhancement of guanylate cyclase activity, or an inhibition of cGMP-specific phosphodiesterase activity.

Cell proliferation is not required in the development of either B-cell (Hämmerling *et al.*, 1975) or T-cell (Scheid *et al.*, 1973) surface markers. In these systems, an increase in cAMP levels appears to function as a differentiation signal. Once a cell has completed a particular differentiation phase, there must occur a further programming process that allows a cell to express the phenotypic markers characteristic of the next phase of the developmental sequence.

5.3. Cyclic AMP and Cyclic GMP as Intracellular Mediators of the Expression of B-Cell Pathways

The expression of B cells is governed by membrane interactions at two different receptor sites. The first site is where antigen binds; the second site is where the T-cell signal is received by B cells. It is reasonable to expect that there exist different intracellular mediators to detect the signals delivered at each of these *two* receptor sites on B cells.

The interaction of haptenic determinants bound to nonimmunogenic carriers with surface immunoglobulin receptors on B cells initiates events that lead to the paralytic pathway or cell inactivation. This interaction at the surface Ig receptors may stimulate adenylate cyclase to increase the intracellular levels of cAMP. The subsequent increase in the ratio of cAMP to cGMP may initiate the biochemical events that constitute the pathway to cell inactivation, and it may be a number of hours before complete inactivation of B cells is observed. High concentrations of extracellular dibutyryl cAMP may inactivate B cells in a similar manner (Watson *et al.*, 1973c).

The T-cell signal delivered to B cells may result in the activation of guanylate cyclases in B cells. This activation would lead to an increase in the intracellular levels of cGMP. A lower intracellular ratio of cAMP to cGMP may lead to the initiation of DNA synthesis, cell division, and maturation to antibody-forming cells. The reason the paralytic response is reversible for some time is to allow B cells receiving the haptenic signal via adenylate cyclase to receive a T-cell signal via guanylate cyclase, and be diverted to the inductive pathway. The proposal that the T-cell signal leads to the activation of guanylate cyclases in B cells is based on three experimental findings: (1) cGMP and LPS stimulate DNA synthesis and immune responses to erythrocyte antigens in T-cell-depleted cultures (Watson, 1974, 1975a,b); (2) LPS diverts B cells from a paralytic to an inductive pathway in the presence of deaggregated human immunoglobulin (Chiller and Weigle, 1973); and (3) all dividing cells appear to have an absolute requirement for a low intracellular ratio of cAMP to cGMP (Watson, 1974; Rudland *et al.*, 1974a,b).

The apparent contradiction—namely, that mitogens activate B cells by the delivery of one type of signal, whereas the inductive stimulus (antigenic plus T-cell signal) activates B cells by the delivery of two types of signals (Bretscher and Cohn, 1970)—is quite simply resolved in terms of an intracellular ratio governing the response of a cell. An intracellular ratio can be altered in a number of ways, e.g., by increasing or decreasing only cAMP or cGMP levels, or by differentially increasing or decreasing both cAMP and cGMP levels. Therefore, a number of stimuli may initiate the activation or inactivation pathways. For example, B-cell mitogens may alter this intracellular ratio by increasing *only* cGMP levels. Provided the cAMP-to-cGMP ratio decreases, a positive pleiotypic response is initiated. The interaction of antigen and the T-cell signal with B cells may elevate both intracellular cAMP and cGMP levels. A positive pleiotypic response is initiated *only* if these increases are differential so that the final ratio between cAMP and cGMP is lowered. The differences observed between the activation of B cells by nonspecific mitogens and that by specific antigens may merely reflect that while positive pleiotypic responses are initiated *only* by a decrease in the intracellular ratio of cAMP to cGMP, the rates of various metabolic components of the response may be regulated by both the ratio between the cyclic nucleotides and their individual concentrations.

5.4. Manipulation of Cyclic Nucleotide Metabolism and the Control of Antibody Synthesis

If the intracellular ratio of cAMP to cGMP controls the expression of the inductive or paralytic pathways in antigen-sensitive cells, then agents that exert selective effects on cyclic nucleotide metabolism may be useful in the manipulation of the immune response. Agents that elevate cAMP levels, such as β-adrenergic agonists, methyl xanthines, and cholera toxin, will tend to inhibit immune responses. In contrast, agents that elevate cGMP levels, such as cholinergic agonists, imidazole, and levamisole, may be mitogenic, or stimulatory to the induction of immune responses, or may have T-cell-replacing activity. There is a potential use for this agents in the regulation of *in vivo* immune responses. Lymphoid cells contain a variety of surface receptors that can be used to influence intracellular cyclic nucleotide levels. To be useful *in vivo,* however, cyclic-nucleotide-enhancing or -inhibiting agents that exert their effects *only* in lymphoid cells are required.

Although such agents are at present unknown, it may be possible to construct them. For example, the conjugation of cholera toxin, or a β-adrenergic agonist, to specific antigens may yield a molecule that binds to lymphoid cells via surface Ig receptors, but inhibits immune responses because of the effects of cholera toxin or the adrenergic agonist via different surface receptors on the same cell. Alternatively, the conjugation of cholinergic agonists or other cGMP-elevating agents to antigens may yield a molecule that binds to lymphoid cells selectively via Ig receptors, but increases intracellular cGMP levels via the conjugated moiety. Such agents that manipulate cyclic nucleotide levels in selective antigen-sensitive cells may be useful in controlling the expression of cells to either inductive or paralytic pathways.

ACKNOWLEDGMENTS

This work was supported by Grant number AI 13383-01 from the National Institutes of Health.

References

Alford, R. H., 1970, *J. Immunol.* **104**:698–703.

Allwood, G., Asherson, G. L., Davey, J. J., and Goodford, P. J., 1971, *Immunology* **21**:509–516.

Amer, M. S., and Byrne, J. E., 1975, *Nature (London)* **256**:421–424.

Andersson, B., and Blomgren, H., 1971, *Cell. Immunol.* **2**:411–424.

Andersson, J., Möller, G., and Sjöberg, O., 1972, *Transplant. Rev.* **11**:131–177.

Bona, C., Damais, C., and Chedid, L., 1974, *Proc. Natl. Acad. Sci. U.S.A.* **71**:1602–1606.

Bösing-Schneider, R., 1975, *Nature (London)* **256**:137–138.

Bourne, H. R., Lichtenstein, L. M., Melmon, K. L., Henny, C. S., Weinstein, Y., and Shearer, G. M., 1974, *Science* **184**:19–28.

Braun, W., and Ishizuka, M., 1971a, *Proc. Natl. Acad. Sci. U.S.A.* **68**:1114–1116.

Braun, W., and Ishizuka, M., 1971b, *J. Immunol.* **107**:1036–1042.

Bretscher, P. A., and Cohn, M., 1970, *Science* **169**:1042–1049.

Burger, M. M., Bombik, B. M., Breckenridge, B. McL., and Sheppard, J. R., 1972, *Nature (London)* **239**:161–163.

Chiller, J., and Weigle, W. O., 1973, *J. Exp. Med.* **137**:740–750.

Chiller, J. M., Skidmore, B. J., Morrison, D. C., and Weigle, W. O., 1973, *Proc. Natl. Acad. Sci. U.S.A.* **70**:2129–2133.

Chiller, J. M., Louis, J. A., Skidmore, B. J., and Weigle, W. O., 1974a, in: *The Immune System* (E. Sercarz and A. Williamson, eds.), pp. 553–567, Academic Press, New York.

Chiller, J. M., Louis, J. A., Skidmore, B. J., and Weigle, W. O., 1974b, in: *Immunological Tolerance* (D. H. Katz and B. Benacerraf, eds.), pp. 373–390, Academic Press, New York.

Claman, H. M., 1963, *J. Immunol.* **91**:833–839.

Cohn, M., 1972, in: *Genetic Control of Immune Responsiveness* (H. O. McDevitt and M. Landy, eds.), p. 436, Academic Press, New York.

Coutinho, A., and Möller, G., 1973, *Nature (London)* **245**:12–14.

Coutinho, A., Gronowicz, E., Bullock, W. W., and Möller, G., 1974, *J. Exp. Med.* **139**:74–92.

Daniel, V., Litwack, G., and Tomkins, G. M., 1973, *Proc. Natl. Acad. Sci. U.S.A.* **70**:76–79.

Davies, A. J. S., Carter, R. L., Leuchars, E., Wallis, V., and Dietrich, F. M., 1970, *Immunology* **19**:945–957.

Diamantstein, T., and Ulmer, A., 1975, *Exp. Cell Res.* **93**:309–314.

Diamantstein, T., Blitstein-Willinger, E., and Schultz, G., 1974, *Nature (London)* **250**:596–597.

Dukor, P., and Hartmann, K. U., 1973, *Cell. Immunol.* **7**:349–356.

Dutton, R. W., 1974, in: *The Immune System, Genes, Receptor, Signals* (E. E. Sercarz, A. Williamson, and F. Fox, eds.), pp. 485–496, Academic Press, New York.

Estensen, R. D., Hadden, J. W., Hadden, E. M., Touraine, F., Touraine, J. L., Haddox, M. K., and

Goldberg, N. D., 1974, in: *Control of Proliferation in Animal Cells* (B. Clarkson and R. Baserga, eds.), pp. 627–635, Cold Spring Harbor Press, Cold Spring Harbor, New York.
Freedman, M. H., Raff, M. C., and Gomperts, B., 1975, *Nature (London)* **255**:378–382.
Golan, D. T., and Borel, Y., 1971, *J. Exp. Med.* **134**:1046–1061.
Golub, E. S., and Weigle, W. O., 1967, *J. Immunol.* **98**:1241–1247.
Gronowicz, E., Coutinho, A., and Möller, G., 1974, *Scand. J. Immunol.* **3**:413–418.
Hadden, J. W., Hadden, E. M., Haddox, M. K., and Goldberg, N. D., 1972, *Proc. Natl. Acad. Sci. U.S.A.* **69**:3024–3029.
Hadden, J. W., Hadden, E., and Goldberg, N. D., 1974, in: *Cyclic AMP, Cell Growth, and the Immune Response* (W. Braun, L. M. Lichtenstein, and C. W. Parker, eds.) p. 237, Springer-Verlag, New York.
Hadden, J. W., Coffey, R. G., Hadden, E. M., Lopez-Corrales, E., and Sunshine, G. H., 1975, *Cell. Immunol.* **20**:98–103.
Hamilton, J. A., and Miller, J. F. A. P., 1973a, *J. Exp. Med.* **138**:1009–1014.
Hamilton, J. A., and Miller, J. F. A. P., 1973b, *Eur. J. Immunol.* **3**:457–460.
Hämmerling, U., Chia, A. F., Abbott, J., and Scheid, M. P., 1975, *J. Immunol.* **115**:1425–1431.
Hershko, A., Mamont, P., Shields, R., and Tompkins, G. M., 1971, *Nature (London)* **232**:206–211.
Hunig, T., Schimple, A., and Wecker, E., 1974, *J. Exp. Med.* **139**:754–760.
Ishizuka, M., Gafin, M., and Braun, W., 1970, *Proc. Soc. Exp. Biol. Med.* **134**:963–967.
Ishizuka, M., Braun, W., and Matsumoto, T., 1971, *J. Immunol.* **107**:1027–1035.
Jaroslow, B. N., and Ortiz-Ortiz, L., 1972, *Cell. Immunol.* **3**:123–132.
Katz, D. H., Paul, W. E., Goidl, E., and Benacerraf, B., 1971a, *J. Exp. Med.* **133**:169–186.
Katz, D. H., Davie, J. M., Paul, W. E., and Benacerraf, B., 1971b, *J. Exp. Med.* **134**:201–223.
Katz, D. H., Hamaoka, T., and Benacerraf, B., 1974, *J. Exp. Med.* **139**:1464–1472.
Krishnaraj, R., and Talwar, G. P., 1973, *J. Immunol.* **111**:1010–1017.
Louis, J. A., Chiller, J. M., and Weigle, W. O., 1973, *J. Exp. Med.* **138**:1481–1495.
Luderitz, O., Westphal, O., Staub, A., and Nikaido, H., 1971, in: *Microbial Toxins* (G. Weinbaum, S. Kadis, and S. J. Ajl, eds.), Vol. 4, p. 145, Academic Press, New York.
MacManus, J. P., and Whitfield, J. F., 1969, *Exp. Cell Res.* **58**:188–191.
MacManus, J. P., Whitfield, J. F., Boyton, A. L., and Rixon, R. H., 1975, *Adv. Cyclic Nucleotide Res.* **5**:719–734.
Maino, V. C., Green, N. M., and Crumpton, M. J., 1974, *Nature (London)* **251**:324–327.
Miller, J. F. A. P., 1961, *Lancet* **2**:748–750.
Mitchell, G. F., Grumet, F. C., and McDevitt, H. O., 1972, *J. Exp. Med.* **135**:126–135.
Mitchison, N. A., 1971, in: *Immunological Tolerance to Tissue Antigens* (N. W. Nisbet and M. W. Elves, eds.), p. 67, Proceedings of the Fourth Symposium of the Charles Salt Research Foundation, London.
Mozes, E., Weinstein, Y., Bourne, H. R., Melmon, K. L., and Shearer, G. M., 1974, *Cell. Immunol.* **11**:57–63.
Nossal, G., and Ada, G., 1971, in: *Antigens, Lymphoid Cells and the Immune Response,* pp. 1–10, Academic Press, New York.
Parker, C. W., Smith, J. W., and Steiner, A. L., 1971, *Int. Arch. Allergy Appl. Immunol.* **41**:40–46.
Pastan, I., and Perlman, R. L., 1971, *Nature (London)* **299**:5.
Paul, W. E., Karpf, M., and Mosier, D. E., 1974, in: *Immunological Tolerance* (D. H. Katz and B. Benacerraf, eds.), pp. 141–158, Academic Press, New York.
Plescia, O. J., Yamamoto, I., and Shinamura, T., 1975, *Proc. Natl. Acad. Sci. U.S.A.* **72**:888.
Rudbach, J. A., 1974, *J. Immunol.* **106**:993–1001.
Rudland, P. S., Gospodarowicz, D., and Seifert, W., 1974a, *Nature (London)* **250**:741, 742.
Rudland, P. S., Seeley, M., and Seifert, W., 1974b, *Nature (London)* **251**:417–419.
Scheid, M. P., Hoffman, M. K., Komuro, K., Hämmerling, U., Abbott, J., Boyse, E. A., Cohen, G. H., Hopper, J. A., Schulof, R. S., and Goldstein, A. L., 1973, *J. Exp. Med.* **138**:1027–1032.
Scher, I., Strong, D. M., Ahmed, A., Knudsen, R. C., and Sell, K. W., 1973, *J. Exp. Med.* **138**:1545–1563.
Schmidtke, J. R., and Dixon, F. J., 1972, *J. Exp. Med.* **136**:392–397.
Schor, S., and Rozengurt, E., 1972, *J. Cell. Physiol.* **81**:339–345.
Schultz, G., Hardman, J. G., Schultz, K., Baird, C. E., and Sutherland, E. W., 1973, *Proc. Natl. Acad. Sci. U.S.A.* **70**:3889–3893.
Seifert, W. E., and Rudland, P. S., 1974, *Nature (London)* **248**:138–140.

Sheppard, J. R., 1972, *Nature (London)* **236**:14–16.
Skidmore, B. J., Chiller, J. M., Morrison, D. C., and Weigle, W. O., 1975, *J. Immunol.* **114**:770–776.
Smets, L. A., 1972, *Nature (London)* **239**:123–124.
Smith, J. W., Steiner, A. L., Newberry, Jr., W. M., and Parker, C. W., 1971, *J. Clin. Invest.* **50**:432–441.
Strong, D. M., Ahmed, A. A., Scher, I., Knudsen, R. C., and Sell, K. W., 1974, *J. Immunol.* **113**:1429–1437.
Sultzer, B. M., and Nilsson, B. S., 1972, *Nature (London) New Biol.* **240**(102):198–200.
Teh, H.-S., and Paetkau, V. H., 1976a, *Cell. Immunol.* **24**:209–219.
Teh, H.-S., and Paetkau, V. H., 1976b, *Cell. Immunol.* **24**:220–229.
Trenkner, E., 1974, *J. Immunol.* **113**:918–924.
Watson, J., 1974, in: *Third ICN–UCLA Symposium on Molecular Biology* (E. E. Sercarz, A. R. Williamson, and C. F. Fox, eds.), pp 511–532, Academic Press, New York.
Watson, J., 1975a, *J. Exp. Med.* **141**:97–111.
Watson, J., 1975b, *Transplan. Rev.* **23**:223–249.
Watson, J., and Riblet, R., 1974, *J. Exp. Med.* **140**:1147–1161.
Watson, J., and Riblet, R., 1975, *J. Immunol.* **114**:1462–1468.
Watson, J., Epstein, R., Nakoinz, I., and Ralph, P., 1973a, *J. Immunol.* **110**:43–52.
Watson, J., Trenkner, E., and Cohn, M., 1973b, *J. Exp. Med.* **138**:699–714.
Watson, J., Epstein, R., and Cohn, M., 1973c, *Nature (London)* **246**:405–409.
Watson, J., Riblet, R., Cohn, M., Skidmore, B. J., Chiller, J. M., and Weigle, W. O., 1975, in: *Role of Mitogens in Immunobiology* (D. Rosenstreict and J. Oppenheim, eds.), Academic Press, New York.
Webb, D. R., Stites, D. P., Perlman, J. D., Luong, D., and Fudenberg, H. H., 1973, *Biochem. Biophys. Res. Commun.* **53**:1002–1008.
Weigle, W. O., 1965, *J. Immunol.* **94**:177–183.
Weinstein, Y., Chambers, D. A., Bourne, H. R., and Melmon, K. L., 1974, *Nature (London)* **251**:352–354.
Weinstein, Y., Segal, S., and Melmon, K. L., 1975, *J. Immunol.* **115**:112–118.
Whitfield, J. F., MacManus, J. P., Franks, D. J., Gillan, D. J., and Youdale, T., 1971, *Proc. Soc. Exp. Biol. Med.* **137**:453–457.
Whitfield, J. F., Rixon, R. H., MacManus, J. P., and Balk, S. D., 1973, *In Vitro* **8**:257–278.
Whitfield, J. F., MacManus, J. P., Boynton, A. L., Gillan, D. J., and Isaccs, R. J., 1974, *J. Cell. Physiol.* **84**:445–458.
Whitney, R. B., and Sutherland, R. M., 1973, *J. Cell. Physiol.* **80**:329–337.
Winchurch, R., Ishizuka, M., Webb, D., and Braun, W., 1971, *J. Immunol.* **106**:1399–1400.
Yamamoto, I., and Webb, D. R., 1975, *Proc. Natl. Acad. Sci. U.S.A.* **72**:2320–2324.

3

Regulation of Alloimmunity by Cyclic Nucleotides

TERRY B. STROM and CHARLES B. CARPENTER

1. Introduction

Lymphocytes express proliferative and cytotoxic responses following stimulation by cells bearing histoincompatible alloantigens. The transplantation antigens of the major histocompatibility gene complex *(HLA, H-2, AgB)* that stimulate the immunoproliferative responses mounted by allogeneic thymus-derived (T) lymphocytes in mixed lymphocyte cultures (MLC) and the graft-vs.-host (GVH) response are closely linked to, albeit separable from, the serologically identifiable specificities (Yunis and Amos, 1971; Schreffler and David, 1975; Cramer *et al.*, 1975). At least two subpopulations of lymphocytes are able to lyse alloantigenic target cells (Cerottini and Brunner, 1974). First, alloimmune cytotoxic T lymphocytes, bearing a receptor for cell-bound, serologically defined alloantigens (Alter *et al.*, 1973; Eijsvoogel *et al.*, 1973), bind to and destroy target cells (lymphocyte-mediated cytotoxicity, LMC). In contrast, nonimmune lymphocytes designated *K cells* that express a receptor for the Fc portion of IgG lyse target cells complexed with IgG anti-target-cell antibodies (antibody-dependent lymphocyte-mediated cytotoxicity, Ab-LMC) (Cerottini and Brunner, 1974; Perlmann *et al.*, 1972). The ability of 3′,5′-cyclic nucleotides to bidirectionally regulate the vigor of these proliferative and cytotoxic cellular responses against allogeneic cells is the subject of this chapter.

2. Cyclic Nucleotides

The pioneering work of Earl Sutherland and his associates, Rall, Butcher, and Robison, demonstrated that the action of glucagon on liver cells in the induction of glycogenolysis was linked to activation by glucagon of the catalytic activity of

---

TERRY B. STROM and CHARLES B. CARPENTER • Immunology Laboratory, Renal Division, Department of Medicine, Peter Bent Brigham Hospital and Harvard Medical School, Boston, Massachusetts 02115.

adenylate cyclase (see Robison *et al.*, 1971). The catalytic effect of adenylate cyclase on adenosine triphosphate (ATP) results in the intracellular formation of cyclic 3′,5′-adenosine monophosphate (cyclic AMP, cAMP). These investigators also determined that the effect of glucagon on glycogenolysis and the formation of cAMP can be amplified by the use of agents that inhibit the ability of phosphodiesterase to degrade cAMP to 5′-AMP. Furthermore, the treatment of liver cells with exogenous cAMP also resulted in enhanced glycogenolysis. The intracellular effects of many polypeptide hormones were subsequently proved to be mediated by cAMP acting as a "second messenger." Recent studies by Nelson Goldberg and his colleagues (see Goldberg *et al.*, 1973) indicated that the other naturally occurring cyclic 3′,5′-nucleotide, cyclic 3′,5′-guanosine monophosphate (cyclic GMP, cGMP), acts as a "second messenger" for certain hormones or neurotransmitters often noted to promote events antagonistic to those mediated by cAMP.

3. Pharmacological Abrogation of Target-Cell Lysis Mediated by Cytotoxic T Lymphocytes

Henney and Lichtenstein (1971) first suggested that cAMP may modulate the specific cytotoxic ability of sensitized T cells on target cells, since isoproterenol and theophylline inhibited the lysis *in vitro* of ^{51}Cr-labeled allogeneic mouse mastocytoma cells by alloimmune C57BL mouse cells during a 6-hr period of interaction between attacking and target cells. We confirmed these observations utilizing attacking cells harvested from Lewis rats sensitized by Lewis × Brown Norway F_1 skin grafts and ^{51}Cr-labeled Brown Norway thymocyte target cells during 4-hr *in vitro* incubations (Strom *et al.*, 1972).

Early experiments indicated that dibutyryl cAMP, a lipid-soluble analogue of cAMP that penetrates cell membranes more readily, causes almost total abolition of rat LMC (Strom *et al.*, 1972). This result stimulated our interest in the simultaneous effects of other agents known to alter intracellular cyclic nucleotide metabolism on LMC and intracellular cyclic nucleotide levels.

3.1. Prostaglandin (PGE_1) Effects

PGE_1 (10^{-4} M), an activator of adenylate cyclase, produces a rapid and sustained rise in lymphocyte cAMP levels, as measured by the cAMP protein assay (Gilman, 1970), that is associated with diminished LMC mounted by PGE_1-treated lymphocyte populations. The effects of PGE_1 on intracellular cAMP levels and cytotoxicity are dose-dependent, parallel, and potentiated by 10^{-3} M aminophylline, an inhibitor of cAMP phosphodiesterase (Strom *et al.*, 1973a).

3.2. β-Adrenergic Effects

Isoproterenol, an activator of adenylate cyclase via stimulation of β-adrenergic receptors, also causes inhibited LMC and elevated cellular levels of cAMP. Again, the actions of this adenylate cyclase activator were potentiated by the phosphodiesterase inhibitor aminophylline (Strom *et al.*, 1973a).

3.3. Cholera Toxin Effects

Since both attacking and target cells were exposed to dibutyryl cAMP, PGE_1, phosphodiesterase inhibitors, and isoproterenol, it was of paramount importance to establish the identity of cells being altered by elevations of cAMP and responsible for diminished LMC. Does cAMP protect the target cell from lysis or diminish the lytic capacity of the cytotoxic T lymphocytes? For this purpose, cholera toxin (1 μg/ml) was interacted separately with attacking or target cells for varying time periods (Figure 1); the cells were washed thrice, and aliquots were tested for cAMP content and cytotoxic capacity. The effect of cholera toxin on adenylate cyclase is long-lived. It also has the interesting property of requiring a lag period before the rise in intracellular cAMP occurs. One can therefore assess cholera toxin effects on cell populations separately, and also demonstrate the temporal relationship between cAMP elevations and effects on cell function. Treatment of target cells with cholera toxin did not protect these cells from LMC. In contrast, preincubation of the attacking cells for 180 min produced a marked inhibition of LMC accompanied by a great increase in cAMP content, whereas shorter preincubation periods were associated with only trivial alterations of cAMP levels or cytotoxicity. Hence, elevated intracellular levels of cAMP inhibit the cytotoxic capacity of cytotoxic T cells (Strom *et al.*, 1973a).

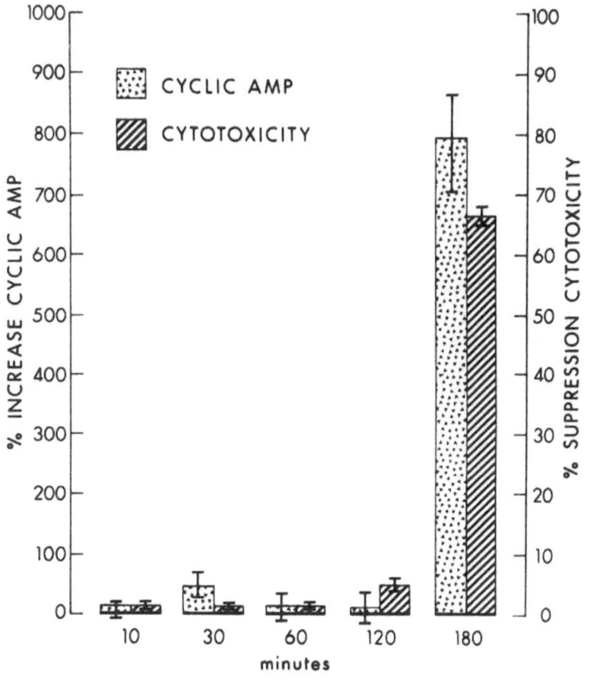

Figure 1. Time course of effects of cholera toxin (1 μg/ml) on LMC (vertical brackets indicate range) and cAMP (vertical brackets indicate S.E.M.). Reproduced from Strom *et al.* (1973a) with permission of the editors.

4. Pharmacological Augmentation of Target-Cell Lysis Mediated by Cytotoxic T Lymphocytes

Goldberg *et al.* (1973) proposed that many cell systems are regulated bidirectionally by the opposing actions of cAMP and cGMP. Whereas β-adrenergic activation produces elevations in cellular cAMP levels, cholinergic stimulation results in activation of guanylate cyclase and the intracellular accumulation of cGMP. The contrasting effects of glucagon, an adenylate cyclase activator, and insulin, an activator of guanylate cyclase, are similarly explained. The question whether lymphocyte function may be governed bidirectionally by cAMP and cGMP was assessed by studying the effects of agents capable of increasing cGMP on LMC.

4.1. Cholinergic Stimulation

The cholinergic agonists acetylcholine (ACh) and carbamylcholine produce augmented cell lysis that is totally dependent on optimal conditions of cholinomimetic concentration and the duration of attacking cell preincubation (Strom *et al.*, 1972, 1973a). Unsensitized cells do not injure target cells in the presence of cholinergic agonists (and the absence of anti-target-cell antibodies); however, the addition of the cholinergic agonist ACh or carbamylcholine at 10^{-9}–10^{-13} M to mixtures of sensitized spleen cells and target cells results in augmented cell lysis. The cholinomimetic augmentation of target-cell lysis by cytotoxic T lymphocytes is not observed if the attacking cells are preincubated with carbamylcholine for more than 6 min before the introduction of the target cells, or if the agonist is added after both attacking and target cells are mixed. In other words, an attacking cell–cholinomimetic interaction period of 1–6 min prior to the addition of target cells is crucial to the expression of enhanced effector-cell function (Figure 2). Effective doses of carbamylcholine fail to alter lymphocytic levels of cAMP (Figure 2).

Cholinergic receptors have been classically designated as either muscarinic or nicotinic. ACh and carbamylcholine are universal cholinergic agonists; however, muscarinic and nicotinic receptors are discriminatorily identified by the use of other agents that selectively stimulate or block these receptors. The cholinergic receptor of cytotoxic T lymphocytes is muscarinic in type, since atropine, a specific muscarinic antagonist, is a much more potent inhibitor of cholinergic-induced augmented cell lysis than the nicotinic inhibitors: α-bungarotoxin, *d*-tubocurarine, decamethonium, and hexamethonium (Strom *et al.*, 1974).

4.2. Insulin Stimulation

Physiologic concentrations of insulin (10^{-8}–10^{-11} M) mimic the effect of cholinergic agonists on LMC, since insulin-induced augmentation is also completely dependent on a short period of preincubation of the attacking cells with insulin. Atropine, a muscarinic antagonist that ablates cholinergic-induced augmentation of LMC, is unable to inhibit the effect of insulin on LMC; therefore, the action of insulin is not mediated via stimulation of the lymphocyte muscarinic receptor (Strom *et al.*, 1975a).

4.3. Imidazole Effects

Imidazole treatment of unsensitized splenic attacking cells does not cause these nonimmune cells to lyse target cells. However, imidazole, an agent known to stimulate cAMP phosphodiesterase and inhibit cGMP phosphodiesterase in broken cell preparations, is able to augment alloimmune LMC. The addition of imidazole at 10^{-7} M to attacking cell suspensions 2 min prior to the introduction of the target cells increased LMC by 50% and was associated with depleted intracellular levels of cAMP (Strom *et al.*, 1973a). Hadden *et al.* (1975) subsequently demonstrated that this concentration of imidazole does elevate spleen lymphocyte concentrations of cGMP. Therefore, the ratio of intracellular cGMP to cAMP is sharply increased by imidazole.

4.4. Cyclic GMP Stimulation

Since the stimulation of various tissues by cholinergic agonists or insulin results in increased cellular concentrations of cGMP, it was of crucial importance to assess the effects of cGMP on LMC. The results show clearly that the lipid-soluble analogue 8-bromo cGMP produces a dose-dependent augmentation of LMC (Strom *et al.*, 1973a).

The elimination of B lymphocytes (Strom *et al.*, 1973a, 1975a) or macrophages (Helderman and Strom, 1977a) from alloimmune attacking cell populations does not alter the action of insulin, ACh, carbamylcholine, imidazole, or 8-bromocyclic GMP on LMC. Since ligand and attacking cell preincubation is required for

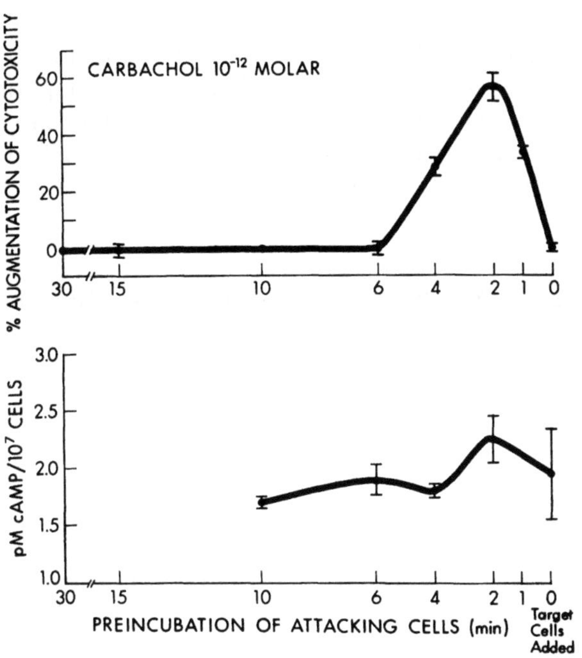

Figure 2. Effects of carbamylcholine (carbachol), 10^{-12} M, on LMC (vertical brackets indicate range) and concomitant levels of cAMP (vertical brackets indicate S.E.M.). Reproduced from Strom *et al.* (1973a) with permission of the editors.

enhanced LMC, the action of these agonists on LMC must result from an effect on attacking T lymphocytes. T–T cell cooperation has not been discerned during the *in vitro* effector phase of LMC; consequently, the augmentation of LMC induced by insulin, ACh, carbamylcholine, imidazole, and 8-bromo cGMP is most probably due to a time-dependent action of these agents on the cytotoxic T lymphocytes.

5. Pharmacological Abrogation of K-Cell-Mediated Lysis of Antibody-Coated Target Cells (Antibody-Dependent Lymphocyte-Mediated Cytotoxicity)

Since dibutyryl cAMP was found to inhibit Ab-LMC, the effects of adenylate cyclase activators and phosphodiesterase inhibitors on cytotoxicity and cellular levels of cAMP were tested in this other *in vitro* model of cell-mediated effector function (Carpenter *et al.*, 1974).

5.1. Prostaglandin Effects

The prostaglandins E_1, F_2, and A, all adenylate cyclase activators, produce a dose-dependent suppression of Ab-LMC. The addition of theophylline to prostaglandins during attacking and target cell interaction results in an additive inhibition of cytotoxicity (Garovoy *et al.*, 1975).

5.2. Cholera Toxin Effects

If attacking cells are preincubated with 1 μg cholera toxin/ml for varying time periods and then washed, it can be shown that incubation periods producing maximum rises in cellular cAMP levels also result in maximum suppression of Ab-LMC. Therefore, there is direct evidence that elevated intracellular cAMP levels inhibit the ability of K cells to lyse antibody-coated target cells (Garovoy *et al.*, 1975).

6. Pharmacological Augmentation of K-Cell-Mediated Lysis by Cyclic GMP

8-Bromo cGMP causes a significant augmentation of lysis at a concentration of 5×10^{-6} M, i.e., the same concentration that maximally boosts T-cell-mediated lysis (Garovoy *et al.*, 1975).

7. Modulation of Graft-vs.-Host Proliferation by Cyclic Nucleotides

Chronic GVH disease was produced by the intraperitoneal injection of 50×10^6 Balb/c murine spleen cells into 6-week-old (Balb/c × A/J) F_1 mice. After a total of four spleen cell immunizations at weekly intervals, the recipient spleens are harvested 4–5 weeks following the last injection and studied for their rate of spontaneous blastogenesis (proliferation) *in vitro*. Triplicate samples of 10^7 spleen cells are placed in culture media, and after 20 hr of culture, the cells are pulsed with thymidine-methyl-H^3 ($[^3H]TdR$) and harvested 4 hr later. The spleen cells harvested

TABLE 1. Pharmacological Modulation of Alloimmune Proliferative Responses

Agent	GVH	MLC
Dibutyryl cAMP	↓	↓
PGE_1	↓	↓
Aminophylline	↓	↓
PGE_1 + aminophylline	↓↓	↓↓
Cholera toxin	↓↓	Not done
Acetylcholine	↑	↑
Carbamylcholine	↑	Not done
8-Bromo cGMP	↑	↑
Imidazole	↑	Not done

from mice undergoing chronic GVH disease demonstrated a higher rate of proliferation than normal Balb/c × A/J F_1 spleen cells (Strom *et al.*, 1975b). Stimulation of GVH spleen cells, but not normal cells, with cholinergic agonists, 8-bromo cGMP (Strom *et al.*, 1975b), and imidazole (Strom, unpublished observations) results in augmented [^{3}H]TdR incorporation (Table 1), while dibutyryl cAMP or PGE_1 produces a dose-dependent inhibition of [^{3}H]TdR incorporation. Cholera toxin also blunts proliferation. The effects of PGE_1 and theophylline are additive (Table 1). These data strongly suggest that alloimmune proliferation produced during GVH disease is bidirectionally regulated by cyclic nucleotides (Strom *et al.*, 1975b).

8. Modulation of Mixed Lymphocyte Culture Proliferation by Cyclic Nucleotides

8.1 Modulation *in Vitro*

Recent experiments performed in our laboratory (Lundin, unpublished observations) demonstrate that the proliferative response of Lewis lymphocytes cultured with histoincompatible, mitomycin-C-treated Brown Norway rat lymphocytes during the MLC is also subject to modulation by cyclic 3′,5′-mononucleotides (Table 1). Dibutyryl cAMP, PGE_1, and theophylline inhibit rat MLC. As expected, the addition of theophylline and prostaglandin to the MLC causes more potent suppression than addition of either agent singly. Previous studies had also indicated that the presence of exogenous cAMP throughout the culture period inhibits the MLC (Estes *et al.*, 1971; Kook and Trainin, 1975). In contrast, the addition of ACh or 8-bromo cGMP to rat MLC results in enhanced proliferation (Lundin, unpublished observations).

8.2. Modulation *in Vivo*

Zurier and Quagliata (1971) demonstrated that *in vivo* PGE_1 administration suppressed delayed hypersensitivity skin reactions. Subsequently, the effect of agents known to elevate lymphocyte levels of cAMP was studied during the development of alloimmunity. Quagliata *et al.* (1973) observed that low doses of PGE_1, ranging from 100 to 200 μg/day and given subcutaneously at 12-hr intervals, did not prolong the survival of A/J murine skin grafts in CBA mice; however, these doses of prostaglandin did synergistically potentiate the ability of procarbazine hydrochloride to prolong skin graft survival. The intracellular levels of lymphocyte cAMP in control and treated animals were not ascertained during this study. A modest albeit statistically significant prolongation of hamster-to-rat cardiac grafts was achieved by the subcutaneous administration of 2 mg PGE_1/kg per day to the recipients (Kakita *et al.*, 1975). *In vivo* administration of cholera toxin by intraperitoneal (Henney *et al.*, 1973) or intravenous (Warren *et al.*, 1974) injection resulted in suppression of some elements of alloimmunity. Henney *et al.* (1973) found that intraperitoneal injection of 1 μg cholera toxin into C57BL/6 mice resulted in a marked elevation of splenic leukocyte cAMP levels that persisted for 3 days. These investigators further observed that the development of splenic or lymph node cytotoxic T lymphocytes at day 11 following sensitization with DBA/2 murine tissues, mastocytoma cells, or skin allografts was markedly suppressed by the administration of cholera toxin; however, cholera toxin disappointingly failed to prolong skin transplant survival. The production of anti-DBA hemagglutinating antibodies was also inhibited by cholera toxin. Since the cytotoxic capacity of spleen and draining lymph node was tested only on day 11 postsensitization, it is possible that a burst appearance of cytotoxic T lymphocytes appeared earlier than day 11 and these effector cells played some role in the rejection process. Alternatively, the cytolytic capacity of peripheral blood or intragraft killer cells that were not assayed may have been unaltered by cholera toxin treatment. Finally, it is possible albeit unlikely that killer cells do not exercise an important role in the rejection of skin transplants.

Warren *et al.* (1974) found that 1 μg cholera toxin i.v. on day 6 and 0.5 μg on day 9 prolonged the mean survival of C57BL/6 skin grafts in Balb/c hosts from 13 to 18 days. This study also reported that a single injection of 2 μg cholera toxin caused elevations of cAMP content in splenic leukocytes that persisted for 3 days. The failure of cholera toxin to prolong skin transplant survival in the Henney *et al.* (1973) study is probably related to differences in mouse strains or the route of cholera toxin administration employed.

We (Strom *et al.*, 1977) observed that daily intravenous administration of aminophylline from 0 to 7 days posttransplantation does promote an increased survival rate of nephrectomized Lewis rats grafted with Lewis × Brown Norway F_1 renal allografts despite severe graft dysfunction on days 7–10 postgrafting. The concomitant injection of aminophylline and prostaglandin analogues results in excellent renal graft function at 1 week posttransplantation and long-term transplant survival. Although the prostaglandin analogues administered to transplant recipients have been proved to stimulate lymphocyte adenylate cyclase *in vitro*, the effect of these agents on *in vivo* cyclic nucleotide metabolism is as yet unknown.

9. Discussion

The ability of sensitized cytotoxic lymphocytes to destroy target cells bearing donor alloantigens is regulated by cAMP and cGMP. The capacity of nonimmune T-independent lymphocytes bearing a receptor for the Fc portion of IgG to lyse target cells complexed with IgG anti-target-cell antibody is similarly modulated by cyclic 3′,5′-nucleotides. The ability of cytotoxic T cells to lyse target cells is inhibited by a variety of agents that have been demonstrated to elevate lymphocyte cAMP levels, including prostaglandins, isoproterenol, aminophylline, cholera toxin, and dibutyryl cAMP, whereas imidazole, cholinergic stimulation, insulin, or addition of 8-bromo cGMP enhances LMC. Either adenylate cyclase activators (isoproterenol, prostaglandin, or cholera toxin) or methylxanthines, which increase intracellular cAMP by protecting cAMP from breakdown, inhibit LMC and Ab-LMC. The combination of adenylate cyclase activators and methylxanthines causes an additive attenuation of LMC or Ab-LMC associated with a synergistic increase in cAMP. The inverse relationship between cAMP and cytotoxicity (LMC or Ab-LMC) in systems in which the attacking cells alone are treated with cholera toxin is decisive evidence that elevations of attacking lymphocyte cAMP levels suppress their ability to kill target cells.

In contrast, 8-bromo cGMP, a lipid-soluble analogue of cGMP, enhances the ability of effector cells that mediate LMC and Ab-LMC to destroy target cells. Furthermore, cholinergic agonists and insulin, agents that elevate cGMP, presumably via activation of guanylate cyclase (George *et al.,* 1970; Kuo *et al.,* 1972; Illiano *et al.,* 1973: Goldberg *et al.,* 1974), also enhance LMC. The augmentation of LMC by insulin and cholinergic agonists is mediated by the activation of separate plasma membrane receptors, since atropine, a muscarinic antagonist, blocks the cholinergic, but not the insulin-induced, augmentation of lysis.

Imidazole, an agent that decreases lymphocyte levels of cAMP, also enhances LMC. Recent investigations have demonstrated that imidazole and its derivative levamisole elevate human and murine lymphocyte levels of cGMP (Hadden *et al.,* 1975), in addition to decreasing cAMP. Thus, the ratio of cGMP to cAMP is altered in a manner that facilitates lymphocyte effector function. Both imidazole and levamisole enhance the proliferative responses of lymphocytes to phytohemagglutinin (Hadden *et al.,* 1975). Levamisole and tetramisole have been demonstrated to potentiate a variety of *in vivo* immune responses in mice, rats, and humans (Renoux and Renoux, 1971, 1972a,b; Tripodi *et al.,* 1973; Lods *et al.,* 1975; Spreafico *et al.,* 1975). The therapeutic effect of levamisole on human tumor resistance is currently under study using a double-blind protocol. A total of 111 patients with primary pulmonary carcinomas were administered levamisole or placebo as an adjunctive therapy to surgery. The levamisole-treated group (51 patients) had 10 recurrences and 7 deaths after 1 year of follow-up, whereas the placebo group (60 patients) sustained 20 recurrences of tumor and 12 deaths. Since levamisole lacks tumoricidal effects *in vitro,* it is likely that this agent augments tumor immunity in man (Study Group for Bronchogenic Carcinoma, 1975). That *in vivo* immunopotentiation may be produced by a variety of agents that alter cyclic nucleotide metabolism is further supported by the provocative observation that transfer factor causes elevations of cGMP within monocytes (Sandler *et al.,* 1975).

A brief preincubation of the attacking cell population with carbamylcholine (see Figure 2), insulin, imidazole, or 8-bromo cGMP prior to the introduction of target cells is a prerequisite for cholinergic enhancement of LMC, an effect consistent with the transient increases in cGMP known to occur with carbamylcholine, insulin, or imidazole stimulation. Since these agents do not alter LMC when preincubated with the target cells, pharmacological augmentation of LMC is apparently the result of an effect on the attacking cells alone. Similarly, isoproterenol, prostaglandin, and cholera toxin attenuate LMC only when the attacking cells are preincubated with agents and at a time when cAMP levels are elevated. Taken together, these data indicate that the levels of cAMP and cGMP within the attacking cells at the moment of initial contact with target cells determine the extent of cytotoxicity.

Other investigators (Gale and Zighelboim, 1975) demonstrated that human polymorphonuclear (PMN) leukocytes that bear an Fc receptor are able to lyse antibody-coated tumor cells. The ability of these PMN effector cells is also governed bidirectionally by their intracellular cyclic nucleotides: cAMP inhibits lysis, whereas cGMP enhances target-cell destruction. That cytotoxic T lymphocytes, K cells, and cytotoxic PMNs may utilize common mechanisms in target cell destruction is further suggested by the common requirement for divalent cations (Cerottini and Brunner, 1974; Garovoy *et al.*, 1975; Gale and Zighelboim, 1975), microtubules (Strom *et al.*, 1973b; Gale and Zighelboim, 1975), and energy (Strom *et al.*, 1975c).

The precise mechanisms of cell-mediated cytotoxicity are unknown; however, attacking and target cell attachment is a prerequisite for lysis in all the systems outlined above. The mechanism by which cytotoxic T lymphocytes destroy target cells is the most rigorously studied cytolytic system. Three stages of this lytic mechanism have been isolated (Martz, 1975). First, cytotoxic T lymphocytes form firm adhesions with target cells; second, a lethal injury is delivered to the target cell; and finally, the target cell lyses in a process that does not require the continued presence of viable attacking cells. Henney (1973) reported data that indicate that the second stage of lysis is inhibited by elevations in cellular cAMP. Since our data (Strom *et al.*, 1973a, 1975a) indicate that cyclic nucleotides alter an early step in the lytic process and the data of others provide evidence that the motility of T and B lymphocytes (Schreiner and Unanue, 1975) and PMNs (Estensen *et al.*, 1973) are bidirectionally modulated by cyclic nucleotides, we would speculate that increased attacking-cell levels of cGMP increase cell motility and enhance the opportunity for attacking and target cell adhesion. In contrast, cellular accumulations of cAMP inhibit attacking and target cell interaction. It is likely that multiple alterations in cell behavior regulated by the cyclic nucleotides account for changes in cell-mediated cytotoxicity.

The ability of cGMP to enhance and of cAMP to inhibit the proliferative response made by lymphoid cells encountering allogeneic cells demonstrates that both phases of cell-mediated alloimmunity, proliferative (recognition) and cytotoxic (effector), are regulated by cyclic nucleotides. These data are in concert with the mounting evidence that cGMP promotes proliferative events and cAMP opposes blastogenesis, as first proposed by Hadden *et al.* (1972a).

Fragmentary evidence gathered from several laboratories has indicated that the expression of lymphocyte cell receptors for ligands such as histamine and insulin change as a function of lymphocyte activation. As previously noted, insulin augments the effector function of cytotoxic T lymphocytes (Strom *et al.*, 1975a), whereas histamine, an activator of leukocyte adenylate cyclase (Bourne *et al.*, 1971), inhibits LMC produced by sensitized murine lymphocytes (Henney *et al.*, 1972). Consequently, the functional appearance or disappearance of specific lymphocyte receptors for agonists that activate adenylate cyclase (Bourne *et al.*, 1974) or guanylate cyclase constitutes a potential and intriguing mechanism for governing lymphocyte function. Obviously, a cell lacking specific receptors for insulin or histamine will not be directly influenced by alterations in concentration of these naturally occurring substances.

The distribution of insulin receptors among mononuclear leukocytes is incompletely defined (see Chapter 17). Recent studies indicate that peripheral blood mononuclear leukocytes prepared by passage through glass-bead columns (Hadden *et al.*, 1972b) or by ficoll–hypaque gradient separation (Gavin *et al.*, 1972; Olefsky and Reavan, 1974) bear insulin receptors. In contrast, rat splenic lymphoid cells (Krug *et al.*, 1972) or human peripheral blood lymphocytes (Olefsky and Reavan, 1974) prepared by filtration through nylon-wool columns do not specifically bind insulin. The primary consequence of passing mononuclear leukocytes through nylon wool is deletion of B lymphocytes (Eisen *et al.*, 1972) and macrophages (Handwerger and Schwartz, 1974). Subsequently, Schwartz *et al.* (1975) demonstrated that 85–90% of the insulin-binding cells found among human, ficoll–hypaque prepared peripheral mononuclear leukocytes are monocytes and not lymphocytes. Whereas nonactivated peripheral T lymphocytes lack insulin receptors, stimulated T lymphocytes appear to express a receptor for insulin. Krug *et al.* (1972) demonstrated that insulin receptors are revealed on the membranes of lymphocytes prepared by nylon-wool filtration during, but not before, activation by concanavalin A. Since physiologic concentrations of insulin augment LMC produced by nylon-wool-filtered effector cells, alloimmune T lymphocytes also appear to develop an insulin receptor. This concept has been formally proven (Helderman and Strom, 1977a) since nylon wool effluent, T-enriched spleen cells obtained from rats transplanted with histoincompatible skin grafts develop specific insulin-binding receptor sites whereas normal T cells or T cells obtained following syngeneic transplantation lack insulin receptors. The T-cell insulin receptor site is of similar affinity ($K_d \simeq 1$ nM) to the insulin receptor expressed upon liver and fat cells. Other data suggest that activated B cells also express an insulin receptor following activation with alloantigens or mitogens (Helderman and Strom, 1977b).

Plaut *et al.* (1975) reported that the cytolytic efficiency of murine splenic lymphocytes obtained 7–9 days after alloimmunization is unaffected by histamine *in vitro*, whereas our data show insulin to be effective at this time. From day 11 onward following allogeneic mastocytoma sensitization, histamine has an increasing ability to inhibit LMC. It would appear that early, alloimmune T lymphocytes (days 6–9 postsensitization) reveal an insulin receptor that allows the cGMP "go" signal to be transmitted, whereas the cells participating in the later immune response are more responsive to a cAMP-induced "turnoff" mechanism. Such dynamic changes on the lymphocyte membrane have obvious implications regarding acceleration of early immune events and exertion of negative control influences at a time when substantial tissue injury has been achieved. A further understanding of the regulatory influences of cyclic nucleotides on the immune response may allow rational and safe methods for pharmacological manipulation of the immune response. Indeed, immunomodulation has already been achieved *in vivo* utilizing agents demonstrated to alter lymphocytic concentrations of cyclic 3′,5′-nucleotides.

ACKNOWLEDGMENTS

This work was supported by N.I.H. grants AM-15579, CA-16937, and The Leukemia Research Foundation, T.B.S. is the recipient of a N.I.H. Research Career Development Award. C.B.C. is an investigator of the Howard Hughes Medical Institute.

References

Alter, B. J., Schendel, D. J., Bach, M. L., Bach, F. H., Klein, J., and Stimpfling, J. H., 1973, *J. Exp. Med.* **137**:1303–1309.

Bourne, H. R., Melmon, K. L., and Lichtenstein, L. M., 1971, *Science* **173**:743–745.

Bourne, H. R., Lichtenstein, L. M., Melmon, K. L., Henney, C. S., Weinstein, Y., and Shearer, G. M., 1974, *Science* **184**:19–28.

Carpenter, C. B., Garovoy, M. R., Strom, T. B., and Merrill, J. P., 1974, *Lymphocyte Recognition and Effector Mechanisms*—II (F. Daguillard, ed.), pp 351–354, Academic Press, New York.

Cerottini, J. C., and Brunner, K. T., 1974, *Adv. Immunol.* **18**:68–132.

Cramer, D. B., Shonnard, J. W., and Gill, T. J., 1975, *J. Immunogenet.* **1**:421–428.

Eijsvoogel, V. P., DuBois, R., Melief, C. J. M., Zeylemaker, W. P., Raat-Koning, L., and DeGroot-Kooy, L., 1973, *Transplant. Proc.* **5**:415–420.

Eisen, S. A., Wedner, H. J. and Parker, C. W. 1972, *Immunol. Commun.* **1**:571–577.

Estensen, R. D., Hill, H. R., Quie, P. G., Hogan, N., and Goldberg, N. D., 1973, *Nature (London)* **245**:458–460.

Estes, G., Solomon, S. S., and Norton, W. L., 1971, *J. Immunol.* **107**:1489–1492.

Gale, R. P., and Zighelboim, J., 1975, *J. Immunol.* **113**:1793–1800.

Garovoy, M. R., Strom, T. B., Kaliner, M., and Carpenter, C. B., 1975, *Cell Immunol.* **20**:197–204.

Gavin, J. R. III, Roth, J., Jen, P., and Freychet, P., 1972, *Proc. Natl. Acad. Sci. U.S.A.* **69**:747–751.

George, W. J., Polson, J. B., O'Toole, A. B., and Goldberg, N. D., 1970, *Proc. Natl. Acad Sci. U.S.A.* **66**:398–403.

Gilman, A. G. 1970, *Proc. Natl. Acad. Sci. U.S.A.* **67**:305–312.

Goldberg, N. D., Haddox, M. K., Hartle, D. K., and Hadden, J. W., 1973, in: *Proceedings of the Fifth International Congress of Pharmacology,* Vol. 5, pp. 146–183, S. Karger, Basel.

Goldberg, N. D., Haddox, M. K., Estensen, R., White, J. G., Lopez, C., and Hadden, J. W. 1974, in: *Cyclic AMP, Cell Growth and the Immune Response* (W. Braun, L. M. Lichtenstein, and C. W. Parker, eds.), pp. 247–262, Springer-Verlag, New York.

Hadden, J. W., Hadden, E. M., Haddox, M. K., and Goldberg, N. D., 1972a, *Proc. Natl. Acad. Sci. U.S.A.* **69**:3024–3027.

Hadden, J. W., Hadden, E. M., Wilson, E. E., Good, R. A., and Coffey, R. G., 1972b, *Nature (London) New Biol.* **235**:174–177.

Hadden, J. W., Coffey, R. G., Hadden, E. M., Lopez-Corrales, E., and Sunshine, G. H., 1975, *Cell. Immunol.* **20**:98–103.

Handwerger, B. S., and Schwartz, R. H., 1974, *Transplantation* **18**:544–548.

Helderman, J. H., and Strom, T. B., 1977a, *J. Clin. Invest.* **59**:338–344.

Helderman, J. H., and Strom, T. B., 1977b, *Clin. Res.* **25**:484 (abst).

Henney, C. S., 1973, *Transplant Rev.* **17**:37–70.

Henney, C. S., and Lichtenstein, L. M., 1971, *J. Immunol.* **107**:610–612.

Henney, C. S., Bourne, H. R., and Lichtenstein, L. M. 1972, *J. Immunol.* **108**:1526–1534.

Henney, C. S., Lichtenstein, L. M., Gillespie, E., and Rolley, R. J., 1973, *J. Clin. Invest.* **52**:2853–2857.

Illiano, G., Tell, G. P. E., Siegel, M. I., and Cuatrecasas, P., 1973, *Proc. Natl. Acad. Sci. U.S.A.* **70**:2443–2447.

Kakita, A., Blanchard, J., and Fortner, J. G., 1975, *Transplantation* **20**:439–442.

Kook, A. I., and Trainin, N., 1975, *J. Immunol.* **115**:8–14.

Krug, U., Krug, F., and Cuatrecasas, P., 1972, *Proc. Natl. Acad. Sci. U.S.A.* **69**:2604–2608.

Kuo, J., Lee, T., Reyes, P. O., Walton, K. G., Connelley, T. E., Jr., and Greengard, P., 1972, *J. Biol. Chem.* **247**:16–22.

Lods, J. C., Dujardin, P., and Halpern, G., 1975, *Ann. Allergy* **34**:210–212.

Martz, E., 1975, *J. Immunol.* **115**:261–267.

Olefsky, J., and Reavan, G. M., 1974, *J. Clin. Endocrinol. Metab.* **38**:554–560.

Perlmann, P., Perlmann, H., and Wigzell, H., 1972, *Transplant Rev.* **13**:91–114.

Plaut, M., Lichtenstein, L. M., and Henney, C. S., 1975, *J. Clin. Invest.* **55**:856–874.

Quagliata, R., Lawrence, V. J. W., and Phillips-Quagliata, J. M., 1973, *Cell. Immunol.* **6**:457–465.

Renoux, G., and Renoux, M., 1971, *C. R. Acad. Sci. Paris Ser. D* **272**:349–350.

Renoux, G., and Renoux, M., 1972a, *C. R. Acad. Sci. Paris Ser. D* **274**:3320–3322.

Renoux, G., and Renoux, M., 1972b, *J. Immunol.* **106**:761–765.

Robison, G. A., Butcher, R. W., and Sutherland, E. W., 1971, *Cyclic AMP,* Academic Press, New York.
Sandler, J. A., Smith, T. K., Manganiello, V. C., and Kirkpatrick, C. H., 1975, *J. Clin. Invest.* **56**:1271–1279.
Schreffler, D. C., and David, C. S., 1975, *Adv. Immunol.* **20**:125–195.
Schreiner, G. F., Jr., and Unanue, E. R., 1975, *J. Immunol.* **114**:802–808.
Schwartz, R. H., Bianco, A. R., Kahn, C. R., and Handwerger, B. S., 1975, *Proc. Natl. Acad. Sci. U.S.A.* **72**:474–478.
Spreafico, F., Vecchi, A., Mantovani, A., Poggi, A., Franchi, G., Anaclerio, A., and Garattini, S., 1975, *Eur. J. Cancer* **11**:555–563.
Strom, T. B., Diesseroth, A., Morganroth, J., Carpenter, C. B., and Merrill, J. P., 1972, *Proc. Natl. Acad. Sci. U.S.A.* **69**:2995–2999.
Strom, T. B., Carpenter, C. B., Garovoy, M. R., Merrill, J. P., Austen, K. F., and Kaliner, M., 1973a, *J. Exp. Med.* **138**:381–388.
Strom, T. B., Garovoy, M. R., Carpenter, C. B., and Merrill, J. P., 1973b, *Science* **181**:171–173.
Strom, T. B., Sytkowski, A. J., Carpenter, C. B., and Merrill, J. P., 1974, *Proc. Natl. Acad. Sci. U.S.A.* **71**:1330–1333.
Strom, T. B., Bear, R. A., and Carpenter, C. B., 1975a, *Science* **187**:1206–1208.
Strom, T. B., Hirsch, M. S., Black, P. J., Carpenter, C. B., and Merrill, J. P., 1975b, *Transplant. Proc.* **7**:305–307.
Strom, T. B., Garovoy, M. R., Bear, R. A., Gribik, M., and Carpenter, C. B., 1975c, *Cell. Immunol.* **20**:247–256.
Strom, T. B., Carpenter, C. B., Cragoe, E. J., Norris, S., Devlin, R., and Perper, R. J., 1977, *Transplant. Proc.* **9**:1075–1079.
Study Group for Bronchogenic Carcinoma, 1975, *Br. Med. J.* **53**:461–464.
Tripodi, D., Parks, L. C., and Brugmans, J., 1973, *N. Engl. J. Med.* **289**:254–257.
Warren, K. S., Mahmond, A. A. F., Boros, D. L., Rall, T. W., Mandel, M. A., and Carpenter, C. C. J., 1974, *J. Immunol.* **112**:996–1007.
Yunis, E. J., and Amos, D. B., 1971, *Proc. Natl. Acad. Sci. U.S.A.* **68**:3031–3035.
Zurier, R. B., and Quagliata, F., 1971, *Nature (London)* **234**:304–305.

4

Regulation of Polymorphonuclear Leukocyte, Macrophage, and Platelet Function

LOUIS J. IGNARRO

1. Introduction

During the past decade, cyclic AMP (cAMP) has been considered to be the principal intracellular regulator or modulator of biological function. Recent advances in the fields of cyclic nucleotides and biological regulation have made it clear, however, that a second cyclic nucleotide, cyclic GMP (cGMP), serves an important, and perhaps obligatory, function in the bioregulation of cellular processes (Goldberg *et al.*, 1973a,b). Following the initial demonstrations of cGMP in mammalian urine and tissues (Ashman *et al.*, 1963; Goldberg *et al.*, 1969; Ishikawa *et al.*, 1969), George *et al.* (1970) provided the first insight as to the possible importance of endogenous cGMP in biological function by demonstrating that the decrease in cardiac contractility mediated by acetylcholine (ACh) is associated with a concomitant and rapid accumulation of cardiac cGMP. Since these initial studies on the heart, numerous reports on the role of cGMP in biological regulatory mechanisms have appeared.

Much of the work involving cGMP suggests that it may function to mediate or signal cellular processes that are ultimately antagonistic or opposite in direction to those mediated by cAMP (Goldberg *et al.*, 1974). The initial studies of George *et al.* (1970) provided the basis for proposing the *dualism* or *Yin–Yang* hypothesis of biological control (Goldberg *et al.*, 1973b), which constitutes a type of control mechanism mediated through dual, opposing actions of cGMP and cAMP in

LOUIS J. IGNARRO • Department of Pharmacology, Tulane University School of Medicine, New Orleans, Louisiana 70112.

bidirectionally regulated systems. Some of the best examples of the dualism theory of biological control were provided by studies on circulating blood cells such as polymorphonuclear leukocytes, lymphocytes, macrophages, basophilic leukocytes, and platelets, and on related fixed-tissue cells such as mast cells. Highlights of the work conducted with polymorphonuclear leukocytes, mononuclear phagocytes, and platelets will be presented in this chapter.

2. Polymorphonuclear Leukocytes (Neutrophils)

2.1. Physiologic Functions

The primary physiologic or pathophysiologic functions of neutrophils include phagocytosis and killing of microorganisms, chemotaxis, and lysosomal enzyme secretion. Normally, following phagocytosis, lysosomes fuse with the phagosome to form a phagolysosome. Secretion of lysosomal enzymes into the extracellular environment does occur during phagocytosis, and can also occur in the absence of particle ingestion (Figure 1). The biological consequence of intracellular lysosomal enzyme release is microbial digestion, while the biological consequence of extracellular enzyme release is tissue injury. Tissue injury occurs because of the presence within human neutrophil lysosomes of enzymes capable of catalyzing the breakdown of connective tissue. Such enzymes include collagenase, elastase, and one or more neutral proteases capable of degrading the proteoglycan matrix of cartilage (see Ignarro, 1975, for a review). Neutrophils migrate toward sites of tissue injury (chemotaxis), accumulate there, phagocytize any ingestable particulate material, and secrete their lysosomal contents. Under these pathophysiologic conditions, lysosomal enzyme discharge proceeds primarily through one of two mechanisms: ''regurgitation during feeding'' (Weissman *et al.*, 1971a) or ''reverse endocytosis'' (Weissmann *et al.*, 1972). In the former instance, release occurs during phagocytosis; in the latter instance, release occurs in the absence of phagocytosis during neutrophil adherence to nonphagocytizable immune complexes.

2.2. *In Vitro* Cell Model Systems

Many different *in vitro* model systems that can be used to quantitate phagocytosis, lysosomal enzyme secretion, and motility have been described. The systems pertaining to phagocytosis were reviewed recently by Stossel (1975). Most of the studies on phagocytosis discussed in this chapter employ serum-treated zymosan particles. In most cases, particle ingestion has been quantitated by oil-immersion phase-contrast microscopy. Latex particles, starch particles, radiolabeled bacteria, and immune complexes have also been used.

Lysosomal enzyme discharge has been measured in both phagocytic and nonphagocytic cell systems. The phagocytic systems named above are quite conducive to the measurement of enzyme release. Immobilized immune reactants used to study nonphagocytic enzyme release include heat-aggregated human IgG or antigen–antibody complexes attached to solid surfaces such as cellulose fiber filter disks, collagen–ferritin biopolymer membranes, or hyaline cartilage disks (Henson, 1971; Hawkins, 1971; Oronsky *et al.*, 1973; Ignarro, 1974a,c). Soluble macromolecules such as activated complement components provoke lysosomal enzyme

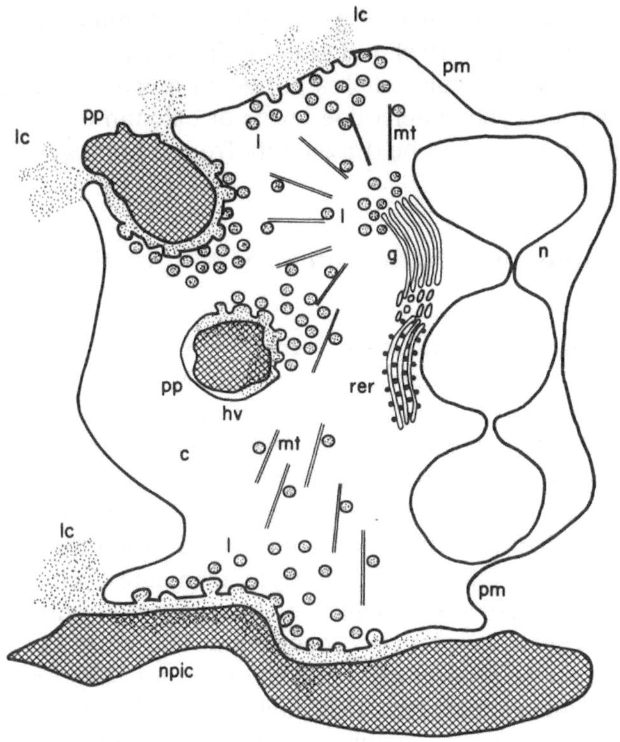

Figure 1. Diagrammatic representation of a neutrophil (polymorphonuclear leukocyte) interacting with immune reactants. During cell contact with phagocytizable particles, lysosomes may translocate from the Golgi to the phagosome or to the cell periphery and merge with the membranes of either completely or incompletely internalized heterophagic vacuoles. In the latter case, lysosomal contents are discharged into the extracellular environment. Lysosomal enzyme secretion may also proceed by translocation of lysosomes to, and their direct fusion with, the plasma membrane, which occurs particularly at the site of adherence to a nonphagocytizable immune complex. Translocation of lysosomes is directed or oriented by the microtubular system. (lc) Lysosomal contents; (pm) plasma membrane; (pp) phagocytizable particle; (l) lysosome; (mt) microtubule; (g) Golgi; (n) nucleus; (rer) rough endoplasmic reticulum; (hv) heterophagic vacuole; (c) cytosol; (npic) nonphagocytizable immune complex.

release when they make contact with neutrophil surfaces (Goldstein *et al.*, 1973; Becker *et al.*, 1974). Another nonphagocytic model of enzyme release entails the use of a fungal metabolite, cytochalasin B, that inhibits phagocytosis but yet allows lysosomal enzyme release to occur during cell contact with particulate or soluble immune reactants (Zurier *et al.*, 1973a).

Neutrophil chemotaxis and motility have been quantitated primarily by modifications of the method of Boyden (1962). In this test system, neutrophils are placed on one side of a chamber divided by a millipore filter (approximately 5-μm pore size), and a chemotactic stimulus is placed on the opposite side. After incubation at 37°C, the number of cells that have migrated to the opposite side of the chamber is determined.

The homogeneity of cell populations employed in the pertinent studies has been variable. Mixed leukocytes as well as purified neutrophils have been used. Neutrophils have been isolated and purified by techniques involving ficoll–hypaque gradients (Böyum, 1967) and siliconized glass-bead column chromatography (Rabinowitz, 1964; Ignarro *et al.*, 1974a). These methods yield leukocyte preparations containing over 95% neutrophils. Such a purification procedure becomes essential when one is measuring cyclic nucleotide levels or calcium influx, since meaningful conclusions, in most cases, can be drawn only from a homogeneous population of cells.

2.3. Bioregulation and Pharmacological Modulation of Neutrophil Function

Extensive progress has been made during the past five years on the elucidation of biological factors that affect neutrophil function. Much of this progress was made possible because of the rapid unraveling of the mechanisms by which cGMP and cAMP mediate and control cell function in general. One of the most important initial experiments on the involvement of cAMP in neutrophil function was reported by Scott (1970), who showed that epinephrine and prostaglandin E_1 (PGE_1) increased cAMP formation by human leukocyte homogenates. Soon thereafter, Bourne and Melmon (1971) reported that human leukocyte adenylate cyclase activity could be stimulated by epinephrine, norepinephrine, isoproterenol, and PGE_1, but not by phenylephrine, glucagon, or adrenocorticotropin. The latter study also suggested the presence of separate β-adrenergic and PG receptor sites on the plasma membrane surfaces of human leukocytes. In a similar study, Bourne *et al.* (1971) showed that PGE_1 and E_2, but not $F_{1\alpha}$, stimulated human leukocyte adenylate cyclase and cAMP accumulation. Moreover, theophylline, a phosphodiesterase inhibitor, enhanced the effect of PGE_1 and E_2. These investigators also demonstrated that PGE_1 and theophylline could inhibit the capacity of human leukocytes to kill, *in vitro, Candida albicans,* an effect that is also elicited by dibutyryl cAMP. The stimulatory effect of PGE_1 and E_2 on human leukocyte adenylate cyclase was reconfirmed by Polgar *et al.* (1973), who also showed that $PGF_{2\alpha}$ elicited a similar stimulatory effect. Thus, the foundation for a cAMP involvement in human granulocyte function was established by the identification of hormone-responsive, cAMP-synthesizing systems associated with human leukocytes.

A direct effect on human leukocyte function of added cAMP and agents that were reported to stimulate leukocyte cAMP accumulation was firmly established by Weissmann and his co-workers. cAMP, dibutyryl cAMP, theophylline, and PGE_1 inhibited the immunologic discharge of lysosomal enzymes from mixed human leukocytes (May *et al.*, 1970; Weissmann *et al.*, 1971a,b).

A pharmacological agent that influences lysosomal enzyme release from neutrophils may interfere with one or more steps leading to release. Motility of neutrophils, adherence between cells and particulate immune reactants, phagocytosis, merger or fusion of lysosomes with heterophagic vacuoles or plasma membrane, and translocation of lysosomes to the site of fusion are all potential targets for the effects of pharmacological agents (Weissmann *et al.*, 1975a). That they are may present a problem to the investigator who desires to examine the detailed effects of hormones on only one neutrophil function independent of any other cellular function, unless he is able to separate or distinguish one cellular process from the others. By making use of the fungal metabolite cytochalasin B, which is known to interfere with microfilament function, the process of phagocytosis of particulate immune reactants can be inhibited without affecting the independent process of lysosomal enzyme release (Zurier *et al.*, 1973a). Thus, the effects of agents on lysosomal enzyme release can be examined independently of their possible additional effects on phagocytosis. Although dibutyryl cAMP, theophylline, and PGE_1 were reported to inhibit divalent-cation-dependent granulocyte adhesion to glass surfaces (Bryant and Sutcliffe, 1974), such drug effects on leukocyte adhesion to immobilized immune reactants have not as yet been demonstrated. Unpublished observations in this laboratory indicate that cholinergic agents, catecholamines, PGs, and glucocorticosteroids do not significantly influence adhesion of purified human neutrophils to either cellulose fibers or hyaline cartilage, coated with heat-aggregated human IgG, at 37°C in calcium-containing media during the first 30 min of cell contact. In any event, the use of soluble immune reactants such as certain activated components of complement has eliminated the need to consider drug influences on particle–cell adherence (Goldstein *et al.*, 1973). Elimination of the process of motility does not appear to be crucial, because in most if not all cases, the reaction vessels are agitating and the neutrophils are therefore making contact with surfaces at predictable and controllable frequencies. Thus, the investigator is left with two possible sites of action: translocation of lysosomes and their merger or fusion with the plasma membrane. Inhibition of lysosomal enzyme release from cytochalasin-B-treated human neutrophils, in which enzyme release was provoked by either particulate or soluble immune reactants, was obtained with cAMP, dibutyryl cAMP, phosphodiesterase inhibitors, epinephrine, histamine, and various PGs (Zurier *et al.*, 1973a,b, 1974; Goldstein *et al.*, 1973). These investigators attributed the inhibitory effect of cAMP on lysosomal enzyme release to an interference with microtubule assembly and function, an interference that limits the translocation of lysosomes to, and their subsequent fusion with, the plasma membrane (Hoffstein *et al.*, 1974; Weissmann *et al.*, 1975a).

Studies from this laboratory first indicated a stimulatory effect of cGMP, analogues of cGMP, and pharmacological agents that elevate cGMP levels in other tissues on the immunologic discharge of lysosomal enzymes from human granulocytes (Ignarro, 1973). In the same study, cAMP and two of its analogues, as well as catecholamines and theophylline, all inhibited lysosomal enzyme release. The finding that the effect of cGMP and cholinergic agents was opposite to that of cAMP and catecholamines provided the basis for our hypothesis that cGMP and cAMP mediate opposing actions on lysosomal enzyme release, thereby endowing the human neutrophil with the capacity to exercise a bidirectional control of cell function (Ignarro and George, 1974a). In the first report (Ignarro, 1973) and in the two that followed (Ignarro, 1974a,b), separate β-adrenergic and muscarinic receptors were identified on the plasma membranes of neutrophils by analyzing the effects of specific adrenergic and cholinergic receptor antagonists. Similar results were obtained in a calcium-requiring, nonphagocytic model system in which cells were allowed to come in contact with nonphagocytizable, aggregated human IgG (Ignarro, 1974a). Thus, opposing actions of cGMP and cholinergic agents, on one hand, and cAMP and catecholamines, on the other, were demonstrated in the absence of phagocytosis. Again, similar results were observed in the absence of phagocytosis by using soluble immune reactants (Ignarro and George, 1974b; R. J. Smith and Ignarro, 1975). Thus, in agreement with the findings of Zurier *et al.* (1974), who employed cytochalasin-B-treated human neutrophils, studies from this laboratory revealed that cyclic nucleotides and autonomic neurohormones are capable of modulating lysosomal enzyme release by affecting intracellular mechanisms that are independent of phagocytosis and are most likely related to lysosome translocation to and fusion with the plasma membrane.

Studies from this laboratory have demonstrated not only direct effects of added cyclic nucleotides and tissue hormones on human neutrophil function, but also changes in the neutrophil concentrations of cyclic nucleotides provoked by the tissue hormones. It is clear that pharmacological agents that cause the accumulation of cGMP and cAMP in neutrophils also cause enhancement and inhibition, respectively, of lysosomal enzyme release (Ignarro and George, 1974a,b; Ignarro *et al.*, 1974a,b; R. J. Smith and Ignarro, 1975; Ignarro and Cech, 1975). Agents that provoke cGMP accumulation and lysosomal enzyme release include muscarinic agonists, $PGF_{2\alpha}$, diavalent cation ionophores, and various particulate and soluble immune reactants, all of which require the presence of calcium. Agents that elevate cAMP levels and inhibit enzyme release include catecholamines, several PGs and theophylline. Glucocorticosteroids also inhibit lysosomal enzyme release, but this effect is associated with an inhibition of cGMP accumulation, rather than an increase in cAMP levels (Ignarro and Cech, 1975; George *et al.*, 1975).

Perhaps the most important interaction is that between neutrophils and immune reactant, which results in release of lysosomal enzymes and a concomitant accumulation of cGMP without influencing cAMP levels. Calcium is required for both cellular events (Ignarro and George, 1974b). Indeed, calcium influx is associated temporally with immune-reactant-mediated lysosomal enzyme secretion and cGMP accumulation (R. J. Smith and Ignarro, 1975). We have postulated that calcium entry into the neutrophil is the initial signal for enzyme release, providing the stimulus for cGMP accumulation and the consequent secretion of lysosomal contents (R. J. Smith and Ignarro, 1975). In support of this hypothesis is the finding that a divalent-cation ionophore, A23187, increases the permeability of the neutrophil plasma membrane to calcium, and also provokes, in succession, cGMP accumulation and lysosomal enzyme release (R. J. Smith and Ignarro, 1975).

Cyclic nucleotides also affect functions of neutrophils other than secretion. For example, convincing evidence exists that cAMP, and pharmacological agents that elevate cAMP levels, inhibit phagocytosis (Bourne *et al.*, 1971; Stossel *et al.*, 1972; Cox and Karnovsky, 1973; Ignarro *et al.*, 1974a; Ignarro and Cech, 1975). PGE_1, E_2, A_1, and $F_{2\alpha}$, as well as cAMP, inhibited phagocytosis by guinea pig polymorphonuclear leukocytes (Cox and Karnovsky, 1973). In an experimental system in which purified human neutrophils were incubated with a high particle/cell ratio of rheumatoid-arthritic-serum-treated zymosan particles, cAMP and catecholamines inhibited phagocytosis, whereas cGMP and cholinergic agents elicited no effect (Ignarro *et al.*, 1974a). In a subsequent study, however, in which the particle/cell ratio was reduced to values yielding phagocytic rates of only 40% of maximum, cGMP and cholinergic agonists stimulated particle ingestion (Ignarro and Cech, 1976). Thus, at maximum phagocytic rates (high particle/cell ratios), enhancement of particle ingestion by cGMP cannot be demonstrated. On the other hand, inhibition of phagocytosis by cAMP and catecholamines was evident at both low and high particle/cell ratios. Experiments with specific receptor antagonists revealed that muscarinic and β-adrenergic receptors mediate enhancement and inhibition, respectively, of both phagocytosis and lysosomal enzyme release (Ignarro and Cech, 1976).

Cyclic nucleotides also affect the motility of human polymorphonuclear leukocytes. The leukotactic response of neutrophils was stimulated by cGMP and pharmacological agents that elevated cGMP levels (Estensen *et al.*, 1973). In contrast, cAMP and agents that elevated cAMP levels in neutrophils inhibited neutrophil motility (Tse *et al.*, 1972; Estensen *et al.*, 1973; Rivkin *et al.*, 1975). In a more detailed study, a variety of pharmacological agents known to elevate cGMP and cAMP levels, respectively, in human neutrophils were observed to enhance and inhibit the chemotactic response of these cells to a bacterial factor (Hill *et al.*, 1975). In a model of human-neutrophil-mediated, antibody-dependent cellular cytotoxicity, cGMP facilitated, whereas cAMP inhibited, this cytotoxic response (Gale and Zighelboim, 1974).

It is clear that cGMP and cAMP are associated with and elicit stimulatory and inhibitory effects, respectively, on several neutrophil functions. The opposing influences of cGMP and cAMP on at least four distinct functions of neutrophils constitute strong evidence for a bioregulatory role of cyclic nucleotides in human neutrophil function.

2.4. Relationship Between *in Vitro* and *in Vivo* Findings

Adrenergic mechanisms, *in vivo,* have been implicated in the regulation of the inflammatory process. Epinephrine and norepinephrine were postulated by Spector and Willoughby over ten years ago to function as naturally occurring, local, antiinflammatory neurohormones (see Ignarro, 1975, for a review and bibliography of the following statements). Inhibitors of the enzymatic degradation of catecholamines produced antiinflammatory effects in experimental animal models of thermal and chemical injury. Moreover, precursors of epinephrine (dopa and dopamine) reduced swelling *in vivo,* and epinephrine elicited antiinflammatory effects in several different animal models of acute and chronic inflammation. Whether or not the catecholamines elicit their *in vivo* effect by inhibiting neutrophil function is unknown. In this regard, however, it is of interest that β-adrenergic receptor antagonists, which inhibited the effect of catecholamines on neutrophil function *in vitro,* also inhibited the beneficial action of catecholamines *in vivo.*

A pathophysiologic role for PGs in the modulation of inflammation is evident, although controversy exists as to whether these tissue hormones exert primarily pro- or antiinflammatory actions (Ignarro, 1975). It was first demonstrated that aspirin and indomethacin inhibit PG biosynthesis by Vane and his colleagues, who suggested that this inhibition was the mechanism of antiinflammatory action of these drugs (Vane, 1971; J. B. Smith and Willis, 1971; Ferreira *et al.*, 1971). Several reports have illustrated, however, that PGs elicit marked antiinflammatory effects *in vivo*. For example, PGE_2 (Aspinall and Cammarata, 1969) and PGE_1 (Zurier and Quagliata, 1971) elicit strong antiarthritic effects in adjuvant polyarthritis in rats. Additionally, PGE_1 inhibits acute edema and retards lysosomal enzyme release from leukocytes at the site of inflammation (Zurier *et al.*, 1973c). There is much *in vitro* evidence to support an antiinflammatory action of PGs. PGs of the E, A, or F series inhibit neutrophil functions such as lysosomal enzyme secretion (Zurier *et al.*, 1973b; Ignarro, 1975), phagocytosis (Cox and Karnovsky, 1973), adhesion to rigid surfaces (Bryant and Sutcliffe, 1974), and chemotaxis (Rivkin *et al.*, 1975).

Inhibitory effects of PGs on neutrophil function are associated with elevations of cellular cAMP levels (Ignarro, 1975).

In several models of acute edema, cAMP and theophylline were reported to elicit antiinflammatory effects (Ichikawa *et al.*, 1972). These effects are consistent with their *in vitro* inhibitory effects on neutrophil function. A decrease in the cAMP concentration of mixed exudate leukocytes in a model of delayed hypersensitivity in guinea pigs was reported (Yamamoto *et al.*, 1975). A recent report (Deporter *et al.*, 1976) indicated that endogenous polymorphonuclear leukocyte cGMP and cAMP levels increased and decreased, respectively, during onset of pyrophosphate-induced pleurisy in rats. On the other hand, as the swelling subsided, cGMP and cAMP levels returned toward normal. These *in vivo* data support the earlier *in vitro* data with purified polymorphonuclear leukocytes (Ignarro and George, 1974a).

Glucocorticosteroids are potent antiinflammatory agents that also inhibit certain functions of neutrophils, such as lysosomal enzyme release (Wright and Malawista, 1973; Ignarro, 1974c,d; Ignarro and Cech, 1975). The inhibitory actions of glucocorticoids on neutrophils resemble those of cAMP and pharmacological agents that cause cAMP to accumulate in these granulocytes. Despite this resemblance, however, the glucocorticoids do not trigger cAMP accumulation; instead, they inhibit the accumulation of neutrophil cGMP during cell contact with particulate or soluble immune reactants (Ignarro and Cech, 1975). Certain glucocorticosteroids can inhibit the accumulation of cGMP in other tissues as well, such as the heart (George *et al.*, 1975).

2.5. Theoretical Considerations and Future Directions

The experiments discussed above illustrate that the Yin–Yang or dualism concept of biological control, as proposed originally by Goldberg *et al.* (1973b) for various tissues, also applies to the polymorphonuclear leukocyte. Most of the experiments have been conducted with human cells, although some evidence exists to support this regulatory concept in granulocytes from the guinea pig (Weissmann *et al.*, 1975b) and the rabbit (Rivkin *et al.*, 1975). Many of the studies indicated that calcium is required and plays a crucial role in triggering several neutrophil functions, including lysosomal enzyme release, phagocytosis, and motility (Woodin and Wieneke, 1963; Ignarro, 1974a; Ignarro and George, 1974b; Ignarro *et al.*, 1974a; R. J. Smith and Ignarro, 1975; Becker *et al.*, 1974; Wilkinson, 1975). Lysosomal enzyme release from neutrophils can be regarded as a secretory process, since release of granule contents is a selective exocytotic process. Just as calcium serves as the link in stimulus–secretion coupling in many secretory processes (Rubin, 1970), it may also serve as the link for lysosomal enzyme secretion from neutrophils (R. J. Smith and Ignarro, 1975). Accumulation of calcium within neutrophils might be facilitated by the presence, at up to 30 times the concentration in the extracellular environment, of potential calcium-binding molecules such as phosphate, nucleotides, amino acids, and reducing sugars (Woodin, 1968). This possibility may account for the earlier findings that relatively large amounts of calcium can accumulate within viable polymorphonuclear leukocytes (Woodin and Wieneke, 1963). Calcium influx may activate neutrophil guanylate cyclase, which would then result in the biosynthesis of cGMP (Ignarro and George, 1975). Calcium activation of guanylate cyclase and cGMP accumulation in other tissues has been reported

(Hardman *et al.*, 1971; L. E. White *et al.*, 1973; Schultz *et al.*, 1973; Ferrendelli *et al.*, 1973). Figure 2 is a schematic representation of the possible mechanisms by which lysosomal enzyme secretion from neutrophils is regulated. A recent study (Goldstein *et al.*, 1975) indicated, in contrast to our findings (R. J. Smith and Ignarro, 1975), that a specific soluble immune reactant, derived from fresh serum by treatment of the latter with zymosan particles, did not require extracellular calcium to stimulate lysosomal enzyme release from human neutrophils. The apparent discrepancy may be attributed to the fact that the cells had been pretreated with cytochalasin B, an agent known to interfere with microfilament function. In agreement with our findings, calcium was required for lysosomal enzyme release from polymorphonuclear leukocytes provoked by a soluble bacterial factor (Becker *et al.*, 1974).

Another point of interest is the finding that immune reactants (particulate, immobilized surfaces, or soluble) had to be in contact with the neutrophil plasma

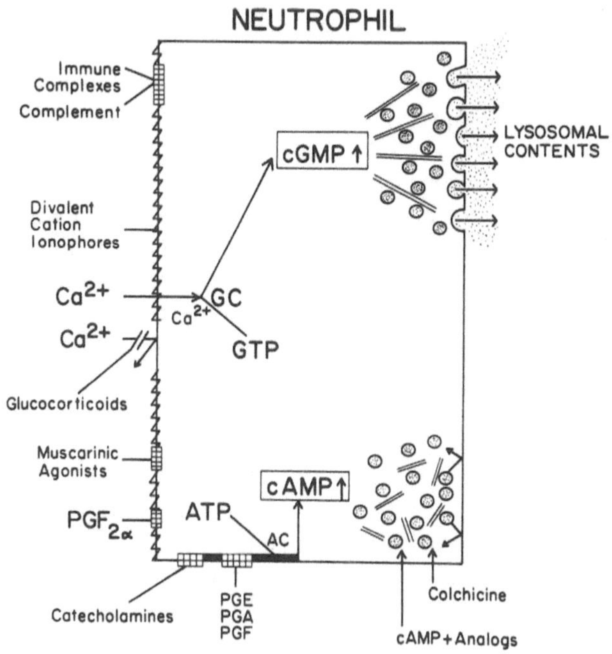

Figure 2. Schematic representation of the hypothetical bioregulation of lysosomal enzyme secretion from neutrophils (polymorphonuclear leukocytes). During cell contact with a soluble or insoluble immune reactant, or a divalent-cation ionophore, the plasma membrane undergoes an increase in permeability to divalent cations such as calcium. Elevated intracellular levels of calcium then stimulate guanylate cyclase (GC) and thereby cause cGMP to accumulate. cGMP may then provoke, via undefined mechanisms, the assembly of microtubules so that the lysosomes can translocate to the periphery of the cell. In the presence of enhanced membrane permeability to calcium, muscarinic agonists and $PGF_{2\alpha}$ promote further calcium influx and cGMP accumulation and secretion. Direct addition of cGMP also promotes lysosomal enzyme secretion. On the other hand, glucocorticosteroids inhibit calcium influx and cGMP accumulation and secretion. Catecholamines, certain PGs, cAMP, and colchicine inhibit secretion. The first two types of agent stimulate adenylate cyclase (AC) and the accumulation of cAMP (without interfering with calcium influx or cGMP accumulation), which may then either promote disassembly or inhibit assembly of microtubules.

membrane for hormones to affect further the intracellular levels of cyclic nucleotides and lysosomal enzyme secretion (Ignarro and George, 1974b; R. J. Smith and Ignarro, 1975). Similarly, when cytochalasin-B-treated neutrophils were used, cholinergic agents elicited no effect on enzyme secretion unless an immune reactant was also present (Weissmann *et al.*, 1975a). PGE_1, cholera enterotoxin, isoproterenol, histamine, and theophylline each elevated neutrophil cAMP levels much more dramatically in the presence than in the absence of zymosan particles (Zurier *et al.*, 1974). Known divalent-cation ionophores did not require the presence of an immune stimulus to elevate cGMP levels and release lysosomal enzymes (R. J. Smith and Ignarro, 1975). Thus, we postulated that most immune reactants that provoke lysosomal enzyme secretion from neutrophils function as divalent-cation ionophores (R. J. Smith and Ignarro, 1975).

Most of the pharmacological agents tested on neutrophil function thus far elicit a unidirectional or monophasic effect. One exception appears to be $PGF_{2\alpha}$, which produces a concentration-dependent biphasic effect on lysosomal enzyme secretion from human neutrophils. At higher concentrations (10^{-5}–10^{-6} M), $PGF_{2\alpha}$ enhances lysosomal enzyme secretion, but at lower concentrations (10^{-6}–10^{-8} M), the exact opposite effect on secretion is observed (Ignarro, 1975). It is of interest in this regard that the higher concentrations of $PGF_{2\alpha}$ cause the accumulation of both cGMP and cAMP in neutrophils, whereas the lower concentrations cause only cAMP to accumulate (Ignarro, 1975). Further studies on this interesting biphasic effect should be applied to other tissues as well.

Analysis of the effects of new pharmacological tools on neutrophil physiology and biochemistry should help to unravel some of the remaining puzzles. Recent studies with phorbol myristate acetate (PMA), a potent inflammatory and tumor-promoting agent, indicate that this substance provokes lysosomal enzyme release from polymorphonuclear leukocytes (Estensen *et al.*, 1974b; Weissmann *et al.*, 1975b), increases oxygen consumption by leukocytes (Repine *et al.*, 1974), stimulates fibroblast and lymphocyte proliferation (Estensen *et al.*, 1974a), stimulates platelet aggregation, secretion, and cGMP accumulation (J. G. White *et al.*, 1973), and elevates mouse fibroblast cGMP levels (Estensen *et al.*, 1974a). Levamisole is an imidazole analogue that elicits immunopotentiating effects in animals (Renoux and Renoux, 1971). Like imidazole, levamisole reduces cAMP but elevates cGMP levels in some lymphoid tissues (Hadden *et al.*, 1975a). Thus, the imidazole agents might be expected to elicit cGMP-like or cholinergic effects. Indeed, both levamisole and imidazole were reported to augment phytohemmagglutinin-induced proliferation of human lymphocytes, mouse thymocytes, and T-cell-enriched splenocytes (Hadden *et al.*, 1975a). Both agents elevate cGMP levels and lower cAMP levels in these cells. These pharmacological agents may operate by influencing cyclic nucleotide phosphodiesterase activity, since imidazole was reported to stimulate and inhibit, respectively, cAMP and cGMP phosphodiesterase activities in brain (Goldberg *et al.*, 1970). Levamisole was reported to increase neutrophil chemotaxis and, correspondingly, to induce cGMP accumulation (Anderson *et al.*, 1976; Wright *et al.*, 1976). Future studies on the influence of imidazole analogues on the physiology and biochemistry of neutrophils should contribute further to our overall understanding of the role of these cells in inflammation. Further, as other pharmacological agents and cellular constituents that might influence neutrophil function are identified, their effects on cyclic nucleotide metabolism and related cellular events should be examined. Such agents include the recently discovered lymphocyte factors or lymphokines (see Chapter 10), polypeptides such as tuftsin that are known to influence neutrophil function (Nishioka *et al.*, 1972), and the new potent precursors and analogues of PGs (endoperoxides and thromboxanes).

3. Mononuclear Phagocytes (Macrophages)

3.1. Physiologic Functions

Mononuclear phagocytes, which include peripheral blood monocytes and tissue macrophages such as liver Kupffer cells and alveolar macrophages), play an important physiologic role in the development and progression of the immune response. Tissue macrophages originate from the bone marrow. During differentiation, monocytes acquire characteristics unique to a particular tissue localization, i.e., alveolar vs. peritoneal macrophages. The participation of mononuclear phagocytes in both the afferent and efferent limbs of the immune response results from certain properties of these cells, such as phagocytosis of a wide spectrum of foreign materials, degradation of macromolecules, and their capacity to respond to certain products from lymphocytes. Mononuclear phagocytes possess functional receptors on their plasma membranes that recognize the Fc region of IgG, certain complement components, and denatured proteins.

Phagocytosis by mononuclear phagocytes is important in providing host resistance to many infections. These cells ingest and destroy numerous organisms and other foreign materials, and cells derived from immunized animals (activated phagocytes) exhibit an enhanced capacity to perform this function (Mackaness, 1964). Recent studies indicated that immune activation of macrophages requires the interaction of T lymphocytes specifically sensitized with the appropriate antigenic substance (Mackaness, 1969). The possible mechanisms involved are discussed in Chapter 5.

Like polymorphonuclear leukocytes, mononuclear phagocytes contain lysosome granules, the contents of which can be extruded extracellularly during cell contact with phagocytizable and nonphagocytizable immune complexes (Weissmann *et al.*, 1971b,c; Ackerman and Beebe, 1975). Mononuclear phagocytes also possess the capacity to mobilize themselves toward an ingestible substance. Unlike phagocytic leukocytes, macrophages possess the capacity to pinocytize soluble protein and fluid droplets. In general, in contrast to the neutrophil, the macrophage has a much wider spectrum of substances that it can endocytose. Release of lysosomal contents from macrophages during cell contact with appropriate immune complexes can, and probably does, lead to local tissue injury and connective tissue degradation as a consequence of the properties of the released lysosomal enzymes (Huffer, 1973; Rojas-Espinosa *et al.*, 1975).

3.2. *In Vitro* Cell Model Systems

Numerous *in vitro* model systems have been described to measure phagocytosis, pinocytosis, motility, and lysosomal enzyme release. For the most part, these testing systems are similar to those already discussed for polymorphonuclear leukocytes. Phagocytosis has been quantitated by enumeration of ingested particulate material such as zymosan, latex, erythrocytes, and denatured proteins. Heat-aggregated, ^{125}I-labeled bovine serum albumin has proved to be convenient because of the ease of quantitation of ingested radiolabel, and because degradation of the ingested protein can be estimated easily (Weissmann *et al.*, 1971c). Procedures for the quantitation of pinocytosis have been developed (Cohn and Ehrenreich, 1969; Schwartz *et al.*, 1972). Lysosomal enzyme release from macrophages has been estimated in much the same manner as for neutrophils (Weissmann *et al.*, 1971b,c; Ackerman and Beebe, 1975). Selective release of lysosomal contents occurs during cell contact with phagocytizable material. Various lysosomal marker enzymes have been measured, including β-glucuronidase, aryl sulfatase, acid phosphatase, and cathepsins (Weissmann *et al.*, 1971c). Motility of mononuclear phagocytes has been measured by relatively simple migration techniques (Pick *et al.*, 1970).

Methods for the isolation and purification of mononuclear phagocytes depend on the location of the desired cell type. Peritoneal macrophages have been isolated primarily from the guinea pig and the mouse after an intraperitoneal injection of light mineral oil (Remold *et al.*, 1970) or sterile thioglycollate medium (Weissmann *et al.*, 1971b). Alveolar macrophages have been isolated from the rabbit and the guinea pig by pulmonary lavage techniques (Myrvik *et al.*, 1962), and human mononuclear phagocytes have been obtained from peripheral blood by use of ficoll–hypaque gradients (Böyum, 1968).

3.3. Pharmacological Modulation of Macrophage Function

Although considerable progress has been made with polymorphonuclear leukocytes, much less information on bioregulatory mechanisms is available for mononuclear phagocytes. In 1971, Weissmann and co-workers reported that phagocytosis of undigestible particles causes selective release of lysosomal enzymes from purified mouse peritoneal macrophages. cAMP and dibutyryl cAMP inhibited lysosomal enzyme release but not phagocytosis, whereas colchicine and vinblastine inhibited both processes. The specificity of this effect for cAMP was clouded, however, by the finding that cGMP (5×10^{-3} M) and 2′,3′-cAMP elicited the same effect. Moreover, 5′-AMP inhibited both lysosomal enzyme release and phagocytosis (Weissmann *et al.*, 1971c). In additional experiments in which phagocytosis of heat-aggregated, ^{125}I-labeled bovine serum albumin by peritoneal macrophages was studied, cAMP and dibutyryl cAMP (5×10^{-3} M) inhibited ingestion (Weissmann *et al.*, 1971c). Further, low concentrations of cAMP (10^{-8}–10^{-10} M) and cGMP (10^{-10} M) enhanced phagocytosis. Once again, however, specificity was a problem, since 10^{-10} M 5′-AMP and 5′-GMP each enhanced phagocytosis. Similarly, theophylline, cAMP, and 5′-AMP profoundly inhibited phagocytosis of sheep red blood cells (SRBC) by peritoneal macrophages (Lima *et al.*, 1974). Although cAMP was reported to inhibit uptake of denatured protein particulates (Weissmann *et al.*, 1971b), Seyberth *et al.* (1973) showed that phagocytosis of latex particles by alveolar macrophages was associated with a concomitant accumulation of cAMP. Similarly, Sandler *et al.* (1975a) reported that cAMP, but not cGMP, accumulated in adherent human mononuclear phagocytes (macrophages) during cell exposure to latex particles. The finding that phagocytosis by macrophages is associated with a marked cAMP accumulation is difficult to understand in view of the reports that cAMP inhibits phagocytosis. Differences in species, cell homogeneity, and type of particulate material employed could explain the apparent discrepancy. It is clear that meaningful conclusions can be drawn only from experiments conducted with purified macrophages (especially when using peripheral blood), since cell contact between purified lymphocytes and latex particles provoked cAMP accumulation (Manganiello *et al.*, 1971).

Working with rabbit alveolar macrophages, Schmidt-Gayk *et al.* (1975) reported that catecholamines, theophylline, papaverine, and PGE_1, A_1, $F_{1\alpha}$, and $F_{2\alpha}$ elevated the levels of cAMP in the absence of ingestible material. Latex particles slightly stimulated cAMP accumulation. In the same study, a cAMP-dependent protein kinase was identified in alveolar macrophages, thus suggesting an intracellular function for cAMP. Increases in hexosemonophosphate shunt activity accompanied phagocytosis of latex particles, and the accumulation of cAMP immediately preceded the increase in the metabolic rate. Interestingly, the addition of dibutyryl cAMP resulted in enhanced metabolic activity and phagocytosis. Thus, these investigators suggested that the effects of cAMP on macrophage function are opposite to those on neutrophil function. Recall, however, that cAMP and agents that elevate cAMP levels were reported to inhibit peritoneal macrophage phagocytosis (Weissmann *et al.*, 1971b,c). Possibly, marked differences between alveolar and peritoneal mononuclear phagocytes exist with respect to the effects, and possible regulatory role, of cAMP. Moreover, species differences may present a further problem, since guinea pig alveolar macrophages did not respond at all to cAMP, cGMP, theophylline, neurohormones, or PGs (Ackerman and Beebe, 1975).

Phagocytosis of SRBC by mouse peritoneal macrophages was increased by imidazole and levamisole (Lima *et al.*, 1974), agents that reduce cAMP levels and elevate cGMP levels in certain tissues (Hadden *et al.*, 1975a). One of the first reports on cGMP levels in macrophages was that of Sandler *et al.* (1975a), which indicated that serotonin and its analogues markedly elevated the levels of cGMP but not cAMP in purified, adherent human mononuclear phagocytes. Unfortunately, no analyses of function were conducted in this study. In a similar report, serotonin, carbamylcholine, and ascorbic acid elevated the levels of cGMP and also stimulated mononuclear cell chemotaxis (Sandler *et al.*, 1975b). The findings that reduction of cAMP levels or generation of cGMP, or both, enhances phagocytosis by macrohages (Weissmann *et al.*, 1971c), as well as migration or chemotaxis of these cells (Sandler *et al.*, 1975b), suggest that a bioregulatory mechanism involving cAMP and cGMP may be operational in mononuclear as well as polymorphonuclear leukocytes. In support of this concept are the findings that cAMP, dibutyryl cAMP, isoproterenol, and chlorphenesin all inhibit migration of guinea pig peritoneal exudate cells (Pick, 1972).

The mechanism by which migration-inhibitory factor (MIF) retards macrophage motility is not well understood. cAMP and agents known to elevate levels of cAMP (such as catecholamines, aminophylline, and the PGEs) consistently prevented MIF activity on guinea pig peritoneal macrophages (Koopman *et al.*, 1973). In other words, cAMP blocked the inhibition of migration by MIF. Yet, in the absence of MIF, these agents actually inhibited peritoneal macrophage migration (Pick, 1972). It must be recalled that cGMP and agents that elevate cGMP levels were reported to enhance macrophage chemotaxis (Sandler *et al.*, 1975b; Wright *et al.*, 1976). More experimental work is needed to clarify the roles played by cyclic nucleotides in macrophage functions (see Chapter 5 and 10 for further discussion).

3.4. Theoretical Considerations and Future Directions

Although cyclic nucleotides, neurohormones, PGs, and lymphocyte factors all affect macrophage function, precise bioregulatory control mechanisms cannot be identified at this time. Very little *in vivo* work has been reported for macrophages. Studies of this nature are essential if we are to understand how the functions of mononuclear phagocytes are regulated and modulated in the host. Additional *in vitro* experiments should be conducted with the objective of comparing peritoneal, alveolar, and peripheral blood mononuclear phagocytes with regard to their functional, biochemical, and immunologic responsiveness to immune reactants, lymphocyte factors, divalent cations, divalent-cation ionophores, cyclic nucleotides, neurohormones, PGs, and other tissue hormones and pharmacological agents. Careful measurements of cGMP and cAMP levels, metabolic activity, phagocytosis, lysosomal enzyme release, migration, calcium influx, transport of other ions, phospholipid transport and metabolism, microtubule integrity, and lysosome translocation and merger should be made. The potent effects of the soluble lymphocyte mediators or lymphokines on macrophage function should be examined more closely at the level of the plasma membrane with regard to calcium mobilization, alteration of cyclic nucleotide levels, and metabolic events. Correlations should be sought between functional and biochemical or metabolic activation by these soluble factors. Indeed, such an approach is being undertaken by Hadden and co-workers (see Chapter 5). For example, MIF-containing fractions were reported not only to inhibit migration, but also to induce proliferation of macrophages, effects that were partially reproduced or enhanced by cGMP, ACh, and imidazole (Hadden *et al.*, 1974). Thus, MIF may be a hormone with multiple effects on macrophage function, the effects being mediated by cGMP. Additional experiments (Hadden *et al.*, 1975b) revealed that the mitogenic factor of the lymphocyte soluble mediator fraction might be distinct from the MIF. It is also of interest that macrophages themselves contain soluble active factors that can influence lymphocyte function. For example, such a factor was reported to stimulate DNA synthesis in lymphocytes if the lymphocytes were cultured in the presence of cGMP or with various mitogens (Diamantstein and Ulmer, 1975) that are thought to elevate cGMP levels. Thus, once again, cGMP appears to play a role in mediating a function of peripheral blood cells.

4. Platelets

4.1. Physiologic Functions

Platelets play an important role in the response of tissue to injury. Platelet hemostasis is a physiologic component of the inflammatory process, whereas thrombosis represents a pathophysiologic response to tissue injury. The relationship between platelets and inflammation was reviewed by Mustard and Packham (1970). Briefly, when blood vessels and their endothelial lining are injured, blood platelets adhere to adjacent collagen fibers, basement membranes, and other connective tissue components, thereby triggering a series of platelet reactions that result in the formation of either a beneficial hemostatic plug or a potentially detrimental intravascular thrombus. Platelet adherence is followed by release from these cells of granule constituents that, in turn, interact with platelets to provoke aggregation (platelet–platelet adherence) and further release of granule contents. Platelet aggregation and the release reaction are triggered by platelet adherence to or contact with various materials, including collagen, other connective tissue components, immune complexes, latex particles, viruses, bacteria, thrombin, other proteases, certain tissue hormones, and divalent-cation ionophores. The platelet release reaction affects microcirculatory function because the granule constituents released are pharmacologically active. Substances are stored in two types of granules: the dense body and the α-granule. The substances released from the dense bodies include vasocative amines (serotonin, histamine, catecholamines), nucleotides (ADP, ATP), clotting factors and other platelet proteins, and cations. Lysosomal enzymes and other proteins are released from the α-granule. The platelet release reaction also accompanies phagocytosis of small particulate materials.

Details of the steps leading to platelet aggregation and release were reviewed by Zucker (1974) and Mustard and Packham (1970). The first step in the platelet reaction is adherence of the cell to collagen or other particulate materials, which results in stimulation of the release from platelets of ADP and other granule constituents. The released ADP, and perhaps other substances, then provokes platelet aggregation. Platelet aggregation stimulates further discharge of granule contents into the extracellular environment. The platelet release reaction, and therefore platelet aggregation, requires calcium. This requirement is true of a variety of substances that induce the platelet release reaction, such as collagen, immune complexes, ADP, epinephrine, thrombin, and others (discussed by Becker and Henson, 1973). The discharge of platelet granule constituents is regarded as a secretory process because it is a calcium-requiring event not accompanied by release of soluble cytoplasmic constituents. Often, the initial platelet release reaction and aggregation are followed by a second wave of aggregation and the accompanying release reaction, due to the explosive discharge of ADP during the initial phase of aggregation.

4.2. *In Vitro* Cell Model Systems

The principal functions of platelets are aggregation and the release of granule constituents, both of which are markedly affected by a variety of endogenous and pharmacological agents. Platelet-rich plasma is usually employed, and is prepared by low-speed centrifugation of blood containing citrate as an anticoagulant. Platelet aggregation is commonly measured *in vitro* by a photometric technique (aggregometry), which was first developed by Born (1962). Briefly, platelet-rich plasma is stirred gently at 37°C as a path of light is directed through it and recorded. Increased transmission of light indicates platelet aggregation. The platelet release reaction can be monitored by measuring the discharge of one or more granule substances into the incubation medium. Commonly, radiolabeled 5-HT (serotonin) is added to the blood, and following preparation of platelet-rich plasma, the latter is preincubated at 37°C to facilitate uptake of the biogenic amine into the dense granules (Spaet and Zucker, 1964; Salzman and Levine, 1971). Release of radiolabeled amine from platelets into the incubation medium, provoked by added agents, can then be quantitated easily. Release of other biogenic amines, lysosomal enzymes, and clotting factors can also be measured (Becker and Henson, 1973).

Changes in platelet volume are often determined, a determination that can be made by use of a Coulter counter (Salzman *et al.*, 1969). Translocation of calcium between platelets and the extracellular environment, which may be the initial trigger of the platelet release reaction, was studied by using $^{45}CaCl_2$ and divalent-cation ionophores (Massini and Lüscher, 1974).

4.3. Bioregulation and Pharmacological Modulation of Platelet Function

A great number of reports have appeared recently on the effects of cyclic nucleotides, and agents that affect cyclic nucleotide levels, on platelet function (see Haslam, 1975, for a review). Historically, the first reported study on cAMP and platelet function was that of Marcus and Zucker (1965), who demonstrated that platelet aggregation could be weakly inhibited by cAMP. Several years elapsed before this original finding was confirmed and extended to include the more potent analogue, dibutyryl cAMP (Marquis *et al.*, 1969; Salzman and Levine, 1971). Dibutyryl cAMP was also shown to inhibit the platelet release reaction (Salzman, 1970; Salzman and Levine, 1971). The more potent action of dibutyryl cAMP in comparison with that of cAMP can be attributed to the lipophilicity of the former and its enhanced uptake by the platelets (Salzman and Levine, 1971), whereupon it may function as does intracellular cAMP. Following the demonstration of adenylate cyclase activity in platelets, numerous tissue hormones were reported to alter platelet adenylate cyclase activity. For example, PGE_1 (Butcher *et al.*, 1967; Wolfe and Shulman, 1969) and glucagon (Zieve and Greenough, 1969) were reported to stimulate, whereas thrombin, norepinephrine, epinephrine, and serotonin inhibited (Zieve and Greenough, 1969), platelet adenylate cyclase activity. Adenylate cyclase activity was also inhibited by collagen, but not by ADP (Salzman and Levine, 1971). The latter investigators showed that the inhibitory effect of epinephrine was blocked by phentolamine (an α-adrenergic receptor antagonist), but not by propranolol (a β-adrenergic receptor antagonist). Caffeine was reported to inhibit platelet phosphodiesterase activity (Marquis *et al.*, 1969). Consistent with the findings cited above is the report that platelet cAMP levels can be reduced, although only slightly, by epinephrine and collagen, and elevated by PGE_1 and caffeine (Salzman and Weisenberger, 1972). Again, in line with these findings, platelet phosphodiesterase activity was reported to be stimulated by agents (ADP, collagen, thrombin, epinephrine) that induce the platelet release reaction (Salzman and Weisenberger, 1972). All the data reported up to 1972 were thus consistent with the hypothesis that platelet release and aggregation are provoked or favored by a decrease, and inhibited by an elevation, of platelet cAMP.

The inhibitory effect of dibutyryl cAMP on platelet aggregation and the release reaction was demonstrated against several different agents that provoke these reactions, including ADP, epinephrine, collagen, and thrombin (Salzman and Levine, 1971). Dibutyryl cAMP inhibited the "primary phase" of platelet aggregation, which is provoked by ADP and epinephrine, although this phase is probably independent of the release reaction and is unaffected by agents (i.e., aspirin, phenylbutazone) that selectively impair the "secondary phase" of platelet aggregation and release. To explain the intracellular actions of cAMP in platelets, Salzman and Weisenberger (1972) sought and found a cAMP-dependent protein kinase in soluble and particulate fractions derived from platelets. Similar observations were made by Marquis *et al.* (1971). The presence of both cytoplasmic and membrane-bound protein kinase activity in human platelets was confirmed more recently by Bishop and Rozenberg (1975). Further, cAMP stimulated whereas ADP inhibited enzyme activity. In this same study, calcium (10 mM) was observed to inhibit cAMP-dependent and -independent protein kinase activity. The soluble protein kinase was inhibited to a greater extent than was the particulate enzyme. In view of the knowledge that cAMP inhibits platelet aggregation and that calcium is required for platelet function, it was reasonable to speculate that inhibition of protein kinase activity by calcium might be a component of the mechanism by which calcium signals or triggers platelet release and aggregation (Bishop and Rozenberg, 1975). In support of this view are the reports (Feinman and Detwiler, 1974; Massini and Lüscher, 1974) that divalent-cation ionophores promote calcium influx in platelets and provoke the platelet release reaction. Thus, the opposing actions of calcium and cAMP on platelet function are reflected in their opposing effects on platelet protein kinase activity.

As indicated earlier, considerable experimental evidence exists that cAMP is the intracellular mediator of inhibition of platelet function by PGE_1 and glucagon. Further studies have illustrated that isoproterenol and adenosine, which inhibit platelet function, also activate platelet adenylate cyclase and elevate intracellular cAMP levels (reviewed by Haslam, 1973). On the other hand, certain inducers of platelet aggregation such as epinephrine and ADP have been found to reduce the accumulation of cAMP provoked by PGE_1. Solid evidence for inhibition of adenylate cyclase or activation of phosphodiesterase by epinephrine and ADP is weak or lacking. Whereas an increase in platelet cAMP almost certainly mediates inhibition of platelet release and aggregation, a decrease in cAMP does not, by itself, mediate these platelet functions, since considerable aggregation can occur with cAMP levels well above basal levels (reviewed by Haslam, 1973).

If a decrease in platelet cAMP levels does not mediate the platelet release reaction and aggregation, then what does? In view of the evidence that cGMP may mediate the secretion of granule contents from both polymorphonuclear leukocytes (discussed in Section 2.3) and certain histamine-containing cells (Kaliner *et al.*, 1972), Goldberg *et al.* (1974) and Haslam and McClenaghan (1974) studied the effects of collagen on human platelet cGMP levels. The results showed that collagen caused an increase in platelet cGMP, which preceded and was quantitatively related to the subsequent platelet aggregation. ADP, epinephrine, and PMA were also shown to elevate cGMP levels in platelets (Goldberg *et al.*, 1974; Haslam *et al.*, 1975a). The presence of guanylate cyclase within platelets was also established (Haslam *et al.*, 1975b). Haslam and McClenaghan (1974) also showed that aspirin, which is a strong inhibitor of the platelet release reaction, reduced the basal levels of platelet cGMP, thereby reducing the final elevated cGMP level produced by the subsequent addition of collagen. These investigators believed that this mechanism could account for the fact that aspirin markedly inhibits release and aggregation provoked by low but not high concentrations of collagen. Aspirin did not affect cAMP levels in platelets (Ball *et al.*, 1970). Thus, the results are consistent with the hypothesis (Goldberg *et al.*, 1974; Haslam and McClenaghan, 1974) that cGMP mediates or potentiates the platelet release reaction.

Following the demonstration that epinephrine and collagen each induced the accumulation of cGMP in human platelets, which was associated with and actually preceded platelet aggregation (Glass *et al.*, 1973), Goldberg *et al.* (1974) determined that the elevations in cGMP levels were extremely marked (up to 9-fold), and occurred within 2 sec of exposure of platelets to epinephrine. This explosive elevation of cGMP levels, which occurred prior to platelet aggregation and returned to basal levels by 60 sec, was unaffected by PGE_1 or isoproterenol, agents that elevate cAMP levels and inhibit platelet aggregation. Further, the second wave of platelet aggregation, which occurred at 90–120 sec, was immediately preceded by a 3-fold elevation of cGMP levels. Little or no decrease in cAMP levels accompanied these cellular events. These data clearly support the view that intracellular cGMP mediates platelet aggregation provoked by epinephrine and collagen, and considerably weaken the view that reduced cAMP levels trigger aggregation.

A reinvestigation of the concept that inducers of platelet aggregation cause a concomitant and meaningful decrease in platelet cAMP levels was recently conducted by Haslam (1975). In short, with various methods employed to assess cAMP concentrations in platelets, several inducers of platelet aggregation failed to produce measurable changes in nucleotide levels, although inhibition of adenylate cyclase activity was observed in certain instances. In the same study, an increase in human platelet cGMP (up to 4-fold) in response to ADP or collagen was associated with both platelet aggregation and the initiation of the release reaction. These data, obtained by prelabeling techniques, were similar to those reported earlier in which direct nucleotide measurements were conducted (Glass *et al.,* 1973; Goldberg *et al.,* 1974). In addition, experiments with dog platelets revealed that the muscarinic receptor agonist carbachol caused platelet aggregation and release of serotonin (Haslam, 1975), a finding that is in agreement with an earlier report (Chuang *et al.*, 1974). In the experiment reported by Haslam, elevated cGMP levels occurred during primary and secondary aggregation along a time course that was consistent with a mediating role for cGMP in either process. The results with ACh, however, were less consistent. Although extracellular calcium was required for carbachol- and ACh-induced cGMP elevations in platelets, aggregation and some release nevertheless occurred, presumably because of mobilization of intracellular calcium stores. These findings led the author (Haslam, 1975) to suggest that in the canine platelet, elevated cGMP levels may play a secondary role to calcium ions in potentiating the platelet release reaction. This view would be consistent with a hypothesis linking intracellular calcium to the stimulation of cGMP synthesis and the consequent mediation of the platelet release reaction and the accompanying aggregation. Such a hypothesis would then be very similar to that invoked for human neutrophils, in which calcium was suggested to serve as the link in the stimulus–secretion coupling mechanism (R. J. Smith and Ignarro, 1975). A schematic representation of this hypothesis on the bioregulation of platelet function is illustrated in Figure 3.

PGs may play an important role in the modulation or regulation of platelet function. Although PGE_1 is a potent inhibitor of platelet aggregation, it is not synthesized by platelets and is not found in sufficient concentrations *in vivo* to affect platelet function (discussed by De Gaetano, 1975). Recently, however, PGD_2 was found *in vitro* to be more potent than PGE_1 in inhibiting platelet aggregation and stimulating adenylate cyclase activity (J. B. Smith *et al.*, 1974). These investigators suggested that PGD_2 is synthesized in platelets from the cyclic endoperoxide precursors of PGs. On the other hand, one or more other cyclic endoperoxide intermediates apparently accumulate, transiently, in platelets and trigger the release reaction and aggregation (Hamberg and Samuelsson, 1974; Willis, 1974a). This reaction is blocked by aspirin (Willis, 1974a). PGE_2 sensitizes platelets to the

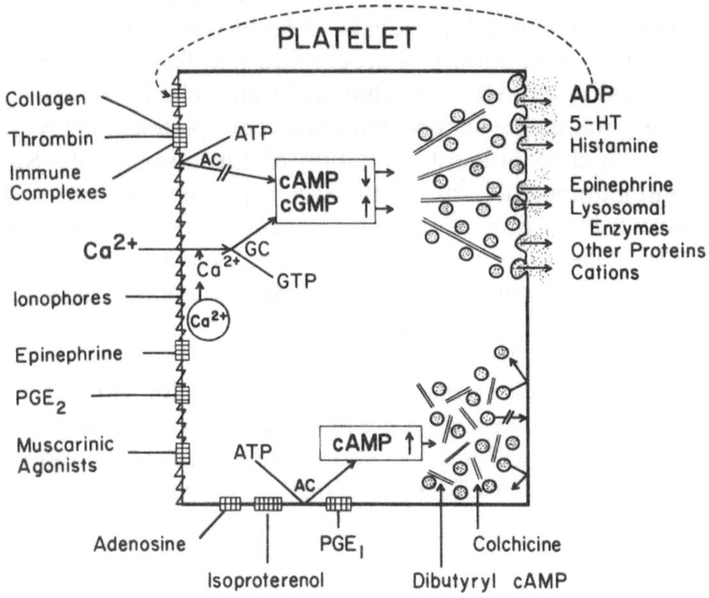

Figure 3. Schematic representation of the hypothetical bioregulation of the platelet release reaction. The hypothesis for platelets is very similar to that for neutrophils (Figure 2). Various inducers of platelet aggregation may promote calcium influx as well as translocation of intracellular stores of calcium, the result being guanylate cyclase (GC) stimulation and cGMP accumulation. These inducers may also inhibit adenylate cyclase (AC) and reduce cAMP levels. The combination of reduced cAMP and elevated cGMP levels promotes the secretion of granule contents, whereupon released ADP provokes platelet aggregation and further secretion. Muscarinic agonists, epinephrine, and PGE_2 (via distinct receptors) enhance or induce platelet secretion and aggregation by similar mechanisms. On the other hand, adenosine, isoproterenol, PGE_1, cAMP, and colchicine inhibit the platelet release reaction. The first three agents stimulate adenylate cyclase and thereby allow cAMP to accumulate and inhibit secretion and further aggregation. As with neutrophils, the state of integrity of the microtubules may be influenced by the intracellular levels of cGMP and cAMP.

aggregating action of the cyclic endoperoxide intermediate(s) (Willis, 1974b). *In vivo* evidence that PG synthesis is central to thrombosis derives from the finding that an intravenous injection of arachidonate or cyclic endoperoxide intermediates into animals causes platelet aggregation and death (Willis, 1974a). Recently, Vargaftig and Chignard (1975) suggested that human platelets interact with added arachidonic acid to form distinct pharmacologically active materials possessing similar lipoperoxide structures. Generation of some, but not all, of these lipids can be inhibited by cAMP and agents that elevate platelet cAMP levels, such as PGE_1 or isoproterenol (in the presence of an α-adrenergic receptor antagonist). These investigators hypothesized that PGs are formed during platelet aggregation, and that they exercise a modulating or regulating role in platelet function.

4.4. Relationship Between *in Vitro* and *in Vivo* Findings

Intravenous infusion of cAMP in man inhibits platelet aggregation (Mannucci and Pareti, 1974). This finding, together with those on PGs discussed earlier, suggests that a concerted effort should be made toward developing more potent and selective inhibitors of platelet aggregation, which may be useful as antithrombotic drugs. Drugs that elevate platelet cAMP levels or inhibit PGE_2 synthesis may possess clinical value as antithrombotic agents (Didisheim *et al.*, 1974). Although PGE_1, which elevates platelet cAMP levels, is rapidly destroyed *in vivo,* it is useful in preventing platelet aggregation in stored blood and for preparing aggregate-free platelet concentrates for transfusion (Shio and Ramwell, 1972). The phosphodiesterase inhibitor dipyridamole was reported to increase platelet survival time (Harker and Slichter, 1970) and to prevent formation of thromboemboli (Sullivan *et al.*, 1971). Aspirin and indomethacin may be useful in preventing myocardial infarction and reducing intravascular fibrin deposition (discussed by De Gaetano *et al.*, 1974; De Gaetano, 1975). One major problem for clinical investigators in this field is that most, if not all, of the antiaggregating drugs studied thus far possess other pharmacological effects (on blood flow and on the inflammatory process) that may interfere with the desirable clinical response. It is therefore clear that more potent and selective inhibitors of platelet aggregation are desired for clinical use. Now that more information is being amassed on the bioregulation of platelet function, such as the modulatory roles of cGMP and calcium, novel chemical compounds should be developed on the basis of their effects on cGMP metabolism and calcium translocation in human platelets.

4.5. Theoretical Considerations and Future Directions

The experimental evidence thus far suggests that both calcium and cGMP are intimately involved in mediating or modulating platelet aggregation and release of granule constituents. Although platelet-aggregating agents promote calcium influx and elevate cGMP levels, the precise interrelationship between calcium and cGMP and the mechanism by which either agent provokes platelet aggregation is not understood. As discussed previously, extracellular calcium is required for elevations of platelet cGMP, although aggregation may proceed, to some extent, in the absence of extracellular calcium, presumably because of a mobilization of intracellular stores of calcium. Studies should be designed and conducted to ascertain the functional consequences of manipulations of the intracellular concentrations of either calcium or cGMP in the absence of the other. For example, the effects of calcium might be assessed in platelets deprived of cGMP. Although specific methods to accomplish this assessment have not been reported, advantage can be taken of the knowledge that aspirin reduces platelet cGMP levels and inhibits aggregation and release. Pharmacological agents that inhibit calcium influx in platelets should be sought and studied for their effects on platelet function and cGMP levels.

Both α- and β-adrenergic receptors have been identified in the plasma membrane of platelets (discussed by Haslam, 1973). It appears that both receptors interact with adenylate cyclase, α-receptors inhibiting and β-receptors activating the membrane-bound enzyme. Isoproterenol interacts primarily with β-receptors, whereas epinephrine interacts with both sites. Antagonists of α-receptors (phentolamine) potentiate the effect of epinephrine on β-receptors, whereas β-receptor antagonists (propranolol) enhance its effect on α-receptors. The precise nature of the α-receptor on platelets is unknown, although many investigators have suggested that α-adrenergic receptors, as well as β-adrenergic receptors, occupy distinct positions on the adenylate cyclase enzyme. Since epinephrine promotes platelet aggregation (which can be inhibited by α-receptor antagonists) and elevates cGMP levels, the α-receptor on platelets may represent a part of a cellular process connected with elevating cGMP levels, rather than simply reducing cAMP levels.

The effects of adrenergic receptor antagonists on cGMP levels in platelets interacting with inducers of aggregation and release should be examined in more detail. More specifically, the relationship, if any, between α-adrenergic receptor interaction and guanylate cyclase activation or cGMP-specific phosphodiesterase inhibition in platelets should be explored.

Future studies of the properties of platelet plasma membrane components and their interaction with calcium and inducers of platelet aggregation should contribute much to our understanding of the bioregulation of platelet function. Along these lines, the role of membrane phospholipids in the platelet release reaction was explored in some detail (Schick and Yu, 1974). These investigators found that phospholipase-C-induced phospholipid hydrolysis caused the selective release of certain platelet granule constituents without provoking release of cytosol components, and postulated that phosphatidylcholine may be situated near the membrane receptor and may function to modulate the platelet release reaction. The effects of collagen, ADP, epinephrine, and other inducers of platelet aggregation on membrane phospholipid mobilization and metabolism were not studied. Such studies, in addition to experiments designed to ascertain calcium binding to, and passage through, membrane phospholipid components, should be considered. As new inducers of platelet aggregation are disclosed, they should be examined for their influence on phospholipid structure, calcium translocation, and cyclic nucleotide metabolism. A recent example is PMA which was first shown to induce platelet aggregation and subsequently demonstrated to elevate platelet cGMP levels (Estensen *et al.*, 1974b). PMA elicits similar stimulatory effects on function and cGMP levels in several other types of blood cells (discussed in Section 2.5). Another interesting observation was that hydrocortisone inhibited platelet aggregation induced by ADP, collagen, thrombin, or endotoxin (Nelson and Taylor, 1975). These *in vitro* findings support the clinical effectiveness of glucocorticoids in certain kinds of shock. The influence of glucocorticoids on platelet membrane phospholipids, calcium influx, and cyclic nucleotide metabolism has not been explored.

Although a considerable amount of work has been conducted on platelet physiology and pharmacology, the precise mechanisms responsible for the bioregulation or modulation of platelet function have not yet been clearly identified. Perhaps an experimental approach can be taken to study the changes in characteristics of the platelet plasma membrane during interaction with modulators of platelet function, and during the platelet release reaction and aggregation. Further, since the platelet release reaction is an important, if not obligatory, cellular event preceding aggregation, the role of microtubules in the release reaction as well as the effects of inducers and inhibitors of release on microtubule integrity should be explored.

5. Summary and Conclusions

The studies on polymorphonuclear leukocytes, mononuclear phagocytes, and platelets discussed above provide evidence in support of the view (Ignarro, 1974d, 1975) that the autonomic nervous system and portions of the endocrine system are capable of influencing the functions of these cells. Moreover, it appears that cyclic nucleotides play a biological role in influencing, modulating, or regulating the principal functions of these cells. In polymorphonuclear leukocytes and platelets, cGMP is associated with provokation or enhancement, whereas cAMP is associated with inhibition, of cell function. Less definitive data are available for mononuclear phagocytes, although some studies have suggested that similar roles for cGMP and cAMP may exist in certain types of mononuclear phagocytes. The findings that two distinct cyclic nucleotides may be involved in mediating opposing influences on the functions of these cells support the dualism or Yin–Yang hypothesis of biological control proposed originally by Goldberg *et al.* (1973b).

To postulate such bioregulatory mechanisms for the cyclic nucleotides, it is necessary to demonstrate that each of the nucleotides plays a role as a distinct second messenger in mediating the biologic effects of an appropriate first messenger. This demonstration may be based on certain criteria set forth originally by Sutherland and co-workers. First, the cyclic nucleotide or a close structural analogue should elicit biological effects similar to those of the first messenger. In the neutrophil, cGMP and numerous agents that elevate neutrophil cGMP levels stimulate, whereas cAMP and agents that elevate neutrophil cAMP levels inhibit, several functions. In the platelet, cAMP elicits effects similar to those of agents that elevate platelet cAMP levels. Any direct effect of cGMP on platelet function has not been substantiated to date. Certain, but not all, experiments with macrophages revealed that cGMP and agents that elevate cGMP levels stimulate, whereas cAMP and agents that elevate cAMP levels inhibit, certain functions.

Second, the first messenger should elevate the concentration of the appropriate cyclic nucleotide in the specific cell type in question (this may or may not be accompanied by a reduction in the level of the other cyclic nucleotide). Further, the time of appearance of cyclic nucleotide accumulation should precede that of the biological effect on the cell. This criterion has been satisfied for both cGMP and cAMP in polymorphonuclear leukocytes, mononuclear phagocytes, and platelets.

Third, both the biological effects and the corresponding elevation of cyclic nucleotide levels induced by the first messenger should be potentiated, or at least enhanced, in the presence of a phosphodiesterase inhibitor. This approach has been used primarily for cAMP because much more information is available on cAMP phosphodiesterase than on cGMP phosphodiesterase. Moreover, most of the phosphodiesterase inhibitors employed enhance the biological effects of cAMP and not those of cGMP. The third criterion, with respect to cAMP, has been satisfied for polymorphonuclear leukocytes, mononuclear phagocytes, and platelets.

Fourth, the specific enzyme systems for biosynthesis (and degradation) of the cyclic nucleotides should be present, and they should be affected in the appropriate direction by the first messenger in question. Unfortunately, not much progress has been made in this area, especially with regard to the properties of, and hormonal effects on, both guanylate cyclase and phosphodiesterases. Adenylate cyclase and its stimulation by various agents that elevate cAMP levels have been demonstrated in neutrophils and platelets. In addition, certain agents that may reduce cAMP levels and elevate cGMP in platelets were reported to inhibit adenylate cyclase activity. Guanylate cyclase has been identified in human neutrophils and platelets, but effects of hormones or other agents that affect cell function have not been reported. Although some reports on platelet phosphodiesterase have appeared, similar studies on neutrophil and macrophage enzymes are lacking. Virtually nothing is known about the existence of distinct cGMP or cAMP phosphodiesterases in these cells, much less about the influence of specific agents on the activities of such enzymes.

Thus, the experimental evidence to date supports the concept that cGMP and cAMP function to mediate opposing influences on, and thereby regulate, the principal functions of neutrophils, platelets, and perhaps macrophages. Additional work will be necessary to achieve a more adequate understanding of the precise biochemical mechanisms by which intracellular cyclic nucleotides modulate the functions of these cells. The recent studies on calcium, its requirement for and mobilization during various functions of blood cells, represent an area of fruitful research. As discussed earlier, much of the available data support the view that calcium serves as a link in the stimulus–secretion coupling mechanism that signals the release of granule constituents from neutrophils, platelets, and possibly macrophages. Evidence also exists that calcium is required for the accumulation of cGMP in neutrophils and in other tissues. Although several reports have indicated that calcium stimulates guanylate cyclase activity, the precise relationship between intracellular calcium and cGMP accumulation is not well understood.

Another point of interest relating to polymorphonuclear leukocytes is that cGMP and agents that elevate cGMP levels stimulate, whereas cAMP and agents that elevate cAMP levels inhibit, not one, but at least four different leukocyte functions. That is, several independent functions of a single cell type may be signaled or mediated by a common intracellular second messenger. These findings indicate that several different neutrophil functions might be initiated concomitantly in response to a single stimulus such as an immune reactant. Such a situation would not be surprising, since concurrent stimulation of motility, metabolic energy production, secretion of granule contents, and phagocytosis would most certainly aid the neutrophil in performing its physiologic and pathophysiologic functions in inflammation and bacterial infections. Similarly, it might be reasonable that cAMP accumulation should simultaneously turn off the same neutrophil functions. Therefore, given the appropriate environmental conditions, a specific first messenger may be capable of influencing the magnitude of numerous neutrophil functions. Such a bioregulatory system would be very efficient in that only one intracellular messenger is required to modulate several different but cooperative functions of a single cell. This concept may apply also to the macrophage and the platelet.

References

Ackerman, N. R., and Beebe, J. R., 1975, *J. Pharmacol. Exp. Ther.* **193**:603–613.

Ashman, D. F., Lipton, R., Melicow, M. M., and Price, T. D., 1963, *Biochem. Biophys. Res. Commun.* **11**:330–334.

Aspinall, R. L., and Cammarata, P. S., 1969, *Nature (London)* **224**:1320, 1321.

Ball, G., Brereton, G. G., Fulwood, M., Ireland, D. M., and Yates, P., 1970, *Biochem. J.* **120**:709–718.

Becker, E. L., and Henson, P. M., 1973, *Adv. Immunol.* **17**:93–193.

Becker, E. L., Showell, H. J., Henson, P. M., and Hsu, L. S., 1974, *J. Immunol.* **112**:2047–2054.

Bishop, G. A., and Rozenberg, M. C., 1975, *Biochim. Biophys. Acta* **384**:112–119.

Born, G. V. R., 1962, *Nature (London)* **194**:927–929.

Bourne, H. R., and Melmon, K. L., 1971, *J. Pharmacol. Exp. Ther.* **178**:1–7.

Bourne, H. R., Lehrer, R. I., Cline, M. J., and Melmon, K. L., 1971, *J. Clin. Invest.* **50**:920–929.

Boyden, S. V., 1962, *J. Exp. Med.* **115**:453–466.

Böyum, A., 1967, *Scand. J. Clin. Lab. Invest. Suppl.* **97**:77–89.

Böyum, A., 1968, *Scand. J. Clin. Lab. Invest. Suppl.* **21**:77–89.

Bryant, R. E., and Sutcliffe, M. C., 1974, *J. Clin. Invest.* **54**:1241–1244.

Butcher, R. W., Scott, R. E., and Sutherland, E. W., 1967, *Pharmacologist* **9**:172.

Chuang, H. Y. K., Shermer, R. W., and Mason, R. G., 1974, *Res. Commun. Chem. Pathol. Pharmacol.* **7**:333–346.

Cohn, Z. A., and Ehrenreich, B. A., 1969, *J. Exp. Med.* **129**:201–225.

Cox, J. P., and Karnovsky, M. L., 1973, *J. Cell Biol.* **59**:480–490.

DeGaetano, G., 1975, *Pharmacol. Res. Commun.* **7**:301–309.
De Gaetano, G., Vermylen, J., Donati, M. B., Dotremont, G., and Nichielsen, P., 1974, *Br. Med. J.* **2**:301–303.
Deporter, D. A., Dieppe, P., and Willoughby, D. A., 1976, *Agents Actions* **6**:476–478.
Diamantstein, T., and Ulmer, A., 1975, *Nature (London)* **245**:418–419.
Didisheim, P., Kazmier, F. J., and Fuster, V., 1974, *Thromb. Diath. Haemorrh.* **32**:21–34.
Estensen, R. D., Hill, H. R., Quie, P. G., Hogan, N., and Goldberg, N. D., 1973, *Nature (London)* **245**:458–460.
Estensen, R., Hadden, J. W., Hadden, E. M., Touraine, F., Touraine, J. L., Haddox, M. K., and Goldberg, N. D., 1974a, in *Cold Spring Harbor Symp: Regulation of Proliferation in Animal Cells* (B. Clarkson and R. Baserga, eds.), pp. 627–634, Cold Spring Harbor Laboratory, New York.
Estensen, R. D., White, J. G., and Holmes, B., 1974b, *Nature (London)* **248**:347–348.
Feinman, R. D., and Detwiler, T. C., 1974, *Nature (London)* **249**:172–173.
Ferreira, S. H., Moncada, S., and Vane, J. R., 1971, *Nature (London) New Biol.* **231**:237–239.
Ferrendelli, F. A., Kinscherf, D. A., and Chang, M. M., 1973, *Mol. Pharmacol.* **9**:445–454.
Gale, R. P., and Zighelboim, J., 1974, *J. Immunol.* **113**:1793–1800.
George, W. J., Polson, J. B., O'Toole, A. G., and Goldberg, N. D., 1970, *Proc. Natl. Acad. Sci. U.S.A.* **66**:398–403.
George, W. J., Busuttil, R. W., and Ignarro, L. J., 1975, *Pharmacologist* **17**:269.
Glass, D. B., White, J., Haddox, M. K., and Goldberg, N. D., 1973, *Pharmacologist* **15**:156.
Goldberg, N. D., Dietz, S. B., and O'Toole, A. G., 1969, *J. Biol. Chem.* **244**:4458–4466.
Goldberg, N. D., Lust, W. D., O'Dea, R. F., Wei, S., and O'Toole, A. G., 1970 in: *Advances in Biochemical Psychopharmacology* (P. Greengard and E. Costa, eds.), Vol. 3, pp. 67–87, Raven Press, New York.
Goldberg, N. D., O'Dea, R. F., and Haddox, M. K., 1973a, in: *Advances in Cyclic Nucleotide Research* (P. Greengard and G. A. Robison, eds.) pp. 155–223, Raven Press, New York.
Goldberg, N. D., Haddox, M. K., Hartle, D. K., and Hadden, J. W., 1973b, in: *Proceedings of the Fifth International Congress of Pharmacology,* Vol. 5, pp. 146–169, S. Karger, Basel.
Goldberg, N. D., Haddox, M. K., Estensen, R., White, J. G., Lopez, C., and Hadden, J. W., 1974, in: *Cyclic AMP, Cell Growth, and the Immune Response* (W. Braun, L. M. Lichtenstein, and C. W. Parker, eds.), pp. 247–262, Springer-Verlag, New York.
Goldstein, I. M., Brai, M., Osler, A. G., and Weissmann, G., 1973, *J. Immunol.* **111**:33–37.
Goldstein, I. M., Hoffstein, S. T., and Weissmann, G., 1975, *J. Immunol.* **115**:665–670.
Hadden, J. W., Leu, R., Goldberg, N. D., and Hadden, E. M., 1974, *Fed. Prc. Fed. Am. Soc. Exp. Biol.* **33**:745.
Hadden, J. W., Coffey, R. G., Hadden, E. M., Lopez-Corrales, E., and Sunshine, G. H., 1975a, *Cell. Immunol.* **20**:98–103.
Hadden, J. W., Sadlik, J. R., and Hadden, E. M., 1975b, *Nature (London)* **257**:483–485.
Hamberg, M., and Samuelsson, B., 1974, *Proc. Natl. Acad. Sci. U.S.A.* **71**:3400–3404.
Hardman, J. G., Beavo, J. A., Gray, J. P., Chrisman, T. D., Patterson, W. D., and Sutherland, E. W., 1971, *Ann. N. Y. Acad. Sci.* **185**:27–35.
Harker, L. A., and Slichter, S. J., 1970, *N. Engl. J. Med.* **283**:1302–1305.
Haslam, R. J., 1973, *Ser. Haematol.* **6**:333–350.
Haslam, R. J., 1975, in: *Ciba Found. Symp.: Biochemistry and Pharmacology of Blood Platelets* (J. Knight, ed.), pp. 121–151.
Haslam, R. J., and McClenaghan, M. D., 1974, *Biochem. J.* **138**:317–320.
Haslam, R. J., Davidson, M. M. L., and McClenaghan, M. D., 1975a, *Nature (London)* **253**:455–457.
Haslam, R. J., McClenaghan, M. D., and Adams, A., 1975b, in: *Advances in Cyclic Nucleotide Research* (G. I. Drummond, P. Greengard, and G. A. Robison, eds.), Vol. 5, pp. 821, Raven Press, New York.
Hawkins, D., 1971, *J. Immunol.* **107**:344–352.
Henson, P. M., 1971, *J. Immunol.* **107**:1535–1546.
Hill, H. R., Estensen, R. D., Quie, P. G., Hogan, N. A., and Goldberg, N. D., 1975, *Metabolism* **24**:447–456.
Hoffstein, S., Zurier, R. B., and Weissmann, G., 1974, *Clin. Immunol. Immunopathol.* **3**:201–217.
Huffer, W. E., 1973, *Lab. Invest.* **29**:304–309.
Ichikawa, A., Nagasaki, M., Umezu, K., Hayashi, H., and Tomita, K., 1972, *Biochem. Pharmacol.* **21**:2615–2626.

Ignarro, L. J., 1973, *Nature (London) New. Biol.* **245**:151–154.
Ignarro, L. J., 1974a, *Arthritis Rheum.* **17**:25–36.
Ignarro, L. J., 1974b, *J. Immunol.* **112**:210–214.
Ignarro, L. J., 1974c, *J. Immunol.* **113**:298–308.
Ignarro, L. J., 1974d, *Agents Actions* **4**:241–258.
Ignarro, L. J., 1975, in: *Lysosomes in Biology and Pathology* (J. T. Dingle and R. T. Dean, eds.), Vol. 4, pp. 481–523, American Elsevier Publishing Co., New York.
Ignarro, L. J., and Cech, S. Y., 1975, *J. Cyclic Nucleotide Res.* **1**:283–292.
Ignarro, L. J., and Cech, S. Y., 1976, *Proc. Soc. Exp. Biol. Med.* **151**:448–452.
Ignarro, L. J., and George, W. J., 1974a, *Proc. Natl. Acad. Sci. U.S.A.* **71**:2027–2031.
Ignarro, L. J., and George, W. J., 1974b, *J. Exp. Med.* **140**:225–238.
Ignarro, L. J., and George, W. J., 1975, *Pharmacologist* **17**:270.
Ignarro, L. J., Lint, T. F., and George, W. J., 1974a, *J. Exp. Med.* **139**:1395–1414.
Ignarro, L. J., Paddock, R. J., and George, W. J., 1974b, *Science* **183**:855–857.
Ishikawa, E., Ishikawa, S., Davis, J. W., and Sutherland, E. W., 1969, *J. Biol. Chem.* **244**:6371–6376.
Kaliner, M., Orange, R. P., and Austen, K. F., 1972, *J. Exp. Med.* **136**:556–567.
Koopman, W. J., Gillis, M. H., and David, J. R., 1973, *J. Immunol.* **110**:1609–1614.
Lima, A. O., Javierre, M. Q., Dias da Silva, W., and Camara, D. S., 1974, *Experientia* **30**:945,946.
Mackaness, G. B., 1964, *J. Exp. Med.* **120**:105–120.
Mackaness, G. B., 1969, *J. Exp. Med.* **129**:973–992.
Manganiello, V., Evans, W. H., Stossel, T. P., Mason, R. J., and Vaughan, M., 1971, *J. Clin. Invest.* **50**:2741–2744.
Mannucci, P. M., and Pareti, F. I., 1974, *J. Lab. Clin. Med.* **84**:828–838.
Marcus, A. J., and Zucker, M. B., 1965, in: *Physiology of Blood Platelets* pp. 53, Grune and Stratton, New York.
Marquis, N. R., Vigdahl, R. L., and Tavormina, P. A., 1969, *Biochem. Biophys. Res. Commun.* **36**:965–972.
Marquis, N. R., Vigdahl, R. L., and Tavormina, P. A., 1971, *Fed. Proc. Fed. Am. Soc. Exp. Biol.* **30**:423.
Massini, P., and Lüscher, E. F., 1974, *Biochim. Biophys. Acta* **372**:109–121.
May, C. D., Levine, B. B., and Weissmann, G., 1970, *Proc. Soc. Exp. Biol. Med.* **133**:758–763.
Mustard, J. F., and Packham, M. A., 1970, *Pharmacol. Rev.* **22**:97–187.
Myrvik, Q. N., Leake, E. S., and Oshima, S., 1962, *J. Immunol.* **89**:745–751.
Nelson, W. R., and Taylor, G. A., 1975, *Scand. J. Haematol.* **15**:35–44.
Nishioka, K., Constantopoulos, A., Satoh, P. S., and Najjar, V. A., 1972, *Biochem. Biophys. Res. Commun.* **47**:172–179.
Oronsky, A. L., Ignarro, L. J., and Perper, R. J., 1973, *J. Exp. Med.* **138**:461–472.
Pick, E., 1972, *Nature (London) New Biol.* **238**:176, 177.
Pick, E., Brostoff, J., Krejci, J., and Turk, J. L., 1970, *Cell. Immunol.* **1**:92–109.
Polgar, P., Vera, J. C., Kelley, P. R., and Rutenburg, A. M., 1973, *Biochim. Biophys. Acta* **297**:378–383.
Rabinowitz, Y., 1964, *Blood* **23**:811–828.
Remold, H. G., Katz, A. B., Haber, E., and David, J. R., 1970, *Cell. Immunol.* **1**:133–145.
Renoux, G., and Renoux, M., 1971, *C. R. Acad. Sci. Paris Ser. D* **272**:349–350.
Repine, J. E., White, J. G., Clawson, C. C., and Holmes, B. M., 1974, *J. Lab. Clin. Med.* **83**:911–920.
Rivkin, I., Rosenblatt, J., and Becker, E. L., 1975, *J. Immunol.* **115**:1126–1134.
Rojas-Espinosa, O., Arce-Paredez, P., Dannenberg, A. M., and Kamenetz, R. L., 1975, *Biochim. Biophys. Acta* **403**:161–179.
Rubin, R. P., 1970, *Pharmacol. Rev.* **22**:389–428.
Salzman, E. W., 1970, *Fed. Proc. Fed. Am. Soc. Exp. Biol.* **29**:316.
Salzman, E. W., and Levine, L., 1971, *J. Clin. Invest.* **50**:131–141.
Salzman, E. W., and Weisenberger, H., 1972, in: *Advances in Cyclic Nucleotide Research* (P. Greengard, R. Paoletti, and G. A. Robison, eds.), Vol. 1, pp. 231–247, Raven Press, New York.
Salzman, E. W., Ashford, T. P., Chambers, D. A., Neri, L. L., and Demptster, A., 1969, *Am. J. Physiol.* **217**:1330–1338.
Sandler, J. A., Clyman, R. I., Manganiello, V. C., and Vaughan, M., 1975a, *J. Clin. Invest.* **55**:431–435.
Sandler, J. A., Gallin, J. I., and Vaughan, M., 1975b, *J. Cell Biol.* **67**:480–484.
Schick, P. K., and Yu, B. P., 1974, *J. Clin. Invest.* **54**:1032–1039.
Schmidt-Gayk, H. E., Jakobs, K. H., and Hackenthal, E., 1975, *J. Reticuloendothel. Soc.* **17**:251–261.

Schultz, G., Hardman, J. G., Schultz, K., Baird, C. E., and Sutherland, E. W., 1973, *Proc. Natl. Acad. Sci. U.S.A.* **70**:3889–3893.

Schwartz, S. L., Evans, D. E., Lundin, J. E., and Bond, J. C., 1972, *J. Pharmacol. Exp. Ther.* **183**:370–377.

Scott, R. E., 1970, *Blood* **35**:514–516.

Seyberth, H. W., Schmidt-Gayk, H., Jakobs, K. H., and Hackenthal, E., 1973, *J. Cell Biol.* **57**:567–571.

Shio, H., and Ramwell, P. W., 1972, *Science* **175**:536–538.

Smith, J. B., and Willis, A. L., 1971, *Nature* (*London*) *New Biol.* **231**:235–237.

Smith, J. B., Silver, M. J., Ingerman, C. M., and Kocsis, J. J., 1974, *Thromb. Res.* **5**:291–299.

Smith, R. J., and Ignarro, L. J., 1975, *Proc. Natl. Acad. Sci. U.S.A.* **72**:108–112.

Spaet, T. H., and Zucker, M. B., 1964, *Amer. J. Physiol.* **206**:1267–1274.

Stossel, T. P., 1975, *Semin. Hematol.* **12**:83–116.

Stossel, T. P., Mason, R. J., Hartwig, J., and Vaughan, M., 1972, *J. Clin. Invest.* **51**:615–624.

Sullivan, J. M., Harken, D. E., and Gorlin, R., 1971, *N. Engl. J. Med.* **284**:1391–1394.

Tse, R. L., Phelps, P., and Urban, D., 1972, *J. Lab. Clin. Med.* **80**:264–274.

Vane, J. R., 1971, *Nature* (*London*) *New Biol.* **231**:232–235.

Vargaftig, B. B., and Chignard, M., 1975, *Agents Actions* **5**:137–144.

Weissmann, G., Zurier, R. B., Spieler, P. J., and Goldstein, I. M., 1971a, *J. Exp. Med.* **134**:149s–165s.

Weissmann, G., Dukor, P., and Zurier, R. B., 1971b, *Nature* (*London*) *New Biol.* **231**:131–133.

Weissmann, G., Dukor, P., and Sessa, G., 1971c, in: *Immunopathology of Inflammation* (B. Forscher and J. C. Houck, eds.), pp. 107–117, Excerpta Medica, The Netherlands.

Weissmann, G., Zurier, R. B., and Hoffstein, S., 1972, *Am. J. Pathol.* **68**:539–559.

Weissmann, G., Goldstein, I., Hoffstein, S., and Tsung, P. K., 1975a, *Ann. N. Y. Acad. Sci.* **253**:750–762.

Weissmann, G., Goldstein, I., Hoffstein, S., Chauvet, G., and Robineaux, R., 1975b, *Ann. N. Y. Acad. Sci.* **256**:222–232.

White, J. G., Goldberg, N. D., Estensen, R. D., Haddox, M. K., and Rao, G. H. R., 1973, *J. Clin. Invest.* **52**:89a.

White, L. E., Ignarro, L. J., and George, W. J., 1973, *Pharmacologist* **15**:157.

Wilkinson, P. C., 1975, *Exp. Cell Res.* **93**:420–426.

Willis, A. L., 1974a, *Prostaglandins* **5**:1–25.

Willis, A. L., 1974b, *Science* **183**:325–327.

Wolfe, S. M., and Shulman, N. R., 1969, *Biochem. Biophys. Res. Commun.* **35**:265–272.

Woodin, A. M., 1968, in: *The Biological Basis of Medicine* (E. E. Bittar and N. Bittar, eds.), Vol. 2, pp. 373–396, Academic Press, New York.

Woodin, A. M., and Wieneke, A. A., 1963, *Biochem. J.* **87**:487–495.

Wright, D. G., and Malawista, S. E., 1973, *Arthritis Rheum.* **16**:749–758.

Wright, D. G., Kirkpatrick, C. H., and Gallin, J. I., 1976, in: *Modulation of Host Immune Resistance in the Prevention or Treatment of Induced Neoplasia* (M. Chirigos, ed.), Fogarty International Center Proceedings No. 28, U.S. Government Printing Office, Washington, D.C., in press.

Yamamoto, S., Dunn, C. J., Capasso, F., Deporter, D. A., and Willoughby, D. A., 1975, *J. Pathol.* **117**:65–73.

Zieve, P. D., and Greenough, W. B., 1969, *Biochem. Biophys. Res. Commun.* **35**:462–466.

Zucker, M. B., 1974, in *The Inflammatory Process* (B. W. Zweifach, L. Grant, and R. T. McCluskey, eds.), Vol. 1, pp. 511–543, Academic Press, New York.

Zurier, R. B., and Quagliata, F., 1971, *Nature* (*London*) **234**:304,305.

Zurier, R. B., Hoffstein, S., and Weissmann, G., 1973a, *Proc. Natl. Acad. Sci. U.S.A.* **70**:844–848.

Zurier, R., Hoffstein, S., and Weissmann, G., 1973b, *J. Cell Biol.* **58**:27–41.

Zurier, R. B., Hoffstein, S., and Weissmann, G., 1973c, *Arthritis Rheum.* **16**:606–618.

Zurier, R. B., Weissmann, G., Hoffstein, S., Kammerman, S., and Tai, H. H., 1974, *J. Clin. Invest.* **53**:297–309.

5

Molecular Aspects of Macrophage Activation and Proliferation

JOHN W. HADDEN and ARTHUR ENGLARD

1. Introduction

The importance of macrophages as effectors of cell-mediated immunity to a variety of microorganisms, particularly to facultative intracellular parasites, is well established. Recent evidence indicates that macrophages are important participants in the host's reaction to engraftment and to spontaneous or induced neoplasia. The effectiveness of macrophages in these aspects of host resistance appears to depend on a process of activation by which monocyte-derived macrophages acquire a nonspecific enhancement of microbicidal and tumoricidal capacity. While this process of activation has been extensively analyzed *in vivo,* it is only recently that it has been examined *in vitro* and its mechanisms have been probed. This chapter, in attempting to develop what is known about this process, is admittedly premature in its presentation, since the specific mechanisms of macrophage activation have yet to be clarified.

2. Macrophage Activation *in Vivo*

One striking feature of acquired cellular resistance to infection is the lack of specificity in its expression. This lack was first observed by Pullinger (1936), who noted that simultaneous inoculation of guinea pigs with *Mycobacterium tuberculosis* and *Brucella abortus* prevented infection by the latter organism. Henderson (1964) found that guinea pigs infected with *Br. suis* possessed a high degree of resistance to *Bacillus anthracis* and a lesser degree of resistance to *Pasteurella*

JOHN W. HADDEN and ARTHUR ENGLARD • Laboratory of Immunopharmacology, Memorial Sloan-Kettering Cancer Center, New York, New York 10021.

pestis and *Myco. tuberculosis*. Guinea pigs infected with *Myco. tuberculosis*, however, developed a pronounced nonspecific resistance to infection with *Br. suis*. Subsequently, it was shown that tuberculous animals were resistant to *Past. pestis* (Girard and Grumbach, 1958), to *Salmonella enteritidis* (Howard *et al.*, 1959), and to *Staphylococcus aureus* (Dubos and Schaedler, 1952). Similarly, mice infected with *Br. abortus* were resistant to *Listeria monocytogenes* (Mackaness, 1964), and mice resistant to *Sal. typhimurium* were also resistant to *Listeria* and vice versa (Blanden *et al.*, 1966). In the study by Blanden *et al.* (1966), it was shown that the peritoneal macrophages from the *Salmonella*-resistant mice could inhibit the growth of *Listeria in vitro.* Coppel and Youmans (1969a) found that mice immunized with *Myco. tuberculosis* became resistant to *Listeria* and *Klebsiella.* In another study (Coppel and Youmans, 1969b), it was shown that mice that had been immunized with bacillus Calmette-Guerin (BCG) 14 weeks earlier were slightly resistant to infection with *Listeria,* but 3 days after a second injection of BCG, they became highly resistant. Likewise, nonspecific resistance that had declined after primary exposure to *Listeria* or *Mycobacteria* could be evoked again by reexposure to the homologous organism.

This characteristic of nonspecificity not only operates among appropriate bacteria, but also extends across phyla. Thus, mice that become immune to the intracellular protozoan *Besnoitia jellisoni* also acquire resistance against *L. monocytogenes*, *Sal. typhimurium*, *Br. melitensis*, meningovirus, and *Toxoplasma gondii* (Ruskin and Remington, 1968). The *in vivo* activity was accompanied by enhanced killing of ingested microorganisms by macrophages in culture. Similarly, mice primarily infected with *Listeria*, *Besnoita*, or *Toxoplasma* were resistant to challenge with the fungus *Cryptococcus neoformans* (Gentry and Remington, 1971), mice infected with *Toxoplasma* and *Besnoitia* developed resistance to *Myco. leprae* (Krahenbuhl *et al.*, 1974), and mice injected with *Trichinella spiralis* developed decreased susceptibility to *Listeria* (Cypress *et al.*, 1974). Even more striking is the finding that macrophages from mice undergoing graft-vs.-host reactions had a heightened capacity to destroy *Listeria* and *Salmonella* (Blanden, 1969).

The cell responsible for the destruction of facultative intracellular parasites is the macrophage. When macrophages were removed from mice that were immune to *L. monocytogenes,* they were shown to prevent the growth of ingested *Listeria* in culture (Mackaness, 1962). When nonimmune mice are injected with lymphocytes from mice immune to *L. monocytogenes,* they become resistant to lethal doses of this organism. However, depletion of macrophage precursors by X-irradiation of the recipient mice prevented the development of resistance to *Listeria* in the mice (Tripathy and Mackaness, 1969). These experiments and others indicate that acquired cellular resistance involves a heightened nonspecific microbicidal power of macrophages, that this power declines with increasing time after immunization, and that nonspecific resistance can be specifically recalled by reexposure to the original organism. The macrophages with a heightened nonspecific microbicidal capacity are referred to as *activated macrophages* (Nelson, 1972).

2.1. Characteristics of Activated Macrophages

The activated macrophage is larger (Blanden, 1968) and much more complex morphologically than the nonactivated macrophage. It has a marked propensity to spread on glass, a property that has been related to its enhanced capacity for phagocytosis (North, 1968). The content of acid hydrolases (Saito and Sutter, 1965; Dannenberg *et al.*, 1963), the digestive capacity (Blanden, 1968), the mitotic rate (Khoo and Mackaness, 1964; North, 1969a, b, 1970), and ruffled membrane activity (Nathan *et al.*, 1971) are all increased. Blanden (1968) showed that peritoneal macrophages from mice infected with BCG had a much more extensive cytoplasm with numerous mitochondria. Phase-dense granules were rarely present in normal macrophages, but were numerous in the macrophages from immunized animals. Pinocytosis, as judged by the incidence of phase-lucent vesicles, was also markedly increased in these macrophages. Using electron microscopy, Blanden (1968) found a more extensive Golgi apparatus and more mitochondria and electron-opaque bodies (presumably lysosomes) in the activated macrophage.

2.2. Relationship between Macrophage Activation and Delayed Hypersensitivity

An important relationship has been observed between the development of cellular immunity to infection after a primary infection with *Listeria* as seen by macrophage activation and delayed hypersensitivity. The host's antibacterial response and the emergence of delayed hypersensitivity were shown to be coincident events (Mackaness, 1962, 1969), indicating that both are manifestations of the immune response.

2.3. Cells Involved in the Passive Transfer of Immunity

Although the activated macrophage seems to be the effector cell in the destruction of facultative intracellular parasites, it lacks the immunologic properties that would permit the passive transfer of immunity (Turk and Polak, 1967). Passive transfer of immunity has been accomplished, however, with lymph node, thoracic duct, and spleen cells (Frenkel, 1967; Allen, 1962; Mackaness, 1969; McGregor and Koster, 1971). The study by Mackaness (1969) showed that the transfer of immunity with spleen cells allowed the recipient to develop macrophages similar to those described by Blanden (1968) as activated. Nonspecific resistance to facultative intracellular parasites could not be transferred with lymphocytes alone (Mackaness, 1967, 1968); concomitant challenge of the recipient with the antigen used to immunize the donor was necessary. This finding indicated that resistance conferred with immune lymphoid cells was specific for the infective agent, and that the generalized antimicrobial properties that develop are dependent on the interaction between the sensitized lymphocyte and the organism or antigen that elicited the sensitization. The interaction of specific antigen with lymphocyte is then followed by an interaction between lymphocyte and macrophage, resulting in the activation of the latter. This form of cellular immunity is thus specific in its elicitation, but nonspecific in its expression.

Treatment of immune spleen cells with antilymphocyte globulin (ALG) (Mackaness and Hill, 1969) or antitheta serum (Lane and Unanue, 1972; North, 1973; Youdim *et al.*, 1973) completely abolished their ability to passively transfer immunity to *Listeria*. Zinkernagel *et al.* (1974) injected antithymocyte serum into mice challenged with a sublethal dose of *Listeria*, and found that it resulted in an increase in the number of bacteria in the liver and spleen as compared with controls. In addition, Pearson and Osebold (1973, 1974) found that such treatment increased the mortality rate of the animals. Youdim *et al.* (1973) found that resistance to *Listeria* and delayed hypersensitivity could be transferred to neonatally thymectomized or lethally irradiated mice by bone marrow, spleen, and lymph node cells from syngeneic immune mice. *In vitro* treatment with antitheta serum and complement abolished the capacity of spleen and bone marrow cells from immune donors to transfer delayed hypersensitivity to irradiated hosts, indicating that the T lymphocyte is required for the transfer. Thus, while cellular immunity is specific in its elicitation and nonspecific in its expression, the specific component is the T lymphocyte, and the nonspecific component is the macrophage.

2.4. Macrophage Proliferation in Association with Cellular Immunity

It has been shown that there is striking proliferation of macrophages in inflammation (Spector and Lykke, 1966; Spector and Willoughby, 1968; Mariano and Spector, 1974). *In vivo* studies have shown that the emergence of activated macrophages following challenge by sublethal doses of facultative intracellular parasites is preceded by a period of vigorous proliferation of peritoneal macrophages and Kupffer cells. Mackaness (1962) observed that the onset of both *Listeria* killing and delayed hypersensitivity was associated with the appearance of numerous macrophages undergoing mitosis. The number of peritoneal macrophages engaged in the process of replication, following a second challenge of antigen, was significantly higher than controls (Forbes and Mackaness, 1963). In a subsequent study, Khoo and Mackaness (1964) studied the proliferative activity of peritoneal macrophages in mice systemically infected with *Listeria* or *Brucella*. A gross difference was found in the time course of infection caused by these organisms, but in both, the percentage of DNA-synthesizing cells rose progressively to a peak 3 days after the bacterial population in the spleens had reached a maximum. During a secondary *Listeria* infection, the cellular response occurred sooner and was more intense. In each case, the onset of macrophage proliferation coincided with the appearance of delayed hypersensitivity and decrease in the bacterial population.

In a series of experiments, North (1969a,b, 1970) found that in mice infected with either *Listeria* or BCG, there was initially an intense proliferation of splenic lymphoid cells followed by proliferation of macrophages in both the liver and spleen, and a subsequent production of macrophages with increased metabolic and bactericidal activity. These properties coincided with increased ability of the peritoneal macrophages to spread on glass and to phagocytize polystyrene particles, and with the onset and intensity of delayed hypersensitivity. It was also shown that following infection with *Listeria*, there occurs a substantial accumulation of migratory macrophages in the liver. These cells had the characteristics of blood monocytes, and their appearance in infective foci of the liver corresponds to the expression of a high level of antimicrobial immunity in the organ. Indications were that the macrophages that express immunity to *Listeria* are those derived from circulatory blood monocytes, and that the proliferation of Kupffer cells was not essential for expression of immunity in the liver.

In another series of experiments (Shima *et al.*, 1972; Ando and Dannenberg, 1972; Dannenberg *et al.*, 1972; Ando *et al.*, 1972), the degree of activation of macrophages in tuberculous lesions produced by BCG was measured by their content of the lysosomal enzyme β-galactosidase. It was shown that the bactericidal capacity of the macrophages correlated with an increased content of β-galactosidase, and that the onset of killing and delayed hypersensitivity was preceded by an increase in division of the recently arrived blood monocytes.

The cell responsible for this macrophage division was shown to be the T lymphocyte (North, 1973; North and Mackaness, 1973; Blanden and Langman, 1972). These studies showed that the transfer of anti-*Listeria* immunity to normal mice with spleen cells from immunized syngeneic mice resulted in a striking increase in the replication of macrophages in recipient mice prior to the onset of immunity. Incubation of the spleen cells with antitheta serum and complement abolished the ability of the recipient macrophages to divide and become activated. T-cell-deficient mice were also shown to have a reduced capacity to develop antimycobacterial immunity (North, 1973, 1974). The reduced capacity to develop antitubercular immunity was associated with a reduced ability to show increased lymphoid and macrophage proliferation in response to the infection. These properties, however, could be restored with syngeneic T cells.

Convincing evidence has been presented that immunity to facultative intracellular parasites depends on the emergence of a population of macrophages with enhanced bactericidal capacity, and that this activation is preceded by T-cell-dependent division of lymphocytes and macrophages.

3. Macrophage Activation *in Vitro*

In vitro studies in which lymphocytes from immune animals were added to macrophages from nonimmune animals support the *in vivo* findings discussed in Section 2. Patterson and Youmans (1970) found that splenic lymphocytes from mice immunized with an attenuated strain of *Mycobacteria,* when added to normal mouse peritoneal macrophages in tissue culture, induced them to inhibit the multiplication of a virulent strain. Krahenbuhl and Remington (1971) obtained similar results using splenic lymphocytes from guinea pigs sensitized to *Toxoplasma* and cultured with normal guinea pig macrophages in the presence of *Toxoplasma* antigens. Following coculture, these macrophages were shown to be highly resistant to *Listeria* infection. Simon and Sheagren (1971, 1972a, b) similarly found that guinea pig lymphocytes immunized with BCG conferred resistance to *Listeria* infection on normal guinea pig macrophages. It was shown that the cell responsible for this *in vitro* macrophage activation was the T lymphocyte, because treatment of *Toxoplasma*-sensitive spleen cells (Krahenbuhl *et al.,* 1973) or *Listeria*-sensitive peritoneal cells (Cole, 1975) with antilymphocyte globulin and complement abolished their ability to activate normal macrophages *in vitro.*

3.1. Interaction between Lymphocyte and Macrophage

A popular explanation to account for macrophage activation is the release of soluble mediators, previously called *lymphokines,* from sensitized lymphocytes (Bloom, 1971; David and David, 1972); several of these mediators are known to affect macrophages. Although the *in vivo* actions of the lymphokines are not known, extensive work has been done on the *in vitro* effects of these lymphocyte products on macrophage activation. Mooney and Waksman (1970) found that the supernatants from tuberculin- or human-serum-albumin-sensitized lymph node cells incubated in the presence of either antigen could confer such properties as increased adherence to glass and increased ameboid activity of macrophages. Patterson and Youmans (1970) showed that lymphocytes from mice immunized against *Mycobacteria* elaborate a factor that when cultured with the *Mycobacteria* activates normal macrophages to kill virulent tubercle bacilli. Godal *et al.* (1971) observed that when supernatants from mixed lymphocyte cultures of genetically different rabbits were added to normal macrophages, they conferred on the macrophages the ability to inhibit the intracellular multiplication of *Mycobacteria*. T. Jones and Youmans (1973) found that supernatants capable of activating macrophages could be obtained from sensitized lymphocytes stimulated with antigen both *in vivo* and *in vitro*, suggesting that the production of lymphocyte mediators of macrophage activation was not an artifact of the *in vitro* culture method.

Borges and Johnson (1975) found that *Toxoplasma* multiplication was identical in monocytes from subjects with established *Toxoplasma* immunity and nonimmune subjects, but was significantly inhibited in cells from both sources if the monocytes were preincubated with immune lymphocytes and *Toxoplasma* antigen. Supernatants prepared from *Toxoplasma*-immune lymphocytes incubated with *Toxoplasma* antigen were also effective in inducing, in monocytes, the ability to inhibit *Toxoplasma* multiplication. This finding is in contrast to the report that normal mice peritoneal macrophages could not be activated by exposure to supernatant from such an interaction to inhibit the growth of *Toxoplasma* (J. C. Jones *et al.*, 1975). Peritoneal macrophages from *Toxoplasma*-immunized mice, however, could be activated by the procedures described above to inhibit *Toxoplasma* growth.

The first association of lymphokines with macrophage activation was made by Nathan *et al.* (1971) and Adams *et al.* (1971). The latter authors cultured tuberculin-sensitive guinea pig peritoneal exudate cells with purified protein derivative, and found that supernatant samples of the experimental cultures had migration-inhibitory factor (MIF) activity. MIF is a lymphokine first described by Bloom and Bennett (1966) and David (1966). In the MIF-containing cultures, the macrophages became larger, adhered to culture vessels more than controls, and developed increased acid phosphatase, lysosomes, Golgi profiles, ribosomes, and rough endoplasmic reticulum. Nathan *et al.* (1971) demonstrated that fractions that contained MIF, chemotactic factor, and lymphotoxin (all three are lymphokines) increased the adherence, phagocytosis, spreading, motility, and hexose monophosphate shunt activity of normal peritoneal macrophages. In a subsequent study, Nathan *et al.* (1973) tested whether the lymphocyte factor responsible for activation of the macrophage corresponds to either MIF, macrophage chemotactic factor, or lymphotoxin. Supernatants obtained from guinea pig lymphocytes sensitized to bovine γ-globulin (BGG) and incubated in the presence of BGG were fractionated on Sephadex G-100, and a fraction containing MIF, lymphotoxin, and chemotactic factor was obtained. On the basis of Sephadex G-100 chromatography, cesium chloride density-gradient centrifugation, and neuraminidase sensitivity, the activating factor could not be distinguished from MIF, but could be distinguished from lymphotoxin and chemotactic factor. The MIF-rich fraction was then shown to activate macrophages by enhancing their bacteriostatic ability against *Listeria* challenge (Fowles *et al.*, 1973; Leibowitch and David, 1973; Englard and Hadden, unpublished observations).

3.2. Activation of Macrophages to Kill Tumor Cells

A number of studies have shown that activated macrophages kill tumor cells. Alexander and Evans (1971) showed that macrophages treated with endotoxin as well as its low-molecular-weight, polysaccharide-free hydrolysis product, Lipid A, or double-stranded RNA become cytotoxic to lymphoma cells. Meltzer *et al.* (1975) found that peritoneal macrophages from mice immune to BGG became cytotoxic to syngeneic tumor cell lines, but not to normal cells. Similarly, peritoneal macrophages from mice injected with killed *Corynebacterium granulosum* were rendered cytotoxic to tumor cells, but not to normal cells (Bâsić *et al.*, 1975). It was shown that whole bacteria are not necessary for the activation of macrophages, but preparations extracted from *Mycobacteria* were able to render macrophages cytotoxic to tumor cells (Juy and Chedid, 1975; Lamensans *et al.*, 1975).

Recent experiments by Piessens *et al.* (1975) showed that supernatants containing MIF activity could activate macrophages to kill tumor cells. There was no correlation, however, between the degree of MIF activity of the supernatants used to activate the macrophages and the subsequent degree of macrophage tumoricidal capacity. Churchill *et al.* (1975) similarly activated macrophages to kill tumor cells with MIF-rich Sephadex fractions.

3.3. Macrophage Replication *in Vitro*

The question as to the mechanism by which T lymphocytes mediate macrophage division has recently been investigated *in vitro*. Godal *et al.* (1971) found that supernatants from a mixed lymphocyte culture (MLC) could induce macrophage replication *in vitro*. Hadden *et al.* (1974a) found that MIF-rich supernatants, from BGG-sensitive lymphocytes incubated with BGG, induce guinea pig macrophages to proliferate *in vitro*. Subsequently, Wynne *et al.* (1975) and Adolphe *et al.* (1975) found that they could initiate *in vitro* proliferation of mouse peritoneal macrophages by addition of inflammatory exudate material to their monolayers. The macrophages began to divide at day 4, and exhibited properties of activation, i.e., increased phagocytosis, acid phosphatase activity, and cytoplasmic organelles. The results of a recent study by Hadden *et al.* (1975a) showed that a mitogenic factor present in MIF-rich supernatants causes significant increases in tritiated thymidine incorporation and DNA synthesis in cultured macrophages. The activity inducing macrophage replication was termed *macrophage mitogenic factor* (MMF). Its molecular weight was shown to be in the same range as MIF (35,000–60,000), but MIF activity could be separated by vacuum dialysis. MMF may thus be the missing link between the interaction of T lymphocytes and macrophages to produce division and activation of macrophages.

3.4. Current Studies on the Relationship of Macrophage Division and Activation *in Vitro*

The reason one would suspect that MMF is the lymphocyte-produced macrophage activator is that it is found in the same molecular-weight range as MIF on Sephadex G-100, and until now, MIF had been thought to be responsible for macrophage activation (Nathan *et al.*, 1973; Fowles *et al.*, 1973). That MIF activity can be removed from supernatants by vacuum dialysis, but the mitogenic activity cannot, and that macrophage proliferation appears to be a prerequisite *in vivo* for activation, suggests that it is highly possible that the same stimulus that induces proliferation also activates the macrophages.

Employing Sephadex G-100 fractions containing MMF and depleted of MIF by prior vacuum dialysis, we examined the effect of MMF on the activation of mineral-oil-induced nonimmune guinea pig peritoneal macrophages (Englard and Hadden, unpublished observations). As the assay for activation, we employed a modification of the listericidal assay of Fowles *et al.* (1973). In this assay, monolayers of macrophages are exposed to MMF for varying periods of time in LabTek® chambers, as previously described for the MMF assay (Hadden *et al.,* 1975a). The monolayers are then subjected to a 30-min exposure to virulent *L. monocytogenes* organisms at an approximate ratio of 10 bacteria/macrophage. The monolayers are then washed 8 times, and the number of phagocytized bacteria is confirmed visually by gram staining. At the onset of incubation following the pulsed exposure to the bacteria, approximately 30–40% of the macrophages have ingested an average of two organisms; over the ensuing 6 hr of incubation, the ingested bacteria will replicate in the normal macrophage with a doubling time of 2 hr. When macrophages have been pretreated with MMF for 4–6 days, they inhibit this replication of *Listeria* and proceed to digest them as judged by disintegration of the bacteria visualized by gram staining. Table 1 summarizes the data of a typical experiment.

Employing this experimental model, we also observed that crude supernatants from human macrophages and phytohemagglutinin-(PHA)-stimulated lymphocytes show macrophage-activating activity as well as MMF and colony-stimulating factor (CSF) activity. CSF is a leukocyte product necessary for the information and growth of granulocytic and monocytic cells (Bradley and Metcalf, 1966; Metcalf, 1969).

The work of Stanley *et al.* (1976) suggested that a fibroblast-produced factor [macrophage growth factor (MGF) of mol. wt. 60,000] having MMF activity also contains CSF activity, which is apparently indistinguishable from the MMF activity. Employing Sephadex G-100 fraction of supernatants from antigen-stimulated lymphocytes and controls, we found that the peak of MMF activity (mol. wt. ≈50,000) corresponds to that of macrophage-activating potential, and that the fractions (mol. wt. >100,000) rich in CSF activity and devoid of MMF do not

TABLE 1. Effect of Macrophage Mitogenic Factor on Macrophage Activation[a]

	Time 0[b]		After 6 hours[c]	
Macrophages	Macrophages that have ingested *Listeria* (%)	Average number of *Listeria*/ macrophage	Macrophages that contain *Listeria* (%)	Average number of *Listeria*/ macrophage
MMF[d]	41 ± 5.67	1.58 ± 0.38	13.67 ± 3.28	1.44 ± 0.37
R control[d]	33 ± 4.93	0.96 ± 0.24	32 ± 2.08	6.51 ± 0.38
MEM control[e]	35 ± 6.23	1.42 ± 0.32	30 ± 4.93	6.68 ± 1.69

[a]Data are presented as means ± S.E.M.
[b]*L. monocytogenes* was added to the macrophage monolayers for 30 min, after which the nonphagocytosed bacteria were removed. Time 0 represents the bacterial counts after removal of the nonphagocytosed bacteria.
[c]After the noningested bacteria were removed, fresh media were added to the monolayers, and they were placed in a 37°C incubator for 6 hr.
[d]Preparation is described in Hadden *et al.* (1975a).
[e]Media control.

activate macrophages. These results suggest that lymphocyte-produced MMF is distinct from CSF, and that MMF (not CSF) is the activator of macrophage bactericidal capacity. It is noteworthy that macrophage activation induced by MMF occurs late in this system (5 days) following the peak of replication of the macrophages, and we conclude tentatively that this form of activation represents a proliferation-dependent differentiation step of the macrophage. Experiments are in progress to relate this biological response of the macrophage to that of tumoricidal capacity, and to ascertain the role of lysosomal enzyme accumulation in these events.

Employing this system, we found that a second form of activation occurs that can be observed as early as 3 hr. We observed that a *Listeria*-derived factor similar to that described by Petit and Unanue (1974) will produce macrophage activation characterized by both increased phagocytosis and *Listeria* killing after 24 hr of incubation. We also observed that levamisole, an immunopotentiator that *in vivo* acts to increase macrophage listericidal capacity (Renoux and Renoux, 1976), will increase macrophage phagocytosis of *Listeria*, with a slight effect of enhancing killing.

4. Mechanism of Action of Macrophage Mitogenic Factor

In Chapter 1, we outlined the characteristics of lymphocyte modulation by agents that act to increase cellular levels of cyclic 3′,5′-guanosine monophosphate (cGMP) and the characteristics of the action of lectin mitogens in inducing lymphocyte proliferation by increasing cGMP and inducing calcium influx. To summarize briefly, a number of agents, including levamisole, will augment mitogen-induced lymphocyte proliferation without themselves being mitogenic, and this action is correlated with the ability of these agents to increase cellular levels of cGMP. On the other hand, mitogenic agents such as PHA, concanavalin A, and calcium ionophore (A23187, Lilly), while they induce cGMP accumulation, also induce calcium influx. These observations point to a role of cGMP in the positive regulation of lymphocyte function and, with calcium, in the initiation of lymphocyte proliferation.

Employing these concepts derived from the lymphocyte to our work with macrophages, we observed that agents that increase cGMP levels, such as acetylcholine, imidazole, and 8-bromo cGMP itself, augment the basal proliferation of macrophages (Hadden *et al.*, 1974b). Similarly, MMF and the *Listeria*-derived factor act to increase macrophage levels of cGMP (Hadden *et al.*, unpublished observations), and levamisole, a derivative of imidazole, also acts to increase cGMP levels in macrophages (Wright *et al.*, 1977), as it does in lymphocytes (Hadden *et al.*, 1975b).

On the basis of these preliminary experiments, we conclude tentatively that GMP fulfills a role in the regulation of the macrophage that is comparable to that of the lymphocyte, and that the action of agents that induce macrophage proliferation and activation will be mediated by calcium influx and GMP accumulation.

5. Lysosomal Enzyme Induction in the Mediation of Macrophage Activation

In vivo studies have shown that agents that activate macrophages cause an increase in lysosomes and lysosomal enzyme activity in macrophages. Saito and Sutter (1965) found increased levels of acid phosphatase, cathepsins, and β-glucuronidase in peritoneal macrophages following injection of live BCG. The time of appearance of the increased enzyme levels corresponded to the time that others (Mackaness, 1964) showed activated macrophages to appear in the peritoneal cavity of mice following BCG injection. Ando *et al.* (1972) showed that increases in β-galactosidase correlate with increased ability of infiltrating macrophages to kill BCG. Injections of killed BCG were found to induce macrophages with increased levels of lysozyme (Myrvik, *et al.*, 1962; Cohn and Weiner, 1963; Heise *et al.*, 1965) and acid phosphatase (Heise *et al.*, 1965). Blanden (1968) showed that peritoneal macrophages from mice injected with BCG contain increased numbers of phase-dense granules, presumably lysosomes, and that the appearance of the lysosomes corresponded to the appearance of other properties associated with activated macrophages.

In vitro studies using lymphocyte products to activate macrophages have produced conflicting results. Remold and Mednis (1972, 1975) showed that the addition of MIF-rich Sephadex fractions from BGG-stimulated lymphocytes produced a decrease in the activities of the lysosomal enzymes, acid phosphatase, cathepsin D, and β-glucuronidase in nonimmune guinea pig macrophages after 3 days of culture. It is after 3 days that the MIF-rich fractions were shown to confer increased bactericidal properties on macrophages (Fowles *et al.*, 1973). Similarly, Pantalone and Page (1975) showed that lymphokine-rich supernatants from human peripheral blood lymphocytes stimulated by PHA, when incubated with mouse peritoneal macrophages, cause a decrease in cellular β-glucuronidase, acid phosphatase, β-galactosidase, and β-*N*-acetylglucosaminidase. However, there were increased levels of these enzymes in the media after 2 days of culture, indicating that the macrophages were indeed stimulated to produce increased levels of lysosomal enzyme, but were releasing them into the surrounding media. This phenomenon of release of lysosomal enzyme might well be related to the tissue damage that accompanies inflamation and delayed hypersensitivity reactions.

On the other hand, Adams *et al.* (1971) found that MIF-rich supernatants produce an increase in lysosomes and acid phosphatase activity in guinea pig peritoneal macrophages. Poulter and Turk (1975a,b) and Nath *et al.* (1973) also showed that MIF-rich fractions produce an increase in acid phosphatase after 3 days of incubation with peritoneal macrophages. McDaniel *et al.* (1976) recently reported that a factor obtained from human lymphoid cell lines, which activates macrophages to kill tumor cells, also causes an increase in acid phosphatase activity in the macrophages.

The effects of lymphocyte products on the levels of lysosomal enzymes in macrophage and their relationship to the enhanced bactericidal capacity of the macrophage therefore remains to be clarified.

While the *in vivo* studies have shown that activated macrophages have an increased content of lysosomes, the *in vitro* studies have produced conflicting results. It should be pointed out that the increases in lysosomes found *in vivo* were in peritoneal macrophages activated by the injection of bacteria into the peritoneal cavity. It was shown that ingestion of digestible substances by macrophages induces the synthesis of lysosomal enzymes (Dannenberg *et al.*, 1963) in these cells. It is therefore possible that the increase in lysosomes found in the *in vivo* activated macrophages is due to phagocytosis of bacteria, and is not a property intrinsic to the activation process. The *in vitro* studies did not employ phagocytic material. The failure to show increases in lysosomal enzymes following incubation with lymphokines does not warrant the conclusion that increases in lysosomal enzymes do not occur in activated macrophages. In addition, there may be a differential induction of enzymes in activated macrophages; i.e., some may increase, while others may stay at the same level or even decrease. In this light, it is noteworthy that the level of lysozyme, the only lysosomal enzyme with direct bactericidal activity, was not measured in the *in vitro* studies.

While it is suggested by some that lysosomal enzymes are responsible for the killing of ingested bacteria (Thorne *et al.*, 1976), the involvment of these enzymes in the killing of facultative intracellular parasites and the possibility that other bactericidal mechanisms such as peroxidative metabolism (Klebanoff, 1971) are involved in the enhanced bactericidal activity of activated macrophage remains to be elucidated. Further, the relationship of cyclic nucleotide changes and the enhanced bactericidal and tumorcidal ability of activated macrophages remains to be understood.

6. Other Mechanisms of Macrophage Activation

A number of other substances not derived from the immune system have been reported to activate macrophages in one manner or another. For example, the action of lipopolysaccharide, or bacterial endotoxin, was associated with macrophage proliferation (Forbes, 1965) and activation in terms of lysosomal enzyme accumulation (Weiner and Levanon, 1968) and nonspecific tumoricidal capacity (Alexander and Evans, 1971). Extracts of BCG (Juy and Chedid, 1975) and poly A:U (Alexander and Evans, 1971) were also reported to produce similar effects in activating macrophages. The diversity of these agents might imply several different mechanisms to promote macrophage activation; however, several, such as endotoxin and poly A:U, have been previously linked to cyclic nucleotides in the intracellular mediation of their action (see Chapters 2 and 14 for further discussion). It is also noteworthy that the process of phagocytosis can lead to lysosomal enzyme accumulation 48 hr later (Dannenberg *et al.*, 1963), and that the signal for phagocytosis and degranulation, at least in the neutrophil, is linked to calcium influx and cGMP accumulation (Smith and Ignarro, 1975). Further work is required to clarify the mechanisms of actions of these agents and to discern whether single or multiple processes are involved.

7. Summary

It is not known at this time whether the diverse processes ascribed to the activated macrophage are indeed intrinsically related and derived from a common mechanism. From the biological data, derived principally from *in vivo* studies, it would appear that the two fundamental processes are macrophage proliferation and enhanced macrophage bactericidal or tumoricidal capacity or both, and that aspects of morphology, membrane activity, motility, and lysosomal enzyme accumulation are reflective of these processes. For the purposes of this discussion, we have treated these two major processes as coordinate; that is, the induction of replication of the mature macrophage yields a differentiation step that commits the progeny to the activated state. Equally plausible hypotheses are that different macrophage subsets are involved in the two processes, or that for the macrophage, the induction of activation derives from different stimuli and mechanisms than the induction of replication. Further experimentation is required to resolve which of these hypothetical processes is the most appropriate.

Certainly, the current level of understanding of the biological properties of macrophages and of the techniques to study them will allow in the near future a better understanding of these very important effectors of cellular immunity.

References

Adams, D. O., Biesecker, J. L., and Koss, L. G., 1971, *J. Reticuloendothel. Soc.* **9**:595.
Adolphe, M., Fontagne, J., Pelletier, M., and Giround, F. P., 1975, *Nature (London)* **253**:637.
Alexander, P., and Evans, R., 1971, *Nature (London) New Biol.* **232**:76–78.
Allen, W. P., 1962, *J. Exp. Med.* **115**:411.
Ando, M., and Dannenberg, A. M., Jr., 1972, *Lab. Invest* **27**:466–472.
Ando, M., Dannenberg, A. M., Jr., and Shima, K., 1972, *J. Immunol.* **109**:8–19.
Bâsić, I., Milas, L., Grdina, D. J., and Withers, H. R., 1975, *J. Natl. Cancer Inst.* **55**:589–596.
Blanden, R. V., 1968, *J. Reticuloendothel. Soc.* **5**:179–202.
Blanden, R. V., 1969, *Transplantation* **7**:484–497.
Blanden, R. V., and Langmen, R. E., 1972, *Scand. J. Immunol.* **1**:379–391.
Blanden, R. V., Mackaness, G. B., and Collins, F. M., 1966, *J. Exp. Med.* **124**:585–619.
Bloom, B. R., 1971, *Adv. Immunol.* **13**:101–208.
Bloom, B. R., and Bennett, B., 1966, *Science* **153**:80–82.
Borges, J. S., and Johnson, W. D., Jr., 1975, *J. Exp. Med.* **141**:482–496.
Bradley, T. R., and Metcalf, D., 1966, *Aust. J. Exp. Biol. Med. Sci.* **44**:287–299.
Churchill, W. H., Jr., Piessens, W. F., Sulis, C. A., and David, J. R., 1975, *J. Immunol.* **115**:781–786.
Cohn, A. A., and Weiner, E., 1963, *J. Exp. Med.* **118**:991–1019.
Cole, P., 1975, *Infect. Immun.* **12**:36–41.
Coppel, S., and Youmans, G. P., 1969a, *J. Bacteriol.* **97**:114–120.
Coppel, S., and Youmans, G. P., 1969b, *J. Bacteriol.* **97**:127–133.
Cypress, R. H., Lubiniecki, A. S., and Swidwa, D. W., 1974, *Infect. Immun.* **9**:477–479.
Dannenberg, A. M., Jr., 1966, *Bacteriol. Rev.* **32**:85–102.
Dannenberg, A. M., Jr., Walter, P. C., and Kapral, F. A., 1963, *J. Immunol.* **90**:448–465.
Dannenberg, A. M., Jr., Ando, M., and Shima, K., 1972, *J. Immunol.* **109**:1109–1121.
David, J. R., 1966, *Proc. Natl. Acad. Sci. U.S.A.* **56**:72–77.
David, J. R., and David, R. R., 1972, *Prog. Allergy* **16**:300–449.
Dubos, R. J., and Schaedler, R. W., 1957, *J. Exp. Med.* **106**:703–717.
Forbes, I. J., 1965, *J. Immunol.* **94**:37–39.
Forbes, I. J., and Mackaness, G. B., 1963, *Lancet* **2**:1203, 1204.
Fowles, R. E., Fajardo, I. M., Leibowitch, J. L., and David, J. R., 1973, *J. Exp. Med.* **138**:952–964.
Frenkel, J. D., 1967, *J. Immunol.* **98**:1309–1319.
Gentry, L. O., and Remington, J. S., 1971, *J. Infect. Dis.* **123**:22–31.
Girard, G., and Grumbach, F., 1958, *C. R. Soc. Biol.*, **152**:280–282.
Godal, J., Rees, R. J. W., and Lamvik, J. O., 1971, *Clin. Exp. Immunol.* **8**:625–637.
Hadden, J. W., Leu, R., Goldberg, N. D., and Hadden, E. M., 1974a, *Fed. Proc. Fed. Am. Soc. Exp. Biol.* **33**:745.
Hadden, J. W., Johnson, E. M., Hadden, E. M., Coffey, R. G., and Johnson, L. D., 1974b, in: *Immune Recognition* (A. S. Rosenthal, ed), pp. 359–390, Academic Press, New York.
Hadden, J. W., Sadlik, J. R., and Hadden, E. M., 1975a, *Nature (London)* **257**:483–484.
Hadden, J. W., Coffey, R. G., Hadden, E. M., Lopez-Corrales, E., and Sunshine, G. H., 1975b, *Cell. Immunol.* **20**:98–103.
Heise, E. R., Myrvik, W. N., and Leake, E. S., 1965, *J. Immunol.* **95**:125–130.
Henderson, D. W., 1964, *Symp. Soc. Gen. Microbiol.* **14**:241–256.
Howard, J. G., Biozzi, G., Halpern, B. N., Stiffel, C., and Mouton, D., 1959, *Br. J. Exp. Pathol.* **40**:281–286.

Jones, J. C., Len, L., and Hirsch, J. G., 1975, *J. Exp. Med.* **141**:466–482.
Jones, T., and Youmans, G. P., 1973, *Cell. Immunol.* **9**:353–362.
Juy, D., and Chedid, L., 1975, *Proc. Natl. Acad. Sci. U.S.A.* **72**:4109.
Khoo, K. K., and Mackaness, G. B., 1964, *Aust. J. Exp. Biol. Med. Sci.* **42**:607–716.
Klebanoff, S. J., 1971, *Annu. Rev. Med.* **22**:39–62.
Krahenbuhl, J. L., and Remington, J. S., 1971, *Infect and Immun.* **4**:337–343.
Krahenbuhl, J. L., Rosenberg, L. T., and Remington, J. S., 1973, *J. Immunol.* **111**:992–995.
Krahenbuhl, J. L., Levy, L., and Remington, J. S., 1974, *Infect. Immun.* **10**:1068–1071.
Lamensans, A., Chedid, L., Lederer, E., Rosselet, J. P., Gustafson, R. H., Spencer, H. J., Ludwig, B., and Berger, F. M., 1975, *Proc. Natl. Acad. Sci. U.S.A.* **72**:3656–3660.
Lane, F. C., and Unanue, E. R., 1972, *J. Exp. Med.* **135**:1104–1112.
Leibowitch, J., and David, J. R., 1973, *Ann. Immunol. (Paris)* **124C**:441–464.
Mackaness, G. B., 1962, *J. Exp. Med.* **116**:381–406.
Mackaness, G. B., 1964, *J. Exp. Med.* **120**:105–120.
Mackaness, G. B., 1967, *Br. Med. Bull.* **23**:52–54.
Mackaness, G. B., 1968, *Am. Rev. Respir. Dis.* **97**:337–344.
Mackaness, G. B., 1969, *J. Exp. Med.* **129**:973–992.
Mackaness, G. B., and Hill, W. C., 1969, *J. Exp. Med.* **129**:993–1012.
Mariano, M., and Spector, W. G., 1974, *J. Pathol.* **113**:1–19.
McDaniel, M. C., Lavdico, R., and Papermaster, B. W., 1976, *Clin. Immunol. Immunopathol.* **5**:91–104.
McGregor, D. D., and Koster, F. T., 1971, *Cell. Immunol.* **2**:317–325.
Meltzer, M. S., Tucker, R. W., Sanford, K. K., and Leonard, E. J., 1975, *J. Natl. Cancer Inst.* **54**:1177–1184.
Metcalf, D., 1969, *J. Cell. Physiol.* **74**:323–332.
Mooney, J. J., and Waksman, B. H., 1970, *J. Immunol.* **105**:1138–1145.
Myrvik, Q. N., Leake, E. S., and Oshima, S., 1962, *J. Immunol.* **89**:745–751.
Nath, I., Poulter, L. W., and Turk, V. L., 1973, *Clin. Exp. Immunol.* **13**:445–446.
Nathan, C. F., Karnovsky, M. L. and David, J. R., 1971, *J. Exp. Med.* **133**:1356–1376.
Nathan, C. F., Remold, H. G., and David, J. R., 1973, *J. Exp. Med.* **137**:275–290.
Nelson, D. S., 1972, in: *Macrophages and Cellular Immunity* (A. Laskin and H. Lechervalier, eds.), pp. 45–76, Chemical Rubber Co., New Jersey.
North, R. J., 1968, *J. Exp. Med.* **130**:315–326.
North, R. J., 1969a, *J. Exp. Med.* **130**:299–314.
North, R. J., 1969b, *J. Exp. Med.* **130**:315–326.
North, R. J., 1970, *J. Exp. Med.* **132**:521–545.
North, R. J., 1973, *Cell. Immunol.* **7**:166–176.
North, R. J., 1974, *Infect. Immun.* **10**:66–71.
North, R. J. and Mackaness, G. B., 1973, *Infect. Immun.* **8**:68–73.
Pantalone, R. M., and Page, R. C., 1975, *Proc. Natl. Acad. Sci. U.S.A.* **72**:2091–2094.
Patterson, J. R., and Youmans, G. P., 1970, *Infect. Immun.* **1**:600–603.
Pearson, L. D., and Osebold, J. W., 1973, *Infect. Immun.* **1**:479–486.
Pearson, L. D., and Osebold, J. W., 1974, *Infect. Immun.* **9**:127–133.
Petit, J. C., and Unanue, E. R., 1974, *J. Immunol.* **113**:984–992.
Piessens, W. F., Churchill, W. H., and David, J. R., 1975, *J. Immunol.* **114**:293–299.
Poulter, L. W., and Turk, J. L., 1975a, *Cell. Immunol.* **20**:12–24.
Poulter, L. W., and Turk, J. L., 1975b, *Cell. Immunol.* **20**:25–32.
Pullinger, E. J., 1936, *J. Hyg. (Cambridge)* **36**:456–466.
Remold, H. G., and Mednis, A., 1972, Fed. Proc. Fed. Am. Soc. Exp. Biol. **31**:753.
Remold, H. G., and Mednis, A., 1975, *Inflammation* **1**:175–188.
Renoux, G., and Renoux, M., 1976, *Fed. Proc. Fed. Am. Soc. Exp. Biol.* **35**:336.
Ruskin, J., and Remington, J. S., 1968, in: *Antimicrobial Agents and Chemotherapy* (G. Hobby, ed.), pp. 474–477, American Society for Microbiology, Washington, D.C.
Saito, K. and Sutter, E., 1965, *J. Exp. Med.* **121**:727–749.
Shima, K., Dannenberg, A. M., Jr., Ando, M., Chandrasekhar, S., Seluzicki, J. A., and Fabrikant, J. I., 1972, *Am. J. Pathol.* **67**:160–180.
Simon, H. B., and Sheagren, J. N., 1971, *J. Exp. Med.* **133**:1377–1389.
Simon, H. B., and Sheagren, J. N., 1972a, *Cell. Immunol.* **4**:163–174.

Simon, H. B., and Sheagren, J. N., 1972b, *Infect. Immun.* **6**:101–103.
Smith, R. J., and Ignarro, L. J., 1975, *Proc. Natl. Acad. Sci. U.S.A.* **72**:108–112.
Spector, W. G., and Lykke, A. W. J., 1966, *J. Pathol. Bacteriol.* **92**:163–178.
Spector, W. G., and Willoughby, D. A., 1968, *J. Pathol. Bacteriol.* **96**:389–399.
Stanley, E. R., Cifone, M., Heard, P. M., and Defendi, J., 1976, *J. Exp. Med.* **143**:631–647.
Thorne, K. J., Oliver, R. C., and Barret, J. J., 1976, *Infect. Immun.* **14**:555–563.
Tripathy, S. P., and Mackaness, G. B., 1969, *J. Exp. Med.* **130**:17–30.
Turk, J. L., and Polak, L., 1967, *Int. Arch. Allergy Appl. Immunol.* **31**:403–416.
Weiner, E., and Levanon, D., 1968, *Lab. Invest.* **19**:584–590.
Wright, D. G., Kirkpatrick, I. C. H., and Gallin, J. I., 1977, in: *Progress in Cancer Research and Therapy II* (M. A. Chirigos, ed.), pp. 227–234, Raven Press, New York.
Wynne, K. M., Spector, W. G., and Willoughby, D. A., 1975, *Nature (London)* **253**:636, 637.
Youdim, S., Stutman, O., and Good, R. A., 1973, *Cell. Immunol.* **6**:98–109.
Zinkernagel, R. M., Blanden, R. V., and Langman, R. F., 1974, *J. Immunol.* **112**:496–501.

6

Pharmacological Control of Mediator Release from Leukocytes

ELIZABETH GILLESPIE

1. Introduction

Basophils and mast cells are the only two cell types known that are capable of tightly binding IgE antibody to their cell surfaces. Antigen specific for this IgE antibody can, by interacting with it, cause the release of histamine and other mediators of anaphylaxis from these two cell types. The properties and pharmacological control of mediator release from mast cells are described in Chapter 7. This chapter will deal almost exclusively with release from circulating basophils, and will consider largely the properties of histamine release, since much more is known about the release of this substance than about the release of other mediators. Two themes will be stressed: The first is that the release of histamine from basophils is a process of secretion analogous to the secretion (exocytosis) of hormones and enzymes (i.e., endocrine and exocrine secretion). The second is that this release process is negatively modulated by cyclic AMP (cAMP), and that perhaps histamine, which raises cAMP through interaction with histamine *H-2* receptors, plays a special role as a modulator of this response and other immune responses.

2. General Properties of Histamine Release

The release of histamine from basophils can be easily and accurately studied *in vitro* by incubating leukocytes from allergic donors with the antigen to which the donor is sensitive. Cells from nonallergic persons can be passively sensitized with IgE antibody and subsequently stimulated by antigen, or, alternatively, antibody to

ELIZABETH GILLESPIE • Division of Clinical Immunology, The Johns Hopkins University School of Medicine at The Good Samaritan Hospital, Baltimore, Maryland 21239.

IgE can be used to initiate the release process. Following an appropriate incubation period, the cells are centrifuged, and the histamine released into the supernatant is measured by a spectrofluorometric method. This *in vitro* model of immediate hypersensitivity was shown to have clinical validity in that the amount of antigen required to release histamine from the cells of different allergic individuals correlates well with clinical symptoms (Lichtenstein *et al.*, 1966), and drugs, e.g., isoproterenol and theophylline, that alleviate the *in vivo* symptoms inhibit the *in vitro* release process. There is also good correlation between the antigen concentrations required to cause histamine release and those required to give positive skin test results (Lichtenstein *et al.*, 1967).

Early studies established the basic properties of histamine release (Lichtenstein and Osler, 1964). It occurs in isotonic salt solutions, and has a pH optimum close to pH 7.4 and a temperature optimum of 37°C. It requires metabolic energy and has an absolute requirement for calcium ions in the medium. These properties suggested that the release process is not a toxic response, and it was more or less assumed for several years that it is not. Recently, Hastie (1971) directly observed human basophils by phase-contrast microscopy before, during, and after histamine release induced by antigen. He amply confirmed that this release is a specific, not a cytotoxic, release process, in that cells continue to move and behave normally after complete degranulation.

The histamine release process can be divided into two separate steps or stages (Lichtenstein, 1971). This division is made by first incubating cells with antigen in the absence of magnesium and calcium. Under these conditions, histamine release does not occur. The cells are then washed with buffer to remove excess antigen and resuspended in an incubation medium containing both magnesium and calcium. Histamine release occurs during this second incubation in the presence of calcium. In practice, the cells are incubated with antigen at 37°C for 2 min only, since longer incubation times at 37°C lead to desensitization of the cells (see Section 4), and release does not occur even when calcium is added. The "activated" cells remain capable of releasing histamine if they are held at 4°C. The antigen concentration required to produce a given final level of histamine release is higher when the two-stage procedure is used than when antigen is added to the cells in the presence of calcium. This two-stage treatment serves to synchronize release from all cells in the cell population, and permits studies designed to determine where (early or late) in the sequence of events leading to release any given compound exerts its action.

2.1. The Role of Cyclic AMP

The first evidence that cAMP was involved in any antigen-induced release process was provided by Lichtenstein and Margolis (1968), who demonstrated that both isoproterenol and theophylline inhibited the release of histamine from human leukocyte preparations. Isoproterenol, of course, increases the production of cAMP by stimulating β-adrenergic receptors, while theophylline is a known inhibitor of cAMP phosphodiesterase, which breaks down cAMP. This early study, in addition to showing effects of the two compounds separately, demonstrated that they were synergistic in their action. These findings were soon confirmed by other laboratories (Assem and Schild, 1969; Ishizaka *et al.*, 1971) in studies that utilized chopped human and monkey lung preparations. It should be mentioned that these results might have been anticipated, since Schild (1937) had already noted that epinephrine inhibited "anaphylactic" histamine release from guinea pig lung. Many compounds that both raise cAMP levels in leukocytes and inhibit antigen-induced histamine release from basophils have now been identified. These compounds include catecholamines, methyl xanthines, prostaglandins, histamine itself, and cholera enterotoxin. The relationship between increased cAMP levels in whole leukocyte preparations and inhibition of histamine release, which involves only basophils, has been observed repeatedly. That these two parameters correlate perfectly is almost certainly fortuitous, and simply means that basophils have the same receptors as do other, more prevalent, leukocyte cell types.

The effects of agents that raise cAMP levels have been studied and compared with the agents present in the first stage or the second stage of the histamine-release reaction. These agents invariably inhibit release to a much greater extent when they are present during the first stage (Lichtenstein and DeBernardo, 1971). Catecholamines, for example, all inhibit histamine release when present in the first stage in the order: isoproterenol > epinephrine > norepinephrine > phenylephrine. Isoproterenol and epinephrine are effective inhibitors at concentrations as low as 10^{-8} M, whereas when they are present in the second stage, they are ineffective at concentrations up to 10^{-3} M (Bourne *et al.*, 1972). Their inhibitory effect has been shown to be prevented by the β-blocker propranolol, leading to the conclusion that basophils, as well as other leukocytes, have a β-adrenergic receptor.

Prostaglandins of the E series are known to raise cAMP in a variety of tissues. This knowledge led to studies of the effects of these and other PGs on histamine release (Lichtenstein *et al.*, 1972a). These compounds inhibit histamine release when present in the first stage (in the order $E_1 = E_2 > A_1 = A_2 > B_2 > F_{1\alpha} = F_2\alpha \approx 0$), but have no effect when they are added in the second stage. They also raise cAMP levels in leukocyte preparations with the same order of potency. PGs of the E series have both effects at concentrations as low as 10^{-8}–10^{-9} M.

Perhaps the most interesting compound that can inhibit the release of histamine is histamine itself, since this action raises the possibility of feedback control *in vivo*. At a concentration of 10^{-6} M, histamine inhibits histamine release and also raises cAMP levels in leukocyte preparations (Bourne *et al.*, 1971). As with the other agents that raise cAMP, inhibition of histamine release occurs when histamine is present in the first, but not in the second, stage of the process. It appears that histamine acts through a receptor of the *H-2* type, since burimamide and metiamide, which are anti-*H-2* antihistamines (Black *et al.*, 1972), reverse both the effects of histamine (Lichtenstein and Gillespie, 1973). The K_B values for these two drugs were measured and found to be approximately 5 μM for burimamide and 0.5 μM for metiamide (Lichtenstein *et al.*, 1974), values very similar to the K_B's described for *H-2* receptors in other tissues. Several anti-*H-1* antihistamines, including diphenhydramine, chlorpheniramine, promethazine, pyrilamine, and cyclizine, were studied in some detail (Lichtenstein and Gillespie, 1975). None of these compounds reverses the effects of histamine on either histamine release or cAMP levels. Three (diphenhydramine, cyclizine, and promethazine) cause histamine release at millimolar concentrations. At somewhat lower concentrations (1–3×10^{-4} M), diphenhydramine, cyclizine, and chlorpheniramine are capable of inhibiting antigen-induced histamine release, while promethazine, a phenothiazine antihistamine, as well as chlorpromazine and imipramine inhibit release at concentrations of approximately 3 × 10^{-5} M. These inhibitory effects are unlikely to be related to cAMP, since none of these compounds raises cAMP levels in leukocyte preparations. In fact, several of them lower leukocyte levels of this nucleotide modestly.

The concentration of histamine that can inhibit histamine release is such that *in vivo,* where release from different cells is not synchronized, one might speculate that histamine released from one basophil or mast cell might inhibit release from adjacent cells. This possibility of *in vivo* control was studied by Chakrin *et al.* (1974) and found to occur. These investigators studied the release of both histamine and slow-reacting substance of anaphylaxis (SRS-A) in chopped monkey skin and monkey lung challenged with anti-IgE antibody. They were able to demonstrate that metiamide markedly potentiated the release of both mediators.

Another compound that both inhibits histamine release and raises cAMP levels in leukocytes is cholera enterotoxin (Bourne *et al.,* 1973). This compound raises cAMP levels in all tissues that have been studied to date, and does so with a different time course than the catecholamines or PGs. It binds avidly to a monosialoganglioside on the cell membrane within minutes, but takes from 30 to 45 min to increase cAMP levels (Cuatrecasas, 1973a,b). Inhibition of histamine release by this compound follows the same time course (Bourne *et al.,* 1973).

The foregoing presentation makes it clear that the human basophil has a variety of receptors, including β-adrenergic receptors, PG receptors, cholera enterotoxin receptors, and histamine *H-2* receptors. The evidence that cAMP negatively modulates the release of histamine is overwhelming. As already stated, the release of histamine from leukocytes was the first immunologic system shown to be inhibited by cAMP. It has been found in recent years, however, that increases in the cAMP concentration inhibit a variety of other processes thought to be important in the immune response or inflammation or both. These processes include the *in vitro* killing by sensitized lymphocytes of target cells, the release of lysosomal enzymes from neutrophils, interferon production, lymphocyte transformation by various plant mitogens, and plaque formation by mouse B lymphocytes. Bourne and his colleagues recently reviewed the literature on this subject and discussed various lines of evidence supporting the hypothesis that cAMP is a general negative modulator of immunity and inflammation (Bourne *et al.,* 1974). They suggest that cAMP and the various compounds (including histamine) that increase cAMP levels in leukocytes might serve to protect the host from the dangerous consequences of an unregulated immune response.

Several lines of evidence suggest that histamine might have a special role to play not only in regulating its own release from mast cells and basophils, but also in modulating various lymphocyte responses. Plaut *et al.* (1973, 1975) found that cytolytically active mouse splenic lymphocytes have histamine receptors of the *H-2* type that increase in concentration (or activity) after immunization. At 10 days after immunization, histamine inhibited the cytolysis of target cells by lymphocytes by approximately 10%, while 15 days after immunization, inhibition by histamine had increased to 50%. Melmon and his colleagues provided evidence that histamine receptors can also develop on the B lymphocytes responsible for humoral immunity. They found, first of all, that histamine inhibits both direct and indirect plaque formation (sheep red blood cells) by lymphocytes from appropriately sensitized mice, a finding that indicates that these antibody-producing cells have histamine receptors (Melmon *et al.,* 1974) (see Chapter 16). When lymphocytes from normal mice were passed over histamine–RSA–Sepharose columns prior to injection into irradiated recipients, which were then immunized, the ultimate plaque-forming capability of the cells was increased rather than decreased (Schearer *et al.*, 1974). This observation was interpreted as showing that (1) lymphocytes do not have histamine receptors prior to immunization and (2) passage over the histamine–RSA–Sepharose columns possibly removed a small population of lymphocytes that act as suppressor cells.

2.2. Effects of Cyclic GMP

Extensive efforts to implicate cyclic GMP (cGMP) in the control of histamine release from leukocytes have been to no avail. The nucleotide itself, over a wide range of concentrations, as well as carbachol (which raises cGMP levels in many tissues) at concentrations of 10^{-16}–10^{-5} M had no effect whatsoever on the release process (Lichtenstein *et al.*, 1972b). This result is in contrast to chopped lung preparations, in which cGMP and agents that increase intracellular cGMP levels potentiate histamine release. Recently, the effects of cGMP on release from leukocyte preparations in the presence of different calcium concentrations were studied (Gillespie and Lichtenstein, 1975). It was found that when the calcium concentration was suboptimal (0.1 mM rather than 0.6 mM), slight enhancement by both cGMP and the 8-bromo derivative of cGMP was seen with an optimum concentration of 10^{-5} M. This observation is interesting in that it does suggest a role of some sort for cGMP in the secretion process. Presumably, under standard incubation conditions, the nucleotide is already present intracellularly at an optimum concentration, so that adding it has no effect.

2.3. Role of Calcium

As already stated, the release of histamine from human leukocytes has an absolute requirement for extracellular calcium. In the absence of this ion, no release occurs. Maximum release is seen in the presence of calcium at a concentration of 0.6 mM or slightly below, while calcium concentrations above this level do not decrease or further increase the extent of release.

The recent introduction of the calcium ionophore A23187 (Lilly) has permitted further investigation of the role of calcium in secretion. This ionophore is a complex organic molecule with a hydrophobic exterior surrounding a core that has a high affinity for calcium and other divalent cations. It apparently inserts into cell membranes and facilitates the transmembrane movement of calcium and other divalent cations from areas of high to areas of low concentration. Its use in the study of mediator release was introduced by Foreman *et al.* (1973), who showed that ionophore A23187 released histamine from rat peritoneal mast cells. The effects of this ionophore on histamine release from human leukocytes were studied in some detail (Lichtenstein, 1975). It causes histamine release from the cells of both normal and allergic persons in the presence of calcium, but not in its absence. The concentrations of calcium and ionophore required for maximum release are interrelated, making it clear that calcium is indeed the releasing agent. Unlike antigen-induced secretion, ionophore-induced release was not affected to any large extent by cAMP or agents that raise cAMP levels in leukocytes. The effects of dibutyryl cAMP were typical in that they were variable and could be either modest enhancement or modest inhibition. In experiments in which different concentrations of this compound were studied, the lower concentrations used (0.3 mM) enhanced release, while a higher concentration (1 mM) was inhibitory, suggesting a multiplicity of actions. Ionophore-induced release was modulated by agents that affect microtubules (see Section 2.4). It was inhibited by colchicine and enhanced by heavy water (D_2O), although in neither case was the effect as large as that seen when antigen was the releasing agent. When the effects of lanthanum, which inhibits calcium at freely available sites, were studied, inhibition of ionophore-induced release was greater than was inhibition of antigen-induced release. When the relationship between antigen and ionophore was examined, it was found that suboptimal concentrations of the two releasing agents were synergistic in promoting release. These various observations make it clear that antigen and ionophore do not release histamine by identical mechanisms, although it is probable that the two processes have steps in common. It should be pointed out that while it is clear that an influx of calcium ions can cause histamine release, it does not necessarily follow that antigen causes an influx of calcium ions.

A recent study examined the interrelationships between antigen, cAMP, and calcium concentrations as they affect histamine release (Gillespie and Lichtenstein, 1975). When the antigen concentration was high enough to inhibit release, the addition of dibutyryl cAMP reversed this inhibition or potentiated release, and when the calcium concentration was lowered to a suboptimal level (0.1 mM), antigen-excess inhibition occurred at a lower antigen concentration. These observations were explained by supposing that antigen acts by lowering cAMP levels, and that at high antigen concentrations, cAMP levels were decreased both too quickly and to too low a level to permit maximum release. There is no way of explaining the patterns obtained by supposing that antigen acts to increase intracellular calcium levels.

2.4. Role of Microtubules

Colchicine and other agents that disrupt microtubules have now been shown to inhibit a large number of different secretory systems. In all cases, this inhibition by colchicine and related compounds has been interpreted as meaning that an intact microtubule system is necessary for secretion to occur. The first three secretory systems shown to be inhibited by colchicine were insulin release from rat pancreatic β cells (Lacy *et al.*, 1968), histamine release from rat peritoneal mast cells (Gillespie *et al.*, 1968), and histamine release from human leukocytes (Levy and Carlton, 1969). In their studies on human leukocytes, Levy and Carlton (1969) found that colchicine inhibited histamine release in a manner that depended both on the concentration of colchicine and on the time of preincubation with the drug; inhibition increased both with increasing concentrations of colchicine and with increasing preincubation time. These investigators found further that incubation of the cells with colchicine at 0°C led to larger inhibitory effects than did incubation of 37°C. This potentiation by cold is almost certainly due to the fact that colchicine binds only to the free subunits of microtubules, not to the structures themselves, and that treatment with cold causes the breakdown of microtubules to subunits.

Another agent known to interact with microtubules is D_2O. This compound causes the formation of microtubules from tubulin subunits, probably by stabilizing the microtubule structure (or one biochemical form of the structure) (Gillespie, 1975). D_2O was found to enhance the antigen-induced release of histamine from leukocyte preparations, while having no effect in the absence of antigen (Gillespie and Lichtenstein, 1972). It increased release at a concentration as low as 7%, while concentrations of approximately 30% routinely increased antigen-induced release from approximately 30% to 80–90%.

It is not possible to study the effects of colchicine on the two stages of histamine release, since colchicine is essentially irreversible within the short time span of *in vitro* incubations. D_2O, however, is completely reversible in its effects, so it was possible to determine where in the release process it was acting. It was found to have no effect when present during the first stage of the release process, but to enhance release when present in the second stage (Gillespie and Lichtenstein, 1972). This finding is of course, compatible with the idea that the microtubule system is involved in some way in the movement of granules from the interior of the cell toward the membrane, since this granule movement is almost certainly a late event in the overall release process.

Experiments of two different designs were carried out in an attempt to understand the relationship between cAMP and microtubules. The first series of experiments involved incubating cells with either isoproterenol or PGE_2 plus D_2O during the first stage of the incubation only. As has already been described, under these conditions, isoproterenol and PGs inhibit the overall release process, while D_2O, which is washed out and is reversible, has no effect. When the two compounds were present together, D_2O partially reversed the inhibition of release due to isoproterenol or PGE_2. It should be pointed out that D_2O itself had no effect on leukocyte cAMP, nor did it interfere with the increase in cAMP caused by isoproterenol and PG. This experiment can therefore be interpreted only as indicating that D_2O in some way protects the microtubule system (by its stabilizing effect) from the action of cAMP. The second series of experiments, which led to the same conclusion, involved the study of antigen and colchicine. Release was compared under two different conditions: (1) Cells were incubated with antigen at 37°C for 2 min, followed by colchicine for 20 min at 4°C. (2) The order of incubation with the two compounds was reversed, i.e., first colchicine for 20 min at 4°C, followed by antigen for 2 min at 37°C. The different orders of handling of the cells had no effect on control release. It was seen, however, that inhibition due to colchicine was much greater when the cells were exposed to colchicine prior to antigen than when the order of treatment was the reverse. This result indicates that antigen, in the absence of calcium, in some way alters the microtubule system, making it less susceptible to colchicine.

3. Mechanism of Action of Antigen

It is probable that antigen triggers the release of histamine by causing a decrease in the intracellular level of cAMP, which, in turn, permits activation of the microtubule system and possibly has other effects as well. This mechanism of action fits well with the known relationships between cAMP and microtubules

(Gillespie, 1975), and is the only mechanism compatible with many of the experimental observations that have been made. It both predicts and explains, for example, the interaction seen between antigen and colchicine and between agents that raise cAMP levels and D_2O. It also permits easy understanding of the relationships among antigen, cAMP, and calcium that have been described. Methods are not currently available for the purification of basophils, so it has not been possible to determine directly whether antigen lowers cAMP levels in this cell type. It was shown, however, that both compound 48/80 and antigen lower cAMP levels in purified rat mast cell preparations (Sullivan and Parker, 1973; Gillespie, 1973; Kaliner and Austen, 1974).

4. The Phenomenon of Desensitization

It has been known for some time that basophils can become desensitized and no longer react to antigen. This desensitization occurs when cells are exposed to antigen in the absence of calcium at 37°C for periods of time longer than 2–5 min; it also occurs in the presence of calcium when cells are exposed to very low levels of antigens, i.e., levels that are themselves insufficient to cause release. This process of desensitization is probably a biochemical rather than an immunologic phenomenon, since it was shown that the cells of a person sensitive to both antigen E and rye grass Group I will not respond to either antigen when they have been previously exposed to and desensitized by treatment with only one (Lichtenstein, 1971). Cells that have been desensitized to antigen will respond with normal histamine release when exposed to ionophore A23187 (Lichtenstein, 1975). An elegant series of experiments carried out by Baxter and Adamik (1975) dealt with the relationship between activation and desensitization. They presented data indicating that during the release process, activation and desensitization are two independent processes that go on simultaneously. The kinetics of these two separate processes, taken together, dictate the kinetics of histamine release. The mechanism of desensitization is not understood in biochemical terms.

5. Release of Mediators Other Than Histamine

It has been known for some time that IgE-mediated reactions cause the release of other mediators in addition to histamine from mast cells. In 1960, Brocklehurst described the release of SRS-A from sensitized lung tissue from several species (Brocklehurst, 1960), and a few years later, Kay and Austen (1971) reported the release of a factor that was chemotactic for eosinophils from human lung preparations. Recently, these two mediators were shown to be released by antigen and anti-IgE from human leukocyte preparations as well (Grant and Lichtenstein, 1974; Czarnetzki, *et al.*, 1976). Another mediator that to date has been shown to be released only from leukocyte preparations is a kallikrein capable of generating bradykinin from kininogen (Newball *et al.*, 1975).

SRS-A is a low-molecular-weight acidic lipid that appears to contain a sulfate group. Its structure is not known at present. In both mast cells and basophils, SRS-A is not a preformed mediator, but is generated as a result of the antigen–antibody interaction (Kay and Austen, 1971; Grant and Lichtenstein, 1974). Also, in both cell types, there is no correlation between the amount of histamine and SRS-A released from the cells of different persons, although in any given experiment, the time course of release and the concentration of antigen required for optimum release of the two mediators are essentially the same. The pharmacological control of SRS-A generation and release from leukocyte preparations has not been studied as yet. Release from human lung fragments, however, is inhibited by agents that raise cAMP levels (Orange *et al.*, 1971).

Eosinophil chemotactic factor of anaphylaxis (ECF-A) is a low-molecular-weight polypeptide. The release of this mediator from leukocyte preparations by IgE-mediated reactions was only recently described and characterized (Czarnetzki *et al.*, 1976). ECF-A appears not to be preformed in these cells, although chemotactic activity was occasionally found in sonicates of unstimulated leukocytes. The kinetics and response curves to antigen and anti-IgE of ECF-A and histamine release have been compared and found to be very similar. The pharmacological control of ECF-A release from leukocytes has not been studied to date; its release from lung preparations is inhibited by agents that elevate cAMP levels (Wasserman *et al.*, 1974).

The newest mediator found to be released from leukocyte preparations by both antigen and anti-IgE is a proteolytic enzyme that is probably a kallikrein. It is quantitatively studied by measuring the hydrolysis of *p*-toluene sulphonyl-L-arginine methyl ester (TAMe). The kinetics of release of this enzyme are very similar to the kinetics of histamine release, although the absolute percentage release of the two mediators may differ. The discovery of this esterase activity led to experiments that demonstrated that supernatants from leukocytes incubated with antigen were capable of generating bradykinin. It is not presently clear, however, whether or not the esterase activity and kinin-generating activity are due to the same enzyme. The pharmacological control of esterase release has not been studied in any detail, although preliminary experiments indicate that it will be closely similar to the control of histamine release.

During the course of the studies of SRS-A release by IgE-mediated mechanisms just described, it was found that the calcium ionophore A23187 was capable of generating a much larger amount (25 ×) of this activity from leukocytes than was antigen or anti-IgE (Conroy *et al.*, 1976). This observation led to experiments with various cell fractions that demonstrated that ionophore released SRS-A activity from purified polymorphonuclear leukocytes (PMNs) as well as basophil-rich preparations. The SRS-A activity released by ionophore from PMNs appeared to be identical to the SRS-A released by antigen challenge in that both mediators were stable to base hydrolysis, inactivated by arylsulfatase, and had similar elution characteristics on silicic acid and Sephadex LH-20 columns. This observation of SRS-A release from PMNs led to the study of ECF-A release by ionophore A23187, in which, again, ionophore released much more activity from leukocyte preparations than did antigen or anti-IgE. Release of this mediator has now also been shown to occur from PMNs following exposure to ionophore; more important ECF-A release also occurs from this cell type during phagocytosis induced by various zymosan preparations (Czarnetzki *et al.*, 1975). These observations provide evidence that considerable overlap exists between the allergic and inflammatory responses.

6. Summary

The release of histamine and other mediators from leukocyte preparations is a process of secretion that requires energy, calcium ions, and an intact microtubule system. The pharmacological control of this release reaction centers around cAMP. All agents that raise cAMP levels—e.g., catecholamines, PGs, histamine, cholera toxin, and methyl xanthines—inhibit release, and it is probable that antigen initiates the process by lowering its levels.

Several articles dealing with selected aspects of this topic have appeared. The special role of cAMP in negatively modulating many immune reactions was discussed by Bourne *et al.* (1974). The role of microtubules in secretion and the relationship of cAMP and calcium to these structures was considered by Gillespie (1975). The importance of histamine and histamine receptors in controlling immune responses was discussed by Plaut and Lichtenstein (1976) (see Chapter 16), and the concept that the reactions of immediate hypersensitivity and inflammation are interrelated and interdependent was developed and discussed by Lichtenstein (1976) (see Chapter 11).

ACKNOWLEDGMENTS

This is Publication No. 267 from the O'Neill Research Laboratories, The Good Samaritan Hospital, Baltimore.

References

Assem, E. S. K., and Schild, H. O., 1969, *Nature* (*London*) **224**:1028, 1029.
Baxter, J. H., and Adamik, R., 1975, *J. Immunol.* **114**:1034–1041.
Black, J. W., Duncan, W. A., Durant, C. J., Ganellin, C. R., and Parsons, E. M., 1972, *Nature* (*London*) **236**:385–390.
Bourne, H. R., Melmon, K. L., and Lichtenstein, L. M., 1971, *Science* **173**:743–745.
Bourne, H. R., Lichtenstein, L. M., and Melmon, K. L., 1972, *J. Immunol.* **108**:695–705.
Bourne, H. R., Lehrer, R. I., Lichtenstein, L. M., Weissmann, G., and Zurier, R., 1973, *J. Clin. Invest.* **52**:698–708.
Bourne, H. R., Lichtenstein, L. M., Henney, C. S., Melmon, K. L., Weinstein, Y., and Shearer, G. M., 1974, *Science* **184**:19–28.
Brocklehurst, W. E., 1960, *Physiologist* **151**:416–435.
Chakrin, L. W., Krell, R. D., and Mengel, J., 1974, *Agents Actions* **4**:297–303.
Conroy, M. C., Orange, R. P., and Lichtenstein, L. M., 1976, *J. Immunol.* **116**:1667–1681.
Cuatrecasas, P., 1973a, *Biochemistry* **12**:3547–3557.
Cuatrecasas, P., 1973b, *Biochemistry* **12**:3558–3566.
Czarnetzki, B. M., König, W., and Lichtenstein, L. M., 1975, *Nature* (*London*) **258**:725,726.
Czarnetzki, B. M., König, W., and Lichtenstein, L. M., 1976, *Inflammation* **1**:201–215.
Foreman, J. C., Mongar, J. L., and Gomperts, B. D., 1973, *Nature* (*London*) **245**:249–251.
Gillespie, E., 1973, *Experientia* **29**:447, 448.
Gillespie, E., 1975, *Ann. N.Y. Acad. Sci.* **253**:771–779.
Gillespie, E., and Lichtenstein, L. M., 1972, *J. Clin. Invest.* **51**:2941–2947.
Gillespie, E., and Lichtenstein, L. M., 1975, *J. Immunol.* **115**:1572–1576.
Gillespie, E., Levine, R. J., and Malawista, S. E., 1968, *J. Pharmacol. Exp. Ther.* **164**:158–165.
Grant, J. A., and Lichtenstein, L. M., 1974, *J. Immunol.* **112**:897–904.
Hastie, R., 1971, *Clin. Exp. Immunol.* **8**:45–61.
Ishizaka, T., Ishizaka, K., Orange, R. P., and Austen, K. F., 1971, *J. Immunol.* **106**:1267–1273.
Kaliner, M., and Austen, K. F., 1974, *J. Immunol.* **112**:664–674.

Kay, A. B., and Austen, K. F., 1971, *J. Immunol.* **107**:899–902.
Lacy, P. E., Howell, S. L., Young, D. A., and Fink, C. J., 1968, *Nature (London)* **219**:1177–1179.
Levy, D. A., and Carlton, J. A., 1969, *Proc. Soc. Exp. Biol. Med.* **130**:1333–1336.
Lichtenstein, L. M., 1971, *J. Immunol.* **107**:1122–1130.
Lichtenstein, L. M., 1975, *J. Immunol.* **114**:1692–1699.
Lichtenstein, L. M., 1976, in: *Molecular and Biological Aspects of Acute Allergic Reaction* (S. G. O. Johansson, K. Strandberg, and B. Uvnäs, ed.), pp. 233–254, Plenum Publishing Co., London.
Lichtenstein, L. M., and DeBarnardo, R., 1971, *J. Immunol.* **107**:1131–1136.
Lichtenstein, L. M., and Gillespie, E., 1973, *Nature (London)* **244**:287–288.
Lichtenstein, L. M., and Gillespie, E., 1975, *J. Pharmacol. Exp. Ther.* **192**:441–450.
Lichtenstein, L. M., and Margolis, S., 1968, *Science* **161**:902–903.
Lichtenstein, L. M., and Osler, A. G., 1964, *J. Exp. Med.* **120**:507–530.
Lichtenstein, L. M., Norman, P. S., Winkenwerder, W. L., and Osler, A. G., 1966, *J. Clin. Invest.* **45**:1126–1136.
Lichtenstein, L. M., Norman, P. S., and Connell, J. T., 1967, *J. Allergy* **40**:160–167.
Lichtenstein, L. M., Gillespie, E., Bourne, H. R., and Henney, C. S., 1972a, *Prostaglandins* **2**:519–528.
Lichtenstein, L. M., Gillespie, E., and Bourne, H., 1972b, in: *The Biological Role of the Immunoglobulin E System* (k. Ishizaka and D. H. Dayton, eds.), pp. 165–186, National Institure of Child Health and Human Development, National Institutes of Health, Bethesda, Maryland.
Lichtenstein, L. M., Plaut, M., Henney, C., and Gillespie, E., 1974, in: *International Symposium on Histamine H2-Receptor Antagonists* (C. J. Wood and M. Simkins, eds.) pp. 187–198. Research and Development Division, Smith, Kline and French Laboratories, Welwyn Garden City, England.
Melmon, K. L., Bourne, H. R., Weinstein, Y., Shearer, G. M., Kram, J., and Baumiager, S., 1974, *J. Clin. Invest.* **53**:13–21.
Newball, H. H., Talamo, R. C., and Lichtenstein, L. M., 1975, *Nature (London)* **254**:635–636.
Orange, R. P., Austen, W. G., and Austen, K. F., 1971, *J. Exp. Med.* **134**:136S.
Plaut, M., and Lichtenstein, L. M., 1977, in: *Handbook of Experimental Pharmacology* (S. H. Ferreira and J. R. Vane, eds.), Springer-Verlag, New York, in press.
Plaut, M., Lichtenstein, L. M., and Henney, C., 1973, *Nature (London)* **244**:284–287.
Plaut, M., Lichtenstein, L. M., and Henney, C. S., 1975, *J. Clin. Inves.* **55**:856–874.
Schild, H., 1937, *Q. J. Exp. Physiol.* **26**:165–179.
Shearer, G. M., Weinstein, Y., and Melmon, K. L., 1974, *J. Immunol.* **113**:597–607.
Sullivan, T. J., and Parker, C. W., 1973, *Biochem. Biophys. Res. Commun.* **55**:1334–1339.
Wasserman, S. I., Goetzl, E. J., Kaliner, M., and Austen, K. F., 1974, *Immunology* **26**:677–684.

7

Generation, Function, and Disposition of Chemical Mediators of the Mast Cell in Immediate Hypersensitivity

EDWARD J. GOETZL and K. FRANK AUSTEN

1. Introduction

The selective binding of IgE to tissue mast cells and circulating basophils prepares them for direct (antigen-induced) or reversed (anti-IgE-mediated) immunologic activation that leads to the appearance intracellularly of unstored mediators and external secretion of both preformed and newly generated mediators of immediate hypersensitivity (Austen *et al.*, 1974, 1975). The preferential distribution of mast cells in respiratory, dermal, and GI connective tissue with a perivenular localization beneath and within mucous membrane and cutaneous surfaces (Riley, 1959; Brinkman, 1968) and even intraepithelially (Feltkamp-Vroom *et al.*, 1975) makes them readily available for interaction with environmental antigens. Since mast cells possess IgE receptors of great affinity (Ishizaka *et al.*, 1972) and IgE-complex-activatable pathways of diverse mediator formation and secretion, antigenic challenge establishes local concentrations of chemical mediators in the primary target tissues. Mast cells appear to have an extended life span without granule turnover (Padawer, 1974), yet they may accumulate in secretions of a target area (Shioda and Mishima, 1966). Basophils can be prominent at sites of tumor invasion (Dvorak *et al.*, 1973), and have been shown to exhibit directed migration *in vitro* to diverse

EDWARD J. GOETZL and K. FRANK AUSTEN • Departments of Medicine, Harvard Medical School and the Robert B. Brigham Hospital, Boston, Massachusetts 02120.

chemotactic factors, including fragments of complement components and products of stimulated lymphocytes (Kay and Austen, 1972). The continued development of *in vitro* models of immediate hypersensitivity has permitted a detailed examination of the formation and release of mediators by mast cells (Austen and Orange, 1975) and basophils (Lichtenstein *et al.*, 1972; Austen *et al.*, 1975), provided sufficient material for purification and characterization of several mediators, and led to the elucidation of both humoral and cellular regulatory mechanisms that limit or reverse the effects of the chemical mediators (Lichtenstein and Margolis, 1968; Austen *et al.*, 1974; Goetzl *et al.*, 1975).

The mast cell represents the only effector cell of immunologically specific reactions positioned throughout the tissues, and it is therefore likely that it represents an initial level of specific defense. On being activated, it elaborates mediators that alter the microenvironment so as to bring plasma proteins, such as antibody and complement, and phagocytic tissue and peripheral blood cells to the reaction site. Thus, mast-cell activation recruits the essential humoral and cellular ingredients of host defense to a local site in a physiologic response that precedes and is not dependent on extensive tissue injury in dealing with a hostile event. Further, since one of the cells that is specifically recruited is the eosinophil, which has the capacity to inactivate the mast-cell products, this physiologic and immunospecific response is locally contained and terminated.

2. Generation and Release of Chemical Mediators

The events that follow the bridging of mast cell membrane-bound IgE by antigen or anti-IgE and lead to release of chemical mediators reflect activation of cellular biochemical pathways and the influence of exogenous agents acting directly or through alterations in the levels of intracellular cyclic nucleotides. The steps that follow the initial antigen-induced calcium-dependent activation of a serine esterase involve an energy requirement for glucose, an intracellular calcium ion requirement, and a stage that is blocked by elevations in the level of intracellular cyclic AMP (cAMP) (Kaliner and Austen, 1973).

Unstored mediators appear intracellularly with great rapidity, as typified by the formation of the slow-reacting substance of anaphylaxis (SRS-A) in human lung tissue or dispersed cells (Lewis *et al.*, 1974). The intracellular accumulation of SRS-A in human lung fragments or cells is demonstrable within 30 sec of IgE-dependent direct or reversed activation and reaches a plateau by 2–5 min, as assessed by extraction of the tissue or cells after thorough washing. In contrast, the release of SRS-A begins after 2–5 min and does not plateau for 15–30 min, well after the saturation of the intracellular compartment. The cellular and fluid-phase SRS-A are indistinguishable by differential bioassay, parallel purification procedures, and susceptibility to inactivation by arylsulfatase B (Lewis *et al.*, 1974; Wasserman *et al.*, 1975a). That IgE-mediated SRS-A formation is a discrete mast cell process was corroborated by fractionation of human lung cells and the demonstration that SRS-A generation was associated with the fractions containing mast cells and the preformed mediators, histamine and eosinophil chemotactic factor of anaphylaxis (ECF-A) (Paterson *et al.*, 1976).

A variety of inhibitors have either blocked mediator release and spared cellular SRS-A accumulation or suppressed SRS-A generation and release, but not histamine release, implicating additional and independent steps for regulation of intracellular generation of SRS-A. Incubation of human lung fragments with colchicine suppressed anti-IgE-mediated release of histamine and SRS-A without diminishing tissue accumulation of SRS-A relative to controls (Orange, 1974). Exposure of sensitized lung fragments to diisopropyl fluorophosphate (DFP), followed by washing, or to cytochalasin A or B, results in suppression of IgE-mediated SRS-A release with no impairment or even augmentation of histamine release (Kaliner and Austen, 1973; Orange, 1974). Stimulation of sensitized lung fragments with a dose of isoproterenol sufficient to elevate total tissue cAMP 10-fold totally blocked histamine and SRS-A release on antigen challenge, while introduction of carbamyl choline reversed the inhibitory effect of the elevated cAMP on release of histamine, but did not restore the elaboration of SRS-A (Kaliner and Austen, 1974a). Thus, a cholinergic agent overcame the cAMP block of mediator release, presumably by stimulating a rise in intracellular cyclic GMP (cGMP) (Kaliner *et al.*, 1972), but not the inhibition of SRS-A generation. The formation of unstored chemical mediators such as SRS-A by immunologically activated tissue mast cells therefore not only must precede release, but also is separately modulated by regulatory agents that exert their influence at multiple intracellular loci.

3. Characteristics of the Chemical Mediators

The mediators released from basophils, mast cells, or mast-cell-rich tissues by IgE-dependent immunologic reactions may be considered in two categories. The preformed principles include histamine, eosinophil chemotactic factor of anaphylaxis (ECF-A), a neutrophil chemotactic factor (NCF), and heparin, and the unstored factors that cannot be demonstrated by extraction of cells or tissue prior to immunologic activation include SRS-A and a platelet-activating factor (PAF) (Table 1). The unstored mediators are presumably present in a precursor form that can be converted to the active principle by an approximate immunologic reaction or even by nonimmunologic perturbation of the cells. Stimuli that are subthreshold in terms of release of unstored mediators may nonetheless be capable of inducing an appreciable intracellular accumulation (Lewis *et al.*, 1974).

3.1. Histamine

Histamine is formed within basophils and mast cells by enzymatic conversion of L-histidine and is stored within the granules, being bound to the matrix by ionic forces (Schayer, 1965; Bergqvist *et al.*, 1971). Histamine synthesis assessed by incubation of highly purified rat mast cells with radiolabeled L-histidine and pyridoxal-5′-phosphate has a baseline rate of 0.5–1.0% of the total cellular stores of histamine/hr (Sullivan *et al.*, 1975a). The rate of histamine synthesis was increased 2- to 3-fold by the introduction of compound 48/80 to induce histamine release, and was decreased by the addition of millimolar concentrations of theophylline or dibutyryl cAMP, both of which presumably elevate the intracellular levels of cAMP.

The pathobiological effects of histamine include smooth muscle contraction, production of venular leakage of plasma proteins (Majno *et al.*, 1969), and an increase in bronchopulmonary airway resistance concomitant with a reduction in

TABLE 1. Primary Chemical Mediators of Immediate Hypersensitivity

Category	Mediator	Structural characteristics	Assay	Other functions	Inactivation
Preformed	Histamine	β-Imidazolylethylamine (mol.wt. 111)	Contraction of guinea pig ileum *or* Specific radiolabeling by histamine *N*-methyltransferase	Increased vascular permeability Elevation of cAMP Enhancement of eosinophil migration	Histaminase; histamine methyltransferase
	Eosinophil chemotactic factor of anaphylaxis (ECF-A)	Hydrophobic acidic tetrapeptides (mol.wt. 360–390)	Chemotactic attraction of eosinophils	Eosinophil deactivation	Aminopeptidase; carboxypeptidase A
	Neutrophil chemotactic factor (NCF)	Protein (mol.wt. >160,000)	Chemotactic attraction of neutrophils	Neutrophil deactivation	—
	Heparin	Macromolecular acidic proteoglycan (mol.wt. ≈1 million)	Antithrombin activation or metachromasia	Anticoagulation	—
Unstored	Slow-reacting substance of anaphylaxis (SRS-A)	Acidic, sulfur-containing ester (mol. wt.	Contraction of antihistamine-treated guinea pig ileum	Contraction of human bronchiole Increased vascular permeability	Arylsulfatase B
	Platelet-activating factors (PAF)	Lipidlike (mol.wt. ≈300–500)	Release of [^{14}C]5HT from platelets	Aggregation	Phospholipase D (for rat PAF)

compliance (Drazen and Austen, 1974). The capacity of atropine pretreatment to ameliorate the alterations in pulmonary mechanics produced by histamine implicates vagal reflexes, triggered by irritant receptors, in the mediation of the histamine effects (Nadel, 1973; Gold, 1973). While the bronchopulmonary actions of histamine are mediated by *H-1* receptors, the cardiac and gastric effects are *H-2*-dependent (Black *et al.*, 1972); further, the "antiinflammatory" actions of histamine in suppressing mediator release from basophils (Lichtenstein and Gillespie, 1973), lysosomal enzyme release from PMN leukocytes (Zurier *et al.*, 1974), and certain lymphocyte effector functions (Plaut *et al.*, 1973) are each dependent on an *H-2* receptor linked to adenylate cyclase.

One controversial function of histamine, namely, the selective attraction of eosinophils *in vitro*, was recently clarified (Clark *et al.*, 1975). Although the eosinophilotactic activity of histamine in modified Boyden chambers is dependent on a concentration gradient, it differs from the action of other eosinophil chemotactic factors in several ways: the dependence of its expression on a short incubation time and very thin polycarbonate filters, the restricted concentration range exhibiting chemotactic activity, and the demonstration of an inhibitory effect at doses only 2- to 3-fold higher than the peak chemotactic concentration (Clark *et al.*, 1975).

3.2. Eosinophil Chemotactic Factor of Anaphylaxis

ECF-A is a preformed mediator that has been extracted from rat and human leukemic basophils (Goetzl *et al.*, 1974; Lewis *et al.*, 1975), mast-cell-rich human and guinea pig tissues, and isolated rat mast cells, in which it is associated with the granules (Wasserman *et al.*, 1973). The synthetic pathway for formation of ECF-A and the nature of its association with the granules have not been elucidated.

ECF-A obtained by extraction in Tyrode's buffer or IgE-dependent release from human lung tissue or isolated rat mast cells exhibited a molecular weight of approximately 300–500 by filtration on Sephadex G-25 (Kay and Austen, 1971; Wasserman *et al.*, 1973); was inactivated by digestion with subtilisin or pronase, but not with trypsin or chymotrypsin (Wasserman *et al.*, 1974); and was composed of two anodal peaks of activity on high-voltage paper electrophoresis at neutral pH (Goetzl *et al.*, 1974). More detailed analysis of the eosinophil chemotactic activity extracted from human lung tissue by sonication in acidic butanol revealed heterogeneity on initial Sephadex G-25 chromatograms, and thus, material in the molecular-weight range 300–1000 was further purified. This material was preferentially chemotactic for eosinophils, and appeared on Sephadex G-25 and subsequent purification steps in the same region as the bulk of the activity released immunologically (Goetzl and Austen, 1975) and previously designated ECF-A (Kay and Austen, 1971). Following Sephadex G-25 filtration, ECF-A was adsorbed to Dowex-1 and eluted in a broad peak in a pyridine–formic acid gradient over the pH range 3.0–2.2. Subdivision of this peak into two equal bands of activity followed by filtration on Sephadex G-10 and descending paper chromatography resolved two distinct tetrapeptides in low yield but of sufficient purity for structural determination. The more acidic and hydrophobic peptide was Val–Gly–Ser–Glu, and the less acidic and hydrophobic peptide was Ala–Gly–Ser–Glu (Goetzl and Austen, 1975). The alanyl- and valyl-tetrapeptides were synthesized and shown to be chemotactic for human eosinophils with a specificity and potency comparable to those of highly purified natural ECF-A. Prior exposure of eosinophils to synthetic or purified ECF-A gave comparable deactivation, as assessed by subsequent chemotactic unresponsiveness to ECF-A or heterologous stimuli. Peak chemotactic activity was seen at peptide concentrations of 10^{-7}–10^{-6} M, amounting to 0.1–1.0 nmol/chamber, and deactivation could be demonstrated at levels as low as 10^{-10} M (Goetzl and Austen, 1976b).

The inactivation of ECF-A by digestion with aminopeptidase M or carboxypeptidase A and the marginal activity of the COOH-terminal tripeptide supported the necessity for the entire tetrapeptide sequence for full eosinophil chemotactic activity (Goetzl and Austen, 1975). The synthetic NH_2-terminal tripeptide Val–Gly–Ser and Val-amide, which possess neither chemotactic nor deactivating capacity, block the eosinophil chemotactic activity of 10^{-7} M valyl-tetrapeptide when present in the stimulus compartment; 50% mean inhibition required equimolar amounts of NH_2-terminal tripeptide and 10-fold excess of Val-amide (Goetzl and Austen, 1976b). Although the COOH-terminal tripeptide Gly–Ser–Glu was neither chemotactic nor inhibitory when present on the stimulus side with tetrapeptide, pretreatment of eosinophils with a 10^{-8} M concentration substantially deactivated them to an ECF-A stimulus. Thus, the COOH-terminal region of ECF-A has eosinophil-directed deactivating activity, but lacks the NH_2-terminal residue required to allow binding of a nature essential to the expression of chemotactic activity (Goetzl and Austen, 1976b).

3.3. Heparin

Heparin was obtained from preformed stores in purified rat mast cells by extraction with 0.05 N NaOH and 1 N NaCl and by treatment of the mast cells with compound 48/80 (Fillion *et al.*, 1970), and these studies were recently extended to include immunologic release (Yurt *et al.*, 1977a,b). Isolated rat mast cells incubated *in vitro* with ^{35}S-sulfate, washed, and exposed to either heat-inactivated anti-rat light-chain antisera or the calcium ionophore A23187 released 10–15% of the labeled heparin along with histamine. The released heparin and residual heparin, extracted from the mast cells after immunologic challenge, chromatographed together on Dowex-1 with elution in 3 N NaCl, and both filtered in the exclusion volume of Sepharose-6B (Yurt *et al.*, 1976), as assessed by radioactivity and such additional parameters as uptake of azure blue and augmentation of antithrombin activity (Jaques *et al.*, 1949; Odegard *et al.*, 1975). The lower specific activity (cpm/μg) of the released heparin relative to the residual material raised the possibility of immunologic release of macromolecular heparin from a specific subcellular compartment.

3.4. Neutrophil Chemotactic Factor(s)

NCF was originally recognized in the extract of human leukemic basophils as a factor distinct from ECF-A by virtue of its filtration in the exclusion volume of Sephadex G-25 columns and its preferential neutrophil chemotactic activity in modified Boyden chambers (Lewis *et al.*, 1975). Incubation of rat mast cells with rabbit anti-rat light-chain antisera, at dilutions capable of releasing 30–40% of the total histamine, liberated substantial quantities of high-molecular-weight neutrophil chemotactic activity, with corresponding decrements in these activities in extracts of the treated mast cells (Goetzl and Austen, 1976a). Further purification of NCF has revealed an acid pK, since the activity appears in effluents from carboxymethyl–cellulose equilibrated in 0.05 M sodium acetate buffer at pH 5.5.

3.5. Slow-Reacting Substance of Anaphylaxis

SRS-A is not detectable in a preformed state in appreciable amounts in unstimulated human leukemic basophils (Lewis *et al.*, 1975), purified rat mast cells, or mast-cell-rich tissues such as human lung (Lewis *et al.*, 1974) or nasal polyps (Kaliner *et al.*, 1973). IgE-mediated direct or reversed immunologic activation of human lung tissue or dispersed cells (Lewis *et al.*, 1974), and the stimulation by calcium ionophore A23187 of human leukemic basophils (Lewis *et al.*, 1975), results in the accumulation of intracellular SRS-A prior to its appearance in the fluid phase. Both intracellular and released SRS-A resist inactivation by incubation at 37°C in 0.2 N NaOH, adhere to Amberlite XAD-2 in water and elute in 80% ethanol, appear in the ethanol:ammonia:water (6:3:1, vol/vol) wash from silicic acid (Orange *et al.*, 1973; Austen *et al.*, 1974; Lewis *et al.*, 1974), and are inactivated by digestion with arylsulfatase B purified from various sources (Orange *et al.*, 1974; Wasserman *et al.*, 1975a). The latter observation and the finding of a sulfur-containing group in spark-source mass spectrometric analyses of highly purified rat SRS-A have suggested the presence of a sulfate moiety that may also explain the acidic nature of SRS-A (Orange *et al.*, 1973).

SRS-A contracts smooth muscle *in vitro* (Brocklehurst, 1960), with a particularly potent effect on the human bronchiole, increases cutaneous vascular permeability (Orange *et al.*, 1969), and reduces pulmonary compliance by a direct action when injected intravenously into unanesthetized guinea pigs (Drazen and Austen, 1974).

3.6. Platelet-Activating Factor(s)

PAF was originally recognized as being released from rabbit mixed leukocytes interacted with specific antigen, and the basophil sensitized with IgE was established as its source (Siraganian and Osler, 1971; Benveniste *et al.*, 1972; Benveniste, 1974). PAF activities have also been derived by antigen challenge of passively sensitized rabbit and human lung (Bogart and Stechschulte, 1974; Kravis and Henson, 1975), IgE-mediated reversed immunologic reactions of human mixed leukocytes (Benveniste, 1974) and rabbit and human lung tissue (Bogart and Stechschulte, 1974; Kravis and Henson, 1975), antigen challenge of the rat peritoneal cavity passively prepared with hyperimmune rat antisera predominantly containing IgGa antibody (Kater *et al.*, 1976), addition of the calcium ionophore A23187 to human leukemic basophils (Lewis *et al.*, 1975), and prolonged incubation of rabbit or human mixed peripheral leukocytes in alkaline buffer (Benveniste, 1974). Since PAF activity was not recognized in human leukemic basophils prior to stimulation with the calcium ionophore (Lewis *et al.*, 1975), and its content increased during the incubation of mixed rabbit or human leukocytes in alkaline buffer (Benveniste, 1974), it is apparently not a preformed mediator, and resembles SRS-A in this respect.

PAF obtained from rabbit or human mixed leukocytes exhibited cationic characteristics on ion-exchange chromatography, filtered on Sephadex LH-20 with an apparent molecular weight of 1100, and chromatographed on silica gel thin-layer plates in a region staining with phospholipid-specific indicators (Benveniste, 1974; Benveniste *et al.*, 1975). Rat PAF activity, purified by a procedure utilized for SRS-A (Orange *et al.*, 1973), appeared in the ethanol eluate from Amberlite XAD-2 and in the ethanol:ammonia:water eluate from silicic acid along with the SRS-A (Kater *et al.*, 1976). This partially purified rat PAF filtered on Sephadex LH-20 with an apparent molecular weight of 300–500, and was substantially inactivated by phospholipase D from cabbage or eosinophil sources, but not by proteolytic enzymes or phospholipase A or B (Kater *et al.*, 1976). PAF activity is assayed by its capacity to release [^{14}C]5HT or other amines from platelets (Benveniste *et al.*, 1972). Other activities attributed to PAF include the induction of platelet rosettes around rabbit basophils (Benveniste *et al.*, 1972), and aggregation of platelets *in vitro* in the presence of fibrinogen (Benveniste *et al.*, 1975).

4. Modulation of Mediators of Immediate Hypersensitivity

Inhibition or enhancement of the apparent activity of a mediator may result from modulation of its generation or release, changes in receptor binding or in intrinsic responsiveness of target cells or tissues, and alterations of the rate or products of biodegradation. The net effect observed may represent the composite of a variety of mechanisms, and the regulatory process at each level may derive from feedback control by the mediator or a degradation product, the action of another primary mediator, or the involvement of secondary humoral factors or cellular components.

The direct or reversed immunologic challenge of IgE-sensitized tissue or cells leads to a complex sequence of reactions that eventuates in the secretion of histamine and other mediators (Kaliner and Austen, 1973; Austen *et al.*, 1974). A feature of this sequence is the inhibition of generation and release of mediators following the introduction of agents that lead to an elevation of the intracellular level of cAMP (Lichtenstein and Margolis, 1968; Orange *et al.*, 1971; Bourne *et al.*, 1971). β-Adrenergic agonists, cholera enterotoxin, prostaglandins (PGs) E_1 and E_2, and histamine each activate adenylate cyclase to induce elevations in human lung and peripheral leukocyte levels of cAMP, and concomitantly inhibit the immunologic release of mediators from these mixed cell systems. Studies with purified rat mast cells have more directly demonstrated the relationship between elevations in cAMP achieved with either PGE_2 or aminophylline, which inhibits cAMP phosphodiesterase, or both together and suppression of histamine release (Kaliner and Austen, 1974b). That histamine inhibition of mediator release is the result of its interaction with a specific basophil receptor accessible only to histamine is confirmed by the ability of H-2-specific antihistamines to block histamine inhibition without influencing that of β-adrenergic agonists, PGs, or choleratoxin (Lichtenstein *et al.*, 1972). Further, β-adrenergic antagonists did not affect histamine inhibition of mediator release while preventing the inhibitory effects of β-adrenergic agonists (Bourne *et al.*, 1972). The suppressive action of histamine on mediator release was also noted with purified rat mast cells stimulated with compound 48/80 (Sullivan *et al.*, 1975b). It is not yet known whether primary mediators other than histamine can influence immunologically activated release reactions in basophils or mast cells by cyclic-nucleotide-dependent or other mechanisms. Enhancement of immunologic mediator generation and release by cholinergic stimulation (Kaliner *et al.*, 1972; Lewis *et al.*, 1974) has not yet been duplicated by a primary mediator.

A second level of modulation of mediator function in immediate hypersensitivity relates to their interactions with receptors on target cells and to the responsiveness of these cells. Histamine receptors are classified as H-1 and H-2 on the basis of the type of antagonist that blocks the histamine effect (Black *et al.*, 1972). A relatively specific inhibitor of SRS-A, termed FPL55712, has been found to block its contractile activity for smooth muscle *in vitro* (Augstein *et al.*, 1973). The NH_2-terminal and COOH-terminal tripeptides of the ECF-A tetrapeptides both suppressed eosinophil chemotaxis when present in the cell compartment of the Boyden chamber (Goetzl and Austen, 1976b). The NH_2-terminal tripeptides interfered by reversible competition with the tetrapeptides, presumably for binding sites, and the COOH-terminal tripeptide inhibited by irreversibly deactivating the eosinophils. The conversion of ^{14}C-labeled tetrapeptide to a mixture of tripeptides after incubation with extracts of eosinophils or neutrophils suggests that these inhibitory tripeptides may be generated during chemotaxis as one level of the regulation of eosinophil influx at the site of an immediate hypersensitivity reaction.

Other primary mediators are also capable of enhancing or diminishing the responsiveness of a target cell population of eosinophils to ECF-A. Histamine at a weakly chemotactic concentration of 30 ng/ml on the stimulus side synergistically enhanced the chemotactic response of eosinophils to several concentrations of tetrapeptides. In contrast, SRS-A diminished the chemotactic responsiveness of eosinophils to the tetrapeptides. The mechanisms of these opposing actions are not known.

A third level of modulation of mediators in immediate hypersensitivity is biodegradation. The eosinophil, attracted by ECF-A to a focus of an allergic reaction, contains three distinct enzymes that are capable of degrading histamine, SRS-A, and PAF. Histaminase activity, assessed by the oxidative deamination of labeled histamine, resides in eosinophils and neutrophils, but not in mononuclear leukocytes, and is recovered predominantly in a dense granular fraction (Zeiger *et al.*, 1976). The other enzyme responsible for histamine inactivation, namely, histamine methyl transferase, is preferentially contained in monocytes and localized in the cytosol fraction (Zeiger *et al.*, 1976). Eosinophil arylsulfatase B, isolated by sequential gel filtration and ion-exchange chromatography, inactivates SRS-A in a time- and dose-dependent reaction (Wasserman *et al.*, 1975a). The inactivation of SRS-A was attributed to arylsulfatase B, since extensive purification of the enzyme failed to dissociate the 4-nitrocatechol-sulfate-cleaving activity from the SRS-A-inactivating activity. Both activities had a pH optimum of 5.7, and SRS-A competitively inhibited the cleavage of the synthetic substrate (Wasserman *et al.*, 1975a). Although arylsulfatase may be released by eosinophils during phagocytosis (Goetzl *et al.*, 1974), SRS-A inactivation by arylsulfatase B appears to be a function of intact eosinophils, since the degradation of SRS-A is 3- to 4-fold more rapid than that for the same quantity of extracted enzyme and exhibits a pH optimum of 7.4, is not associated with enzyme release, and is suppressed by metabolic inhibitors that do not affect the function of the isolated enzymes (Wasserman *et al.*, 1975b). Eosinophil phospholipase D has been specifically implicated in inactivation of one form of PAF. PAF-inactivating activity copurified in a four-step procedure along with choline-generating activity from a lecithin substrate, and there was reciprocal inhibition of PAF inactivation by lecithin and of choline generation by PAF.

Biodegradation is not wholly dependent on infiltrating cells in the lung. Arylsulfatase B, which predominates over arylsulfatase A in human lung, inactivates SRS-A in a reaction comparable to that for the eosinophil enzyme (Wasserman and Austen, 1976).

5. Summary

The IgE-dependent immunologic activation of mast cells and basophils leads to the generation of SRS-A and PAF(s) and their release with the preformed mediators, histamine, ECF-A, heparin, and NCF(s) (Figure 1). The apparent activity of the mediators may be modulated on at least three levels, namely, regulation of generation and release, alteration of target cell response by modification of receptor binding or cell activation, and inactivation by biodegradation. Of the six primary mediators, only histamine is known to inhibit its own release and that of other mediators by way of an action on H_2 receptors that elevates intracellular levels of cAMP. ECF-A tripeptides, possibly produced by the action of PMN leukocytes on the tetrapeptides, inhibit chemotaxis by blocking eosinophil receptors for ECF-A, as well as by deactivation of the eosinophils. Further, the chemotactic responsiveness of eosinophils is enhanced by histamine and suppressed by the presence of SRS-A. Finally, the eosinophils, which undergo directed migration and may be held at the site of immediate hypersensitivity by deactivation, modulate mediator activity through enzymatic biodegradation of histamine by histaminase, SRS-A by arylsulfatase B, and PAF by way of phospholipase D. Thus, the consequences of

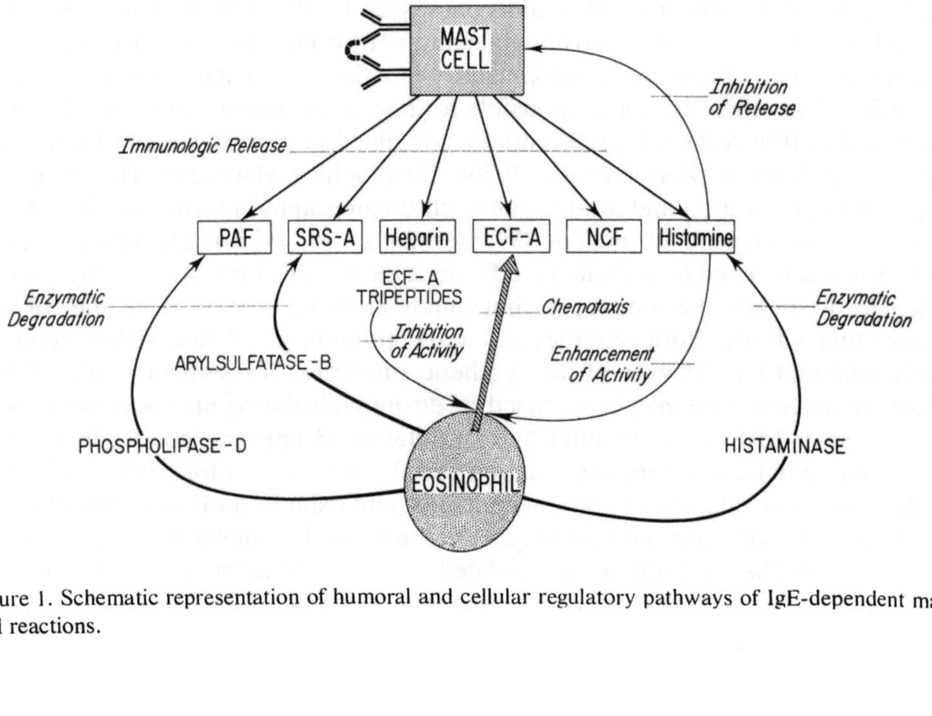

Figure 1. Schematic representation of humoral and cellular regulatory pathways of IgE-dependent mast cell reactions.

mast cell activation are subject to regulatory mechanisms that serve to limit the initial humoral phase of mast cell activation. Presumably, the humoral phase recruits the essential components of a full host response, namely, antibodies, complement, and other humoral factors and cells, to a discrete site of mast cell involvement forming an inflammatory phase. The failure of regulation could shift the IgE-mediated reaction from beneficial humoral and cellular phases to an excessive response, with attendant possibilities for adverse acute and subacute tissue effects.

ACKNOWLEDGMENTS

This work was supported by N.I.H. grants AI-07722 and AI-10356. E.J.G. is an investigator of the Howard Hughes Medical Institute.

References

Augustein, J., Farmer, J. B., Lee, T. B., Sheard, P., and Tattersall, M. L., 1973, *Nature (London) New Biol.* **245**:215–217.

Austen, K. F., and Orange, R. P., 1975, *Am. Rev. Respir. Dis.* **112**:423–436.

Austen, K. F., Lewis, R. A., Stechschulte, D. J., Wasserman, S. I., Leid, R. W., and Goetzl, E. J., 1974, in: *Progress in Immunology II* (L. Brent and J. Holborow, eds.), Vol. 2, pp. 61–71, North-Holland Publishing Co., Amsterdam.

Austen, K. F., Lewis, R. A., Wasserman, S. I., and Goetzl, E. J., 1975, in: *New Directions in Asthma* (M. Stein, ed.), pp. 187–203, American College of Chest Physicians, Park Ridge, Illinois.

Benveniste, J., 1974, *Nature (London)* **249**:581–582.

Benveniste, J., Henson, P. M., and Cochrane, C. G., 1972, *J. Exp. Med.* **136**:1356–1377.

Benveniste, J., Kamoun, P., and Polonsky, J., 1975, *Fed. Proc. Fed. Am. Soc. Exp. Biol.* **34**:985A.

Bergqvist, U., Samuelson, G., and Uvnäs, B., 1971, *Acta Physiol. Scand.* **83**:362–372.

Black, J. W., Duncan, W. A. M., Durant, C. J., Ganellin, C. R., and Parsons, E. M., 1972, *Nature (London)* **236**:385–390.

Bogart, D. B., and Stechschulte, D. J., 1974, *Clin. Res.* **22**:652A.

Bourne, H. R., Melmon, K. L., and Lichtenstein, L. M., 1971, *Science* **173**:743–745.

Bourne, H. R., Lichtenstein, L. M., and Melmon, K. L., 1972, *J. Immunol.* **108**:695–705.

Brinkman, G. L., 1968, *J. Ultrastruct. Res.* **23**:115–123.

Brocklehurst, W. E., 1960, *J. Physiol.* **151**:416–435.

Clark, R. A. F., Gallin, J. I., and Kaplan, A. P., 1975, *J. Exp. Med.* **142**:1462–1476.

Drazen, J. M., and Austen, K. F., 1974, *J. Clin. Invest.* **53**:1679–1685.

Dvorak, H. F., Dvorak, A. M., and Churchill, W. H., 1973, *J. Exp. Med.* **137**:751–775.

Feltkamp-Vroom, T. M., Stallman, P. J., Aalberse, R. C., and Reerink-Brongers, E. E., 1975, *Clin. Immunol. Immunopathol.* **4**:392–404.

Fillion, G. M. B., Storach, S. A., and Uvnäs, B., 1970, *Acta Physiol. Scand.* **78**:547–560.

Goetzl, E. J., and Austen, K. F., 1975, *Proc. Natl. Acad. Sci. U.S.A.* **72**:4123–4127.

Goetzl, E. J., and Austen, K. F., 1976a, in: *Molecular and Biological Aspects of the Acute Allergic Reaction* (S. G. O. Johansson, K. Strandberg, and B. Uvnäs, eds.), pp. 417–435, Plenum, New York.

Goetzl, E. J., and Austen, K. F., 1976b, *J. Exp. Med.* **144**:1424–1437.

Goetzl, E. J., Wasserman, S. I., and Austen, K. F., 1974, in: *Progress in Immunology II* (L. Brent and J. Holborow, eds.), Vol. 4, pp. 41–50, North-Holland Publishing Co., Amsterdam.

Goetzl, E. J., Wasserman, S. I., and Austen, K. F., 1975, *Arch. Pathol.* **99**:1–4.

Gold, W. M., 1973, in: *Asthma: Physiology, Immunopharmacology, and Treatment* (K. F. Austen and L. M. Lichtenstein, eds.), pp. 169–184, Academic Press, New York.

Ishizaka, T., Ishizaka, K., and Tomioka, H., 1972, *J. Immunol.* **108**:513–520.

Jaques, L. B., Monkhouse, F. C., and Stewart, M., 1949, *J. Physiol.* **109**:41–48.

Kaliner, M., and Austen, K. F., 1973, *J. Exp. Med.* **138**:1077–1094.

Kaliner, M., and Austen, K. F., 1974a, in: *Cyclic AMP, Cell Growth, and the Immune Response* (W. Braun, L. M. Lichtenstein, and C. W. Parker, eds.), pp. 163–175, Springer-Verlag, New York.

Kaliner, M., and Austen, K. F., 1974b, *J. Immunol.* **112**:664–674.
Kaliner, M., Orange, R. P., and Austen, K. F., 1972, *J. Exp. Med.* **136**:556–567.
Kaliner, M., Wasserman, S. I., and Austen, K. F., 1973, *N. Engl. J. Med.* **289**:277–281.
Kater, L. A., Goetzl, E. J., and Austen, K. F., 1976, *J. Clin. Invest.* **57**:1173–1180.
Kay, A. B., and Austen, K. F., 1971, *J. Immunol.* **107**:899–902.
Kay, A. B., and Austen, K. F., 1972, *Clin. Exp. Immunol.* **11**:37–42.
Kravis, T. C., and Henson, P. M., 1975, *J. Immunol.* **115**:1677–1681.
Lewis, R. A., Wasserman, S. I., Goetzl, E. J., and Austen, K. F., 1974, *J. Exp. Med.* **140**:1133–1146.
Lewis, R. A., Goetzl, E. J., Wasserman, S. I., Valone, F. H., Rubin, R. H., and Austen, K. F., 1975, *J. Immunol.* **114**:87–92.
Lichtenstein, L. M., and Gillespie, E., 1973, *Nature (London)* **244**:287–288.
Lichtenstein, L. M., and Margolis, S., 1968, *Science* **161**:902–903.
Lichtenstein, L. M., Gillespie, E., and Bourne, H. R., 1972, in: *The Biological Role of the Immunoglobulin E System* (K. Ishizaka and D. H. Dayton, eds.), pp. 165–189, National Institute of Child Health and Development, National Institutes of Health, Washington, D.C.
Majno, G., Shea, S. M., and Leventhal, M., 1969, *J. Cell Biol.* **42**:647–659.
Nadel, J.A., 1973, in: *Asthma: Physiology, Immunopharmacology and Treatment* (K. F. Austen and L. M. Lichtenstein, eds.), pp. 29–38, Academic Press, New York.
Odegard, O. R., Lie, M., and Abildgaard, U., 1975, *Thromb. Res.* **6**:287–294.
Orange, R. P., 1974, in: *Progress in Immunology II* (L. Brent and J. Holborow, eds.), Vol. 4, pp. 29–39, North-Holland Publishing Co., Amsterdam.
Orange, R. P., Stechschulte, D. J., and Austen, K. F., 1969, *Fed. Proc. Fed. Am. Soc. Exp. Biol.* **28**:1710–1715.
Orange, R. P., Kaliner, M. A., and Austen, K. F., 1971, *Fed. Proc. Fed. Am. Soc. Exp. Biol.* **30**:1725–1729.
Orange, R. P., Murphy, R. C., Karnovsky, M. L., and Austen, K. F., 1973, *J. Immunol.* **110**:760–770.
Orange, R. P., Murphy, R. C., and Austen, K. F., 1974, *J. Immunol.* **113**:316–322.
Padawer, J., 1974, *Exp. Mol. Pathol.* **20**:269–280.
Paterson, N. A. M., Wasserman, S. I., Said, J., and Austen, K. F., 1976, *J. Immunol.* **117**:1356–1362.
Plaut, M., Lichtenstein, L. M., Gillespie, E., and Henney, C. S., 1973, *J. Immunol.* **111**:389–394.
Riley, J. F., 1959, *The Mast Cells,* Livingstone, Edinburgh.
Schayer, R. W., 1965, *Fed. Proc. Fed. Am. Soc. Exp. Biol.* **24**:1295–1297.
Shioda, H., and Mishima, K., 1966, *J. Asthma Res.* **3**:323, 324.
Siraganian, R. P., and Osler, A. G., 1971, *J. Immunol.* **106**:1244–1251.
Sullivan, T. J., Seyfried, L. R., and Parker, C. W., 1975a, *Clin. Res.* **23**:298A.
Sullivan, T. J., Parker, K. L., Eisen, S. A., and Parker, C. W., 1975b, *J. Immunol.* **114**:1480–1485.
Wasserman, S. I., and Austen, K. F., 1976, *J. Clin. Invest.* **57**:738–744.
Wasserman, S. I., Goetzl, E. J., and Austen, K. F., 1973, *J. Immunol.* **112**:351–358.
Wasserman, S. I., Goetzl, E. J., Ellman, L., and Austen, K. F., 1974, *N. Engl. J. Med.* **290**:420–424.
Wasserman, S. I., Goetzl, E. J., and Austen, K. F., 1975a, *J. Immunol.* **114**:645–649.
Wasserman, S. I., Goetzl, E. J., and Austen, K. F., 1975b, *J. Allergy Clin. Immunol.* **55**:72.
Yurt, R. W., Leid, R. W., Austen, K. F., and Silbert, J. E., 1977a, *J. Biol. Chem.* **252**:518–521.
Yurt, R. W., Leid, R. W., Spragg, J., and Austen, K. F., 1977b, *J. Immunol.*, in press.
Zeiger, R. S., Yurdin, D. L., and Colten, H. R., 1976, *J. Allergy Clin. Immunol.* **58**:172–179.
Zurier, R. B., Hoffstein, S., Kammerman, S., and Tai, H. H., 1974, *J. Clin. Invest.* **53**:297–309.

8

Plasma Factors: The Hageman-Factor-Dependent Pathways and the Complement Sequence

JOCELYN SPRAGG and K. FRANK AUSTEN

1. Introduction

The Hageman-factor-dependent pathways of coagulation, kinin generation, and fibrinolysis, and the complement sequence have been considerably clarified with regard to physicochemical characterization, mechanisms of activation, the nature of the interactions of the components, the generation of several biological functions during complete activation of the systems, and the modulation of activation and function by amplification or depression. The most complete examination of these systems is afforded by studies with human components, to which this chapter will be confined unless otherwise noted.

2. Hageman-Factor-Dependent Pathways

Human Hageman factor (coagulation Factor XII) is a plasma proenzyme that, being activated, is capable of converting the γ-globulin proenzymes plasma thromboplastin antecedent (PTA, or Factor XI), prekallikrein, and plasma plasminogen proactivator to their respective active forms, activated PTA (PTA_a or XI_a), kallikrein, and plasma plasminogen activator, thereby initiating the three pathways schematically depicted in Figure 1. The physicochemical characteristics of the components of these pathways are given in Table 1.

JOCELYN SPRAGG and K. FRANK AUSTEN • Departments of Medicine, Harvard Medical School and the Robert B. Brigham Hospital, Boston, Massachusetts 02120.

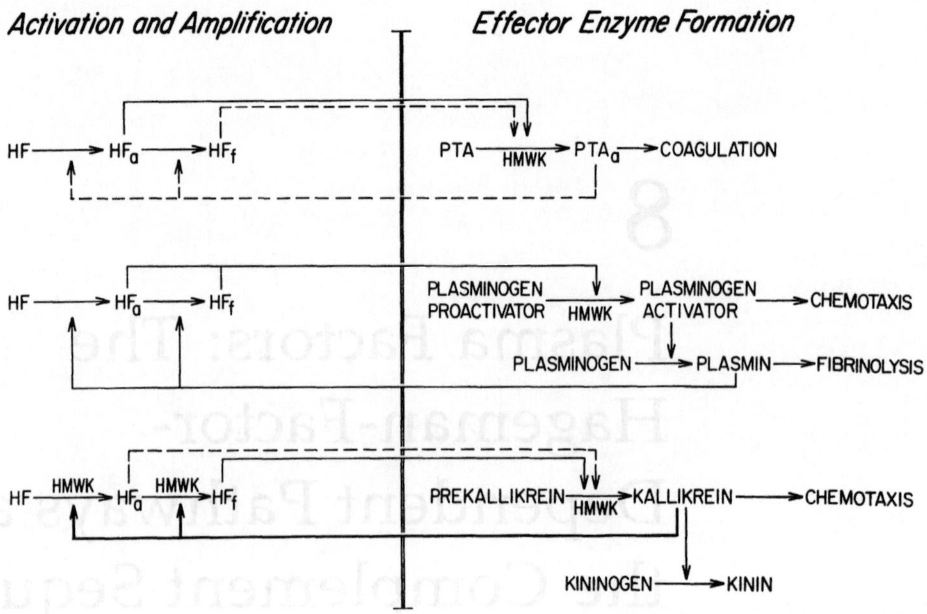

Figure 1. Schematic representation of the activation of the Hageman-factor-dependent enzymes and their functions. All three pathways generate enzymes demonstrating feedback activation of Hageman factor, but kallikrein is the most potent. (HF_a) Intact activated Hageman factor; (HF_f) Hageman factor fragments. High-molecular-weight kininogen (HMWK) is involved in both the function of Hageman factor and its reciprocal activation; although the latter effect has so far been examined only with kallikrein, it might also be expected with plasmin and PTA.

2.1 Hageman Factor, Hageman Factor Fragments, and PF/dil

Activation of Hageman factor can be accomplished by two general mechanisms that normally function in concert. Exposure of Hageman factor to a negatively charged surface such as glass (Margolis, 1958; Ratnoff and Rosenblum, 1958), elastin (Niewiarowski *et al.*, 1965), renal vascular basement membrane (Cochrane *et al.*, 1972a), articular cartilage (Moskowitz *et al.*, 1970), or monosodium urate and calcium pyrophosphate crystals (Kellermeyer and Breckenridge, 1965) leads to binding of the Hageman factor (Niewiarowski *et al.*, 1965; Cochrane *et al.*, 1972a) and activation, presumably by conformational changes, since fragmentation of Hageman factor has not been observed as a result of surface activation in the absence of enzymes. The ability of partially purified collagen to activate Hageman factor (Niewiarowski *et al.*, 1965; Wilner *et al.*, 1968) was recently questioned (Zacharski and Rosenstein, 1975), and may be due to its contamination with mucopolysaccharides (Cochrane, personal communication). Soluble *Escherichia coli* lipopolysaccharide or its negatively charged Lipid A moiety was also shown to bind and activate Hageman factor without fragmentation; high concentrations of the lipopolysaccharide appeared to yield decreased activation and to inhibit the capacity of Hageman factor to be activated by trypsin (Morrison and Cochrane, 1974).

Fluid-phase activation of Hageman factor is accomplished by plasma kallikrein, plasmin, and trypsin, and weakly by PTA, and is associated with cleavage of the Hageman factor into three fragments, the prekallikrein-activating activity being associated with a moiety of molecular weight 28,000 (Revak *et al.*, 1974). Plasmin is the plasma protease that was initially shown to fragment previously activated Hageman factor, thereby generating a fragment with a molecular weight of approximately 30,000 that was capable of converting each of the Hageman factor proenzyme substrates to its active form (Kaplan and Austen, 1971, 1972; Kaplan *et al.*, 1971; Burrowes *et al.*, 1971). Fragmentation of Hageman factor leads to a greater capacity to activate prekallikrein relative to its clot-promoting activity (Kaplan and Austen, 1971; Cochrane and Wuepper, 1971a), and to a decreased isoelectric point (Kaplan *et al.*, 1971) associated with a diminished capacity to bind to negatively charged surfaces (Webster, 1972). Elucidation of the role of Hageman factor in the activation of prekallikrein suggested that various forms of activated Hageman factor may represent PF/dil (Kaplan and Austen, 1971), a permeability factor defined by its generation on the dilution of normal plasma in glass (MacKay *et al.*, 1953; Stewart and Bliss, 1957). This view was confirmed by the capacity of insolubilized anti-Hageman factor to absorb functional PF/dil generated in the classic fashion (Johnston *et al.*, 1974).

The ability of antigen–antibody aggregates to activate Hageman factor, as reflected by kinin generation, was suggested in animal models *in vivo* (reviewed by Spragg *et al.*, 1970; Austen, 1977) and *in vitro* (Davies and Lowe, 1962; Movat and DiLorenzo, 1968; Movat *et al.*, 1968; Epstein *et al.*, 1969; Eisen and Smith, 1970), but primary and secondary events could not be distinguished. These findings were

TABLE 1. Physicochemical Characteristics of Components of the Hageman-Factor-Dependent Systems of Man

Component	Molecular weight G100	Molecular weight SDS	Electrophoretic mobility	pI	Serum concentration (γ/ml)[a]
Hageman factor	110,000	80,000	β	5.8–7.5	29
Active Hageman factor	110,000	80,000	β	5.8–7.5	—
Hageman factor prealbumin fragments	30,000–35,000	28,000	Prealb.	4.4–4.6	—
XI (PTA)	175,000	163,000	γ	8.8–9.4	?
XI_a (PTA_a)	175,000	163,000	γ	8.8–9.4	—
Plasminogen proactivator	100,000	—	γ	8.7–9.0	?
Plasminogen activator	100,000	—	γ	8.6–8.9	—
Plasminogen		83,000	β	6.3–6.8	285
Plasmin		76,000	β	6.1–8.4	—
Prekallikrein	127,000	107,000	γ	8.5–8.9	103
Kallikrein	108,000	107,000	γ	8.5–8.9	—
Kininogen					
High-molecular-weight	175,000		β	} 4.5–4.7	} 675
Low-molecular-weight	80,000	80,000	α		
Bradykinin	1,040 (by composition)		Cathodal	>10	<0.005

[a]Based on immunoassay values for total protein.

supported by early studies employing highly purified reagents (Cochrane and Wuepper, 1971b; Kaplan *et al.*, 1971), but contamination with endotoxins was not excluded, and more recent work failed to demonstrate immunologic activation of human or rabbit Hageman factor (Cochrane *et al.*, 1972b).

Recent studies of surface activation of Hageman factor in the presence of its proenzymes substrates have revealed two critical features, which are presumably operative in the usual complex biological fluids. Although high-molecular-weight kininogen and prekallikrein are not needed for binding of Hageman factor (Revak *et al.*, 1976), they are essential for its efficient activation and function, which under these conditions is associated with release of the active Hageman factor fragment (Griffin and Cochrane, 1976). Although the primary initiating event has not yet been identified, it appears that a trimolecular interaction of Hageman factor, kallikrein, and high-molecular-weight kininogen activates Hageman factor. This factor in turn converts prekallikrein to kallikrein, which amplifies the Hageman factor activation and releases the active Hageman factor fragment (Griffin and Cochrane, 1976). Plasmin can substitute for kallikrein, but is less efficient. The "contact activation cofactor" that is apparently required for PTA activation by Hageman factor (Schiffman and Lee, 1974) may be synonymous with high-molecular-weight kininogen, which has been determined to be a new coagulation trait, variously designated Fitzgerald (Waldman *et al.*, 1975; Saito *et al.*, 1975; Donaldson *et al.*, 1976), Flaujeac (Wuepper *et al.*, 1975), or Williams (Colman *et al.*, 1975). Plasmas from persons with this trait exhibit retarded activation of Hageman factor and its substrates.

2.2. Proenzyme Substrates of Activated Hageman Factor

2.2.1. Plasma Thromboplastin Antecedent and the Intrinsic Coagulation Pathway

Employing either partially or highly purified reagents, several groups have demonstrated the conversion of PTA to its active form, PTA_a, by active Hageman factor or by prolonged incubation with Hageman factor fragments (Ratnoff, 1972; Wuepper, 1972; Heck and Kaplan, 1974; Kaplan *et al.*, 1976). PTA appears to consist of two polypeptide chains held together by disulfide bonds that, on activation by Hageman factor (Kaplan *et al.*, 1976) or trypsin (Wuepper, 1972), undergo intrachain peptide bond cleavage, as determined by reduction and alkylation of the activated molecule.

PTA_a then converts the next factor of the intrinsic pathway to its active enzyme form (IX to IX_a), which, in combination with Factor VIII, phospholipid, and calcium ions, is capable of activating Factor X (Østerud and Rapaport, 1970). The mechanisms of activation and function of Factor VIII in this reaction are not clearly defined, and it has been suggested that prior exposure of Factor VIII to thrombin, possibly generated by the extrinsic pathway, precedes its participation in the complex that activates Factor X (reviewed by Davie and Fujikawa, 1975). Activated Factor X forms a complex with Factor V that, again in the presence of phospholipid and calcium ions, converts prothrombin to thrombin, the enzyme responsible for the fibrinogen-to-fibrin conversion. During the course of this conversion, fibrinopeptides having C-terminal arginine residues are released from the α- and β-chains of fibrinogen (Blömback *et al.*, 1966). Fibrinopeptide B exhibits enhancement of the smooth muscle contracting activity of bradykinin (Osbahr *et al.*, 1964), and is a leukocyte chemotactic factor (Kay *et al.*, 1973). Other functions of thrombin include activation of Factor XIII, which forms intermolecular covalent bonds cross-linking the fibrin monomers; initiation of the platelet release reaction (Davey and Lüscher, 1967); release of C3 anaphylatoxin from the third component of complement (Bokisch *et al.*, 1969); and enhancement of Factor VIII activity, as noted above. In addition to the thrombin-generated fibrinopeptides, there are biologically active plasmin-generated fibrin split products (see Section 2.2.3). For a more detailed account of the interactions leading to clot formation, the reader is referred to the review by Davie and Fujikawa (1975).

2.2.2. Prekallikrein and the Kinin-Generating Sequence

Activated Hageman factor, and to a greater extent Hageman factor fragments, convert plasma prekallikrein to its active enzymatic form, kallikrein (Kaplan and Austen, 1970). The prealbumin "prokininogenase activator" (i.e., prekallikrein activator) purified from rabbit, guinea pig, or human sources (Wuepper *et al.*, 1970; Treloar and Movat, 1970; Movat *et al.*, 1971; Wuepper and Cochrane, 1971) has since also been shown to be a fragment of Hageman factor (Cochrane and Wuepper, 1971a; Soltay *et al.*, 1971). Plasma kallikrein has at least three functions: feedback activation of Hageman factor, chemotaxis of neutrophilic leukocytes, and release of bradykinin from the kininogen substrate.

The feedback activation of Hageman factor by plasma kallikrein was shown both with purified reagents (Cochrane *et al.*, 1972a; Revak *et al.*, 1974) and with plasma from persons who were deficient in prekallikrein (Fletcher factor deficiency) and demonstrated an abnormality of the contact phase of coagulation that was correctable by the addition of highly purified prekallikrein (Wuepper, 1973). The diminished surface-activated chemotactic capacity of this plasma (Weiss *et al.*, 1974) supported the earlier finding, in a study employing purified reagents, that kallikrein was directly chemotactic for human neutrophils (Kaplan *et al.*, 1972). Kallikrein neutrophil chemotaxis is dependent, like other functions of kallikrein, on the integrity of its active enzymatic site (Kaplan *et al.*, 1972); such principles have been termed *active site chemotactic factors* (Goetzl and Austen, 1974).

Kallikrein also acts on a plasma protein substrate, kininogen, to release the biologically active nonapeptide bradykinin (Webster and Pierce, 1963), the functions of which are detailed below. The observations that kininogen existed in two states, a "high-molecular-weight" (mol.wt. 197,000) and a "low-molecular-weight" (mol.wt. 57,000) form, which was less suitable for plasma kallikrein cleavage (Jacobsen, 1966; Jacobsen and Kriz, 1967), does not necessarily imply unique principles under separate genetic control. The following observations are compatible with a single kininogen that may be physiologically present in two forms that have sequential functions: (1) the reactivity to plasma kallikrein of kininogen with a molecular weight of approximately 80,000–90,000 purified under mild conditions (Spragg and Austen, 1971, 1974; Cochrane and Wuepper, 1971b; Wuepper and Cochrane, 1971; Habermann and Jahrreis, 1971); (2) the susceptibility of kininogen to alteration of its apparent physicochemical properties during purification (Spragg and Austen, 1971, 1974; Habermann and Jahrreis, 1971; Londesborough and Hamberg, 1975); (3) the antigenic cross-reactivity of "low"- and "high"-molecular-weight kininogens (Pierce, 1968; Habal *et al.*, 1975); and (4) the high degree of amino acid homology in low- and high-molecular-weight bovine kininogens (Komiya *et al.*, 1972; Suzuki *et al.*, 1973).

The recent reports of persons with a deficiency in which all the Hageman-factor-dependent pathway defects are correctable *in vitro* by the addition of partially (Wuepper *et al.*, 1975) or highly (Colman *et al.*, 1975) purified kininogen have permitted further examination of the functions and multiplicity of kininogens. Fitzgerald, Williams, and Flaujeac plasmas, which fail to correct one another, each demonstrate deficiencies of surface-activated coagulation, fibrinolysis, and kinin generation. PTA_a, but not XII_a, corrected the coagulation defect in Fitzgerald trait plasma; this plasma was shown to lack "contact activation cofactor" (Schiffman *et al.*, 1975), a principle that is similar in size and charge to high-molecular-weight kininogen (Schiffman and Lee, 1975). While the addition of the Hageman factor substrates PTA and plasminogen proactivator, or kininogen of molecular weight 80,000, to Williams plasma partially corrected the surface-activated coagulation and fibrinolytic defects, full correction of all three functions was obtained only on the addition of high-molecular-weight (175,000) kininogen alone (Colman *et al.*, 1975). Flaujeac plasma was also corrected by plasma fractions that eluted from Sephadex at a molecular weight of 170,000 and contained kininogen (Wuepper *et al.*, 1975). Since neither Flaujeac nor Williams plasma show any kininogen antigenically or functionally, these findings support the concept that low- and high-molecular-weight kininogens are related gene products.

The basic nonapeptide bradykinin, which is released from kininogens by plasma kallikrein (Webster and Pierce, 1963; Spragg and Austen, 1971), is a potent hypotensive agent, eliciting both increased capillary permeability and arteriolar vasodilatation. Bradykinin directly contracts a variety of smooth muscle preparations and elicits pain (Erdös, 1966, 1970). Bradykinin and bradykinin analogues have secondary effects, which include the release of histamine from rat peritoneal mast cells (Johnson and Erdös, 1973), a finding that is consistent with the capacity of antihistamine pretreatment to diminish the increase in vascular permeability produced in the skin by bradykinin (Becker *et al.*, 1968).

In guinea pig lung slices, bradykinin produces an accumulation of both 3′,5′-adenosine monophosphate and 3′,5′-guanosine monophosphate; the prevention of the former, but the not latter, by inhibitors of prostaglandin (PG) biosynthesis suggests a role for bradykinin in the formation or function, or both, of PGs (Stoner *et al.*, 1973). Further, in animal models, the vascular-permeability-enhancing effect of bradykinin is augmented by PGs of the E series (Harrison, 1973; Thomas and West, 1973, 1974). Finally, the bronchoconstricting activity of bradykinin in guinea pig lung (Collier, 1976) and the effects of bradykinin on renal blood flow in the isolated perfused dog kidney (McGiff *et al.*, 1976) are diminished by pretreatment with aspirinlike agents, which have been shown to inhibit PG synthesis (Vane, 1971). These data are consistent with mediation by bradykinin-stimulated PGs.

2.2.3. Plasminogen Proactivator and Fibrinolysis

Highly purified plasminogen proactivator, on activation by Hageman factor or Hageman factor fragments, converts plasminogen to plasmin in the absence of streptokinase (Kaplan and Austen, 1972). It also exhibits direct chemotaxis for human polymorphonuclear neutrophilic leukocytes (Kaplan *et al.*, 1973); both functions require the integrity of the active enzymatic site. Although similar in charge and size to plasma prekallikrein, plasminogen proactivator was thought to be distinct from it by chromatographic techniques (Kaplan and Austen, 1972; Cochrane *et al.*, 1973) and by its inhibition by α_2-macroglobulin, but not by the inhibitor of the first component of complement (Schreiber *et al.*, 1973a), which inhibits kallikrein. More recent evidence indicating that plasminogen proactivator activity is associated with prekallikrein (Mandle and Kaplan, 1977; Cochrane, personal communication) is supported by studies showing a lack of prekallikrein-associated plasminogen proactivator in Fletcher-factor-deficient plasma (Mandle and Kaplan, 1977), which lacks prekallikrein (Wuepper, 1972), and suggesting that the activity found in this plasma (Kaplan *et al.*, 1973) is due to an additional factor also present in normal plasma. Studies indicating that kallikrein converts prekallikrein to an altered proenzyme of 10,000 lower molecular weight (Mandle and Kaplan, submitted for publication) serve to identify the plasminogen proactivator originally isolated.

Plasmin, once generated, has the capacity to lyse a fibrin clot; to further activate and fragment Hageman factor (II.A); to convert C1s to its active enzymatic form, $C\bar{1}s$ (Ratnoff and Naff, 1967); to release C3 anaphylatoxin from C3 (Ward, 1967); and to generate from fibrinogen or fibrin products that have anticoagulant, chemotactic, and vascular-permeability-increasing activities (Marder and Shulman, 1969; Barnhart *et al.*, 1971).

2.3. Modulation

2.3.1. Amplification

Amplification of Hageman factor activation by products of the Hageman-factor-dependent pathways, i.e., kallikrein, plasmin, and PTA_a, was noted in Section 2.1 and in Figure 1. A major role of kallikrein in this feedback is indicated by its ability to activate Hageman factor *in vitro* at low concentration (Cochrane *et al.*, 1973) and, especially, by the contact coagulation defect in prekallikrein-deficient plasma, which is overcome by prolonged incubation of the plasma with an activating surface or corrected by reconstitution with purified prekallikrein (Wuepper, 1973). Fragmentation of Hageman factor by plasmin is associated with an increased fluid-phase capacity to activate prekallikrein as compared with PTA (see Sections 2.1 and 2.2.2), thus directing the pathway toward kinin generation and away from coagulation.

2.3.2. Inhibition or Inactivation

Inhibition of the Hageman-factor-dependent system enzymes has been examined with the plasma protease inhibitors α_2-macroglobulin, α-antitrypsin, the inhibitor of the first component of complement (ClINH), and antithrombin III (heparin cofactor). The functions of active Hageman factor (Forbes *et al.*, 1970) or the Hageman factor fragments (Schreiber *et al.*, 1973a) are inhibited by $C\bar{1}INH$, but not by α_2-macroglobulin or α_1-antitrypsin. Both Hageman factor and its fragments are also rapidly inhibited by the antithrombin III–heparin complex (Stead *et al.*, 1976), which in addition inhibits Factors XI_a (Damus *et al.*, 1973), IX_a (Rosenberg *et al.*,

1975), X_a (Seegers *et al.*, 1964; Biggs *et al.*, 1970), and thrombin (Abildgaard, 1968). Factor XI_a is also inhibited by C$\bar{1}$INH (Forbes *et al.*, 1970), an inhibitor of molecular weight 65,000 that is distinguishable from other plasma protease inhibitors (Amir *et al.*, 1972), and α_1-antitrypsin (Heck and Kaplan, 1974), but not by α_2-macroglobulin (Harpel, 1971). In terms of the coagulation pathway, the only reported effect of α_2-macroglobulin is on the protease activity of thrombin (Lanchantin *et al.*, 1966).

In the fibrinolytic pathway, the plasmin-activating and chemotactic functions of plasminogen activator are inhibited by α_2-macroglobulin, but not by α_1-antitrypsin or C$\bar{1}$INH (Kaplan and Austen, 1972; Schreiber *et al.*, 1973a; Goetzl and Austen, 1974). The fibrinolytic activity of plasmin is diminished by all four of the protease inhibitors discussed herein; on a molar basis, the most effective inhibitor appears to be α_2-macroglobulin (Ratnoff *et al.*, 1969; Norman and Hill, 1958; Highsmith and Rosenberg, 1974; Schreiber *et al.*, 1973a).

The kinin-forming pathway is inhibited at the kallikrein level by C$\bar{1}$INH (Gigli *et al.*, 1970; Schreiber *et al.*, 1973b) and α_2-macroglobulin (Harpel, 1970; McConnell, 1972; Schreiber *et al.*, 1973a), both of which also inhibit the chemotactic activity of kallikrein (Goetzl and Austen, 1974). The esteratic and proteolytic activities of kallikrein are inhibited relatively slowly by the antithrombin III–heparin complex (Lahiri *et al.*, 1974; Burrowes *et al.*, 1975). The end product, bradykinin, is inactivated by two serum enzymes, kininase I and II. The first of these, an arginine carboxypeptidase (Erdös and Sloane, 1962) called *carboxypeptidase N*, appears to be the same as the anaphylatoxin inactivator that inactivates human C3a and C5a as well as bradykinin (Bokisch and Müller-Eberhard, 1970). Kininase II is a carboxydipeptidase (dipeptide hydrolase) that appears to be the same as the angiotensin-converting enzyme (Yang *et al.*, 1970, 1971; Engel *et al.*, 1972). The latter is also found in lung and kidney in several mammalian species (Overturf *et al.*, 1975; Yang *et al.*, 1971; Nakajima *et al.*, 1973), and is located in the vascular endothelium (Ryan and Ryan, 1976). *In vivo* animal studies indicate that the lung may be an important tissue site of bradykinin inactivation (Leibowitz *et al.*, 1976; Levine *et al.*, 1973). Additionally, neutrophilic granulocytes contain kininases, but the conditions under which they are released or functional *in vivo* have not been delineated (Erdös and Yang, 1970; Schwab, 1962; Zachariae *et al.*, 1966; Greenbaum and Kim, 1967).

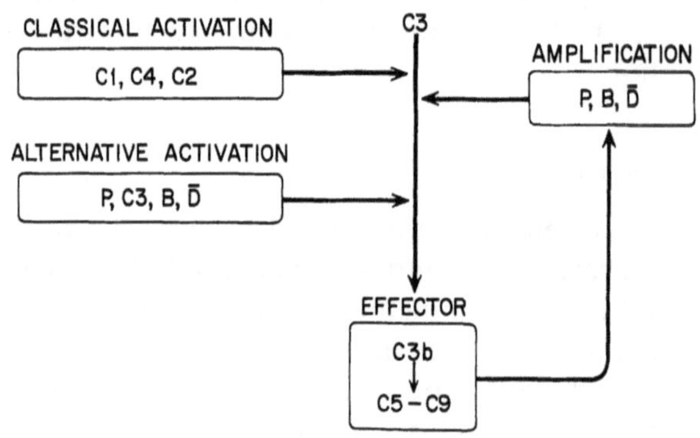

Figure 2. Depiction of the functional divisions involved in the activation, amplification, and function of the complement system. Modified from Fearon and Austen (1977a).

3. Complement

The interactions of the plasma proteins comprising the complement system, like the Hageman-factor-dependent pathways, lead to the generation of active enzymes and a variety of biologically active complexes and cleavage products. Two activation pathways, each initiated by different mechanisms, as well as a common amplification route, lead to the formation of C3 convertase activities (Figure 2), and thereby to activation of the final effector sequence from which most of the biological activities are derived (Figure 3). The focus of this discussion will be on the biological functions; detailed descriptions of the physicochemistry (see Tables 2 and 3) of the proteins and their interactions, synthesis, phylogeny, and human deficiency syndromes are available in recent reviews (Fearon and Austen, 1976, 1977a; Müller-Eberhard, 1975; Colten, 1974; Alper and Rosen, 1974; Ruddy *et al.*, 1972; Gigli and Austen, 1971).

3.1. Convertase Formation

Formation of classical convertase begins with the activation of the first component of complement, C1,* which exists as a trimolecular complex of C1q, C1r, and C1s in the presence of calcium ions (Lepow *et al.*, 1956). Binding to antigen–antibody complexes or to immunoglobulin aggregates of the IgG1, 2, or 3 subclasses or to IgM is achieved through the C1q portion of C1. Such fixation activates C1r to C$\bar{1}$r, which then activates C1s by cleavage of a single peptide bond to a two-chain, disulfide-bridged form (Sakai and Stroud, 1973) capable of activating C4 and C2. Interaction of C$\bar{1}$s with a three-chain protein C4 results in the release of a small peptide, C4a, and the generation of C4b (Schreiber and Müller-Eberhard, 1974), which binds via a labile site to immune complexes or membranes (Müller-Eberhard and Biro, 1963), thereby directing surface deposition of C3 and C5 convertase components. C4b or C4i facilitates C2 cleavage to C2a and C2b by C$\bar{1}$ (Gigli and Austen, 1969a,b), thereby allowing formation of the classical convertase, C4b2a. Via a stable site, C4b binds to immune adherence receptors on erythrocytes (Cooper, 1969), neutrophils (Ross and Polley, 1974), and B lymphocytes (Bokisch and Sobel, 1974). C4b2a together with C3b yields C5 convertase (Müller-Eberhard *et al.*, 1967; Cooper and Müller-Eberhard, 1970). C4a may have smooth-muscle-contracting activity, but this activity has been a variable finding (Budzko and Müller-Eberhard, 1970; Patrick *et al.*, 1970). There are suggestive data from studies of the C$\bar{1}$ inhibitor deficiency disease, hereditary angioedema (reviewed by Lepow, 1971), that a C-kinin may be cleaved from C2. It differs from bradykinin in trypsin sensitivity, amino acid content, and certain of its biological activities (Donaldson *et al.*, 1969; Lepow, 1971).

*The nomenclature for the classical complement components conforms to that agreed on under the auspices of the World Health Organization (1968). The provisional nomenclature for alternative pathway factors is that adopted at the Second International Congress of Immunology, 1974, Brighton, United Kingdom. B (Blum *et al.*, 1959) is the symbol for the protein that has been termed "C3 proactivator" (Götze and Müller-Eberhard, 1971) and "glycine-rich β-glycoprotein" (GBG) (Alper *et al.*, 1973); $\bar{D}$ (Hunsicker *et al.*, 1973) is a protein that has been termed "C3 proactivator convertase" (Müller-Eberhard and Götze, 1972), and P represents properdin (Pillemer *et al.*, 1954). A bar over a letter indicates the activated form of the protein. C3NeF is the abbreviation for C3 nephritic factor (Spitzer *et al.*, 1969), and C3bINA, that for the C3b inactivator (Tamura and Nelson, 1967) or conglutinogen-activating factor (KAF) (Nicol and Lachmann, 1973).

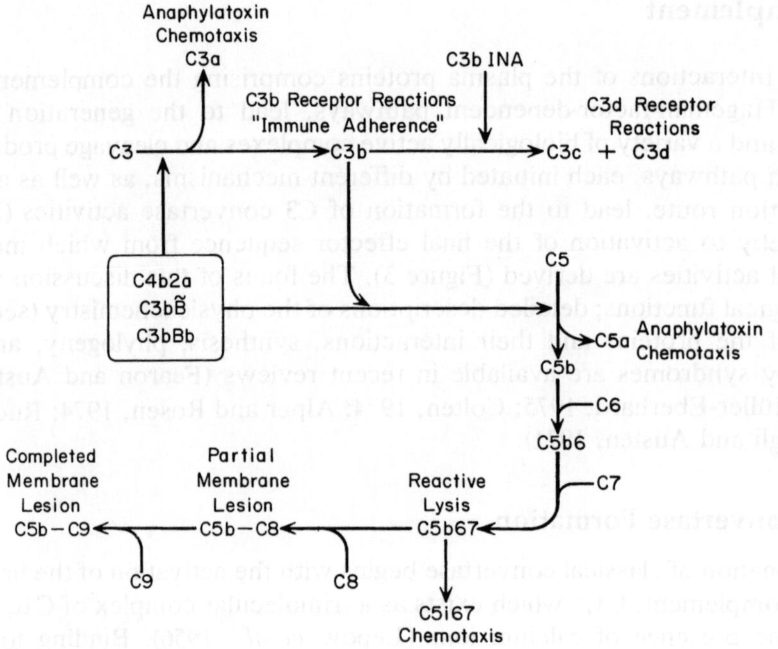

Figure 3. The complement effector sequence and the points at which biological functions are generated. Reproduced from Fearon and Austen (1977a).

TABLE 2. Physicochemical Characteristics of Components of the Complement System of Man

Component	Molecular weight	Electrophoretic mobility	pI	Serum concentration (μg/ml)
C1q	388,000	$\gamma 2$		190
C1r	180,000	β		100
C1s	86,000	$\alpha 2$		120
C4	202,000	$\beta 1$	6.0; 6.4	430
C2	117,000	$\beta 2$	5.5	30
C3	210,000	$\beta 1$	6.3–6.6	1300
Properdin	223,000	$\gamma 2$	>9.7	25
C3NeF	150,000	γ	8.75–8.95	—
B	100,000	$\beta 2$	6.6	240
D	23,500	α	7.4	?
C5	206,000	$\beta 1$	4.1	75
C6	95,000	$\beta 2$	6.0	60
C7	120,000	$\beta 2$	5.6	55
C8	163,000	$\gamma 1$	5.6; 6.5	80
C9	79,000	α	4.7	160

TABLE 3. **Biologically Active Products of the Complement Sequence**

Parent molecule	Cleavage product	Molecular weight	Biological functions
C4	C4a	8,000	Weak smooth muscle contracting activity (?).
	C4b	198,000	Labile site: binds to complexes and membranes; participates in deposition of C3 ($C\overline{42}$) and C5 ($C\overline{423}$) convertases on surfaces. Stable sites: immune adherence; increased efficiency of C2 cleavage by $C\overline{1}$; participation in C42 formation.
	C4i	200,000	Retains stable site functions of C4b.
	C4c	157,000	
	C4d	35,000	
C2	C2a	83,000	Participation in C2 ($C\overline{42}$) and C5 ($C\overline{423}$) convertase formation.
	C2b	37,000	
	C-kinin	>5,000	Increased vascular permeability.
C3	C3a	9,000	Mast cell degranulation: smooth muscle contraction; chemotaxis; increased vascular permeability.
	C3b	171,000	Labile sites: formation of C5 convertases; membrane and complex binding. Stable sites: immune adherence; enhanced phagocytosis; binding to P and B in amplification convertase.
	C3i	171,000	Retains stable site functions of C3b.
	C3c	151,000	
	C3d	27,000	Binds to membrane receptors.
C5	C5a	17,000	Mast cell degranulation; smooth muscle contraction; chemotaxis; increased vascular permeability.
	C5b	163,000	Membrane binding; subunit of C5b6789 cytolytic complex; participation in C5b67 innocent bystander reaction.
	C5i	163,000	Participation in C5i67 chemotaxis.

The alternative, or properdin, pathway generates a C3 convertase independent of C1, C4, and C2 (Pillemer *et al.*, 1954). This pathway is initiated by microbial products, dextrans, inulin, erythrocyte membranes (Pillemer *et al.*, 1954; Poskitt *et al.*, 1973; Burger *et al.*, 1975), or aggregated IgA (Boackle *et al.*, 1974; Soter *et al.*, 1974; Götze and Müller-Eberhard, 1971). In the fluid phase, initial C3 cleavage occurs when native C3 and B are interacted with $\bar{D}$, $\bar{P}$ (Fearon and Austen, 1975b), or C3 nephritic factor (C3Nef) (Daha *et al.*, 1976a). While the trimolecular reaction involving $\bar{D}$ cleaves B as well as C3, implying a convertase constituted of C3bBb, that formed with $\bar{P}$ or C3Nef without $\bar{D}$ contains uncleaved B(C3bB). The combination of at least four principles—C3, B, $\bar{D}$, and $\bar{P}$ or C3Nef—greatly accelerates the overall fluid-phase reaction, and represents the circumstances in complex biological fluids required to overcome the controlling function of the C3b inactivator and B1H. Müller-Eberhard and associates (Medicus *et al.*, 1976) concluded that on a particulate surface, initial C3 cleavage involves C3, B, $\bar{D}$, and an initiating factor, and that properdin activation occurs subsequently and functions only in amplification. More recently, however, Fearon and Austen (1977b,c) have shown that activating surfaces such as zymosan or rabbit erythrocytes protect C3b from inactivation by C3b INA and C3bBb from decay dissociation by B1H (see Section 3.3), and have suggested that activation can be surface deposition and protection of the C3b formed in a continuous low-grad fluid phase reaction involving C3, B, $\bar{D}$, and P.

Once C3b is made available by either the alternative or the classical pathway C3 convertases, factor $\bar{D}$ cleaves factor B in the presence of Mg^{2+} to form the amplification convertase, C3bBb or $C\bar{3}\bar{B}$ (Müller-Eberhard and Götze, 1972; Fearon *et al.*, 1973). The alternative pathway and amplification convertases are stabilized by $\bar{P}$ or C3Nef (Fearon and Austen, 1975a; Daha *et al.*, 1976b). Utilization of C3 and B by the amplification pathway has been found in a person lacking the C3b inactivator (see Section 3.3).

3.2. The Complement Effector Sequence and Generation of Biologically Active Molecules

The cleavage of C3 is followed by C5 cleavage and sequential formation of the terminal pentamolecular complex (Kolb *et al.*, 1972) (see Figure 3). The major product of C3 cleavage, C3b, binds passively to specific receptors on several types of cells via a stable immune adherence site. When neutrophils, monocytes, macrophages, or nonhuman platelets are involved, the energy-dependent steps of phagocytosis or noncytotoxic secretion of certain cellular contents, or both, may occur (Gigli and Nelson, 1968; reviewed by Becker and Henson, 1973). Adherence to bone-marrow-derived lymphocytes by C3b or its C3b inactivator cleavage product, C3d (Ruddy and Austen, 1971), may play a role in B-cell-dependent immunologic function (Pepys, 1974; Dukor *et al.*, 1974). A labile binding site(s) of C3b for membranes, immune complexes, or C3 convertases is necessary for formation of classical or alternative pathway C5 convertase. A cleavage product of C3 with a molecular weight of 9000, C3a, has been identified as an anaphylatoxin with C-terminal arginine; it has histamine-releasing, chemotactic, and weak direct smooth-muscle-contracting activity (Dias de Silva *et al.*, 1967; Bokisch *et al.*, 1969; Bokisch and Müller-Eberhard, 1970). When injected into human skin, C3a elicits a wheal and flare reaction and, at relatively high concentrations, a neutrophil accumulation (Wuepper *et al.*, 1972).

Cleavage of C5 by either C5 convertase results in the formation of a major (C5b) and minor (C5a) cleavage product. C5b, when fixed to a membrane, binds with C6 to continue the cytolytic sequence. Fluid-phase C5b may form a trimolecular complex, C5b67, transiently capable of binding to "innocent bystander" cells, resulting in cytolysis when C8 and C9 are present (the "reactive lysis" mechanism) (Goldman *et al.*, 1972; Thompson and Lachman, 1970). Fluid-phase C5b67 is also chemotactic and retains this activity after decay of the reactive lysis capacity (Ward *et al.*, 1966; Lachmann *et al.*, 1970). The minor fragment, C5a, is an anaphylatoxin peptide with a molecular weight of approximately 17,000 and having a basic C-terminal residue, i.e., lysine or arginine has been reported for hog C5a (Vallota *et al.*, 1973; Johnson *et al.*, 1975). C5a has histamine-releasing and neutrophil chemotactic activities, as well as some direct smooth muscle contracting activity. C5a produces a wheal and flare in human skin at concentrations several logs less than required for C3a. Unlike those of hog C5a, all the activities of human C5a are lost on exposure to autologous anaphylatoxin inactivator (Vallota *et al.*, 1973; Vallota and Müller-Eberhard, 1973).

In the final steps, membrane-bound C5b67 complexes with C8 and C9 to form the cytolytic "attack unit." Although the addition of C8 only generates a cytolytic capacity, as shown in the guinea pig (Stolfi, 1968), its efficiency is enhanced by the presence of C9 (Stolfi, 1968; Kolb *et al.*, 1972). The mechanism by which C5b6789 causes cytolysis is not completely understood, but probably involves insertion of the complex into the cell membrane, resulting in osmotic lysis (Mayer, 1972).

3.3. Modulation

The functions of the complement pathway are modulated in a number of ways, which can be generally grouped as either the effect of proteins external to the pathway, such as the inhibitor of $C\bar{1}$ ($C\bar{1}$INH) or the C3b inactivator (C3bINA), or the inherent alterations in reactivity of the pathway components themselves.

The inhibitor of the first component of complement, $C\bar{1}$INH, was shown to inhibit both isolated $C\bar{1}$s and $C\bar{1}$r (Ratnoff *et al.*, 1969; Gigli *et al.*, 1968), as well as several components of the Hageman-factor-dependent pathways (see Section 2.3.2). $C\bar{1}$ inhibitor forms a firm complex with the light chain of C1s in which the active site is located with no apparent cleavage of $C\bar{1}$s (Harpel and Cooper, 1975). In contrast, the action of C3bINA on C3 involves inactivation and subsequent cleavage without consumption of the inactivator (Ruddy and Austen, 1971); a serum cofactor, B1H, that enhances the activity of C3b inactivator was recently described (Whaley and Ruddy, 1976; Weiler *et al.*, 1976). An additional function of C3b inactivator is inactivation of C4b (Cooper, 1975), which again is augmented by a cofactor (Nagasawa *et al.*, 1976). An inhibitor that diminishes the ability of C1q to activate C1r was recently described (Conradie *et al.*, 1975). The inactivation of two products of the complement pathway, C3a and C5a, is accomplished by the anaphylatoxin inactivator, a serum carboxypeptidase that also inactivates bradykinin (Cochrane and Müller-Eberhard, 1968) (see Section 2.3.2).

The effective activation of the complement sequence is modified at several points by the rapid decay of active intermediates. The loss on fluid-phase activation of the membrane binding sites of C4b, C3b, and C5b and the decay of fluid-phase or bound C4b2a, C4b2a3b, C3bBb, and C3bBb3b represent intrinsic points of control. Certain of these decayed components, such as C5i, although hemolytically inactive, are still capable of fluid-phase binding with the next protein in the sequence, thereby removing it from participation in an effective reaction (Koethe *et al.*, 1973). Points at which effective interactions of the sequence are facilitated are represented by the capacity of C4b2a and C3bBb to be reformed after decay by the presence of additional C2 and $C\bar{1}$ or B and $\bar{D}$, respectively; by the amplification of C3 cleavage through formation of additional C3bBb; and by the stabilization of C3bBb with $\bar{P}$ or C3Nef so as to retard decay and prevent the activity of C3b inactivator (Daha *et al.*, 1976c).

4. Interactions with Other Mediator Systems

The foregoing discussion has indicated several points at which the Hageman-factor-dependent and complement systems may interact, such as the action of plasmin and thrombin on certain complement components, enhancement of bradykinin function by fibrinopeptide B, shared inhibition ($C\bar{1}$INH) or inactivation (anaphylatoxin inactivator) mechanisms, and the generation in both systems of principles having the same functions. Additionally, the elaboration of a function designated Kf, which modifies the action of $C\bar{1}$ on its substrates to permit more efficient utilization of C3, has been associated with the activation of the Hageman-factor-dependent systems (Gigli *et al.*, 1971). Further, both alternative pathway complement components and fibrinogen appear to play a role in the zymosan-induced human platelet release reaction (Zucker *et al.*, 1974).

Interactions of these pathways with cellular systems include the observations that leukocytes contain enzymes that cleave C3 (Hugli *et al.*, 1976) or C5 (Ward and Hill, 1970), that kinin-generating and -inactivating enzymes have been found in leukocytes (Greenbaum and Kim, 1967; Movat *et al.*, 1973), that a kinin-generating enzyme can be recovered after immunologic challenge of human leukocytes (Newball *et al.*, 1975), and that cell-mediated hypersensitivity reactions are associated with fibrin deposition (Colvin *et al.*, 1973).

5. Pharmacological Modulation

Experimentally employed agents that modify the action, activation, or metabolism of the components of the Hageman-factor-dependent and the complement systems have been extensively reviewed (Erdös, 1966, 1970; Davie and Fujikawa, 1975; Becker, 1972; Fearon and Austen, 1975c). Therapeutically useful agents that modulate the Hageman factor systems include, at present, anticoagulants, possibly aspirin, as noted in Section 2.2.3, and a low-molecular-weight (6500) polypeptide, originally isolated from bovine parotid gland and now prepared from bovine lung (aprotinin, Trasylol), that inhibits such proteases as trypsin, plasmin, and plasma and tissue kallikreins, and has found use outside the United States for the treatment of acute pancreatitis, shock, and coagulative and fibrinolytic disorders (Vogel and Zickgraf-Rüdel, 1970). ϵ-Aminocaproic acid (EACA) (Frank *et al.*, 1972) and its analogue, tranexamic acid (Sheffer *et al.*, 1972), have been employed in the treatment of hereditary angioedema on the basis of their inhibition of plasminogen activation. However, studies indicating that EACA also inhibits the generation of $C\bar{1}$ esterase activity (Taylor and Fudenberg, 1964) have been extended by the demonstration that EACA inhibits the intrinsic activation of cell-bound C1 (Soter *et al.*, 1975). The recent finding that methyl testosterone (Sheffer *et al.*, 1977) and synthetic or attenuated androgens (Rosse *et al.*, 1976; Gelfand *et al.*, 1976) are prophylactic in preventing attacks of hereditary angioedema, because their administration increases serum levels of C$\bar{1}$INH and, secondarily, C4, provides a rationale for the use of androgens in the management of this genetic disease of the complement system (Spaulding, 1960). Modulation of C1 activation or function represents at this time the only point in the complement sequence at which clinically useful agents have been employed.

References

Abildgaard, U., 1968, *Scand. J. Clin. Lab. Invest.* **21**:89–91.

Alper, C. A., and Rosen, F. S., 1974, in: *Progress in Immunology II,* Vol. 1 (L. Brent and E. J. Holborow, eds.), pp. 201–208, American Elsevier, New York.

Alper, C. A., Goodkofsky, I., and Lepow, I. H., 1973, *J. Exp. Med.* **137**:424–437.

Amir, J., Ratnoff, O. D., and Pensky, J., 1972, *J. Lab. Clin. Med.* **80**:786–802.

Austen, K. F., 1977, in: *Immunological Diseases* (M. Samter, ed.), 3rd Ed., Little Brown, Boston, in press.

Barnhart, M. I., Sulisz, L., and Bluhm, G. B., 1971, in: *Immunopathology of Inflammation* (B. K. Forscher and J. C. Houck, eds.), pp. 59–65, Excerpta Medica, Amsterdam.

Becker, E. L., 1972, in *Mediators of Inflammation: Mechanisms and Control* (I. H. Lepow and P. A. Ward, eds.), pp. 281–299, Academic Press, New York.

Becker, E. L., and Henson, P. M., 1973, *Adv. Immunol.* **17**:93–194.

Becker, E. L., Mota, I., and Wong, D., 1968, *Br. J. Pharmacol.* **34**:330–336.

Biggs, R., Denson, K. W. E., and Akman, N., 1970, *Br. J. Haematol.* **19**:283–305.

Blömback, B., Blömback, M., Edman, P., and Hessel, B., 1966, *Biochim. Biophys. Acta* **115**:371.

Blum, L., Pillemer, L., and Lepow, I. H., 1959, *Z. Immunitaetsforsch.* **118**:349–357.

Boackle, R. J., Pruitt, K. M., and Mestecky, J., 1974, *Immunochemistry* **11**:543–548.

Bokisch, V. A., and Müller-Eberhard, 1970, *J. Clin. Invest.* **49**:2427–2436.

Bokisch, V. A., and Sobel, A. T., 1974, *J. Exp. Med.* **140**:1336–1347.

Bokisch, V. A., Müller-Eberhard, H. J., and Cochrane, C. G., 1969, *J. Exp. Med.* **129**:1109–1130.

Budzko. D. B., and Müller-Eberhard, H. J., 1970, *Immunochemistry* **7**:227–234.

Burger, R., Hadding, U., Schorlemmer, W., Brade, V., and Bitter-Suermann, D., 1975, *Immunology* **29**:549–554.

Burrowes, C. E., Movat, H. Z., and Soltay, M. J., 1971, *Proc. Soc. Exp. Biol. Med.* **138**:959–966.

Burrowes, C. E., Habal, F. M., and Movat, H. Z., 1975, *Thromb. Res.* **7**:175–183.

Cochrane, C. G., and Müller-Eberhard, H. J., 1968, *J. Exp. Med.* **127**:371–386.

Cochrane, C. G., and Wuepper, K. D., 1971a, *J. Exp. Med.* **134**:986–1004.

Cochrane, C. G., and Wuepper, K. D., 1971b, in: *Sixth International Symposium of Immunopathology* (P. A. Miescher, ed.), pp. 220–235, Benno-Schwabe, Basel.

Cochrane, C. G., Revak, S. D., Aiken, B. S., and Wuepper, K. D., 1972a, in: *Inflammation: Mechanisms and Control* (I. H. Lepow and P. A. Ward, eds.), pp. 119–138, Academic Press, New York.

Cochrane, C. G., Wuepper, K. D., Aiken, B. S., Revak, S. D., and Spiegelberg, H. L., 1972b, *J. Clin. Invest.* **51**:2736–2745.

Cochrane, C. G., Revak, S. D., and Wuepper, K. D., 1973, *J. Exp. Med.* **138**:1564–1583.

Collier, H. O. J., 1976, in *The Chemistry and Biology of the Kallikrein–Kinin System in Health and Disease,* pp. 495–503, Fogarty International Center Proceedings No. 27, U.S. Govt. Printing Office, Washington, D.C.

Colman, R. W., Bagdasarian, A., Talamo, R. C., Scott, C. F., Seavey, M., Guimares, J. A., Pierce, J. V., and Kaplan, A. P., 1975, *J. Clin. Invest.* **56**:1650–1662.

Colten, H. R., 1974, in: *Progress in Immunology II,* Vol. 1 (L. Brent and E. J. Holborow, eds.), pp. 183–190, American Elsevier, New York.

Colvin, R. B., Johnson, R. A., Mihm, M. C., and Dvorak, H. F., 1973, *J. Exp. Med.* **138**:686–698.

Conradie, J. D., Volanakis, J. E., and Stroud, R. M., 1975, *Immunochemistry* **12**:967–971.

Cooper, N., 1969, *Science* **165**:396–398.

Cooper, N. R., 1975, *J. Exp. Med.* **141**:890–903.
Cooper, N. R., and Müller-Eberhard, H. J., 1970, *J. Exp. Med.* **132**:775–793.
Daha, M. R., Fearon, D. T., and Austen, K. F., 1976a, *J. Immunol.* **116**:1–7.
Daha, M. R., Fearon, D. T., and Austen, K. F., 1976b, *J. Immunol.* **116**:568–570.
Daha, M. R., Fearon, D. T., and Austen, K. F., 1976c, *J. Immunol.* **117**:630–639.
Damus, P. S., Hicks, M., and Rosenberg, R. D., 1973, *Nature (London)* **246**:355–357.
Davey, M. G., and Lüscher, E. F., 1967, *Nature (London)* **216**:857, 858.
Davie, E. W., and Fujikawa, K., 1975, *Annu. Rev. Biochem.* **44**:799–829.
Davies, G. E., and Lowe, J. S., 1962, *Int. Arch. Allergy Appl. Immunol.* **20**:235–250.
Dias de Silva, W., Eisele, J. W., and Lepow, I. H., 1967, *J. Exp. Med.* **126**:1027–1048.
Donaldson, V. H., Ratnoff, O. D., Dias de Silva, W., and Rosen, F. S., 1969, *J. Clin. Invest.* **48**:642–653.
Donaldson, V. H., Glueck, H. I., Miller, M. A., Hovat, H. Z., and Habal, F. M., 1976, *J. Lab. Clin. Med.* **87**:327–337.
Dukor, P., Schumann, G., Gisler, R. H., Dierick, M., König, W., Hadding, W., and Bitter-Suermann, D., 1974, *J. Exp. Med.* **139**:337–354.
Eisen, V., and Smith, H. G., 1970, *Br. J. Exp. Pathol.* **51**:328–331.
Engel, S. L., Schaeffer, T. R., Gold, B. I., and Rubin, B., 1972, *Proc. Soc. Exp. Biol. Med.* **140**:240–244.
Epstein, W. V., Tan, M., and Melmon, K. L., 1969, *Ann. N.Y. Acad. Sci.* **168**:173–187.
Erdös, E. G., 1966, *Adv. Pharmacol.* **4**:1–90.
Erdös, E. G. (ed.), 1970, *Handbook of Experimental Pharmacology*, Vol. XXV, Springer-Verlag, Berlin.
Erdös, E. G., and Sloane, E. M., 1962, *Biochem. Pharmacol.* **11**:585–592.
Erdös, E. G., and Yang, H. Y. T., 1970, in: *Handbook of Experimental Pharmacology*, Vol. XXV (E. G. Erdös, ed.) pp. 289–323, Springer-Verlag, Berlin.
Fearon, D. T., and Austen, K. F., 1975a, *J. Exp. Med.* **142**:856–863.
Fearon, D. T., and Austen, K. F., 1975b, *Proc. Natl. Acad. Sci. U.S.A.* **72**:3220–3224.
Fearon, D. T., and Austen, K. F., 1975c, *Ann. N.Y. Acad. Sci.* **256**:441–450.
Fearon, D. T., and Austen, K. F., 1976, *Essays in Medical Biochemistry* **2**:1–35.
Fearon, D. T., and Austen, K. F., 1977a, in: *Immunochemistry* (L. E. Glynn and M. Stewart, eds.), John Wiley and Sons, Chichester, England, in press.
Fearon, D. T., and Austen, K. F., 1977b, *Proc. Natl. Acad. Sci. U.S.A.* **74**:1683–1687.
Fearon, D. T., and Austen, K. F., 1977c, *J. Exp. Med.*, in press.
Fearon, D. T., Austen, K. F., and Ruddy, S., 1973, *J. Exp. Med.* **138**:1305–131.
Forbes, C. B., Pensky, J., and Ratnoff, O. D., 1970, *J. Lab. Clin. Med.* **76**:809–815.
Frank, M. M., Sergent, J. S., Kane, M. A., and Alling, D. W., 1972, *N. Engl. J. Med.* **286**:808–812.
Gelfand, J. A., Sherins, R. J., Alling, D. W., and Frank, M. M., 1976, *N. Engl. J. Med.* **295**:1444–1448.
Gigli, I., and Austen, K. F., 1969a, *J. Exp. Med.* **130**:833–846.
Gigli, I., and Austen, K. F., 1969b, *J. Exp. Med.* **129**:679–696.
Gigli, I., and Austen, K. F., 1971, *Annu. Rev. Microbiol.* **25**:309–332.
Gigli, I., and Nelson, R. A., 1968, *Exp. Cell Res.* **51**:45–67.
Gigli, I., Ruddy, S., and Austen, K. F., 1968, *J. Immunol.* **100**:1154–1164.
Gigli, I., Mason, J. W., Colman, R. W., and Austen, K. F., 1970, *J. Immunol.* **104**:574–581.
Gigli, I., Kaplan, A. P., and Austen, K. F., 1971, *J. Exp. Med.* **134**:1466–1484.
Goetzl, E. J., and Austen, K. F., 1974, in: *Chemotaxis, Biology and Biochemistry* (E. Sorkin, ed.), pp. 218–232, S. Karger, Basel.
Goldman, J. N., Ruddy, S., and Austen, K. F., 1972, *J. Immunol.* **109**:353–359.
Götze, O., and Müller-Eberhard, H. J., 1971, *J. Exp. Med.* **134**:90s–108s.
Greenbaum, L. M., and Kim, K. S., 1967, *Br. J. Pharmacol. Chemother.* **29**:238–247.
Griffin, J. H., and Cochrane, C. G., 1976, *Proc. Natl. Acad. Sci. U.S.A.* **73**:2554–2558.
Habal, F. M., Underdown, B. J., and Movat, H. Z., 1975, *Biochem. Pharmacol.* **24**:1241–1243.
Habermann, E., and Jahrreis, R., 1971, *Arch. Pharmakol.* **269**:101–111.
Harpel, P. C., 1970, *J. Exp. Med.* **132**:329–352.
Harpel, P. C., 1971, *J. Clin. Invest.* **50**:2084–2090.
Harpel, P. C., and Cooper, N. R., 1975, *J. Clin. Invest.* **55**:593–604.
Harrison, R. G., 1973, *Bibl. Anat.* **12**:458–459.
Heck, L. W., and Kaplan, A. P., 1974, *J. Exp. Med.* **140**:1615–1630.

Highsmith, R. F., and Rosenberg, R. D., 1974, *J. Biol. Chem.* **249**:4335–4338.
Hugli, T. E., Taylor, J. C., and Crawford, I. P., 1976, *J. Immunol.* **116**:1737 (abstract).
Hunsicker, L. G., Ruddy, S., and Austen, K. F., 1973, *J. Immunol* **110**:128–138.
Jacobsen, S., 1966, *Br. J. Pharmacol.* **26**:403–411.
Jacobsen, S., and Kriz, M., 1967, *Br. J. Pharmacol. Chemother.* **29**:25–36.
Johnson, A. R., and Erdös, E. G., 1973, *Proc. Soc. Exp. Biol. Med.* **142**:1252–1256.
Johnson, A. R., Hugli, T. E., and Müller-Eberhard, H. J., 1975, *Immunology* **28**:1067–1080.
Johnston, A. R., Cochrane, C. G., and Revak, S. D., 1974, *J. Immunol.* **113**:103–109.
Kaplan, A. P., Meier, H. L., Yecies, L. D., and Heck, L. W., 1976, in: *The Chemistry and Biology of the Kallikrein–Kinin System in Health and Disease*, pp. 237–254, Fogarty International Center Proceedings No. 27, Government Printing Office, Washington, D.C.
Kaplan, A. P., and Austen, K. F., 1970, *J. Immunol.* **105**:802–811.
Kaplan, A. P., and Austen, K. F., 1971, *J. Exp. Med.* **133**:696–711.
Kaplan, A. P., and Austen, K. F., 1972, *J. Exp. Med.* **136**:1378–1393.
Kaplan, A. P., Spragg, J., and Austen, K. F., 1971, in: *Second International Symposium on the Biochemistry of the Acute Allergic Reactions* (K. F. Austen and E. L. Becker, eds.), pp. 279–298, Blackwell Scientific Publications, Oxford.
Kaplan, A. P., Kay, A. B., and Austen, K. F., 1972, *J. Exp. Med.* **135**:81–97.
Kaplan, A. P., Goetzl, E. J., and Austen, K. F., 1973, *J. Clin. Invest.* **52**:2591–2595.
Kay, A. B., Pepper, D. S., and Ewart, M. R., 1973, *Nature (London) New Biol.* **243**:56–57.
Kellermeyer, R. W., and Breckenridge, R. T., 1965, *J. Lab. Clin. Med.* **65**:307–315.
Koethe, S. M., Austen, K. F., and Gigli, I., 1973, *J. Immunol.* **110**:390–400.
Kolb, W. P., Haxby, J. A., Arroyave, C. M., and Müller-Eberhard, H. J., 1972, *J. Exp. Med.* **135**:549–566.
Komiya, M., Kata, H., and Suzuki, T., 1972, *Biochem. Biophys. Res. Commun.* **49**:1438–1443.
Lachmann, P. J., Kay, A. B., and Thompson, R. A., 1970, *Immunology* **19**:895–899.
Lahiri, B., Rosenberg, R., Talamo, R. C., Mitchell, B., Bagdasarian, A., and Colman, R. W., 1974, *Fed. Proc. Fed. Am. Soc. Exp. Biol.* **33**:642A.
Lanchantin, G. F., Plesset, M. L., Friedman, J. A., and Hart, D. W., 1966, *Proc. Soc. Exp. Biol. Med.* **121**:444–449.
Leibowitz, M., Turino, G., and Greenbaum, L. M., 1976, in: *The Chemistry and Biology of the Kallikrein–Kinin System in Health and Disease*, Fogarty International Center Proceedings No. 27, U.S. Government Printing Office, Washington, D.C., in press.
Lepow, I. H., 1971, in: *Biochemistry of the Acute Allergic Reactions* (K. F. Austen and E. L. Becker, eds.), pp. 205–215, Blackwell Scientific Publications, Oxford.
Lepow, I. H., Naff, G. B., Todd, E. W., Pensky, J., Hinz, C. F. Jr., 1956, *J. Exp. Med.* **117**:983–1108.
Levine, B. W., Talamo, R. C., and Kazemi, H., 1973, *J. Applied Physiol.* **34**:821–826.
Londesborough, J. C., and Hamberg, U., 1975, *Biochem. J.* **145**:401–403.
MacKay, M. W., Miles, A. A., Schacter, M., and Wilhelm, D. L., 1953, *Nature (London)* **172**:714–716.
Mandle, R., Jr., and Kaplan, A. P., 1977, *Fed. Proc. Fed. Am. Soc. Exp. Biol.* **36**:329A.
Marder, V. J., and Shulman, N. R., 1969, *J. Biol. Chem.* **244**:2120–2124.
Margolis, J., 1958, *J. Physiol.* **144**:1–22.
Mayer, M. M., 1972, *Proc. Natl. Acad. Sci. U.S.A.* **69**:2954–2958.
McConnell, D. J., 1972, *J. Clin. Invest.* **51**:1611–1623.
McGiff, J. C., Itskovitz, H. D., Terragno, A., and Wong, P. Y.-K., 1976, *Fed. Proc. Fed. Am. Soc. Exp. Biol.* **35**:175–180.
Medicus, R. G., Schreiber, R. D., Götze, O., and Müller-Eberhard, H. J., 1976, *Proc. Natl. Acad. Sci. U.S.A.* **73**:612–616.
Morrison, D. C., and Cochrane, C. G., 1974, *J. Exp. Med.* **140**:797–811.
Moskowitz, R. W., Schwartz, H. J., Michel, B., Ratnoff, O. D., and Astrup, T., 1970, *J. Lab. Clin. Med.* **76**:790–798.
Movat, H. Z., and DiLorenzo, N. L., 1968, *Lab. Invest.* **19**:187–200.
Movat, H. Z., DiLorenzo, N. L., and Treloar, M. D., 1968, *Lab. Invest.* **19**:201–210.
Movat, H. Z., Poon, M. C., and Takeuchi, Y., 1971, *Int. Arch. Allergy Appl. Immunol.* **40**:89–112.
Movat, H. A., Steinberg, S. G., Habal, F. M., and Ranadive, N. S., 1973, *Lab. Invest.* **29**:669–684.
Müller-Eberhard, H. J., 1975, *Annu. Rev. Biochem.* **44**:697–724.
Müller-Eberhard, H. J., and Biro, C. E., 1963, *J. Exp. Med.* **118**:447–460.
Müller-Eberhard, H. J., and Götze, O., 1972, *J. Exp. Med.* **135**:1003–1008.

Müller-Eberhard, H. J., Polley, M. J., and Calcott, M. A., 1967, *J. Exp. Med.* **125**:359–380.
Nagasawa, S., Shiraishi, S., and Stroud, R. M., 1976, *J. Immunol.* **116**:1743 (abstract).
Nakajima, T., Oshima, G., Yeh, H. S. J., Igac, R., and Erdös, E. G., 1973, *Biochem. Biophys. Acta* **315**:430–438.
Newball, H. H., Talamo, R. C., and Lichtenstein, L. M., 1975, *Nature (London)* **254**:635, 636.
Nicol, P. A. E., and Lachmann, P. J., 1973, *Immunology* **24**:259–275.
Niewiarowski, S., Bankowski, E., and Rogowicka, I., 1965, *Throm. Diath. Haemorrh.* **14**:387–400.
Norman, P. S., and Hill, B. M., 1958, *J. Exp. Med.* **108**:639–649.
Osbahr, A. J., Gladner, J. A., and Laki, K., 1964, *Biochim. Biophys. Acta* **86**:535–542.
Østerud, B., and Rapaport, S. I., 1970, *Biochemistry* **9**:1854–1861.
Overturf, M., Wyatt, S., Boaz, D., and Fitz, A., 1975, *Life Sci.* **16**:1669–1681.
Patrick, R. A., Taubman, S. B., and Lepow, I. H., 1970, *Immunochemistry* **7**:217–225.
Pepys, M. B., 1974, *J. Exp. Med.* **140**:126–145.
Pierce, J. V., 1968, *Fed. Proc. Fed. Am. Soc. Exp. Biol.* **27**:52–57.
Pillemer, L., Blum, L., Lepow, I. H., Ross, O. A., Todd, E. W., and Wardlaw, A. C., 1954, *Science* **120**:279–285.
Poskitt, T. R., Fortwengler, H. P., Jr., and Lunskis, B., 1973, *J. Exp. Med.* **138**:715–722.
Ratnoff, O. D., 1972, *J. Lab. Clin. Med.* **80**:704–710.
Ratnoff, O. D., and Naff, G. B., 1967, *J. Exp. Med.* **125**:337–358.
Ratnoff, O. D., and Rosenblum, J. M., 1958, *Am. J. Med.* **25**:160–168.
Ratnoff, O. D., Pensky, J., Ogston, D., and Naff, G. B., 1969, *J. Exp. Med.* **129**:315–330.
Revak, S. D., Cochrane, C. G., Johnston, A. R., and Hugli, T. E., 1974, *J. Clin. Invest.* **54**:619–627.
Revak. S. D., Cochrane, C. G., and Griffin, J. H., 1976, *Fed. Proc. Fed. Am. Soc. Exp. Biol.* **35**:692.
Rosenberg, J. S., McKenna, P. W., and Rosenberg, R. D., 1975, *J. Biol. Chem.* **250**:8883–8888.
Ross, G. D., and Polley, M. J., 1974, *Fed. Proc. Fed. Am. Soc. Exp. Biol.* **33**:759.
Rosse, W. F., Logue, G. I., Silberman, H. R., and Frank, M. M., 1977, *Trans. Assoc. Am. Physicians* **89**:122–132.
Ruddy, S., and Austen, K. F., 1971, *J. Immunol.* **107**:742–750.
Ruddy, S., Gigli, I., and Austen, K. F., 1972, *N. Engl. J. Med.* **287**:489–495, 545–549, 592–596, 642–646.
Ryan, J. W., and Ryan, U. S., 1976, in: *The Chemistry and Biology of the Kallikrein–Kinin System in Health and Disease,* pp. 315–333, Fogarty International Center Proceedings No. 27, Government Printing Office, Washington, D.C.
Saito, H., Ratnoff, O. D., Waldmann, R., and Abraham, J. P., 1975, *J. Clin. Invest.* **55**:1082–1089.
Sakai, K., and Stroud, R. M., 1973, *J. Immunol.* **110**:1010–1020.
Schiffman, S., and Lee, P., 1974, *Br. J. Haematol.* **27**:101–114.
Schiffman, S., and Lee, P., 1975, *J. Clin. Invest.* **56**:1082–1092.
Schiffman, S., Lee, P., and Waldmann, R., 1975, *Thromb. Res.* **6**:451–454.
Schreiber, A. D., Kaplan, A. P., and Austen, K. F., 1973a, *J. Clin. Invest.* **52**:1394–1401.
Schreiber, A. D., Kaplan, A. P., and Austen, K. F., 1973b, *J. Clin. Invest.* **52**:1402–1409.
Schreiber, R. D., and Müller-Eberhard, H. J., 1974, *J. Exp. Med.* **140**:1324–1335.
Schwab, J., 1962, *Nature (London)* **195**:345–347.
Seegers, W. H., Cole, E. R., and Harmison, C. R., 1964, *Can. J. Biochem.* **42**:359–364.
Sheffer, A. L., Austen, K. F., and Rosen, F. S., 1972, *N. Engl. J. Med.* **287**:452–454.
Sheffer, A. L., Fearon, D. T., and Austen, K. F., 1977, *Ann. Int. Med.* **86**:306–308.
Soltay, M. J., Movat, H. Z., and Ozge-Anwar, A. H., 1971, *Proc. Soc. Exp. Biol. Med.* **138**:952–958.
Soter, N. A., Austen, K. F., and Gigli, I., 1974, *J. Invest. Dermatol.* **63**:219–226.
Soter, N. A., Austen, K. F., and Gigli, I., 1975, *J. Immunol.* **114**:928–932.
Spaulding, W. B., 1960, *Ann. Int. Med.* **53**:739–745.
Spitzer, R. E., Valotta, E. H., Forristal, J., Sudora, E., Stitzel, A., Davis, N. C., and West, C. D., 1969, *Science* **164**:436, 437.
Spragg, J., and Austen, K. F., 1971, *J. Immunol* **107**:1512–1519.
Spragg, J., and Austen, K. F., 1974, *Biochem. Pharmacol.* **23**:781–791.
Spragg, J., Talamo, R. C., and Austen, K. F., 1970, in: *Handbook of Experimental Pharmacology,* Vol. XXV (E. G. Erdös, ed.), pp. 531–549, Springer-Verlag, Berlin.
Stead, N., Kaplan, A. P., and Rosenberg, R. D., 1976, *J. Biol. Chem.* **251**:6481–6488.
Stewart, P. B., and Bliss, J. Q., 1957, *Br. J. Exp. Pathol.* **38**:462.
Stolfi, R., 1968, *J. Immunol.* **100**:46–54.

Stoner, J., Manganiello, V. C., and Vaughan, M., 1973, *Proc. Natl. Acad. Sci. U.S.A.* **70**:3830–3833.
Suzuki, T., Kato, H., and Komiya, M., 1973, in: *Proceedings of the Fifth International Congress of Pharmacology: Pharmacology and the Future of Man,* Vol. 5, pp. 296–306, S. Karger, Basel.
Tamura, N., and Nelson, R. A., 1967, *J. Immunol.* **99**:582–589.
Taylor, F. B., Jr., and Fudenberg, H., 1964, *Immunology* **7**:309–331.
Thomas, G., and West, G. B., 1973, *J. Pharm. Pharmacol.* **25**:747–748.
Thomas, G., and West, G. B., 1974, *Br. J. Pharmacol.* **50**:231–235.
Thompson, R. A., and Lachmann, P. J., 1970, *J. Exp. Med.* **131**:629–641.
Treloar, M. P., and Movat, H. Z., 1970, *Fed. Proc. Fed. Am. Soc. Exp. Biol.* **29**:576A.
Vallota, E. H., and Müller-Eberhard, H. J., 1973, *J. Exp. Med.* **137**:1109–1123.
Vallota, E. H., Hugli, T. E., and Müller-Eberhard, H. J., 1973, *J. Immunol.* **111**:294A.
Vane, J. R., 1971, *Nature (London) New Biol.* **231**:232–235.
Vogel, R., and Zickgraf-Rüdel, G., 1970, in: *Handbook of Experimental Pharmacology,* Vol. XXV (E. G. Erdös, ed.), pp. 550–578, Springer-Verlag, Berlin.
Waldmann, R., Rebuck, J. W., Saito, H., Abraham, J. P., Caldwell, J., and Ratnoff, O. D., 1975, Lancet 1:949–950.
Ward, P. A., 1967, *J. Exp. Med.* **126**:189–206.
Ward, P. A., and Hill, J. H., 1970, *J. Immunol.* **104**:535–543.
Ward, P. A., Cochrane, C. G., and Müller-Eberhard, H. J., 1966, *Immunology* **11**:141–153.
Webster, M. E., 1972, in: *Proceedings of the Fifth International Congress of Pharmacology,* p. 248A, S. Karger, Basel.
Webster, M. E., and Pierce, J. V., 1963, *Ann. N.Y. Acad. Sci.* **104**:91–107.
Weiler, J. M., Daha, M. R., Austen, K. F., and Fearon, D. T., 1976, *Proc. Natl. Acad. Sci. U.S.A.* **73**:3268–3272.
Weiss, A. S., Gallin, J. I., and Kaplan, A. P., 1974, *J. Clin. Invest.* **53**:622–633.
Whaley, K., and Ruddy, S., 1976, *J. Exp. Med.* **144**:1147–1163.
Wilner, G. D., Nossel, H. L., and LeRoy, E. C., 1968, *J. Clin. Invest.* **47**:2608–2615.
World Health Organization, 1968, *Bull. WHO* **39**:395.
Wuepper, K. D., 1972, in: *Inflammation: Mechanisms and Control* (I. H. Lepow and P. A. Ward, eds.), pp. 93–117, Academic Press, New York.
Wuepper, K. D., 1973, *J. Exp. Med.* **138**:1245–1355.
Wuepper, K. D., and Cochrane, C. G., 1971, in: *Second International Symposium on the Biochemistry of the Acute Allergic Reactions* (K. F. Austen and E. L. Becker, eds.), pp. 299–320, Blackwell Scientific Publications, Oxford.
Wuepper, K. D., Tucker, E., III, and Cochrane, C. G., 1970, *J. Immunol.* **105**:1307–1311.
Wuepper, K. D., Bokisch, V. A., Müller-Eberhard, H. J., and Stoughton, R. B., 1972, *Clin. Exp. Immunol.* **11**:13–20.
Wuepper, K. D., Miller, D. R., and Lacombe, M. J., 1975, *J. Clin. Invest.* **56**:1663–1672.
Yang, H. Y. T., Erdös, E. G., and Levin, Y., 1970, *Biochim. Biophys. Acta* **214**:374–376.
Yang, H. Y. T., Erdös, E. G., and Levin, Y., 1971, *J. Pharmacol. Exp. Ther.* **177**:291–300.
Zachariae, H., Malmquist, J., and Oates, J. A., 1966, *Life Sci.* **5**:2347–2355.
Zacharski, L. R., and Rosenstein, R., 1975, *Thromb. Res.* **64**:929–931.
Zucker, M. B., Grant, R. A., Alper, C. A., Goodkofsky, I., and Lepow, I. H., 1974, *J. Immunol.* **113**:1744–1751.

9

Prostaglandins in the Regulation of Immune and Inflammatory Responses

FREDERICK A. KUEHL, JR.

1. Introduction

Although the prostaglandins (PGs) were discovered in mammalian systems in the early 1930s (Kurzrok and Lieb, 1930; Goldblatt, 1933; von Euler, 1934) and shown to trigger many biological responses, appreciation of their wide spectrum of activities at the cellular level began only recently. Evidence showing a quantitative relationship between the action of PGs of the E type (PGEs) and increased intracellular levels of cyclic AMP (cAMP) (Kuehl *et al.*, 1970, 1972) explains the ability of these PGs to mimic the actions of many extracellular hormones and stimulators. cAMP has long been recognized to be the intracellular "second messenger" of certain hormone actions. The isolation of a membrane receptor unique to the PGEs (Kuehl and Humes, 1972) and the correlation between their affinity for this receptor and their ability to stimulate cAMP synthesis (Oien *et al.*, 1973) underline the importance of these PGs in cell regulation. Data suggesting that PGs of the F series act at a different receptor site to trigger increases in cyclic GMP (cGMP) levels (Kuehl *et al.*, 1973) are supported by the discovery of a receptor unique to $PGF_{2\alpha}$ in the ovine corpus luteum (Powell *et al.*, 1973). The reports that the contractile action of $PGF_{2\alpha}$ in veins is related to increased cGMP levels (Dunham *et al.*, 1974; Kadowitz *et al.*, 1975) are also consistent with this concept, but the interrelationship between cGMP and $PGF_{2\alpha}$ on the whole, remains to be elucidated further.

That PGEs and $PGF_{2\alpha}$ are the initial stable products formed from PG precursor acids, and that receptors unique to each exist, permits their classification as the primary PGs. Most studies have been confined to these two series. Recent research,

FREDERICK A. KUEHL, JR. • Merck Institute for Therapeutic Research, Rahway, New Jersey 07065.

mostly by Samuelsson and his associates (Hamberg and Samuelsson, 1974; Hamberg *et al.*, 1974), has now focused attention on the endoperoxide intermediates in the formation of these "primary prostaglandins" as well as on a new class of compounds, the thromboxanes (Hamberg *et al.*, 1975). These extremely labile compounds are far more potent than the primary PGs in many respects. However, data to show whether they act at the receptor level or directly on intracellular enzymatic processes remain to be established. In any event, it is necessary to include all these oxidation products of arachidonic acid (AA) in any consideration of "prostaglandins" as they relate to inflammation and the immune responses.

The complicated picture representing the synthesis and metabolism of the oxidation products of AA is shown schematically in Figure 1. The other major precursor acid of PGs, ecosatrienoic acid, which differs from AA in the absence of a double bond at the 5,6 position, has not been fully studied in terms of the exact nature of the intermediates in PG formation. However, this C_{20} acid should give products similar to those derived from AA, differing only in the absence of a 5,6

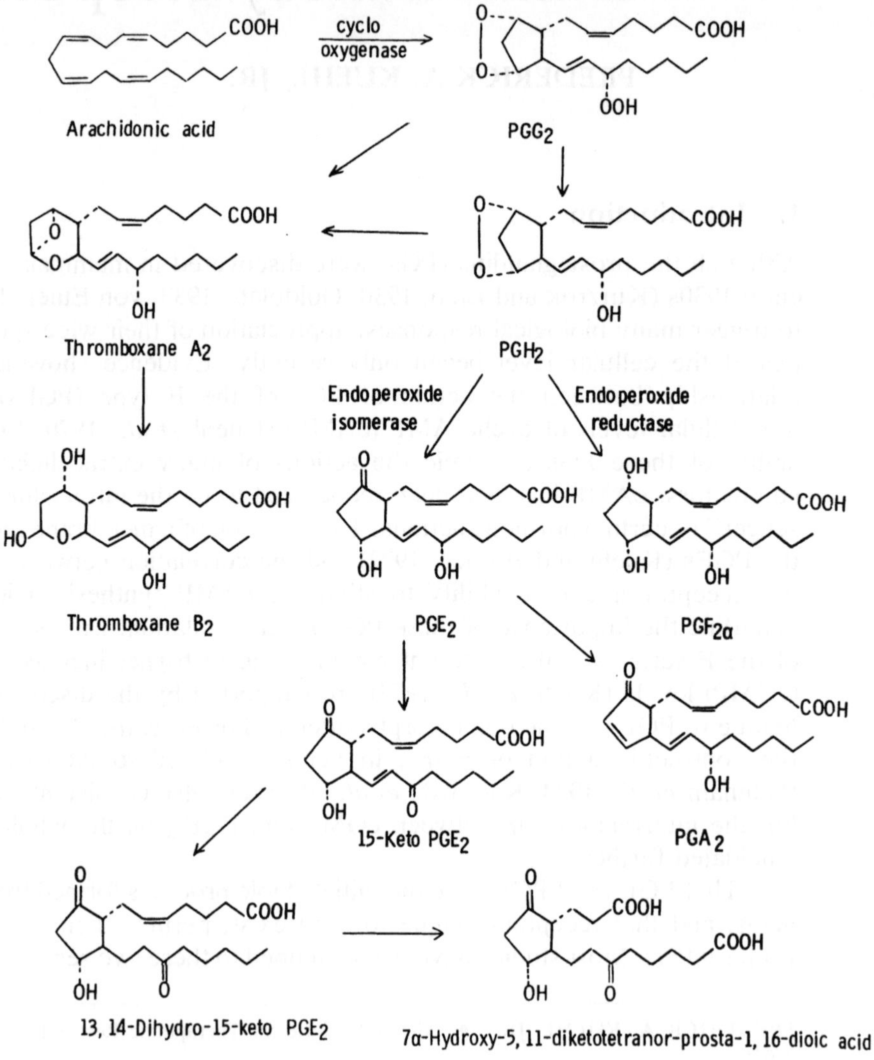

Figure 1. Synthesis and metabolism of prostaglandins and thromboxanes.

double bond. This series is distinguished by having a subscript 1 following the compound designation, as opposed to the products of the AA series, which are identified by the subscript 2 (i.e., PGE_1 vs. PGE_2).

As detailed in Figure 1, the PG precursor, AA, consumes molecular oxygen in the presence of a microsomal enzyme complex, generally referred to as "prostaglandin synthetase," to yield the primary PGs formed via the intermediates PGG_2 and PGH_2. No such conversion takes place with AA bound to phospholipids, the nominal precursor of the free AA pool. The intermediates, PGG_2 and PGH_2, predicted by Samuelsson (1965) to exist prior to their actual isolation were judged to be simply precursors of primary PGs and to play no biological role. However, with the recent isolation of these intermediates and the finding that they are far more active than $PGF_{2\alpha}$ or PGE_2 in eliciting contractile responses or inducing platelet aggregation, respectively (Hamberg and Samuelsson, 1973; Willis, 1974; Hamberg *et al.,* 1975), their function as potential intercellular regulators now must be acknowledged. The report by Hamberg *et al.* (1975) that thromboxane A_2 is the most potent platelet aggregator known, and its identification as the "rabbit-aorta contracting substance," require us to focus on this structure, which has a half-life of less than 1 min in solution. The growing importance of the thromboxanes is evident in the title of a forthcoming series of books on prostaglandins: *Advances in Prostaglandin and Thromboxane Research.* Unfortunately, little is yet known about the role of endoperoxides and thromboxanes as they relate to immunology, but an involvement of some kind seems likely. In Figure 1, the endoperoxide intermediates are converted by endoperoxide isomerase to PGE_1 (Miyamoto *et al.,* 1974). To date, there is no evidence for the existence of an endoperoxide reductase for the formation of PGF, although such an enzyme has been assumed. Since endoperoxide intermediates are readily converted to PGFs in a reducing medium, their chemical conversion in body tissues and fluids is a distinct possibility. The importance of the enzyme that converts PGE to PGF, PGE-9-ketoreductase, is just now beginning to be realized (Lee and Levine, 1974). This enzyme is present in a number of tissues, and is particularly abundant in the kidney. It has the unique property of being reversible, depending on whether cofactor NADP or NADPH is available (Lee and Levine, 1974).

The metabolism of PGEs, PGFs, and PGAs rapidly occurs by a cytosol enzyme(s), 15-hydroxyprostaglandin dehydrogenase, to yield the 15-keto derivative, which is then reduced by a 13,14-reductase to the 13,14-dihydro-15-keto derivative. Although evidence on this point is not clear, it is reasonable to conclude that primary PGs and these metabolites are released from the cell and enter the circulation to be converted by liver enzymes to the tetranorprostanoic acids, which are found in the urine in large amounts compared with the PGs themselves (Hamberg and Samuelsson, 1969). These latter tetranorprostanoic acids, identified for the PGE and PGF series, are believed to represent an accurate measurement of total PG production by the whole body.

2. Biological Function of the Prostaglandins

2.1. Prostaglandins of the E Type

If PGs of the E type function primarily by regulating intracellular cAMP levels, thereby mimicking the action of virtually all extracellular regulators, the key question is, "What is their role in cell regulation?" Since virtually every cell type, with the exceptions of the human red cell and lymphocyte, has the ability to synthesize PGs, and all types examined respond to PG action (Kuehl *et al.*, 1976), it is obvious that PG action must be ubiquitous. It seems unlikely that these substances can serve as hormones in the normal sense, because not only do they fail to survive circulation through the lung, kidneys, and liver, but also they lack target-organ specificity. This lack of specificity is evident from the remarkable similarities of the PGE receptors in the tissues examined (Kuehl, 1976), and no doubt accounts for the failure of administered PGEs and metabolically stable analogues to become important in the drug armamentarium. Despite the desired biological effects of PGEs in isolated systems, their too-wide spectrum of activities throughout the body vitiates their potential as widely useful drugs. The primary PGs (PGEs and $PGF_{2\alpha}$) appear to function as local or intercellular messengers, being formed in one tissue or cell type, and acting on the external receptor of a target cell near the site of formation. Examples of this interplay are the uterine production of $PGF_{2\alpha}$, which exerts a luteolytic action on the ovary in sheep (McCracken *et al.*, 1973), and the formation of PGEs in the kidney inner medulla, which presumably regulate the hemodynamics of the cortex (Herbaczynska-Cedro and Vane, 1973). The recent suggestions by Morley (1974) and Kurland and Moore (1976) that PGs formed by the macrophage act to raise cAMP levels and inhibit macrophage migration-inhibitory factor (MIF) release from the activated lymphocyte and to inhibit the action of colony-stimulating factor on the growth of macrophage precursors are good examples of intercellular interactions in circulating body fluids.

Studies with lipocytes revealed that the PGE receptor is closely related to membranous adenylate cyclase, but that there is no competition between stimulators (epinephrine, glucagon) for the PGE binding site (Oien *et al.*, 1973). A similar pattern of receptor independence has also emerged for the luteal cell PGE and luteinizing hormone receptors (Rao, 1973). Thus, it is necessary to visualize a receptor for PGE different from receptors of other hormones, but nevertheless associated with the same adenylate cyclase. The question whether this PGE receptor is on the inner or outer portion of the cell membrane (as with pituitary and other hormones) is, in terms of PG action, a critical one that remains to be answered. Overall, a large body of evidence supports the concept that primary PGs are formed and released from cells to interact with adjacent target cells, which could indeed include cells of the same type. It is reasonable to expect that the PG effect is terminated by an action of 15-hydroxyprostaglandin dehydrogenase.

2.2. Prostaglandin $F_{2\alpha}$

Although high levels of $PGF_{2\alpha}$ can raise cAMP levels, and thus mimic PGE action, this phenomenon is no doubt due to an interaction with the PGE receptor (Kuehl, 1974). It was not possible to demonstrate any antagonistic action of $PGF_{2\alpha}$ on PGE-induced increases of cAMP. Therefore, in situations in which PGEs and $PGF_{2\alpha}$ have opposing actions, it is necessary to invoke the existence of a receptor unique to $PGF_{2\alpha}$, as well as a mediator other than cAMP. Such a receptor was found in the membrane fraction of the ovine and bovine corpus luteum (Powell *et al.*, 1973), and must be considered specific for $PGF_{2\alpha}$, since $PGF_{1\alpha}$ has only a small fraction of the affinity of the former. The binding characteristics are consistent with the luteolytic actions of these PGs (Oien *et al.*, 1973). Thus, the presence of the 5,6 double bond is an obligatory requirement for PGF action, but not for the PGE series.

The suggestion that cGMP mediates the action of $PGF_{2\alpha}$ (Kuehl *et al.*, 1973) appears to be true in some instances. In the vein, where $PGF_{2\alpha}$ exerts a contractile effect, a rise in cGMP has been observed (Dunham *et al.*, 1974; Kadowitz *et al.*, 1975). The opposing relaxing effect of PGEs is associated with a rise in cAMP levels. Similarly, the opposing leukotactic effects of $PGF_{2\alpha}$ and PGE may also be related to cGMP and cAMP, respectively (Hill *et al.*, 1975). Thus, in situations in which $PGF_{2\alpha}$ counters the action of PGE_1, the opposing actions of the two nucleotides may be related. There is no evidence, however, to show that the luteolytic action of $PGF_{2\alpha}$ is mediated via cGMP.

Overall, it is evident that the relationship between $PGF_{2\alpha}$ and cyclic nucleotides is complex and is a function of the system under study. The receptor for $PGF_{2\alpha}$ does not appear to be ubiquitous, as is that for PGE. However, our understanding of PGF action at the cellular level needs further development.

2.3. Prostaglandins of the A Type

Although the coral, *Plexaura homomalla,* appears to have a unique synthetic pathway not involving endoperoxide intermediates for A-type PGs (Corey *et al.*, 1975), mammalian tissues apparently do not. All evidence thus far indicates that A-type PGs originating in mammalian tissue are derived from PGE, probably mainly by nonenzymatic conversion. Although an 11-dehydrase was described by Polet and Levine (1975) in human plasma, the conversion of PGE to PGA is very small, and the nonenzymatic blank is high. Studies by many groups, including our own, have failed to provide convincing evidence for the enzymatic conversion of AA to PGAs either via PGE or via an independent pathway. The ease with which PGEs are converted by PGAs in isolation procedures at a consistent ratio of about 20:1 casts doubt on the occurrence of an enzymatic formation of PGA in the body.

A-type PGs bind to the lipocyte PGE receptor (1/50th of PGE) and raise cAMP levels in ovarian tissue; there is a close correlation between these two events (Oien *et al.*, 1973). Thus, actions of PGAs can be explained by an interaction with the PGE receptor to raise cAMP levels. The higher potency of PGAs in certain applications *in vivo* (i.e., hypotensive actions) could be attributable to their binding to plasma proteins and consequent resistance to metabolism by the lung and other organs. Unlike other PGs, PGAs are unique in having a highly reactive 1-4 unsaturated carbonyl function capable of interacting covalently with the sulfhydryl group of glutathione, as well as with that of a number of SH-containing proteins (Ham *et al.*, 1975b). It is therefore possible that some effects of PGAs may represent nonspecific interactions with sulfhydryl groups at the enzyme level, and may thus have no physiologic significance.

3. Inflammatory and Immunologic Diseases

3.1. Prostaglandin–Glucocorticoid Interrelationships

The role of PGs in inflammatory diseases has been the subject of much controversy. With the discovery by Vane (1971) and his associates that nonsteroidal antiinflammatory agents such as aspirin and indomethacin are inhibitors of the synthesis of PGs in *in vitro* systems, a role for PGs was implied in those inflammatory diseases in which such drugs are effective. Action of PGs of the E type can be associated with vasodilation, edema, increases in temperature, and pain—components of inflammatory diseases that can be blocked by PG synthetase inhibitors. An extensive study by Ham *et al.* (1972) indicated a good correlation between the ability of nonsteroidal antiinflammatory agents, including active and inactive enantiomorphs, to inhibit PG synthesis *in vitro* with their activity in both the carrageenan paw-edema assay and *in vivo* antiinflammatory assays. Similar studies by other groups confirmed these initial findings, supporting the concept that PGs are causal in inflammatory diseases in which nonsteroidal antiinflammatory agents are effective.

The glucocorticoids have long been shown to be efficacious in many diseases, including conditions involving inflammation. Since these steroids are not effective PG synthetase inhibitors, their potent antiinflammatory activity has been considered to involve mechanisms not including PGs. The ability of corticosteroids to stabilize cell membranes and inhibit the release of proteolytic and hydrolytic enzymes has been considered to be a prime factor in their antiinflammatory activity. Recently, dexamethasone and hydrocortisone were shown to depress the production of PGE_2 and $PGF_{2\alpha}$ by rheumatoid synovial tissue in culture, although the mechanism by which this depression occurs was not defined (Kantrowitz *et al.*, 1975). There have been studies suggesting that corticosteroids may regulate PG transport (Lewis and Piper, 1975) and inhibit induction of PG synthetase (Kuehl *et al.*, 1975); however, these observations have not been confirmed. Recently, Gryglewski *et al.* (1975) demonstrated that corticosteroids inhibit release of PGs from perfused blood vessels and lung tissue. Since PGs are not believed to be stored, but synthesized on demand, release is generally equated with synthesis. Gryglewski and co-workers suggested that the effect of administered hydrocortisone involved a blockade of the release of substrate PG-precursor fatty acids from phospholipid stores. This interpretation was supported by the additional observation that coadministration of AA countered the action of hydrocortisone in depressing PG release. Direct evidence confirming this concept has now been provided at the cellular level by Hong and Levine (1976). These workers found that glucocorticoid pretreatment inhibited the release of AA induced by mechanical agitation, by the action of bradykinin, and by a component of human plasma on transformed NC5 cells. This depression of AA release paralleled a decreased release of PGs resulting from steroid treatment. Interestingly, a phospholipase inhibitor was also shown to inhibit PG production induced by bradykinin; this effect is consistent with an action of such stimulators to cause release of AA from phospholipid pools.

It is now evident from the studies cited above that there is a common denominator in the action of steroidal and nonsteroidal antiinflammatory agents in their ability to depress tissue PG levels. The mechanisms are quite different, however, the first being involved with inhibition of the enzyme PG synthetase and the second relating to substrate availability. On the basis of the many actions of glucocorticoids, it is reasonable to conclude that their action in depressing PG synthesis represents but one of many, and may be secondary to a stabilizing effect on the cell membrane. Additional studies are required to establish the precise mode of action of glucocorticoids in regulating the availability of PG precursor acids.

3.2. Models for Inflammatory Diseases

3.2.1. Topical Inflammation

Exposure to sunlight or ultraviolet (UV) light results in erythema of the skin, an effect well known to humans and also observed for shaved guinea pig and rabbit skin. The recent finding by Snyder and Eaglstein (1974) that indomethacin prevents this erythema even if administered as late as 18 hr after exposure of the skin implies that PGs are important in this process. This interpretation was strengthened by the finding (Kuehl *et al.*, 1975) that there is a significant increase in both PGE and PGF levels in guinea pig skin after exposure to UV light. Consistent with the expectation that this challenge is associated with an increase in the rate of microcirculation, a rise in cAMP but not cGMP levels accompanied this increase in epidermal PG levels. The method by which UV light stimulates PG synthesis is not known. However, isolation of guinea pig microsomes revealed no increased ability to synthesize PGs as a consequence of UV exposure (Kuehl *et al.*, 1975). Thus, it would appear that UV challenge alters availability of PG precursor acids. Such an interpretation is consistent with the effects of irradiation on the release of hydrolytic enzymes from the epidermis (Weissmann and Fell, 1962). The erythema and increase in skin PGs associated with scalding injury to guinea pig skin (Hamberg and Jensson, 1973) may arise through a similar mechanism.

Chemically induced irritation of the skin is accompanied by increases in PG levels (Goldyne *et al.*, 1973; Søndergaard *et al.*, 1974). A rise in PGs as a consequence of immunologic stimulus has also been noted. Both E and F PGs were greater in patients suffering from contact dermatitis (Greaves *et al.*, 1971). Thus, it is evident that increases in PG levels are common to many types of skin diseases associated with an irritation. At present, it is not possible to prove that the source of precursor acids or involved enzymes is in the epidermal tissue or in the invading white cells. However, the presence of AA as a major component of skin phospholipids and the ability of the epidermis to synthesize PGs (Ziboh, 1973; Kuehl *et al.*, 1975) would permit synthesis to be exclusive to the epidermis.

Van Arman (1974) recently described a model for measuring topically active antiinflammatory agents. In his system, the ability of compounds to depress the weight gain induced by topically applied croton oil on the mouse ear is the measure of their antiinflammatory activity. It is of interest that the skin mitogen 12-tetradecanoylphorbol-13-acetate (phorbol myristate acetate, PMA) in an appropriate vehicle elicits the same response (Van Arman and Kuehl, unpublished observation). Since PMA is a component of croton oil, it is reasonable to conclude that it is the prime factor in the croton oil response. PMA increases cGMP levels in many tissues and cell types, including fibroblasts and epidermal cells (Estensen *et al.*, 1974; Voorhees *et al.*, 1974). Interestingly, compounds with a wide range of activities are active in this test system, including PG synthetase inhibitors, glucocorticoids, a PGF antagonist, and some diuretic agents. The action of diuretic agents suggests that water transport and edema may be the major components of weight gain in this model.

3.2.2. Carrageenan Paw Edema

Carrageenan, a sulfated mucopolysaccharide derived from Irish sea moss, produces a characteristic swelling in the rat paw when injected therein. This model, which is considered to relate to human inflammatory diseases, led Winter *et al.* (1962) to the discovery of indomethacin long before this nonsteroidal antiinflammatory agent was known to be a PG synthetase inhibitor. The mechanism by which carrageenan elicits its response has not been rigorously established in terms of PG action for technical reasons. However, development by Willis (1969) of the technique in which carrageenan is introduced into an air bleb in the skin of the rat appears to be relevant to the joint assay. This procedure results in the formation of a blood-free edematous fluid that can be readily examined for cellular and subcellular components. As a consequence of studies with the air bleb, PGs, mainly of the E type, were found to accumulate (Anderson *et al.,* 1971) along with lysosomal enzymes over the 24-hr period following carrageenan injection. This finding led to the suggestion that invading white cells during the process of phagocytosis of the carrageenan particles release enzymes that liberate PG precursor acids from membrane phospholipids. As noted earlier, tissue levels of PGs are generally considered to be regulated by available PG precursor acids, not by alteration in PG synthetase activity. This interpretation is supported by the fact that introduction of phospholipase A alone into the air bleb (Whelan, 1974) caused a marked increase in PG levels. Further support for such an action of invading white cells is evident from studies by Van Arman (1974). He showed that treatment of rats with cyclophosphamide or 6-MP, drugs that acutely lower white cells, gave a direct correlation between the number of white cells and the degree of swelling in carrageenan-induced inflammation in the foot. At present, there is no evidence to delineate the source of PG precursor acids or PG synthetase activity, whether at the white cell or synovial tissue site.

3.2.3. Urate Crystal Edema

Intraarticular introduction of sodium urate crystals into the knee joint of the dog and the rat produces an inflammatory response that is believed to represent a model for human gouty arthritis (Faires and McCarty, 1962; Seegmiller *et al.,* 1962). The antimitotic and antiinflammatory agent colchicine, a drug used for centuries in the treatment of gout, is active in the urate crystal model in rats. Apparently its antimitotic activity is divorced from its antiedema activity (Denko and Whitehouse, 1970). PGs, particularly those of the E type, were shown to enhance urate crystal edema in rats (Denko, 1974a,b), and both these actions of PGE and urate crystals are countered by colchicine. On these grounds, it is reasonable to conclude that the challenge induced by urate crystals is one of increasing the synthesis of PGE in the joint. Since colchicine blocks the action of both PGE and urate crystals in the rat joint (Denko, 1975), it was concluded that this drug is acting counter to the action of PGEs (Denko, 1975); i.e., it is a PG antagonist, not a PG synthetase inhibitor. Consistent with a causal role of PGE in this model is the finding that both the PG synthetase inhibitor indomethacin and PGE antagonists are active in suppressing the inflammatory activity of urate crystals in the dog joint (Beveridge, personal communication). Inconsistent with a causal role are the findings by Rosenthale *et al.* (1972) and by Van Arman (personal communication) that direct injection of relatively large doses of PGE_1 or PGE_2 did not duplicate the effects of urate crystals. Van Arman (1974) was also unable to show colchicine to be active in the dog urate crystal gout model. The recent report by Robinson *et al.* (1975) that colchicine has the ability to stimulate the synthesis of PGE and PGF by a human rheumatic synovium may relate to the antimitotic action of colchicine, and if this stimulation occurs in the urate crystal model, it is necessary to conclude that the anti-PG activity of colchicine predominates to overcome the increase in tissue levels of PGs induced by this drug.

3.2.4. Adjuvant Arthritis

In the aforementioned models, a depression of PG synthesis is consistent with a beneficial action on the diseased state. On the other hand, adjuvant-induced arthritis in rats, a model believed to relate to delayed hypersensitivity, was shown to be suppressed by administration of high nonphysiologic doses of PGE to the intact animal (Zurier and Quagliata, 1971). This dichotomy was rationalized by many as attributable to the ability of PGEs to produce glucocorticoids either by a direct action on the adrenals or indirectly by stimulating the release of ACTH; such effects of PGs were demonstrated by, respectively, Flack *et al.* (1969) and DeWied *et al.* (1969). This interpretation was countered, however, by the subsequent observation that the beneficial effect of added PGE also occurs in adrenalectomized rats (Zurier *et al.*, 1973). It may well be that a feature predominates in this inflammatory model that is not characteristic of the aforementioned ones. When one considers the potential of PGEs to stimulate cAMP accumulation in virtually all cell types plus the evidence that cAMP action is associated with immunosuppression (see Chapters 1–4), it would appear necessary to focus on this aspect of PG action in the adjuvant arthritis model. Another possibility to be considered is that administered PGs may be incapable of mimicking the action of those formed endogenously. Thus, the action of high doses of PGEs may bear little relevance to the role of those formed *in situ* in inflammation.

3.3. Prostaglandins and Leukotaxis

Although Kaley and Weiner (1971) provided evidence that PGEs are chemotactic to rabbit neutrophils, subsequent studies in this regard have been conflicting. Others were unable to demonstrate a chemotactic response by any of a number of PGs examined, including PGE_1 (Diaz-Perez *et al.*, 1974). A single injection of PGE_1 in rats failed to cause any invasion of leukocytes (Arora *et al.*, 1970), although multiple injections of PGE_1 were reported to produce a mononuclear cell invasion in human skin (Søndergaard *et al.*, 1973). On the other hand, Søndergaard and Wolf-Jurgensen (1972), using a skin window technique, were unable to demonstrate any difference in the cellular response from added PGE_1 compared with a simultaneous control. Thus, there is little evidence to suggest that PGE is directly involved in leukotaxis. The recent report that inflammatory symptoms and appearance of PGs, but not the invasion of granulocytes, are blocked by sodium salicylate in urate crystal inflammation is consistent with this interpretation (Glatt and Brune, 1974). The inhibitory action of indomethacin on temperature, swelling, and PGE levels in joints of rabbits challenged intraarticularly with ovalbumin, but not on invasive leukocytes and phosphatase levels, may be interpreted in the same manner (Blackham *et al.*, 1974). The recent report that PGEs and cAMP inhibit leukotactic action of a chemotactic factor from *Escherichia coli*, whereas cGMP and $PGF_{2\alpha}$ enhance the chemotactic response by neutrophils, poses the possibility, however, that PGs acting through cyclic nucleotides may alter actions of known chemotactic agents (Hill *et al.*, 1975). A similar facilitative but opposite action of PGE_2 was indicated by McClatchey and Snyderman (1974), who reported that it enhanced the response of human mononuclear leukocytes to other chemotactic stimuli.

All in all, there is little reason to believe that primary PGs play an important role in chemotaxis, and the failure of PG synthetase inhibitors to block invasive leukocytes suggests that other PG intermediates are not chemotactic agents (Glatt and Brune, 1974; Turner *et al.*, 1975a). A recent report that the product of the lipoxygenase present in platelets, 12-L-hydroxy 5,8,10,14-eicosatetranoic acid (HETE), is chemotactic to human neutrophils and is the sole chemotactic agent produced by incubation of platelets with AA may be very relevant to the process of inflammation (Turner *et al.*, 1975a,b). This finding is particularly interesting, since, unlike the cyclooxygenase that produces thromboxanes, the formation of the chemotactic product (HETE) derived from the reaction of AA with lipoxygenase is not inhibited by indomethacin (Hamberg and Samuelsson, 1975).

3.4. Intercellular Messenger Role of Prostaglandins

Since the actions of PGs on specific cell types involved with inflammatory and immune responses are discussed in detail in other chapters of this book, this subject is discussed only briefly here. In general, in situations in which a cellular response is associated with a rise in cAMP, PGEs will elicit the same response—a fact compatible with the actions of PGEs being mediated via cAMP. The actions of PGFs are either not observed or generally mimic PGE responses weakly. The data in Table 1 summarize the actions of PGs in relevant cells, indicating the ability of these cells to produce and respond to PGs, as well as the systems in which these cells play key roles. Interrelationships among cells in terms of the precise functions of PGs can only be speculated on at this time.

As shown in Table 1, with the possible exception of lymphocytes, all cells involved in immunologic responses have the capacity to synthesize PGEs. These cells include neutrophils, macrophages, synoviocytes, basophils, and eosinophils. On the other hand, every cell type in this category, including stimulated but not unstimulated lymphocytes, has the capacity to respond to exogenous PGEs. This ability to respond to PGEs implies the existence of receptors to PGEs that appear to be located on the external surface of the cell. Thus, the difficulties of establishing which cell types release PGs and which respond to these compounds in mixed cell populations becomes apparent.

The function of leukocytes in inflammation is not well understood, and in fact there is no agreement on the chemotactic mechanism by which they accumulate at the inflammed site. There is a consensus, however, that neutrophils represent the first cell type to arrive at the site of inflammation, and release lysosomal enzymes during phagocytosis that may be instrumental in providing available precursors for PG production. With time, in inflammation of a more chronic nature, macrophages play a more dominant role, and their ability to release PGs led to the concept proposed by Morley (1974) that MIF, derived from activated T lymphocytes, stimulates formation in macrophages of PGEs, which act on the lymphocytes as negative-feedback inhibitors to prevent MIF release. They suggest further that

TABLE 1. Prostaglandin Involvement with Cells in Immune and Inflammatory Responses

Cell type	Action	Functional role	Nucleotide action (see Chapters 1–7)	PGE action	PG synthetase activity	References[a]
T lymphocyte Rat, mouse	Immune cytolysis	Cell-mediated immunity	cAMP inhibits cytolysis and proliferation. cGMP stimulates proliferation.	cAMP resonse	–	2, 12
Man	Interferon production	Cell-mediated immunity	cAMP inhibits.	cAMP response	–	6
B lymphocyte, mouse	Plaque formation on SRBC	Humoral immunity (HI)	cAMP inhibits HI and proliferation. cGMP stimulates (HI) and proliferation.	cAMP response	–	15
Neutrophils	Phagocytosis, release of lysosomal enzymes	Acute inflammation	cAMP inhibits, cGMP stimulates, release of lysosomal enzyme from human neutrophils. cAMP inhibits fusion of PMN granules with plasma membrane.	cAMP response	+	7, 14, 19
Macrophages	Respond to MIF, resulting in increased phagocytosis, PG production, and neutral protease secretion. Release lysosomal enzymes in response to inflammatory stimuli.	Chronic inflammation	cAMP inhibits MIF activity.	cAMP response	+	3, 5, 10, 16
Basophil, human	Histamine release	Immediate hypersensitivity	cAMP inhibits histamine release.	cAMP response	+	11, 13
Mast cell, human	Histamine, SRS-A release	Immediate hypersensitivity	cAMP inhibits.	cAMP response	+	1, 9, 18
Eosinophil	Releases EDI (PGE) to inhibit histamine release from mast cell; also nonphagocytic activity.	Immediate hypersensitivity	?	?	+	4, 8
Synoviocyte, human	Production of synovial fluid?	Inflammation, rheumatoid arthritis	?	Increases cAMP.	+	17

[a] **(1)** Assem and Schild (1969); **(2)** Bourne *et al.* (1972); **(3)** Bray *et al.* (1974); **(4)** Eidinger *et al.* (1962); **(5)** Gemsa *et al.* (1975); **(6)** Henney (1973); **(7)** Hoffstein *et al.* (1974); **(8)** Hubscher (1975); **(9)** Ishizaka *et al.* (1971); **(10)** Koopman *et al.* (1973); **(11)** Lichtenstein and Margolis (1968); **(12)** Lichtenstein *et al.* (1972); **(13)** Lichtenstein *et al.* (1973); **(14)** McCall and Youlton (1973); **(15)** Melmon *et al.* (1974a); **(16)** Myatt *et al.* (1975); **(17)** Newcombe *et al.* (1975); **(18)** Tauber *et al.* (1973); **(19)** Zurier *et al.* (1973, 1974).

under conditions in which the lymphocytes are unresponsive to this negative-feedback action, the macrophages produce excessive amounts of PGs, which produce the symptoms of inflammation. In addition to a release of MIF, lymphocytes also have the capacity of destroying target cells and releasing chemotactic, cytotoxic, and mitogenic agents. In rheumatoid arthritis, which is considered to be an autoimmune disease, the lymphocytes are believed to have lost their ability to distinguish between foreign and host cell types; the result is destruction of the joints.

If one adds to the relationships discussed above the demonstrated ability of synovial cells to produce PGs, it is readily understood why the contribution of each cell type, in terms of PG formation and action, is slow to evolve, and thus is one that requires careful examination. Studies of the actions of added PGEs, PGE antagonists, and PG synthetase inhibitors must be carried out in cell preparations containing at most two distinct cell populations to clarify this complicated picture. Such studies may provide firmer evidence for the roles of each individual cell in the milieu normally encountered at the site of inflammation or of immunologic response.

3.5. Immunosuppressive Role of Prostaglandins

PGs of the E type have been found to elicit immunosuppressive responses by increasing intracellular cAMP levels. In *in vitro* studies, PGEs have been shown to inhibit lysosomal enzyme release from human leukocytes exposed to immune complexes and other particles (Weissmann *et al.*, 1971), inhibit release of IgE-dependent immunoglobulin induced by histamine from human basophils (Lichtenstein *et al.*, 1972), inhibit cytolytic activity of sensitized allogeneic mouse lymphocytes (Lichtenstein *et al.*, 1972), inhibit transformation of human lymphocytes after exposure to phytohemagglutinin (Smith *et al.*, 1971), inhibit lymphokine secretion from sensitized human lymphocytes (Bray *et al.*, 1974), reduce granulocyte adhesion (Bryant and Sutcliffe, 1974), and suppress 19S antibody production by mouse lymphocytes sensitized to sheep red blood cells (SRBC) (Melmon *et al.*, 1974a).

There is a large body of evidence to support the belief that the unabated cell proliferation associated with cancer is due to a suppression of the immunologic response. High levels of PGEs have been found to be present in many cancerous conditions, including neurogenic tumors, pheochromocytomas, and carcinoid and pancreatic tumors (Sandler *et al.*, 1968; Jaffe *et al.*, 1973; Kaplan *et al.*, 1973). A similar high level of PGs was noted in HSDM cells in culture (Levine *et al.*, 1972) and in Maloney sarcoma virus (MSV)-induced tumors in rats (Humes and Strausser, 1974), a level that could in both instances be lowered by indomethacin. Thus, there is generally but not always an increase in PG levels associated with tumor growth in the situations studied. Although one cannot be certain at this time whether PGs are causal or simply a reflection of tissue damage, the *in vitro* effects of PGEs in causing immunosuppression suggest that PGEs may play a similar role *in vivo*, i.e., that tumors secrete large amounts of PGEs and thus allow the tumor to escape immune surveillance. Evidence that this may be the case is strengthened from studies by Humes and Strausser (1974), who showed that indomethacin treatment suppressed the growth of MSV-induced tumors in antilymphocyte-serum-treated mice. Plescia *et al.* (1975) showed that the PGs produced by tumor cells caused mice that bore various types of tumors to be immunologically unresponsive to SRBC. This unresponsiveness, as well as tumor growth *in vivo*, was depressed by treatment with indomethacin.

Since graft rejection represents an immunologic response, PGEs would be expected to be beneficial in preventing this phenomenon. Although PGE_1 had little effect by itself, this PG was found to synergize with and prolong the effect of the immunosuppressive agent procarbazine in lengthening the survival time of A/J tail skin grafts on CBA/J mice (Quagliata *et al.*, 1973). Clearly, this area is one worthy of further study.

4. Summary and Speculation

It is very difficult to evolve a cohesive picture of the role(s) of prostaglandins in inflammatory and immunologic processes if one considers a PGE–receptor-cAMP sequential relationship alone. True, there does appear to be an interrelationship between $PGF_{2\alpha}$ and cGMP in eliciting an effect opposite to PGEs in some instances, but there are few data supporting the concept that the ratio between $PGF_{2\alpha}$ and PGEs is regulatory in many systems related to the subject of this discussion. Yet, the fact remains that it is very difficult to assign the antiinflammatory action of PG synthetase inhibitors only to inhibition of PGE and consequently cAMP. As an alternative, it is possible to turn to other oxidation products of arachidonic acid blocked by PG synthetase inhibitors to explain more satisfactorily the action of such drugs.

As shown in Figure 1, PGG_2, PGH_2, and thromboxane A_2, which are all products of the oxidation of AA, although they are not "primary prostaglandins," are in fact inhibited by the action of indomethacin, since indomethacin blocks the initial step in the sequence (Egan, personal communication). Thromboxane B_2 is less active, and may simply be a metabolic or degradation product of its precursor, thromboxane A_2. There is little evidence in print indicating that thromboxanes can be produced in tissues other than the spleen, lung, leukocytes, and platelets, but such a possibility seems likely. And, of course, since PGG_2 and PGH_2 are intermediates in the formation of PGE_2 and $PGF_{2\alpha}$, they are necessarily present, if only transiently, in all tissues that exhibit PG synthetase activity. If one considers the roles of these compounds in the few instances examined, it is evident that the unstable oxidation products of AA, which we can consider to include PGG_2, PGH_2 and thromboxane A_2, act to oppose the action of PGEs in increasing cAMP levels. PGH_2 was shown to inhibit adenylate cyclase in fat cell ghosts (Gorman *et al.*, 1975); PGG_2, PGH_2, and thromboxanes were all shown to be extremely potent stimulators of the contraction of smooth muscle (Hamberg *et al.*, 1974), a response that was associated with rises in cGMP levels (Goldberg *et al.*, 1975). These labile compounds were also shown to trigger platelet aggregation (Hamberg and Samuelsson, 1973), an effect that was also suggested to relate to increased levels of cGMP (Goldberg *et al.*, 1975). Thus, it is reasonable to conclude that the actions of these compounds are associated with responses triggered by cGMP, which in many instances have been shown to oppose cAMP effects. As noted earlier, the close relationship between the binding of PGEs to membranous receptors (Oien *et al.*, 1976) and the relative stability of such PGs are consistent with an intercellular role of PGEs, wherein they act as local messengers in cell regulation. On the other hand, the ephemeral nature of the labile AA oxidation products would militate against their major role as intercellular messengers. A more likely function of these compounds would be an action within the cells that produce them, and hence a direct action on adenylate and guanylate cyclases. As noted above, PGH_2 inhibits adenylate cyclase in fat cells (Gorman *et al.*, 1975). Direct studies of the action of labile AA products on guanylate cyclase have not been reported. Nevertheless, indirect evidence requires that the action of PG synthetase inhibitors in inflammatory reactions be considered in terms of their ability to depress such oxygenated AA products as well as PGEs, and hence the cGMP as well as cAMP responses. Thus, the action of PG synthetase inhibitors would depend on the nature of the system studied, i.e., on whether cAMP or cGMP predominates or whether the two cyclic nucleotides play mixed roles.

There is general agreement that the heat, pain, and erythema involved in inflammatory responses can be associated with rises in PGE levels, and that these effects are diminished by administration of PG synthetase inhibitors. On the other hand, there are no data to show that such drugs limit the number and nature of invasive leukocytes; in fact, there are data to show that they do not. As noted earlier, there is little evidence that either the primary PGs or their precursors have chemotactic properties, although the latter compounds have not been thoroughly studied in this regard. The apparent requirement for the presence of white cells for the inflammatory response neither excludes nor supports the possibility that removal of PGEs by indomethacin represents the sole antiinflammatory action elicited by the drug in this model. On the other hand, accumulating evidence that release of lysomal enzymes is largely responsible for tissue and joint destruction in inflammation, particularly in chronic inflammation, raises the question why the decrease in PGE levels does not facilitate the destructive process by depressing the inhibitory action of cAMP on enzyme release. Inhibition of PGE synthesis alone would therefore tend to facilitate the release of destructive lysosomal enzymes. Since lymphocyte proliferation and release of lysosomal enzymes have been shown to be associated with rises in cGMP levels (see Chapters 1, 2, and 4), invoking a role for PGG_2, PGH_2, or thromboxane A_2, or any combination thereof, in initiating this response permits one to suggest that PG synthetase inhibitors could also block release of lysosomal enzymes by this mechanism. In fact, it was suggested that the important action of indomethacin is to depress release of lysosomal enzymes (Van Arman, 1974). The recent finding that indomethacin inhibits the release of lysosomal enzymes from macrophages (Finlay *et al.*, 1975) may be interpreted to support this mechanism, although its possible action to increase cAMP levels by its inhibition of cAMP phosphodiesterase cannot be excluded, and this action would be expected to block the release of lysosomal enzymes.

In considering a dual action of PG synthetase inhibitors, it is evident that total blockade of PGG_2 would also completely eliminate the formation of PGEs. It is unreasonable, however, to expect total blockade to be effected by any drug *in vivo*. Furthermore, it must be remembered that endoperoxide isomerase, the enzyme that forms PGEs, may vary depending on the system under study. Such a possibility is suggested by studies in the rat uterus, in which, under estrogen domination (at estrus), PGF is produced almost exclusively, whereas at other times of the cycle, both PGF and PGE can be detected (Ham *et al.*, 1975a). Finally, studies in lymphocytes and other tissues (Melmon *et al.*, 1974b; see Chapter 16; Kuehl *et al.*, 1974) showing that the PG receptor is separate from other receptors that regulate cAMP levels must remind one that cyclic nucleotide levels are surely not determined by PGs alone. Other mediators also play a role. Thus, the assignment of a modulating role to PGs best describes the current beliefs. Obviously, there are many facets to the mechanisms involving inflammation and immunologic diseases, of which PGs are only one. It is evident that our current knowledge of the action of PGs in inflammatory and immunologic diseases represents only the tip of the iceberg of knowledge on this subject.

References

Anderson, A. J., Brocklehurst, W. E., and Willis, A. L., 1971, *Pharmacol. Res. Commun.* **3**:13–19.
Arora, S., Lahiri, P. K., and Sangal, R. K., 1970, *Int. Arch. Allergy Appl. Immunol.* **39**:186–191.
Assem, E. S. K., and Schild, H. W., 1969, *Nature (London)* **224**:1028–1029.
Blackham, A., Farmer, J. B., Radziwonik, H., and Westwick, J., 1974, *Br. J. Pharmacol.* **51**:35–44.
Bourne, H. R., Lichtenstein, L. M., and Melmon, K. L., 1972, *J. Immunol.* **108**:695–705.
Bray, M. A., Gordon, D., and Morley, J., 1974, *Br. J. Pharmacol.* **52**:453P.
Bryant, R. E., and Sutcliffe, M. C., 1974, *J. Clin. Invest.* **54**:1241–1244.
Corey, E. J., Ensley, H. E., Hamberg, M., and Samuelsson, B., 1975, *J. Chem. Soc. Chem. Commun.*, pp. 277–278.
Denko, C. W., 1974a, *Rheumatism* **1**:222–229.
Denko, C. W., 1974b, *Pharmacology* **12**:331–339.
Denko, C. W., 1975, *Pharmacology* **13**:219–227.
Denko, C. W., and Whitehouse, M. W., 1970, *Pharmacology* **3**:229–242.
DeWied, D., Witter, A., Versteeg, H. G., and Mulder, A. A., 1969, *Endocrinology* **85**:561–569.
Diaz-Perez, J. L., Goldyne, M. E., and Winkelmann, R. K., 1974, *Clin. Res.* **22**:575A.
Dunham, E. W., Haddox, M. K., and Goldberg, N. D., 1974, *Proc. Natl. Acad. Sci. U.S.A.* **71**:815–819.
Eidinger, D., Raff, M., and Rose, B., 1962, *Nature (London)* **196**:683–684.
Estensen, R. D., Hadden, J. W., Hadden, E. M., Touraine, J. L., Haddox, M. K., and Goldberg, N. D., 1974, in: *Control of Proliferation in Animal Cells* (B. Clarkson and R. Baserga, eds.), pp. 627–634, Cold Spring Harbor Press, Cold Spring Harbor, New York.
Faires, J. S., and McCarty, D. J. G., 1962, *Lancet* **2**:682–685.
Finlay, C., Davies, P., and Allison, A. C., 1975, *Agents and Actions* **5**:345–354.
Flack, J. D., Jessup, R., and Ramwell, P. W., 1969, *Science* **163**:691–692.
Gemsa, D., Stessemann, L., Menzel, J., and Till, G., 1975, *J. Immunol.* **114**:1422–1424.
Glatt, M., and Brune, K., 1974, *Arch. Pharmacol.* **284**:R21.
Goldberg, N. D., Haddox, M. K., Nicol, S. E., Glass, D. B., Sanford, C. H., Kuehl, F. A., Jr., and Estensen, R., 1975, in: *Advances in Cyclic Nucleotide Research* (G. I. Drummond, P. Greengard, and G. A. Robison, eds.), Vol. 5, pp. 307–330, Raven Press, New York.
Goldblatt, M. W., 1933, *J. Soc. Chem. Ind. London* **52**:1056–1057.
Goldyne, M. E., Winkelmann, R. K., and Ryan, R. J., 1973, *Prostaglandins* **4**:737–749.
Gorman, R. R., Hamberg, M., and Samuelsson, B., 1975, *J. Biol. Chem.* **250**:6460–6463.
Greaves, M. W., Sondergaard, J. S., and McDonald-Gibson, W., 1971, *Br. Med. J.* **2**:258–260.
Gryglewski, R. J., Panczenko, B., Korbut, R., Grodzinska, L., and Ocetkiewicz, K., 1975, *Prostaglandins* **10**:343–348.
Ham, E. A., Cirillo, V. J., Zanetti, M., Shen, T. Y., and Kuehl, F. A., Jr., 1972, in: *Prostaglandins in Cellular Biology* (P. Ramwell and B. Pharris, eds.), pp. 345–352, Plenum Press, New York.
Ham, E. A., Cirillo, V. J., Zanetti, M. E., and Kuehl, F. A., Jr., 1975a, *Proc. Natl. Acad. Sci. U.S.A.* **72**:1420–1424.
Ham, E. A., Oien, H. G., Ulm, E. H., and Kuehl, F. A., Jr., 1975b, *Prostaglandins* **10**:217–229.
Hamberg, M., and Jensson, C., 1973, *Acta Physiol. Scand.* **87**:240–245.
Hamberg, M., and Samuelsson, B., 1969, *J. Am. Chem. Soc.* **91**:2177, 2178.
Hamberg, M., and Samuelsson, B., 1973, *Proc. Natl. Acad. Sci. U.S.A.* **70**:899–903.
Hamberg, M., and Samuelsson, B., 1974, *Biochem. Biophys. Res. Commun.* **61**:942–949.
Hamberg, M., Svensson, J., Wakabayashi, T., and Samuelsson, B., 1974, *Proc. Natl. Acad. Sci. U.S.A.* **71**:345–349.
Hamberg, M., Svensson, J., and Samuelsson, B., 1975, *Proc. Natl. Acad. Sci. U.S.A.* **72**:2944–2948.

Henney, C. S., 1973, *Transplant. Rev.* **47**:37–70.
Herbaczynska-Cedro, K., and Vane, J. R., 1973, *Circ. Res.* **33**:428–436.
Hill, H. R., Estensen, R. D., Quie, P., Hogan, N. A., and Goldberg, N. D., 1975, *Metabolism* **24**:447–456.
Hoffstein, S., Zurier, R. B., and Weissmann, G., 1974, *Clin. Immunol. Immunopathol.* **3**:201–217.
Hong, S. L., and Levine, L., 1976, *Proc. Natl. Acad. Sci. U.S.A.* **73**:1930–1934.
Hubscher, T., 1975, *J. Immunol.* **114**:1389–1393.
Humes, J. L., and Strausser, H. R., 1974, *Prostaglandins* **5**:183–196.
Ishizaka, T., Ishizaka, K., Orange, R. P., and Austin, K. F., 1971, *J. Immunol.* **106**:1267–1273.
Jaffe, B. M., Behrman, H. R., and Parker, C. W., 1973, *J. Clin. Invest.* **52**:398–405.
Kadowitz, P. J., Joiner, P. D., Hyman, A. L., and George, W. J., 1975, *J. Pharmacol. Exp. Ther.* **192**:677–686.
Kaley, G., and Weiner, R., 1971, *Ann. N.Y. Acad. Sci.* **180**:338–350.
Kantrowitz, F., Robinson, D. R., McGuire, M. B., and Levine, L., 1975, *Nature (London)* **258**:737–739.
Kaplan, E. L., Sizemore, G. W., Peskin, G. W., and Jaffe, B. M., 1973, *Surgery* **74**:21–29.
Koopman, W. J., Gillis, M. H., and David, J. R., 1973, *J. Immunol.* **110**:1609–1614.
Kuehl, F. A., Jr., 1974, *Prostaglandins* **5**:325–340.
Kuehl, F. A., Jr., 1976, in: *Molecular Aspects of Hormone Receptor Interactions* (G. Levey, ed.), pp. 385–400. Marcel Dekker, New York.
Kuehl, F. A., Jr., and Humes, J. L., 1972, *Proc. Natl. Acad. Sci. U.S.A.* **69**:480–484.
Kuehl, F. A., Jr., Humes, J. L., Tarnoff, J., Cirillo, V. J., and Ham, E. A., 1970, *Science* **169**:883–886.
Kuehl, F. A., Jr., Humes, J. L., Cirillo, V. J., and Ham, E. A., 1972, in: *Advances in Cyclic Nucleotide Research* (P. Greengard, G. A. Robison, and R. Paoletti, eds.), Vol. I, pp. 493–502, Raven Press, New York.
Kuehl, F. A., Jr., Cirillo, V. J., Ham, E. A., and Humes, J. L., 1973, in: *Advances in the Biosciences* (S. Bergström and S. Bernhard, eds.), pp. 155–172, Pergamon Press, Oxford.
Kuehl, F. A., Jr., Ham, E. A., Zanetti, M. E., Sanford, C. H., Nicol, S. E., and Goldberg, N. D., 1974, *Proc. Natl. Acad. Sci. U.S.A.* **71**:1866–1870.
Kuehl, F. A., Jr., Cirillo, V. J., Zanetti, M. E., Beveridge, G. C., and Ham, E. A., 1976, *Agents and Actions* **6**:165–170.
Kuehl, F. A., Jr., Cirillo, V. J., and Oien, H. G., 1976, in: *Prostaglandins—Chemical and Biochemical Aspects* (S. Karim, ed.), pp. 191–225, Oxford Wiley Interscience, U.K.
Kurland, J. I., and Moore, M. A. S., 1976, *Fed. Proc. Fed. Am. Soc. Exp. Biol.* **35**:251 (abstract).
Kurzrok, R., and Lieb, C. C., 1930, *Proc. Soc. Exp. Biol. Med.* **28**:268–272.
Lee, S.-C., and Levine, L., 1974, *J. Biol. Chem.* **249**:1369–1375.
Levine, L., Hinkle, P. M., Voelkel, E. E., and Tashjian, A. H., Jr., 1972, *Biochem. Biophys. Res. Commun.* **47**:888–896.
Lewis, G. P., and Piper, P. J., 1975, *Nature (London)* **254**:308–311.
Lichtenstein, L. M., and Margolis, S., 1968, *Science* **161**:902–903.
Lichtenstein, L. M., Gillespie, E., Bourne, H. R., and Henney, C. S., 1972, *Prostaglandins* **2**:519–528.
Lichtenstein, L. M., Henney, C. S., Bourne, H. R., and Greenough, W. B., III, 1973, *J. Clin. Invest.* **52**:691–697.
McCall, E., and Youlton, L. J. F., 1973, *J. Physiol.* **234**:99–99P.
McClatchey, W., and Snyderman, R., 1974, *Clin. Res.* **22**:243A.
McCracken, J. A., Barcikowski, B., Carlson, J. C., Gréen, K., and Samuelsson, B., 1973, in: *Advances in the Biosciences* (S. Bergström and S. Bernhard, eds.), Vol. 9, pp. 599–624, Pergamon Press, Oxford.
Melmon, K. L., Bourne, H. R., Weinstein, Y., Shearer, G. M., Kram, J., and Bauminger, S., 1974a, *J. Clin. Invest.* **53**:13–21.
Melmon, K. L., Weinstein, Y., Shearer, G. M., and Bourne, H. R., 1974b, in: *Cyclic AMP, Cell Growth, and the Immune Response* (W. Braun, L. M. Lichtenstein, and C. W. Parker, eds.), pp. 114–134, Springer-Verlag, New York.
Miyamoto, T., Yamamoto, S., and Hayaishi, O., 1974, *Proc. Natl. Acad. Sci. U.S.A.* **71**:3645–3648.
Morley, J., 1974, *Prostaglandins* **8**:315–325.
Myatt, L., Bray, M. A., Gordon, D., and Morley, J., 1975, *Nature (London)* **257**:227–228.
Newcombe, D. S., Ortel, R. W., and Levey, C. S., 1972, *Biochem. Biophys. Res. Commun.* **48**:201–204.

Newcombe, D. S., Ciosek, C. P., Jr., Ishikawa, Y., and Fahey, J. V., 1975, *Proc. Natl. Acad. Sci. U.S.A.* **72**:3124–3128.
Oien, H. G., Mandel, L. R., Humes, J. L., Taub, D., Hoffsommer, R. D., and Kuehl, F. A., Jr., 1973, *Prostaglandins* **9**:985–995.
Oien, H. G., Ham, E. A., Zanetti, M. E., Ulm, E. H., and Kuehl, F. A., Jr., 1976, *Proc. Natl. Acad. Sci. U.S.A.* **73**:1107–1111.
Plescia, O. J., Smith, A. H., and Grinwich, K., 1975, *Proc. Natl. Acad. Sci. U.S.A.* **72**:1848–1851.
Polet, H., and Levine, L., 1975, *J. Biol. Chem.* **250**:351–357.
Powell, W., Hammarström, S., and Samuelsson, B., 1973, *Eur. J. Biochem.* **41**:103–107.
Quagliata, F., Lawrence, V. S. W., and Phillips-Quagliata, J. M., 1973, *Cell. Immunol.* **6**:457–465.
Rao, C. V., 1973, in: *Abstracts of a Symposium on Advances in Chemistry, Biology and Immunology of Gonadotrophins,* p. 67, Bangelor Press, Bangelor.
Robinson, D. R., Smith, H., McGuire, M. B., and Levine, L., 1975, *Prostaglandins* **10**:67–85.
Rosenthale, M. E., Devinis, A., Kasgarich, J., and Singer, S., 1972, *J. Pharm. Pharmacol.* **24**:149–150.
Samuelsson, B., 1965, *J. Am. Chem. Soc.* **87**:3011–3013.
Sandler, N., Karim, S. M. M., and Williams, E. P., 1968, *Lancet* **2**:1053–1055.
Seegmiller, J. E., Howell, R. R., and Malawista, S. E., 1962, *J. Am. Med. Assoc.* **180**:464–475.
Smith, J. W., Steiner, A. L., and Parker, C. W., 1971, *J. Clin. Invest.* **50**:442–448.
Snyder, D. S., and Eaglstein, W. H., 1974, *J. Invest. Dermatol.* **62**:47–50.
Søndergaard, J., and Wolf-Jürgensen, P., 1972, *Acta Derm.-Venereol.* **52**:361–364.
Søndergaard, J., Helin, P., and Jorgensen, H. P., 1973, *J. Pathol.* **109**:239–243.
Søndergaard, J., Greaves, M. W., and Jorgensen, H. P., 1974, *Arch. Dermatol.* **110**:556–558.
Tauber, A. I., Kaliner, M., Stechchutte, D., and Austen, K. F., 1973, *J. Allergy Clin. Immunol.* **51**:106.
Turner, S. R., Tainer, J. A., and Lynn, W. S., 1975a, *Nature (London)* **257**:680–681.
Turner, S. R., Campbell, J. A., and Lynn, W. S., 1975b, *J. Expt. Med.* **141**:1437–1441.
Van Arman, C. G., 1974, *Clin. Pharmacol. Ther.* **16**:900–904.
Vane, J. R., 1971, *Nature (London) New Biol.* **231**:232–235.
von Euler, U. S., 1934, *Arch. Exp. Pathol. Pharmakol.* **175**:78–84.
Voorhees, J. J., Colburn, N. H., Stawiski, M., Duell, E. A., Haddox, M., and Goldberg, N. D., 1974, in: *Control of Proliferation in Animal Cells* (B. Clarkson and R. Baserga, eds.), pp. 635–648, Cold Spring Harbor Press, Cold Spring Harbor, New York.
Weissmann, G., and Fell, H., 1962, *J. Exp. Med.* **16**:365–380.
Weissmann, G., Zurier, R. B., Spieler, P. J., and Goldstein, I. M., 1971, *J. Exp. Med.* **134**:149S–165S.
Whelan, C. J., 1974, *J. Pharm. Pharmacol.* **26**:355–356.
Willis, A. L., 1969, *J. Pharm. Pharmacol.* **21**:126–128.
Willis, A. L., 1974, *Prostaglandins* **5**:1–25.
Winter, C. A., Risley, E. A., and Nuss, G. W., 1962, *Proc. Soc. Exp. Biol. Med.* **111**:544–547.
Ziboh, V. A., 1973, *J. Lipid Res.* **14**:377–384.
Zurier, R. B., and Quagliata, F., 1971, *Nature (London)* **234**:304–305.
Zurier, R. B., Hoffstein, S., and Weissmann, G., 1973, *Arthritis Rheum.* **16**:606.
Zurier, R. B., Weissmann, G., Hoffstein, S., Kammerman, S., and Tai, H., 1974, *J. Clin. Invest.* **53**:297–309.

10

Lymphokines: Physiologic Control and Pharmacological Modulation of Their Production and Action

EDGAR PICK

1. Introduction: What Are Lymphokines?

"Lymphokines"* (LKs) is the common denotation suggested by Dumonde *et al.* (1969) for a loosely related group of soluble materials that are liberated by lymphoid cells cultured *in vitro* and usually recovered from the cell-free culture fluid. They were originally discovered in supernatants of lymphocytes obtained from immunized animals that were cultured in the presence of specific antigen, and subsequently under conditions of nonspecific lymphocyte stimulation by membrane-reactive agents such as plant lectins, antibodies reacting with surface components, and certain bacterial products. It later became apparent that LK-like materials are also produced, under certain conditions, by cells other than lymphocytes. The methods used for the detection and quantitation of LKs are biological, and are based on the ability of a culture supernatant to inhibit the migration of macrophages or polymorphonuclear leukocytes *in vitro,* to act as a chemotactic attractant for a

*A widely used term that is synonymous with "lymphocyte-soluble mediators" or "products of activated lymphocytes."

EDGAR PICK • Department of Human Microbiology, Tel Aviv University Sackler School of Medicine, Tel Aviv, Israel.

variety of cells, to be cytotoxic for certain target cells, to induce lymphocyte proliferation, to inhibit virus multiplication, and other properties.

The tendency to ascribe each biological activity to the presence of a distinct molecule has generated a profusion of LK descriptions without regard to whether a biological effect is actually due to a separate substance or to an unrelated biological activity of the same material. The assumption has been made that LKs are the mediators of cell-mediated immunity in the intact animal and represent a parallel to such classic mediators of immediate-type hypersensitivity as histamine, serotonin, and the kinins. Indeed, the first international meeting dedicated to LKs entitled its proceedings *Mediators of Cellular Immunity*. This ideal symmetry was disturbed, however, by a number of recent experimental findings. It became apparent that cells with no known function in cell-mediated immunity, such as B cells, were nevertheless active LK producers, if adequately stimulated, and that cells of no immunologic relevance, such as fibroblasts and virus-transformed cells, secrete LKs or at least materials indistinguishable from LKs by presently available criteria. In addition to these findings, materials similar to LKs in physicochemical characteristics and conditions of production were discovered to mediate the cooperation between T and B cells, among different T-cell subclasses, and between macrophages and immunocompetent lymphocytes, in a positive (stimulatory) or negative (suppressor) sense. Also, a number of other soluble materials produced by lymphocytes have been described, the inclusion of which in the LK class becomes a problem of semantics. Examples are the colony-stimulating factors (promoting granulocyte and macrophage proliferation and differentiation), the immunoglobulin-binding factor, the lymphocyte chalones, and the procoagulant tissue factor of lymphocyte origin.

It is impossible, at present, to offer a rigorous definition of the term lymphokine, but in this writer's opinion, two categories of lymphocyte-derived materials should be excluded from the LK category: (1) antibodies or antibody fragments in free or antigen-complexed form and (2) all other forms of nonimmunoglobulin antigen receptors (such as the T-cell receptor) in free or antigen-complexed form. The exclusion of this second category does not mean that materials with LK activity may not contain lymphocyte antigen receptors (or other membrane components with or without defined receptor function) as a constituent part of a plurimolecular complex, liberated as such into the culture supernatant. A further point that must be made here is that even though LK-like materials might be of wider occurrence than hitherto believed and might function in a variety of nonimmunologic situations as intercellular messengers, that they do does not mean that they have no role in the mediation of cellular immunity. On the contrary, there is accumulating evidence for such a function.

It is my intention to place the emphasis in this chapter on LKs with a well-defined role in the mediation of the peripheral manifestations of cell-mediated immunity. This is the site at which specific pharmacological modulation of the response might be attempted by methods distinct from those of classic immunosuppression. The LKs that will be discussed in this chapter are: macrophage migration-inhibitory factor (MIF), chemotactic factors, lymphotoxin, and interferon. Only MIF will be discussed in great detail to serve as a model for understanding LK function in general. For additional information concerning these and other LKs, a number of review articles published within the last few years are available (Bloom, 1971; David and David, 1972; Pick and Turk, 1972a; Morley, 1974; Pekarek and Krejci, 1974).

2. Macrophage Migration-Inhibitory Factor (MIF)

The early descriptions of the phenomenon of migration inhibition were based on the use of tissue fragments or unfractionated complex cell mixtures derived from sensitized animals, which were incubated in the presence or absence of specific antigen. It was observed that the *in vitro* migration of cells was inhibited in antigen-containing cultures (see the reviews by Svejcar and Johanovsky, 1961, and David and David, 1972). It was only in 1966 that it became clearly established that antigen-induced migration inhibition is a complex phenomenon composed of two entirely distinct processes: (1) the secretion of a soluble material by lymphocytes present in the tissue fragment or cell mixture and (2) the inhibition of *in vitro* migration of a target-cell population, usually consisting of macrophages or polymorphonuclear leukocytes.

Migration-inhibitory factor was the name given to the material, which was first discovered in culture supernatants of antigen-stimulated lymphocytes of sensitized guinea pigs by Bloom and Bennett (1966) and David (1966). When peritoneal exudate cells are packed in capillary tubes open at one end and these tubes are affixed to the bottom of special chambers, the cells migrate from the capillary in a fanlike manner on the chamber bottom. Addition of MIF-containing supernatants to the chambers inhibits migration, as evident by the smaller size of the area covered by the migrating cells. The inhibitory potency of a certain supernatant is usually expressed as the percentage inhibition of migration.

When soluble antigen is used for lymphocyte stimulation, the control supernatants are supplemented after incubation with the antigen. Comparison of migration areas in MIF-containing supernatants to areas of migration in plain culture medium is definitely inadequate. It is important to realize that when measuring migration areas, we are assessing the combined effect of many factors, among which are intrinsic macrophage motility (which in itself is subject to influence by a number of factors), type of culture medium and of serum added to it, presence of migration-stimulatory factors or migration-inhibitory materials other than MIF, duration and temperature of incubation, type of surface on which the cells migrate, diameter of the capillary tube, and degree of cell compression during centrifugation. Another difficulty is that in the majority of cases, culture supernatants are tested at only one dilution, since the use of serial dilution tests for MIF quantitation is still very limited. An additional problem is that the difference among areas of migration in control and MIF-containing supernatants is maximum after a certain time interval, which varies from experiment to experiment and is unpredictable. These difficulties in quantitation are of special relevance for studies of pharmacological modulation of LK production and action. To circumvent them, the use of serial 2-fold dilution and comparison with MIF standards of known activity has been suggested and should be given more attention (Leu *et al.*, 1972; T. J. Williams *et al.*, 1972; Morley, 1974). The importance of correct statistical evaluation of data has been stressed repeatedly (Morley, 1974), and adequate methods to serve this purpose are given by Bergstrand and Kallen (1973).

2.1. Cellular Origin

MIF is produced by lymphocytes of sensitized animals under conditions of specific antigenic stimulation or by lymphocytes of normal animals exposed to a number of stimuli, including phytomitogens, antilymphocyte serum, antigen–antibody complexes, and certain bacterial products (reviewed by Pick and Turk, 1972a). More recently, it became apparent that MIF is also secreted by established lymphoid cell lines in the absence of overt antigenic stimulation (Granger *et al.*, 1970), by some nonlymphoid cell lines (Papageorgiou *et al.*, 1972; Tubergen *et al.*, 1972), by fibroblasts derived from skin biopsies (Papageorgiou and Glade, 1974), and by cells transformed by both DNA and RNA viruses and by human tumor cell lines (Hammond *et al.*, 1974; Poste, 1975a).

Specific antigen-induced MIF production was obtained with lymphocytes from lymph nodes, the peritoneal exudate, peripheral blood, spleen, and even thymus. It was established, however that the peritoneal lymphocyte is a particularly potent MIF producer (Rosenstreich *et al.*, 1971). Relatively little work has been performed with lymphocyte populations separated by physical methods, but it was found that MIF production in guinea pigs, in response to stimulation by tuberculin or purified protein derivative (PPD), is the property of cells that do not adhere to glass at 37°C (Manheimer and Pick, 1973), and that localize in the lowest density layer on centrifugation in an albumin density gradient (Pick, 1973). With the use of velocity sedimentation at unit gravity, it was found that MIF production in the mouse, in response to tumor antigens, was the property of large, blastlike cells (Gorczynski, 1974).

The original assumption that MIF production is limited to T cells was supported by the finding that spleen cells of thymectomized chickens do not release MIF on exposure to antigen (Morita and Soekawa, 1972), and by the report that the MIF-mediated macrophage disappearance reaction requires T lymphocytes (Sonozaki and Cohen, 1972). It is now well established, however, that MIF production is a property of both T and B cells, if they are adequately stimulated. In the guinea pig, T lymphocytes produce MIF in response to some antigens (Yoshida *et al.*, 1973), while B lymphocytes are responsible for the release of MIF following stimulation by PPD (Bloom *et al.*, 1975; Pick *et al.*, 1975a) and *Escherichia coli* lipopolysaccharide (Yoshida *et al.*, 1973). In humans, both T and B lymphocytes were found to be able to produce MIF when stimulated by at least three different antigens (Rocklin *et al.*, 1974). In the mouse, MIF production by both T cells (Clinton *et al.*, 1974) and B cells (Sugane *et al.*, 1975; Altbaum and Pick, in preparation) has been found.

It is not entirely clear at present whether macrophages are required for antigen-induced MIF production. The finding that PPD-induced MIF production was improved by passing lymph node cells through glass-bead columns at 37°C (Manheimer and Pick, 1973) was taken as indicating that macrophages are not required. Recently, however, evidence was presented by a number of laboratories in support of the opposite idea, namely, that antigen-induced MIF production is possible only with the aid of macrophages (Nelson and Leu, 1975; Ohishi and Onoue, 1975).

2.2. Mechanism of Production

MIF cannot be found in quantities detectable by classic methods in extracts of lymphocytes in the absence of stimulation. MIF activity was detected in lymphocyte extracts after 6 hr (but not after 2 hr) of exposure to specific antigen (Bennett and Bloom, 1967; Svejcar *et al.*, 1968). PPD-stimulated sensitized guinea pig lymphocytes produced MIF for up to 4 days (Bennet and Bloom, 1967). Production of MIF after antigen stimulation in the guinea pig is independent of DNA synthesis (Bloom *et al.*, 1972), but there is recent evidence that in man, T cells producing MIF proliferate, while B cells releasing MIF do not proliferate, in response to antigen (Rocklin *et al.*, 1974). MIF production by continuous cell lines in the absence of stimulation was found to be limited to the S phase (Tubergen *et al.*, 1972) or to the G_1 and early S phases of the cell cycle (Thomas, 1972), and the production was associated with microsomes (Prystowsky *et al.*, 1975).

Antigen-induced MIF production could not be blocked by mitomycin C (Mizoguchi *et al.*, 1973), X-irradiation (Salvin and Nishio, 1972), or *L*-asparaginase (Schlag, 1971), all of which inhibit DNA synthesis by stimulated lymphocytes. Actinomycin D (which suppresses DNA-dependent RNA synthesis) blocks MIF production when added within 6 hr after antigenic stimulation, whereas the protein synthesis inhibitor puromycin blocks MIF production only when present for more than 6 hr from antigenic exposure (David, 1965; Mizoguchi *et al.*, 1973). Further support for the suggestion that MIF represents a protein that is newly synthesized in response to antigenic or nonantigenic stimuli is offered by the radiolabeling studies of Sorg and Bloom (1973). Whether protein synthesis is required for the actual synthesis of the factor itself, or for the synthesis of a protein needed in some way for the transfer of MIF from the cell to the medium, remains to be established.

While the prevalent view is that stimulated lymphocytes are those that release MIF, it has also been suggested that an amplifying mechanism, including recruitment of unstimulated cells, might be at work (Pick and Turk, 1972b).

Little is known about the minimum time of contact between stimulant and lymphocyte required for induction of MIF production. MIF synthesis was consistently induced by a 2-hr pulse of sensitized guinea pig lymphocytes with PPD (Pick, unpublished observation). It is also well established that insoluble or insolubilized stimulants are effective MIF inducers, as exemplified by the successful use of bacillus Calmette-Guerin (BCG) or Sepharose-linked concanavalin A (Con A) (Pick, 1972b; Friedrich *et al.*, 1975) for this purpose.

Further information about the mechanism of MIF secretion is offered by the finding that MIF production is blocked by agents that increase the intracellular concentration of cyclic AMP (cAMP) (Pick, 1974) and by the microfilament-blocking drug cytochalasin B (Pick, 1974; Ben-Sasson and Rosenthal, 1975). On the other hand, there seems to be no involvement of microtubules in the process of MIF secretion (Pick, 1974). The effect of various pharmacological agents on MIF production is discussed in more detail in Section 6.1.

2.3. Characterization and Isolation

2.3.1. Methods

No complete purification of MIF has been achieved, and there is controversy over the biochemical characteristics of the partially purified materials. Both stimulated and unstimulated lymphocyte culture supernatants contain a number of materials, as evident from polyacrylamide gel electrophoretic analysis and detection of bands by protein staining or radioactivity measurement. Characterization of MIF is made even more difficult by the now widely accepted finding that supernatants of unstimulated lymphocytes also contain a material with MIF activity. It is not entirely clear whether the MIF present in stimulated lymphocyte supernatants represents only a larger amount of the material also present in control supernatants or a distinct substance released only by stimulated cells. It is also possible that stimulated lymphocyte supernatants contain both specific (stimulant-induced) and nonspecific inhibitory materials. It is important to emphasize that there is no proof for the assumption that the migration-inhibitory activity of whole supernatants is due to a single, homogeneous molecule. After the first step of most fractionation procedures, MIF activity is found spread over a relatively wide molecular-weight range, and the reduction in molecular-weight range with subsequent purification steps raises the question whether the final product can account for all the activity present in the unfractionated supernatant. The methodology of MIF purification is further complicated by the difficulty in distinguishing between losses of activity due to destruction of a single homogeneous material by enzymatic or other degradation or adsorption to surfaces and losses due to selective degradation of some molecules with MIF activity and retention of activity by other molecules. The lack of a strictly quantitative nonbiological assay for MIF makes its detection during fractionation procedures difficult. This difficulty is accentuated by the fact that culture supernatants do contain migration-stimulatory materials that might cofractionate with MIF and cancel out its activity in the assay system. To minimize such effects, it is wise to test materials derived from fractionation of MIF-containing supernatants after dilution in control supernatant, not in plain culture medium, to ensure that lack of migration caused by a certain fraction is actually due to the presence of an inhibitor, not to the lack of a promoting factor.

2.3.2. Characteristics of Guinea Pig MIF

I shall discuss the properties of guinea pig MIF in some detail, since it is the best characterized. In a few instances, it will be compared with MIFs of other animal species and with MIF-like factors released by lymphoid and nonlymphoid cell lines and virus-infected cells.

(a) Dialysis. It is established that prolonged dialysis of MIF-containing supernatants against isotonic solutions at 4°C results in no loss of activity; however, vacuum dialysis does result in loss of activity (Hadden *et al.*, 1975). No data are available concerning the dialyzability of MIF in the presence of low pH, high-molarity salt, or other dissociating condition.

(b) Heat Stability. Guinea pig MIF was reported to be stable at 56°C for at least 30 min (David, 1966); however, Ashworth *et al.* (1975) claimed considerable loss of activity after 20 min at 56°C. Loss of activity at 56°C was also reported for sheep MIF generated *in vivo* (Hay *et al.*, 1973). MIF-containing supernatants can be kept for prolonged periods when frozen at −20 or −70°C, but it was claimed that human MIF, while stable at 56°C, loses potency when stored at −20°C (Bartfeld and Atoynatan, 1970). Mouse MIF is also stable at 56°C, and claims were made for both loss (Kuhner *et al.*, 1975) and maintenance (Altbaum and Pick, in preparation) of activity at 80°C. MIF produced by continuous cell lines was heat-stable at 56°C, and in some cases (MIF from HeLa cells and simian virus [sv 40]-transformed mouse 3T3 cells), activity was left unchanged after heating at 80°C (Papageorgiou *et al.*, 1972; Poste, 1975b).

(c) Sensitivity to Enzymes. The biological activity of guinea pig MIF was destroyed by treatment with chymotrypsin and neuraminidase, but only partially destroyed by trypsin (Remold and David, 1971). It was unaffected by RNAse and DNAse. Sensitivity of guinea pig MIF to neuraminidase could not be confirmed by Ashworth *et al.* (1975), and further studies are required to settle this question. It is of interest that human MIF loses its activity when exposed to chymotrypsin, but not when exposed to neuraminidase (Rocklin *et al.*, 1972). Mouse MIF (Kuhner *et al.*, 1975; Altbaum and Pick, in preparation) and MIF produced by human lymphoid cell lines (Papageorgiou *et al.*, 1972) or by HeLa cells and sv-40-transformed mouse 3T3 cells (Poste, 1975b) were all found to be sensitive to chymotrypsin. The conclusion to be drawn from these experiments is that guinea pig MIF is most probably a glycoprotein containing sialic acid, or possibly a molecule bound to a glycoprotein carrier acting as a protector.

(d) Salt Precipitation. Dumonde *et al.* (1972) found that guinea pig MIF is precipitated by ammonium sulfate between 50 and 80% saturation. This finding might be important in any studies in which separation of MIF from antibody or antigen–antibody complexes is desired.

(e) Molecular Weight. It is generally agreed that even the largest MIF molecules are smaller than immunoglobin G, and the extreme limits of molecular weights reported are 12,000 and 82,000. Such heterogeneity may be due to totally different materials with similar biological activity, to one basic unit in various polymeric forms, or to limited enzymatic degradation of a larger molecule. There are indications that the molecular weight of a certain MIF might differ with the nature of the lymphocyte stimulant. For instance, guinea pig MIF induced by *o*-chlorobenzoyl–bovine γ-globulin (BGG) was estimated to be in the molecular-weight range of 35,00 –67,000 by gel filtration on Sephadex G-100 (Remold *et al.*, 1970), while MIF induced by tuberculin PPD was estimated to be 25,000 (Bloom and Jimenez, 1970), and that induced by BGG ranged from 56,000 to 82,000 (Dumonde *et al.*, 1972). In one report, a molecular weight of 12,000 was claimed for part of the MIF induced by stimulation with PPD (Yoshida and Reisfeld, 1970). MIF induced by Con A was found to be even more heterogeneous than MIF induced by a particular antigen, ranging between molecular weights of 23,000 and 67,000 (Remold *et al.*, 1972). It should be noted here that the different results obtained using identical separation methods might be due in part to different ways of evaluating MIF activity in a certain fraction. When the presence of MIF is assessed by comparing macrophage migration in a supernatant fraction with that in plain culture medium, MIF activity is found in numerous fractions (Sorg and Bloom, 1973). MIF appears more restricted when the term is limited to fractions of stimulated lymphocyte supernatants that are more inhibitory than the corresponding fractions of control supernatants (Remold *et al.*, 1970).

The molecular weights of MIF preparations obtained in other animal species are similar to those reported for guinea pig MIF. A molecular weight of 23,000 was reported for antigen-induced human MIF (Rocklin *et al.*, 1972), while mouse MIF induced by antigen or mitogen was found to have a molecular weight of 35,000–67,000 (Kuhner *et al.*, 1975). No difference was found in the molecular dimensions of MIF produced by T or B cells, either in the guinea pig (Yoshida *et al.*, 1973) or in man (Rocklin *et al.*, 1974). MIF released by human lymphoid and nonlymphoid cell lines was found to have a molecular weight between 12,400 and 25,000 (Papageorgiou *et al.*, 1972). MIF produced by monkey kidney cell cultures infected with sv 40 was reported to have a molecular weight between 45,000 and 65,000 (Flanagan *et al.*, 1973), while rodent cell lines transformed by the same virus produced MIF with a molecular weight close to 25,000 (Poste, 1975b).

Nothing is known about the molecular structure of MIF, with the exception of some data suggesting the existence in human MIF of disulfide bonds, the integrity of which is essential for biological activity (Bartfeld and Atoynatan, 1971). In contrast, very recent evidence suggests that guinea pig MIF treated with the disulfide-bond-disrupting agents 2-mercaptoethanol and dithiothreitol and high concentrations of the denaturing chemicals urea and guanidine hydrochloride maintains full activity on removal of these agents by dialysis (Kotkes and Pick, 1976).

(f) Charge. Determination of the electrical charge of MIF is based on fractionation by ion-exchange chromatography, polyacrylamide gel electrophoresis, and isoelectric focusing. Bloom and Bennett (1970) and Dumonde *et al.* (1972) reported that guinea pig MIF is eluted from DEAE–cellulose by buffers of a molarity used to elute serum α-globulins and albumin. A different conclusion was drawn from studies employing polyacrylamide gel electrophoresis, MIF being recovered from fractions containing molecules that migrated faster than albumin (Remold *et al.*, 1970). The identification of guinea pig MIF with a prealbumin was questioned, however, by Sorg and Bloom (1973), who expressed doubts about the suitability of the methods of Remold and co-workers for determination of charge. Sorg and Bloom (1973), using preparative isoelectric focusing, found a migration-inhibitory material, predominant in stimulated cultures, with an isoelectric point of 5.3 which represents a lower charge than albumin, and could correspond to the material of α-globulin mobility recovered by ion-exchange chromatography. Human MIF has a mobility identical to that of albumin (Rocklin *et al.*, 1972), while mouse MIF was found to migrate in the region of β-globulins (Kuhner *et al.*, 1975). It is possible that charge heterogeneity is due to various amounts of sialic acid bound to a single protein core.

(g) Glycoprotein Nature. The sensitivity of guinea pig MIF to neuraminidase pointed to its glycoprotein nature and the presence of sialic acid as an essential part of the molecule. On isopycnic centrifugation in a cesium chloride gradient, guinea pig MIF was found to have a slightly greater buoyant density than simple proteins, which is in accordance with MIF being a glycoprotein with a small percentage of sugar (Remold and David, 1971). Additional support for the glycoprotein nature of MIF is offered by the finding that the activity of guinea pig MIF is totally abolished by treatment with 0.02 M sodium periodate for 90 min at 4°C (Pick, unpublished observation). Strong evidence for the presence of sugar in guinea pig MIF is also represented by the recent findings of Kotkes and Pick (1976) that MIF binds to Con A covalently linked to sepharose, and can be specifically eluted from it by methyl-α-D-glucopyranoside. Preliminary data also indicate that rabbit antisera against partially purified guinea pig MIF agglutinate human group A red cells, a reaction that can be partially blocked by *N*-acetyl-D-galactosamine and *N*-acetyl-D-glucosamine (Pick, in preparation). In contrast to these data, human MIF appears to be resistant to neuraminidase, and behaves like a simple protein on isopycnic centrifugation (Rocklin *et al.*, 1972).

(h) Antigen Requirement and Antigen-Binding Property. It has been claimed that the migration-inhibitory activity of some MIF preparations is dependent on or potentiated by the presence of specific antigen used for inducing the production of the mediator (reviewed by David and David, 1972). MIF with such properties has been described in guinea pigs, humans, sheep, and mice. Progress in the characterization of MIF, indicating a size considerably smaller than immunoglobulin, as well as the existence of many nonantigenic stimuli for MIF production, makes the task of offering an explanation for the role of antigen in MIF action difficult. Some authors claimed antigen amplification of the activity of partially purified MIF preparations of a size smaller than immunoglobulin, and conditions have been described that favor the production of antigen-dependent MIF, such as the use of low antigen concentrations or prolonged culture intervals. The only argument in support of the existence of antigen-dependent MIF is based on augmentation of activity on addition of specific antigen. One proof of the existence of such MIF would be based on the demonstration of antigen-binding by purified MIF. While it is difficult to be certain that the usual partially purified MIF samples are free of traces of the inducing antigen, it has never been shown that MIF can specifically bind antigen, and MIF cannot be removed from supernatants by passage through columns capable of specifically retaining antigen (Yoshida *et al.*, 1972).

(i) Antigenicity. In the absence of highly purified preparations, it is impossible to define the antigenic properties of MIF. There have been, however, several successful attempts at producing antibodies against partially purified MIF. Yoshida *et al.* (1975a) produced a rabbit anti-guinea pig MIF antibody that was capable of binding not only MIF, but also macrophage chemotactic factor and skin reactive factor. It is interesting that an antiserum prepared against guinea-pig-lymphocyte-derived MIF was able to bind MIF released by sv-40-infected monkey kidney cells, indicating at least partial antigenic identity (Yoshida *et al.*, 1975b). There is some evidence for lack of cross-reaction between guinea pig lymphotoxin and MIF, since an antiserum to lymphotoxin was incapable of neutralizing MIF (Gately *et al.*, 1975). It is also of interest that classic heterologous antilymphocyte serum did not neutralize MIF in the mouse (Ranlov and Hardt, 1970) or rabbit (Pekarek *et al.*, 1971). Recent preliminary work also indicates that there is no relationship between Ia antigens and MIF in the mouse (Sorg and Hämmerling, 1975).

(j) Isolation. No standard procedure for MIF purification has yet been established. The most common sequence in use at present is the following: (1) dialysis of culture supernatants against distilled water to eliminate the bulk of salts; (2) concentration by freeze–drying; (3) fractionation based on molecular weight, using gel filtration; and (4) further fractionation of material, within a certain molecular-weight range, by a method that separates molecules of different charge. The most common of these methods is preparative polyacrylamide gel electrophoresis, but isoelectric focusing may become the method of choice.

Due to difficulties encountered with classic physicochemical methods of fractionation, other approaches are being introduced. These approaches are based on one form or other of affinity chromatography, and can be classified in three categories. The first is based on the property of guinea pig MIF to bind to a fucose-containing receptor on macrophages (Remold, 1973). This observation served as the basis for the method of Fox and MacSween (1974), who found that MIF will bind to a column of fucosamine bound to agarose beads, and could be recovered by elution with a solution of L-fucose. A second approach, based on the fact that guinea pig MIF is a glycoprotein, is that of Kotkes and Pick (1976), who adsorbed MIF from supernatants onto Con A covalently bound to agarose, and eluted it subsequently with methyl-α-D-glucopyranoside. The third approach which has not yet been fully exploited, depends on the availability of specific anti-MIF antibody. Anti-MIF immunoadsorbent columns will become increasingly popular in the future, and have already been used as an intermediate step in MIF purification by Geczy *et al.* (1975).

2.4. Mechanisms of Action

It is usually assumed that one of the main effects of MIF is the one to which it owes its name, namely, the impairment of macrophages motility. Although there is direct evidence from microcinematographic studies that individual macrophages move slower on agar, incorporating MIF (Salvin *et al.*, 1971), the effects of MIF on other cellular functions that result in reduced migration of cells packed into a capillary must be given consideration. The most notable is a possible effect on the macrophage membrane that results in increased cell–cell adherence. The clearest morphological expression of this effect is the occurrence of macrophage aggregates in cell suspensions exposed to MIF (Lolekha *et al.*, 1970).

2.4.1. Mechanism of Macrophage Motility

Cultured macrophages exhibit a gliding-type movement associated with ruffled membrane activity occurring at the leading edge of the cell, with the rest of the cell moving in a relatively rigid manner (Bhisey and Freed, 1971). Movement is performed with the aid of actinlike microfilaments, which appear as a network situated beneath the plasmalemma and are most prominent in the area of the cell attached to a surface (Reaven and Axline, 1973). More centrally, there is an area of microfilaments organized as oriented bundles penetrated by an array of microtubules, some of which reach the plasma membrane. More microtubules are seen radiating from the centrioles toward the cell periphery. The microfilament-blocking agent cytochalasin B stops ruffled membrane activity and effectively blocks macrophage migration from capillaries (Pick and Abrahamer, 1973). On the other hand, treatment of macrophages with the microtubule-disrupting drugs colchicine and vinblastine sulfate causes a change in motility from the usual gliding, directional type to a random, amoeboid type (Bhisey and Freed, 1971). Colchicine-treated macrophages become very motile and develop pseudopodlike processes and cytoplasmic streaming. Addition of 10^{-5}–10^{-7} M colchicine or vinblastine sulfate to the chamber fluid in the capillary migration system causes an impressive increase in the migration area (Pick and Abrahamer, 1973).

It was found that alveolar macrophages migrate faster than peritoneal ones, and mineral-oil-induced peritoneal macrophages migrate faster than unstimulated cells (Pollock *et al.*, 1971). Migration was blocked by the glycolytic inhibitors iodoacetic acid and L-deoxyglucose, but not by the oxidative phosphorylation inhibitors potassium cyanide and dinitrophenol (Pollock and Vazquez, 1971).

Macrophage migration occurs best at 37°C, and is not influenced by subtoxic doses of puromycin, cycloheximide, or actinomycin D (Pick and Manheimer, 1974). It was also found that *in vitro* migration is enhanced by increasing serum concentrations, by removal of calcium and magnesium from the culture medium, and by certain polyanions, such as dextran sulfate. Treatment of macrophages with proteolytic enzymes, such as trypsin or pronase, also results in enhanced migration (Pick and Manheimer, 1974).

Exogenous cAMP and some agents that increase the level of endogenous cAMP block macrophage migration (Pick, 1972a; Pick and Manheimer, 1974). The most effective inhibition was caused by dibutyryl cAMP, by the cyclic nucleotide phosphodiesterase inhibitor theophylline, and by the adenylate cyclase stimulator isoproterenol. The phenomenon is not a general one, since some very potent activators of macrophage adenylate cyclase, such as prostaglandin E_1 and cholera toxin, do not inhibit macrophage migration. These effects of cAMP on macrophage motility are paralleled by reports of very similar inhibitory actions of the nucleotide on fibroblast locomotion (Johnson *et al.*, 1972), on antiimmunoglobulin-stimulated B-lymphocyte motility (Schreiner and Unanue, 1975), and on the spontaneous movement of neutrophils (Rivkin *et al.*, 1975). Conversely, cyclic GMP (cGMP) occasionally stimulated macrophage migration, but the cholinergic drugs acetylcholine and carbamylcholine, which increase the cellular level of cGMP in most tissues, were without effect (Pick and Manheimer, 1974; Kotkes and Pick, 1975a). However, stimulation of macrophage migration could be induced by ouabain, by a mechanism independent of the effects of the drug on sodium–potassium transport (Leu *et al.*, 1973), and to a moderate degree by the competitive inhibitor of adenylate cyclase, α, β-methylene ATP (Pick, unpublished observation). While there is little doubt that cyclic nucleotides have a central role in the regulation of macrophage motility (see Sections 2.4.3 and 6.3), the intracellular target for cAMP is unknown. The following possibilities can be considered: (1) cAMP influences cell movement or membrane topography or both via its effect on the state of polymerization of microtubules; (2) it influences microfilament function; or (3) it modulates the properties of the cell surface, possibly by influencing the formation of microvilli (Willingham and Pastan, 1975a).

2.4.2. Receptor for MIF

Bartfeld and Atoynatan (1969) were the first to show clearly that treatment of macrophages with trypsin made them insensitive to the effect of MIF. The ability to be inhibited by MIF was recovered by culturing the trypsinized cells in normal medium for 20 hr. These authors also found that MIF could be removed from solution by absorption with macrophages. The most straightforward explanation for these findings is that MIF binds to a trypsin-sensitive structure on the macrophage membrane that might represent a specific MIF receptor. The evidence for the existence of a receptor for MIF was strengthened by the finding that macrophages exposed to MIF for a brief interval were prevented from migrating when subsequently transferred to regular culture medium (Leu *et al.*, 1972; Manheimer and Pick, 1973). MIF could bind to macrophages at both 4 and 37°C, in both the presence and the absence of serum. When binding was effected at 4°C, however, macrophages were inhibited only when the cells were incubated in culture medium at 37°C before being packed into capillaries (Manheimer and Pick, 1973). Pulse exposure to MIF for 2 hr at 37°C was found to be optimal for maximum inhibition of migration; prevention of pinocytosis during pulse exposure by sodium azide did not influence the outcome of the test (Manheimer and Pick, 1973). Leu *et al.* (1972) also confirmed that during pulse exposure, MIF was removed from supernatants by both viable and dead macrophages, optimally at 37°C. Trypsinized macrophages lost their absorptive capacity (Leu *et al.*, 1972).

Considerable uncertainty exists about the different responsiveness of peritoneal and alveolar macrophages to MIF. While Leu *et al.*, (1972) reported that in the guinea pig, alveolar cells were unresponsive, Bartfeld and Atoynatan (1970) described inhibition by MIF of human alveolar cells. The macrophage receptor in one animal species is usually able to react with MIF produced by lymphocytes of different species, although quantitative differences and cases of unresponsiveness occur (Svejcar *et al.*, 1971).

Our knowledge of the nature of MIF receptors was considerably broadened by the finding by Remold (1973) that α-L-fucose is an essential component of the receptor, at least in the guinea pig, The effect of MIF could be prevented by the presence of free α-L-fucose, acting as a competitive inhibitor, by the treatment of target macrophages with α-L-fucosidase, and by their pretreatment with *Lotus* agglutinin, which binds to fucose on the cell surface. It is interesting that both mitogen-induced guinea pig lymphocyte MIF and MIF produced by mouse 3T3 cells transformed by SV 40 were found to act on guinea pig macrophages via a fucose-containing receptor (Poste, 1975b). The ability of guinea pig MIF to bind to a fucose-containing receptor was the rationale behind the methods of MIF purification based on binding to agarose-linked fucosamine (Fox and MacSween, 1974) or frozen–thawed macrophages (Braunstein *et al.*, 1974), followed by elution with fucose solutions.

The relationship of the MIF receptor to macrophage receptors for IgG, IgM, C3, opsonized bacteria, phytomitogens, and chemically altered or aged red cells remains to be explored.

2.4.3. How Does MIF Act?

In dealing with this question, the point must be made that while inhibition of macrophage migration is the effect that has been studied the most, it might not represent the biologically relevant action of MIF. There is therefore full justification for investigating effects of MIF on macrophages (and possibly other target cells) that are not strictly related to the phenomenon of migration inhibition. The use of unfractionated MIF-containing supernatants makes it impossible to determine whether different activities are caused by MIF or by other unrelated materials.

Even if we limit ourselves to migration inhibition itself, a number of possible mechanisms can be held responsible. The following mechanisms have been proposed: (1) MIF acts as a passive divalent agglutinating agent. (2) It potentiates spontaneous agglutination by modifying the electrical surface charge, by increasing the number of microvilli, by removing a surface component that normally prevents cell aggregation, or by activating a membrane glycosyltransferase. (3) It blocks a metabolic process or enzyme essential for migration (glycolysis, ATPase, cAMP generation or degradation) or an essential membrane transport system (Na^+ and K^+

pump, Ca^{2+} flux, sugar transport). (4) It inhibits microfilament function. (5) It modifies the state of polymerization of microtubules. (6) It competes with a migration-enhancing factor present in serum. (7) It induces secretion by macrophages of an autoinhibitory or autoaggregating material.

The simplest approach to understanding the mechanism of action of MIF is the morphological one. At the light-microscopic level, the most frequently reported effects of MIF-containing supernatants or partially purified MIF are inhibition of macrophage spreading on surfaces (during the first hour of incubation), rounding up and loss of pseudopodia (after 24 and 48 hr of incubation), and increased cell adherence and spreading with the formation of long pseudopods and stimulated motility (between 48 and 72 hr of incubation). Aggregation of macrophages has also been repeatedly reported. MIF-induced inhibition of migration and cell aggregation are reversible, even in the continued presence of MIF. This "escape" phenomenon is an intrinsic property of the macrophages, and is not due to progressive destruction of MIF. The changes in macrophage physiology that occur 48–72 hr after exposure to MIF and that represent in part a reversion of the early changes induced by MIF are categorized as phenomena of "macrophage activation." These changes are discussed in Section 3 and in Chapter 5, but it should be realized that the separation of early and late changes in the macrophage is probably artificial, especially if we assume that they are all caused by MIF itself.

At the ultrastructural level, surprisingly few typical changes induced by MIF have been reported. Smyth and Weiss (1970) found an increase in the number of microvilli, especially among the aggregated cells, and Dvorak *et al.* (1972) described the loss of the glycoprotein cell coat material that is normally attached to the outer surface of the macrophage membrane. The latter authors suggested that the absence of the cell coat might favor intercellular adherence and clumping. In general, morphological studies of MIF-treated cells suggest that an alteration in cell-surface properties of macrophages is responsible for inhibition of migration. It is remarkable that no change in the number of repartition of microfilaments and microtubules was noticed in such cells, but further studies, using improved fixation methods, are warranted.

Modified surface properties might be at the basis of the change in electrophoretic mobility (Caspary, 1972), the reduced macrophage spreading (Fauve and Dekaris, 1968), the inhibition of macrophage adherence (Halliday and Miller, 1972) and the increased resistance to detachment (Weiss and Glaves, 1975), which have all been described as occurring early during the MIF–macrophage interaction. The only biochemical correlate to these alterations is the enhanced uptake of glucosamine by MIF-treated macrophages (Hammond *et al.,* 1975). It is not entirely clear what part of the increased uptake is due to incorporation in membrane-associated and other cell material and what part to increased sugar transport across the membrane. Incorporation of glucosamine into membrane-associated material might represent an effort to repair the loss of the glycoprotein cellcoat caused by MIF. On the other hand, that uptake of the nonmetabolized 2-deoxyglucose was also enhanced in cultures of sensitized peritoneal exudate cells cultured with antigen (Hammond *et al.,* 1975) and in purified macrophages exposed to MIF (Pick, in preparation) suggests that increased active membrane transport plays a role.

A second approach to the study of MIF action was to investigate whether MIF possesses enzymatic properties, which might affect macrophage membrane components. Havemann *et al.* (1972) reported that human MIF is inactive in the presence of some antiproteases and diisopropylfluorophosphate (DFP), and suggested that MIF is an esterase with serine as an essential component. Such a protease might act on the macrophage or on a serum component present in the culture medium. Similar results were obtained with MIF released by mouse 3T3 cells transformed by sv 40, which was inactivated by inhibitors of trypsinlike enzymes and by DFP (Poste, 1975a). On the other hand, guinea pig MIF was active in the presence of DFP (David and Becker, 1974), and it seems unlikely that proteolytic potency is a general property of MIF. Treatment of macrophages with trypsin or pronase does not inhibit but actually enhances their spontaneous migration (Pick and Manheimer, 1974).

Further information concerning the mechanism of MIF action was obtained when it was found that pretreatment of macrophages with a variety of esterase inhibitors, including DFP, soybean trypsin inhibitor, and plasma esterase inhibitor enhances MIF activity (Remold, 1974; Remold and Rosenberg, 1975). This finding suggests that the action of MIF might be controlled by macrophage esterases, possibly by inactivating MIF itself.

Recently, numerous attempts have been made to elucidate the intracellular biochemical machanism by which MIF influences macrophages. It is unlikely that MIF acts merely as a passive agglutinin, bridging receptors on adjacent cells, since the macrophage is an active participant in the process, as was clearly shown by the abolishment of MIF-induced migration inhibition (Pick and Manheimer, 1974), macrophage aggregation (Lolekha and Gotoff, 1971), and reduction of electrophoretic mobility (Caspary, 1972) by inhibitors of protein synthesis such as puromycin. The results of pulse exposure experiments make it unlikely that the action of puromycin is simply to impair the renewal of MIF receptors. Alternatively, puromycin may block the synthesis by the macrophage of a material with an essential role in migration inhibition. Although there is evidence for increased production and release by MIF-treated macrophages of collagenase (L. M. Wahl *et al.*, 1975) and other lysosomal enzymes (Pantalone and Page, 1975), these phenomena occur only after prolonged incubation with MIF, and are more related to macrophage activation than to migration inhibition *per se*. Most studies of enzyme levels in MIF-treated macrophages were done on cells exposed to the mediator for longer than 48 hr, and are discussed in Section 3 and Chapter 5. The significance of early changes in the activity of succinate dehydrogenase and glucose-6-phosphate dehydrogenase in macrophages incubated with MIF, which were described by Nath *et al.* (1973), is difficult to evaluate at present. There are no reports on an effect of MIF on ATPase and cation transport, while the enhanced sugar transport mentioned before is a late event.

The striking similarity between the effects of exogenous cAMP and cAMP-generating agents and that of MIF on macrophage migration was at the basis of the hypothesis that MIF affects macrophages by influencing cAMP metabolism in a manner similar to that of a number of hormones. The effect of drugs that affect cAMP on the MIF-induced inhibition of migration was therefore studied. Drugs that decrease cAMP levels in other tissues, such as insulin, nicotinic acid, and imidazole, were found to have no effect on MIF action (Pick and Manheimer, 1973). Other drugs that were reported to decrease cAMP are adenosine (and 2-chloroadenosine) (Haslam and Lynham, 1972) and α,β-methylene ATP (Krug *et al.*,

1973). The former inhibited migration and potentiated MIF, while the latter promoted migration and did not affect MIF. On the other hand, some drugs that elevate cAMP levels in macrophages were found to effectively block MIF activity. These drugs included the phosphodiesterase inhibitor theophylline and the adenylate-cyclase-activating β-adrenergic drugs isoproterenol and epinephrine (Koopman *et al.*, 1973; Pick and Manheimer, 1974). The same drugs also reversed the inhibition of macrophage migration caused by soluble antigen–antibody complexes, suggesting a basic mechanism common to MIF and complex-induced phenomena (Kotkes and Pick, 1975a, b).

The finding that drugs that elevate cAMP antagonize MIF action is difficult to reconcile with the MIF-mimicking effect of the same drugs when added to normal macrophages. The solution to this problem can be helped only by direct measurements of cAMP levels and of the activities of enzymes regulating this level in macrophages exposed to MIF. Preliminary data originating from several laboratories indicate that: (1) MIF does not induce increases in cAMP levels of macrophages within the first 20 min of stimulation (Higgins *et al.*, 1973; Hadden, personal communication). (2) At later times, the level of cAMP tends to be lower in macrophages treated with MIF than in cells treated with control supernatants or medium. Slight but significant differences could be detected after 6 hr (Higgins *et al.*, 1973) or even 1–2 hr of incubation (Pick, in preparation). (3) On the other hand, MIF increased the activity of macrophage adenylate cyclase without a concomitant increase in cellular levels of cAMP, after 24–28 hr of exposure of whole cells to the mediator (Higgins *et al.*, 1973; Remold-O'Donnell and Remold, 1974). (4) Exposure of macrophages to MIF for 1–2 hr makes the cells refractory to the cAMP-generating effect of the adenylate cyclase activators PGE_1, isoproterenol, and cholera toxin. Refractoriness lasts for at least 6 hr, develops in the presence of theophylline and of protein synthesis inhibitors, and is not due to the release of an inhibitor into the culture medium (Pick *et al.*, 1975b). At present, it is difficult to shape these findings into a unified scheme, but most data are compatible with a late stimulation of adenylate cyclase by MIF, which results in little change or even a decrease in the total cellular content of cAMP, due to the refractoriness described above or to some other compensatory feedback mechanism. The blocking effect of cAMP generators could be due to desensitization of adenylate cyclase and prevention of its activation by MIF, although the MIF-antagonizing effect of theophylline is not explained by such a hypothesis. Such an explanation is supported by the finding that preexposure of macrophages to isoproterenol or aminophylline made them refractory to MIF, whereas the same drugs were ineffective when added to cells that were first pulsed with MIF (Kotkes and Pick, 1975a). It was also suggested that adenylate cyclase activation by MIF might be effected via the stimulation of prostaglandin (PG) synthesis (Remold-O'Donnell and Remold, 1974). This suggestion seems unlikely, since the PG synthesis inhibitors indomethacin and acetylsalicylic acid did not prevent MIF action (Kotkes and Pick, 1975a). A possible role for cGMP has not yet been thoroughly investigated, but no change in MIF activity was caused by exogenous cGMP or by two agents reported to raise cGMP concentrations, acetylcholine and carbamylcholine (Pick and Manheimer, 1974; Kotkes and Pick, 1975a). Mediation by cGMP was proposed, however, for a macrophage-proliferation factor that is produced by stimulated lymphocytes and that has a similar molecular weight but is distinct from MIF (Hadden *et al.*, 1974a, 1975).

A further unsolved problem is that of the mechanism by which changes in cAMP levels (whether general or localized) influence macrophage behavior. A role for cAMP has been implied in the regulation of cell motility, adhesiveness, shape, and agglutinability by plant lectins. Increased cAMP levels were found to increase the adhesion of fibroblasts to a substrate (Johnson and Pastan, 1972), and to promote extension of cellular processes, which are then unable to retract (Willingham and Pastan, 1975b). Extension of processes is mediated by increased assembly of microtubular subunits, which in turn is promoted by rises in cellular cAMP, while retraction of processes is inhibited, probably via the blocking action of cAMP on microfilament function (Willingham and Pastan, 1975b). An increase in levels of cAMP in fibrobasts results in cells that are spread out and firmly attached to their substrate, characteristics that are strikingly similar to those of macrophages exposed to MIF for longer intervals. On the other hand, it is possible that MIF modulates elevations in cAMP resulting from cell–cell contact. In mouse fibroblasts, however, an increase in microvilli was associated with reduced cAMP levels (Willingham and Pastan, 1975a), and such abundance of microvilli was described in MIF-treated macrophages (Smyth and Weiss, 1970). We can therefore conclude that the mechanism of MIF action is still unknown. It can be concluded, however, that it is unlikely that cAMP acts as the second messenger of MIF action. The decrease in macrophage cAMP levels caused by MIF and the MIF-induced unresponsiveness to adenylate cyclase stimulators are probably secondary, compensatory events, only indirectly related to inhibition of migration. The nature of the true second messenger is unknown, but there is indirect evidence pointing toward cGMP and Ca^{2+} (Pick and Grunspan-Swirsky, in preparation).

3. Macrophage Activation

Macrophage activation is defined as the enhancement of a number of macrophage functions, and is illustrated most specifically by an increased ability to destroy bacteria, which is essentially nonspecific in its final effects. The typical example of macrophage activation *in vivo* is that occurring soon after infection of mice with *Listeria monocytogenes,* which is expressed by increased numbers of peritoneal macrophages showing an increased tendency to spread out on glass, an abundance in mitochondria and lysosomes, and an enhanced capacity to phagocytize and destroy bacteria. It is not known how specific lymphocyte–antigen interaction *in vivo* is translated into macrophage activation, but evidence is accumulating from *in vitro* studies showing that the link between the two stages of the reaction is via a lymphokine produced by antigen-stimulated lymphocytes.

Most studies of macrophage activation by lymphokines have been performed by using supernatants of antigen- or mitogen-stimulated lymphocytes containing MIF or partially purified MIF-rich fractions of such supernatants. It is therefore natural that no clear relationship, except a temporal one, can be drawn between alterations in macrophage metabolism linked to inhibition of migration and those related to activation. Macrophages in monolayers exposed to MIF-rich supernatants or fractions for 72 hr showed enhanced adherence to surfaces, were markedly spread out, and demonstrated increased ruffled membrane movement (Nathan *et al.,* 1971). These changes were accompanied by an enrichment in vacuoles and lysosomal granules. A fact of interest is that the latent period of 48 hr of contact with MIF required before most manifestations of macrophage activation become evident can be considerably shortened if the target cells are kept in culture for 24–48 hr before being exposed to MIF. Activation also occurs more rapidly when macrophages are cocultured with sensitized lymphocytes and antigen. The reason is unknown, but the finding suggests the existence of lymphocyte-derived activating factors other than MIF, which might be absent from culture supernatants because of their lability.

Of direct relevance to *in vivo* events is the enhanced capacity of activated macrophages to phagocytize some but not all of particles. Nathan *et al.* (1971) reported a moderately increased ability of MIF-activated guinea pig macrophages to engulf mycobacteria, but only a modest increase in phagocytosis of starch, while Meade *et al.* (1974) found a markedly enhanced pinocytosis of colloidal gold. Similarly activated human monocytes demonstrated a rapid increase in phagocytosis of latex particles (Schmidt *et al.*, 1973), but reduced phagocytosis of aggregated protein was also demonstrated (Remold and Mednis, 1972). Of even greater importance is the assessment of the capacity of activated macrophages to inhibit the growth of and to kill bacteria. Fowles *et al.* (1973) found that LK-activated macrophages exhibit a 2- to 10-fold increase in bacteriostatic ability for *Listeria,* and attributed this activation to MIF.

Finally, two other phenomena have been linked to the process of LK-induced macrophage activation. The first is the proliferation of mature macrophages after exposure to antigen-stimulated sensitized lymphocyte supernatants for 2–8 days (Godal *et al.*, 1971; Hadden *et al.*, 1975). The responsible LK (macrophage mitogenic factor) appears to be distinct from MIF, and might be responsible for the macrophage proliferation that occurs in delayed hypersensitivity reactions to facultative intracellular pathogens. The second, possibly related, phenomenon is the induction by LKs of macrophage fusion with the formation of giant cells (Godal *et al.*, 1971; Galindo *et al.*, 1974). The relative importance of endomitosis and actual fusion remains to be determined. The relationship of LKs to macrophage activation is discussed in detail in Chapter 5.

4. Evidence for a Role of MIF *in Vivo*

A central point in all discussion on MIF is the function of the mediator in immunologic reactions *in vivo*. There is reasonably good evidence for MIF acting as an essential link in the development of the mononuclear infiltrate that follows the interaction of sensitized lymphocytes with antigen *in vivo*. There is also some evidence for MIF being involved in the pathogenesis of more complex granulomatous reactions to a number of pathogens. Evidence for an *in vivo* role of MIF comes from two sources, which are discussed below.

4.1. Administration of MIF to Animals

It is difficult to separate the effect of MIF, when administered to animals, from that of other LKs, since no studies have been performed with rigorously purified MIF.

4.1.1. Skin Reactive Factor

Most reports deal with the effects of the intradermal injection of MIF-containing supernatants and the local inflammatory reaction that results. The term *skin reactive factor* (SRF) is being used to denote the material(s) responsible for the complex inflammatory response in the skin, the main components of which are increased vascular permeability and a perivascular infiltrate composed of mononuclear cells or a mixture of mononuclear cells and granulocytes. The general chemical characteristics of SRF appear to be very similar to those of MIF, but it is probable that various components of skin inflammation are produced by distinct factors, and that there is little justification for considering SRF a separate LK. The cellular origin, mechanism of production, and action mechanism of SRF were described by Bennett and Bloom (1968), Pick *et al.* (1969, 1970), Maillard *et al.* (1972), and others. As indicated above, the SRF-induced inflammatory reaction might represent a combination of the effects of mononuclear and neutrophil chemotactic factors and MIF, but the increased vascular permeability is probably caused by a separate substance. That the action of SRF is enhanced by the addition of plasma or serum indicates that SRF might induce the production of a second mediator that affects vascular permeability (Maillard *et al.*, 1972). This final mediator might well be a kinin, with the implication that SRF acts as a kinin generator distinct from kallikrein. This implication is suggested by the inhibition of SRF activity by kinin antagonists such as meclofenamate and its enhancement by kininase inhibitors such as diethyl-dithiocarbamate. The considerable inhibition of SRF action by hexadimethrine bromide and protamine sulfate suggests the involvement of Hageman factor (see Chapter 8).

The relationship of SRF (or some components of SRF) to MIF is further complicated by contradictory reports on the effect of anti-LK antisera on the two mediators. Yoshida *et al.* (1975a) found that an antiserum to MIF-rich supernatant fractions will bind MIF and SRF, but Geczy *et al.* (1975), using an anti-LK antibody prepared by a different technique, found selective binding of MIF only.

4.1.2. Other *in Vivo* Effects of MIF

An effect that has been known for a long time is the macrophage disappearance reaction. Injection of MIF-containing culture supernatants into the peritoneal cavities of normal guinea pigs was found to cause a reduction in the number of peritoneal macrophages (Sonozaki and Cohen, 1971). This reduction is probably due to macrophage clumping and increased adherence to the lining of the peritoneal cavity. It was later found that intravenous injection of MIF-containing supernatants into normal animals also results in a marked reduction in the number of circulating monocytes (Yoshida and Cohen, 1974). This finding suggests that the reduction in peripheral blood monocytes that occurs after intravenous administration of antigen is mediated by MIF released *in vivo*. It is of interest to note that the peripheral monocytopenia that follows MIF injection into sensitized recipients results in the suppression of delayed reactions to the intradermal injection of specific antigen.

Repeated injection of MIF-containing supernatants into the joint resulted in the development of chronic synovitis, characterized by synovial effusion, hyperplasia, and mononuclear infiltration (Andreis *et al.*, 1974).

A special place is occupied by the recent reports on the use of locally injected LK-containing preparations in the treatment of tumors. The growth of a syngeneic transplantable tumor in guinea pig skin could be prevented by the local injection of purified MIF (Bernstein *et al.*, 1971). In a certain number of cases, supernatants derived from phytohemagglutinin-stimulated human lymphocyte cultures or continuous lymphoblastoid cell lines caused temporary regression of cutaneous tumors in man (May-Levin *et al.*, 1972; Papermaster *et al.*, 1974). It is reasonable to assume that tumor destruction in these situations is due to the local accumulation and immobilization of macrophages, followed by their activation. Such activated macrophages are selectively cytotoxic for tumor cells (Piessens *et al.*, 1975).

4.2. Detection of MIF Produced *in Vivo*

MIF has been detected in the blood, lymph, and several tissue reaction sites in animals and humans. MIF was first described in the sera of immunized and antigen-challenged animals by Krejci *et al.* (1968), this report being followed by a number of articles reporting the detection of MIF in serum after antigen challenge (Yamamoto and Takahashi, 1971; Salvin *et al.*, 1973) or in the serum of humans with lymphoproliferative disorders (Cohen *et al.*, 1974). MIF was also released into the efferent lymph of lymph nodes following the injection of antigen into the corresponding drainage area (Hay *et al.*, 1973).

Of even greater interest is the detection of MIF at sites of immune tissue reactions. Lymphocytes that were recovered from human kidney allografts in the process of being rejected produced MIF when placed in culture (Hattler *et al.*, 1973). MIF was found in supernatants of cultures of rheumatoid synovial tissue (Stastny *et al.*, 1973), and in culture fluids of schistosome egg granulomas exposed *in vitro* to soluble egg antigens (Boros *et al.*, 1973). It was disappointing, however, to find that extracts of delayed hypersensitivity skin reaction sites had no MIF activity, but possessed good SRF-like activity (Cohen *et al.*, 1973). It therefore appears that by present methods, proof of MIF production in complex tissues *in vivo* can be obtained only when these tissues are explanted *in vitro* and allowed or induced to continue synthesis in culture.

5. Physiologic Control of MIF

There are few data available concerning the physiologic control of MIF production and action. It is inconceivable, however, that MIF could perform any function *in vivo* in the absence of adequate feedback regulation.

Data discussed in Section 2.2 indicate that MIF secretion is probably regulated by the intracellular level of cAMP. An increase in this level will depress production, while the lowering of cellular cAMP acts as a stimulus for synthesis. A regulatory role for cAMP in a number of secretory systems has been described. This role includes the release of histamine, slow-reacting substance of anaphylaxis, and lysosomal enzymes, and the production of lymphotoxin. A regulatory role for the nucleotide in the extent of cell proliferation has been repeatedly suggested (see Chapter 1). It might well be that in these cells, the cellular level of cAMP regulates both DNA synthesis and MIF synthesis. The level of cAMP in MIF-producing lymphocytes could be elevated by a number of factors normally present *in vivo*. These factors include β-adrenergic stimulants such as epinephrine and rapidly acting mediators of inflammation such as histamine and the PGs. Histamine was found to block MIF secretion (Rocklin, 1975), and feedback inhibition of MIF synthesis by PGs released by MIF-treated macrophages was recently reported (Morley *et al.,* 1975). In contrast to the role played by cAMP, it would appear that cGMP may be associated with augmentation of MIF production, since acetylcholine, which increases cGMP in lymphocytes, augments MIF production (Hadden *et al.*, 1974b).

Other regulatory factors that were found capable of inhibiting MIF by unknown mechanisms are the naturally occurring immunoregulatory α-globulin (Davis *et al.*, 1971), lymphocyte chalones (Houck *et al.,* 1973), serum factors (Ward and Rocklin 1975), and, in the opinion of some but not all authors, the glucocorticosteroids (S. M. Wahl *et al.,* 1975). Definite proof for their function *in vivo* is still lacking, but it is reasonable to assume that the amount of MIF produced following antigenic stimulation of the whole animal is continuously controlled by such factors and others present in the lymphoid microenvironment. The relationship of physiologic regulators to materials that might be responsible for the suppression of MIF production in diseases such as mucocutaneous candidiasis is of great interest.

6. Pharmacological Modulation of MIF

The knowledge that has accumulated concerning the mechanisms of MIF production and action should lead to the development of drugs and other agents able to suppress or promote MIF function. Since MIF is thought to play a central role in the development of cell-mediated immunity, it is hoped that drugs able to influence MIF will also modify immune reactions *in vivo*.

6.1. Influencing Production

The border between physiologic and pharmacological modulators of MIF production is not a sharp one. Glucocorticosteroids, immunoregulatory α-globulin, and the chalones, which were discussed in Section 5, can be considered pharmacological agents, but it is difficult to know how much of their immunosuppressive activity *in vivo* is actually due to depression of MIF production. MIF synthesis is inhibited by agents that increase the cellular level of cAMP, as best illustrated by the suppressive effects of the phosphodiesterase inhibitor theophylline and of chlorphenesin (Pick, 1973). The latter drug is probably an activator of adenylate cyclase, and was reported to block the IgE-mediated histamine release from lung (Malley and Baecher, 1971) and the production of SRF by mitogen-stimulated lymphocytes (Pick *et al.,* 1970). It is of interest that chlorphenesin was found to depress delayed hypersensitivity reactions in guinea pigs (Berger *et al.,* 1969). Agents elevating cAMP also inhibit the production of leukocyte inhibitory factor by mitogen-stimulated human lymphocytes (Lomnitzer *et al.,* 1976a). Recently, attention was focused on the potent, long-acting adenylate cyclase activator cholera toxin. This agent was found to stimulate adenylate cyclase in human and mouse mononuclear cells (Bourne *et al.,* 1973) and in purified guinea pig peritoneal macrophages (Pick *et al.,* 1975b). Cholera toxin was found to inhibit MIF secretion by antigen-stimulated guinea pig lymphocytes, down to a concentration of 1 ng/ml (Pick, in preparation). Different results were reported by Henney *et al.*, (1974), who found no significant effect of cholera toxin, theophylline, or dibutyryl cAMP on MIF synthesis, while PGE_1 was sometimes inhibitory. The mechanism of toxin-induced inhibition is unknown, and may be related directly to elevation of cAMP levels and to the inhibition of RNA and protein synthesis that has been described in toxin-treated mouse spleen cells (Sultzer and Craig, 1973). The inhibitory effect of cholera toxin on the production of MIF was in marked contrast to the moderate direct macrophage-migration-blocking effect of toxin and its inability to interfere with MIF action. The effect on mediator synthesis could serve as an explanation for the pronounced suppressive effect of cholera toxin injected into mice on dermal reactions to schistosome egg antigens, granuloma formation around schistosome eggs, and MIF secretion by granulomas from livers of schistosome-infected animals (Warren *et al.*, 1974). The significance of cholera toxin as an immunosuppressive agent is further stressed by the finding that it also depresses histamine release, mitogen-induced lymphocyte stimulation, hemolytic plaque formation, and the binding of SRBC to T cells in humans and T-cell-mediated cytolysis.

Another agent that was found to block MIF synthesis is cytochalasin B (Pick, 1973). It was later reported that this inhibition is effective only when the drug is present during the first 2 hr of exposure to antigen, indicating that it blocks an event that follows soon after antigen recognition (Ben-Sasson and Rosenthal, 1975). It has been suggested that cytochalasin B interferes with the macrophage–lymphocyte interaction required for the induction of MIF synthesis, but this suggestion seems unlikely, since MIF production by purified lymphocytes was also blocked by the drug (Pick, 1973).

Little is known about the effect of specific antisera on MIF production. Pekarek *et al.* (1971) reported that heterologous antilymphocyte serum blocked the antigen-induced release of MIF in the absence of a cytotoxic effect on lymphocytes. A finding of considerable theoretical importance is the inhibition of MIF production by specific alloantisera, under conditions that do not result in prevention of antigen-binding (Ben-Sasson *et al.*, 1974).

A number of agents that affect membrane function were also tested, and it was reported that chloroquine and ouabain were without effect (Ben-Sasson and Rosenthal, 1975). This finding is in accordance with the previously recorded inability of chloroquine to block SRF production (Pick *et al.*, 1970). As mentioned earlier, there are contradictory results concerning the effect of glucocorticosteroids. Inhibition of MIF synthesis was reported by S. M. Wahl *et al.* (1975), in contradiction to earlier findings that production of the mediator is not diminished by hydrocortisone (Balow and Rosenthal, 1973). The situation is further complicated by the fact that hydrocortisone was found to induce the formation by human lymphocytes of a factor that stimulates cell migration *in vitro* (Stevenson, 1973).

Niridazole, which was initially used as an antischistosomal agent, was found to block granuloma formation around schitosome eggs and delayed hypersensitivity reactions to soluble antigens, and to prolong skin allograft survival across the *H-2* area (Mahmoud *et al.*, 1975). It was found that all actions of niridazole are caused by a metabolite of the drug present in the blood and excreted in the urine. When niridazole was added *in vitro* to lymphocytes of sensitized animals or such cells were taken from drug-treated animals, antigen-induced MIF formation was found to be normal. Addition to the lymphocytes of serum from niridazole-treated animals suppressed MIF production, however, indicating that a metabolite of the drug is responsible for the inhibitory effect (Daniels *et al.*, 1975). Also of interest is the finding that antigen-induced DNA synthesis was normal in cultures in which MIF production was blocked. The intracellular mechanism by which the niridazole metabolite interferes with MIF synthesis is unknown.

6.2. MIF Neutralization

At present, there are three possible approaches to pharmacological neutralization of MIF. One could make use of the natural MIF inactivator that was found in serum (Ward and Rocklin, 1975). Progress in its fractionation might lead to the production of large quantities of MIF inactivator, with a potential use as a peripheral immunosuppressive agent in humans. That the same serum fraction will inactivate MIF, monocyte chemotactic factor, and complement-derived and bacterial chemotactic factors might generate problems, and the production of material with better specificity might be required.

The second approach is to make use of chemical means of MIF inactivation. This approach was discussed in detail in Section 2.3, but in the light of the pronounced resistance of MIF to drastic denaturing procedures, there is little hope of finding specific MIF-inactivating agents that can be administered *in vivo* in quantities high enough to result in blood concentrations similar to those found to inactivate MIF *in vitro*. However, Bartfeld and Atoynatan (1971) reported that treatment of MIF with 0.01 M *N*-acetylcysteine and cysteine resulted in the disappearance of MIF activity and of skin inflammatory (SRF) activity. These authors mention preliminary findings of reduced delayed hypersensitivity reactions in cysteine-fed guinea pigs, and suggest that an increased level of cysteine compounds may be the reason for deficient cellular immunity in uremic patients.

The third approach is based on the development of specific antibodies directed against MIF. Yoshida *et al.* (1975a) used an original approach for the production of such antibody by immunizing rabbits with a partially purified lymphocyte supernatant fraction that was freed of components other than MIF by passage through a column of agarose-immobilized antibody directed against control lymphocyte supernatant. Passage of MIF-containing supernatants through columns of agarose-immobilized anti-MIF resulted in the loss of MIF activity. The same treatment also removed macrophage chemotactic and skin reactive activity. Of special interest is the finding that local injection of anti-MIF into the skin partially prevented the development of delayed hypersensitivity reactions in immunized animals.

Geczy *et al.* (1975) recently reported the production of a precipitating antibody against MIF, purified by gel filtration and polyacrylamide electrophoresis. Passage of MIF-containing supernatant through immunoabsorbent columns prepared with this antibody resulted in the loss of MIF, but apparently not of mitogenic factor and SRF. When injected intradermally into sensitized animals, this antiserum also blocked the development of delayed reactions. The antibody was not cytotoxic for T cells and did not prevent rosette formation by T cells, and can therefore be distinguished from antilymphocyte serum and specific anti-T antisera. These results are encouraging and justify further research for developing antisera of high specificity that can be administered by the systemic route. Such antisera might be more effective than antilymphocyte serum because of their lack of effect on the inductive phase of immunity, a lesser degree of general immunosuppressive capacity, and an evanescent action, which would allow their use for short periods (e.g., during an allograft rejection crisis). That anti-MIF prepared against lymphocyte-derived MIF cross-reacts with virus-induced MIF opens the way for preparing large quantities of MIF for immunization under standardized conditions.

6.3. Interference with MIF Action

Pharmacological means of preventing MIF action can be classified under the following categories: (1) agents that promote macrophage migration; (2) agents that interfere with the function of microtubules; (3) agents that affect the MIF receptor on macrophages or interfere with binding of MIF to the receptor; (4) inhibitors of proteolysis; (5) agents that act on cAMP metabolism; and (6) agents of unknown action mechanism.

Macrophage migration is promoted by a serum component of yet undetermined nature, some polyanions, treatment of macrophages with proteolytic enzymes, and by lack of Ca^{2+} and Mg^{2+} in the medium (Pick and Manheimer, 1974). While the serum component that promotes macrophage migration has not been identified, similar factors that promote fibroblast migration were isolated from serum (Lipton *et al.*, 1971) and from the culture medium in which sv-40-transformed cells were grown (Bürk, 1973). The migration-promoting effect of polyanions such as dextran sulfate is probably linked to an increase in surface charge, resulting in reciprocal repulsion of the cells. Promotion of migration by enzymatic treatment of the macrophage membrane and by removal of divalent cations is of little importance from a pharmacological point of view, since they represent situations difficult to achieve *in vivo*. Migration is also promoted under certain conditions by the ATPase inhibitor ouabain (Leu *et al.*, 1973), and the recent report that the migration of human monocytes is enhanced by ascorbic acid, via stimulation of the hexose monophosphate shunt, is of interest (Goetzl *et al.*, 1974). No data are available about the response of macrophages to MIF in the presence of the latter two agents.

Colchicine and vinblastine were found to be very potent migration promoters in a wide concentration range (10^{-5}–10^{-7} M) (Pick and Abrahamer, 1973). The loss of MIF responsiveness by drug-treated cells and the relatively widespread clinical use of both drugs make them good candidates for *in vivo* use as suppressors of cell-mediated immune responses. On the other hand, it appears that the very same drugs have no effect on human polymorphonuclear cell migration and do not block the action of leukocyte-migration- inhibitory factor (Lomnitzer *et al.*, 1976b).

Another way of interfering with MIF action is at the level of macrophage receptor–MIF interaction. This interference can be achieved by damaging macrophage receptors with proteolytic enzymes, by enhancing the activity of macrophage-bound esterase, by inhibition of macrophage protein synthesis, and by the use of competitive inhibitors such as α-L-fucose and fucose-containing glycoproteins or the fucose-binding *Lotus* lectin. Among these methods, drugs that are of possible practical importance for development are the agents that are able to block the MIF-enhancing plasma esterase inhibitors described by Remold and Rosenberg (1975). For instance, it was found that heparin binds to the esterase inhibitor antithrombin–heparin cofactor, forming a complex that is prevented from binding to the macrophage, probably because of its highly negative charge. This effect may increase MIF inactivation and explain in part the blocking effects of heparin on cell-mediated immune reactions *in vivo* (Cohen *et al.*, 1967). A second category of compounds of possible practical importance are fucose-containing molecules (blood group substance H, bovine submaxillary mucin) that are able to bind to MIF (Fox *et al.*, 1974) or alternatively *Lotus* lectin, which is capable of reacting with the macrophage receptor and preventing MIF binding (Poste, 1975b). The development of sugar-containing synthetic compounds of little antigenicity, based on the fucose model in the guinea pig, for use as MIF inhibitors *in vivo* is a challenging prospect. An alternative possibility is the development of biologically inactive MIF analogues capable of binding to macrophages and occupying the MIF receptor. With progress in the purification of MIF, it is certain that chemically modified MIF will be developed with intact macrophage-binding capacity but no migration-inhibitory ability.

As discussed in Section 2.4.3, there are several reports indicating that MIF acts as a protease. While this finding could not be universally confirmed, it might be worthwhile to consider the use of antiproteases for counteracting MIF action. Two such inhibitors, Trasylol and ϵ-aminocaproic acid (EACA), are of special interest, since they are in clinical use in humans. Care should be exercised in their application, however, since the inhibition of macrophage-bound esterases by such compounds can result in an enhancement of MIF activity. Also, the MIF-antagonizing effect of EACA, which was attributed exclusively to its antiproteolytic action, appears to be mediated by a different mechanism, probably via an interaction with MIF receptors (Houck and Chang, 1975).

A central place among MIF antagonists was recently taken by drugs that affect the cellular concentration of cAMP. It was demonstrated by two laboratories that agents that elevate macrophage cAMP levels counteract MIF action (Koopman *et al.*, 1973; Pick and Manheimer, 1974; Kotkes and Pick, 1975a). Effective inhibition of MIF was found with the adenylate cyclase activators isoproterenol, epinephrine, and norepinephrine. The MIF-blocking effect of the β-adrenergic agents isoproterenol and epinephrine could be reversed by β-antagonists, and that of the α-adrenergic agent norepinephrine, by α-antagonists. A certain cross-inhibition was found (α-antagonists also block the effect of β-adrenergic agents), however, and remained unexplained. Not all adenylate cyclase activators block MIF action. As mentioned before, contradictory results were obtained with PGE_1 and PGE_2, some authors reporting inhibition of MIF (Koopman *et al.*, 1973), and other authors finding no such effect (Pick and Manheimer, 1974; Morley *et al.*, 1975). The total lack of effect on MIF action of the very potent adenylate cyclase activator cholera toxin is also difficult to understand. MIF action was successfully reversed, however, by the phosphodiesterase inhibitor theophylline, at concentrations that have no or only a slight direct inhibitory effect on macrophages ($1-2 \times 10^{-4}$ M). While it was claimed that the MIF-antagonizing effects of the drugs named above can be reproduced by exogenous dibutyryl cAMP (Koopman *et al.*, 1973), an enhancing effect on MIF activity was found in another laboratory (Pick, unpublished). As discussed in Section 2.4.3, the reversal of MIF action by drugs that elevate macrophage cAMP has yet to be explained, and is probably linked to the phenomenon of nonspecific desensitization of cells to adenylate cyclase stimulators described by R. J. Ho and Sutherland (1971). In any case, the observation that certain cAMP-raising agents block MIF action suggests that *in vivo* manipulations with these agents might also do so.

In the light of the many situations in which an antagonism was found between the cellular effects of cAMP and cGMP, the influence of drugs that elevate cGMP levels was investigated. Acetylcholine and carbamylcholine were found to have no influence on MIF activity, but proof is lacking for an actual effect of these drugs on macrophage cGMP levels (Kotkes and Pick, 1975a). Interestingly, levamisole, a derivative of imidazole that increases cGMP levels in lymphocytes and macrophages (Hadden *et al.* 1975; Wright *et al.*, 1976), increases phagocytosis and chemotaxis of macrophages (Wright *et al.*, 1976), thus suggesting that cGMP may play a role in MIF actions.

Finally, the effect of agents working through an unknown mechanism of action, as illustrated by the glucocorticosteroids, should be mentioned. Hydrocortisone was reported to suppress the action of MIF (Balow and Rosenthal, 1973) and that of macrophage-aggregating factor, which is probably identical with MIF (Weston *et al.*, 1973). It has been suggested that the inhibitory action of the steroid is mediated via the inhibition of macrophage protein synthesis, the inhibition of proteolysis, or the induction of the synthesis of a protein that modifies membrane transport, but there is no good evidence in support of any of these propositions.

It may be appropriate to end this section by mentioning the pharmacological means of suppressing the vascular-permeability-increasing action of SRF, although it is probable that the actual mediator responsible for this effect is different from MIF. No specific inhibitor of SRF is available, and all drugs that affect SRF act on secondary mediators probably produced under the influence of SRF. As mentioned before, it is assumed that these mediators are kinins. Meclofenamate, which blocks the effects of kinins, blocks SRF action, and diethyldithiocarbamate, which protects kinins by antagonizing kininases, enhances the inflammatory effect of SRF (Maillard *et al.*, 1972). Marked inhibition of SRF activity was also found with the Hageman factor antagonists polybrene and protamine sulfate. The moderate inhibitory effect detected with heparin and Warfarin also suggest the participation of Hageman factor, and may be related to the suppressive effects of the two drugs on delayed hypersensitivity reactions *in vivo* (Cohen *et al.*, 1967). It is interesting to note that the PG synthesis inhibitors indomethacin and sodium salicylate, as well as hydrocortisone, had no influence on SRF-induced skin inflammation.

7. Physiologic Control and Pharmacological Modulation of Other Lymphokines

The intricate regulatory mechanisms that govern the production and action of MIF, as well as the many possibilities for pharmacological modulation of this mediator, were described in detail not because it is believed that MIF occupies a special place among lymphokines, but because it is the one that has been studied the most. In this section, I would like to describe possible pharmacological approaches to the modulation of synthesis and action of lymphokines other than MIF. I have chosen among these the chemotactic lymphokines, lymphotoxins, and interferons produced by stimulated lymphocytes. This choice is a biased one, the rationale behind it being that emphasis is placed on lymphokines active at the effector end of the immune response.

7.1. Chemotactic Lymphokines

Stimulated lymphocytes of a variety of animal species produce soluble materials that are chemotactic for macrophages, neutrophils, eosinophils, and basophils. Although chemical characterization is less advanced than that of MIF, we are probably dealing with distinct molecular entities, each of which is specific for a certain target cell. LKs chemotactic for macrophages (Ward *et al.*, 1970), neutrophils (Ramseier, 1967; Ward *et al.*, 1970), eosinophils (Cohen and Ward, 1971), and basophils (Ward *et al.*, 1975) have been detected in cultures of lymphocytes of guinea pigs, chickens, and humans as the result of stimulation by specific antigen or histoincompatible cells, mitogens, antigen–antibody complexes, antigen–antibody–complement complexes, the isolated fragment C3b, and antiimmunoglobulin. As far as macrophage chemotactic LK is concerned, it has been established that it can be produced by both T and B cells, if they are appropriately stimulated (Altman and Kirchner, 1972; S. Wahl *et al.*, 1974b). Macrophage chemotactic LK can be detected in supernatants as early as 8 hr after stimulation of cultures, and its formation is independent of DNA synthesis. In the guinea pig, it is a protein that is stable at 56°C, of a molecular weight close to and smaller than albumin, and with an electrophoretic mobility identical to that of albumin (Ward *et al.*, 1970). It therefore appears to be distinct from MIF (which migrates faster than albumin) and from the only partially characterized neutrophil chemotactic LK (which migrates slower than albumin). Human macrophage chemotactic LK is a smaller molecule (mol. w. 12,500) that is sensitive to trypsin and pepsin and unaffected by neuraminidase, demonstrates heterogeneity on isoelectric focusing, and is antigenically distinct from C3 and C5 (Altman *et al.*, 1975). There seems to be no difference in physicochemical properties between macrophage chemotactic LKs released by human T and B lymphocytes. Guinea pig macrophage chemotactic LK was reported to act equally well on homologous and heterologous target cells (Ward *et al.*, 1970), but considerable species specificity was later reported with similar LKs from chickens, humans, and even guinea pigs (S. M. Wahl *et al.*, 1974a). It is of interest to note that the presence of MIF does not affect the chemotactic responsiveness of macrophages to chemotactic LK (Ward *et al.*, 1970). Both macrophages and basophils respond chemotactically to C5a, and it was recently found that preincubation of basophils with antigen- or mitogen-stimulated human lymphocyte culture supernatants augments their response to the chemotactic influence of C5a (Boetcher and Leonard, 1973).

There is ample evidence for the participation of chemotactic LKs in immunologic events *in vivo*. As mentioned earlier, extracts prepared from skin sites of delayed hypersensitivity reactions contain macrophage chemotactic LK (Cohen *et al.*, 1973), and both macrophage and neutrophil chemotactic LKs were detected in the supernatants of cultures of lymphocytes recovered from an allografted rejected kidney (Hattler *et al.*, 1973). Macrophage chemotactic LK was also found in homogenates of kidneys undergoing a local graft-vs.-host reaction (Ward and Volkman, 1975), and could be partially purified from peritoneal fluid taken from sensitized guinea pigs after intraperitoneal challeange with antigen (Postlethwaite and Snyderman, 1975).

Little is known about modulation of the production of chemotactic LKs. Hydrocortisone was found to inhibit the antigen- and mitogen-induced release of macrophage chemotactic LK by human and guinea pig lymphocytes (S. M. Wahl, 1975). L-Asparaginase, while it effectively blocked mitogen-induced DNA synthesis, did not influence the production of chemotactic LK (Rühl *et al.*, 1974).

The mechanism of action of chemotactic LKs is poorly understood in comparison with the information available concerning the way in which cells respond to complement-derived and other chemotactic stimuli, but it is unlikely that the two mechanisms are essentially different. The classic chemotactic response of neutrophils is inhibited by lysosomal stabilizers such as glucocorticosteroids and quinolines (chloroquine) by a direct effect on the responding cell. Lysosomal labilizers such as vitamin A enhance the chemotactic response, possibly by an effect on the cell membrane. Chemotaxis is also suppressed by the microtubule disruptive drugs colchicine and vinblastine, by the clinically used antiinflammatory drug phenylbutazone, and by the ATPase inhibitor ouabain (these data concerning drug effects on chemotaxis were reviewed by Ward, 1971). To this author's knowledge, the effect on LK-mediated chemotaxis of the agents named above has not been investigated. The chemotactic response of neutrophils and monocytes was enhanced by ascorbic acid and levamisole, probably by stimulation of cellular accumulation of cGMP (Goetzl *et al.*, 1974: Sandler *et al.*, 1975; Anderson *et al.*, 1976; Wright *et al.*, 1976). Chemotaxis of neutrophils to complement-derived stimuli was blocked by synthetic esterase inhibitors and plasma α-globulins, and very recently it was found that chemotactically directed movement of neutrophils was blocked by the cholesterol-specific θ toxin, but not by phospholipase C. On the other hand, the chemotactic response of monocytes was blocked by phospholipase C, but not by θ toxin. These latter data suggest that the interaction of chemotactic factors with membrane lipids (cholesterol, phospholipids) might be of prime importance in initiating directional movement, and that the reactive lipid is different in neutrophils and macrophages (Wilkinson, 1975). A recent report also indicates interaction among complement-mediated chemotaxis and LKs. This interaction is illustrated by the finding that a macrophage acid proteinase is able to release C5a from C5 (Snyderman *et al.*, 1972). C5a is chemotactic for both neutrophils and macrophages, and it is conceivable that macrophages activated by MIF release proteinases that, by inducing the formation of C5a, amplify the accumulation of phagocytic cells at the site of inflammation.

There is an increasing amount of evidence for regulation of chemotactic responses by cyclic nucleotides. cGMP and agents that increase cGMP levels in leukocytes (PMA, carbamylcholine) was found to promote neutrophil chemotaxis toward an *E. coli* filtrate, while cAMP decreased chemotactic responsiveness (Estensen *et al.*, 1973). In contrast, cAMP inhibited neutrophil motility and chemotaxis (Rivkin *et al.*, 1975).

The response of human monocytes to macrophage chemotactic LK was found to be considerably reduced by incubation of the cells with herpes simplex or influenza virus, under conditions in which cell viability was not affected (Kleinerman *et al.*, 1974). This mechanism might be responsible for the impaired cell-mediated immunity seen in some viral infections. Also of interest is the recent finding that tumor cells produce a factor that prevents the accumulation of polymorphonuclears at sites of inflammation, and it has been suggested that this results from the inactivation of or competition with chemotactic factors (Fauve *et al.*, 1974).

Two distinct serum components that are able to irreversibly inactivate bacterial and complement-derived chemotactic factors were recently described (Till and Ward, 1975). It was also shown that these serum factors inactivate macrophage chemotactic LK and MIF, but it remains to be seen whether we are in fact dealing with the same inactivator (Ward and Rocklin, 1975). There is also evidence for the existence of a serum inhibitor of chemotaxis and leukocyte motility, and for the presence in plasma of a natural antagonist to this factor. Defects in chemotactic responsiveness might be brought about by increased levels of inhibitor or the absence of its antagonist (Soriano *et al.*, 1973). The effect of such serum modulators on the responsiveness of cells to chemotactic LKs has not been investigated.

7.2. Lymphotoxins

Lymphotoxins (LTs) are soluble materials released by lymphocytes in culture as the result of mitogenic or specific antigenic stimulation that have a deleterious effect on a number of target cells *in vitro*. The phenomenon was first described by Ruddle and Waksman (1968) and by Granger and Williams (1968). LTs are produced by lymphocytes of mice, guinea pigs, rats, cats, hamsters, and humans following stimulation by mitogens such as phytohemagglutinin (PHA) and Con A and, when derived from sensitized animals, by specific antigen. LT production by lymphoid cell lines has also been reported. Cytotoxic factors, distinct from LTs, are also produced by normal or antigen-stimulated macrophages, and are apparently responsible for a variety of effects ranging from frank cytotoxicity to inhibition of cell proliferation.

Damage to target cells is assessed by morphological observation and cell counts; by measuring the uptake of labeled amino acids, thymidine, 2-deoxyglucose, or inositol; by the release of ^{51}Cr from prelabeled cells; and by uptake of rubidium. Considerable confusion is caused by the use of terms such as "proliferation-inhibition factor" and "cloning-inhibition factor" for materials that are not clearly distinguishable from LTs, their names being merely descriptive of the assay system used for their detection. It is very probable that the same material demonstrates apparently different activities, provided the concentration of material and the type of target cell are varied. At high concentrations, LTs cause cell destruction, at lower concentrations, permanent inhibition of growth, and at very low concentrations, a temporary growth inhibition (Jeffes and Granger, 1975).

Release of LTs starts 2 or 3 days after exposure to the stimulants and proceeds by an energy-requiring process, as shown by the need for a temperature of 37°C and by the inhibition of secretion by 2,4-dinitrophenol and puromycin. LT secretion does not require DNA synthesis, and is inhibited by glucocorticosteroids (T. W. Williams and Granger, 1969b). A surprising recent finding is the requirement for the continuous presence of the stimulatory mitogen for LT secretion; removal of free and cell-bound mitogen results in the cessation of LT production (Daynes and Granger, 1974). Little is known about the properties of lymphocytes that produce LTs; in the mouse, there is evidence for T cells being responsible for LT production following stimulation by PHA and pokeweed mitogen (Shacks *et al.,* 1973). Whether the T cell is actually secreting the mediator or only cooperating in the production of LT by another cell is not known. LT is definitely secreted by established human lymphoid lines that also produce immunoglobulin.

The physicochemical properties of LTs vary from animal species to species, but certain common characteristics are evident. All LTs are proteins and have a molecular weight ranging between 35,000 and 150,000 (guinea pig LT has a molecular weight around 50,000, mouse LT is close to 100,000, and human LT has been reported to be heterogeneous and contain molecules with a molecular weight of 80,000–150,000). There is some evidence that guinea pig LT is a glycoprotein, but unlike MIF, it is insensitive to neuraminidase. Guinea pig LT is destroyed by chymotrypsin; human LT is inactivated by pronase, but both human and mouse LT seem to be resistant to trypsin. Most LTs are destroyed by heating to 80–100°C, and are stable to (human LT) or partially destroyed by (guinea pig LT) heating to 56–60°C. Only mouse LT is unusual in remaining active after heating to 100°C. The elecrophoretic mobility of LTs varies; guinea pig LT moves with albumin, while human LT migrates in the area of β- and α_2-globulins. Of great significance is the finding from several laboratories that LT is distinct from MIF, interferon, and mitogenic factor.

The mechanism of action of LTs is only partially known. It is well established that LTs are nonspecific toxic agents that affect a variety of target cells, but great differences in susceptibility to LTs are commonly found. Discrepancies in the literature concerning the same target cell are probably due to a different origin of the cell line, conditions of exposure to LT, and concentration of LT. LTs are different from chalones, which are characterized by a strict target specificity for the type of cell that is also producing the chalone. The relationship of classic LT to LKs that are toxic for yeast cells and prevent the multiplication of bacteria remains to be determined.

The following facts are known about the way in which LTs act: (1) LTs are apparently bound to the target cells. (2) Alternatively, they might act via a lipid component of serum. (3) The action of LTs on some target cells is prevented by polyanions such as DNA, RNA, and polyvinylpyrrolidone (T. W. Williams and Granger, 1969a, but is not influenced by possible substrates such as albumin, denatured hemoglobin, mixtures of phospholipids, and some amino sugars or by chelating agents such as EDTA and EGTA (Peter *et al.,* 1973). (4) LT action is accelerated by the presence of 2,4-dinitrophenol, puromycin, cycloheximide, and actinomycin D (T. W. Williams and Granger, 1969a), but is unchanged by lysozyme and hyaluronidase (Peter *et al.,* 1973). (5) Exposure to LTs does not induce alterations in glycolysis, oxidative phosphorylation, or the Na^+–K^+ pump, and lysolecithin is not involved. While the exact sequence of events is unknown, it appears that their primary action is a lytic one on the plasma membrane, with failure of repair and a compensatory increase in RNA synthesis, early shutdown of DNA synthesis, and finally cell destruction. Alternative views have also been expressed; it has been claimed that inhibition of DNA synthesis is the primary event, and that this inhibition is not mediated by an action of LTs on the cell membrane.

Of central importance for the relevance of pharmacological modulation of LTs is the question whether LTs play a role in the mediation of cell-mediated immunity *in vivo*. It has been repeatedly claimed that LTs are not involved in lymphocyte-mediated direct cytotoxicity, since the mediator could not be detected in supernatants of actively cytolytic cultures. This view was challenged when it became apparent that cytolysis by immune lymphocytes involves a secretory process (Plaut *et al.*, 1973), and that an antiserum to LT partially blocks target-cell destruction by immune lymphocytes and antibody-dependent lymphocyte cytotoxicity (cited by Walker and Lucas, 1974). Also, a direct correlation between the susceptibility of target cell line mutants to LTs and to cytolysis by immune or mitogen-stimulated lymphocytes was reported (Namba and Waksman, 1975; Kramer and Granger, 1975). It is therefore possible that the absence of LTs in supernatants of cytotoxic lymphocyte cultures is due to rapid binding of LTs to target cells. Specificity of the lytic process would be ensured by the fact that in immune cytolysis, the target cells serve both as inducers of LT production and at the same time, by their proximity to the producing lymphocytes, as natural targets for the mediator produced. The role of LTs in cell-mediated cytotoxicity is nevertheless far from being established, and was recently questioned by Henney *et al.* (1974), who were able to dissociate LT production and cell lysis by inhibitors of protein synthesis, by drugs that elevate cAMP levels, and by microtubule-disruptive agents.

Pharmacological modulation of LTs can act at three levels: inhibition of production, neutralization of the product, and prevention of its action. Production of LTs by antigen-stimulated lymphocytes is inhibited by cytochalasin B, which affects microfilaments (Yoshinaga *et al.*, 1972). The inhibition is reversible, and is not mediated by interference with binding of antigen. Mitogen-induced LT production is blocked by agents that elevate the cellular level of cAMP and by dibutyryl cAMP itself (Lies and Peter, 1973; Prieur and Granger, 1975). Inhibition is reversible and affects a process following triggering by mitogen. Among agents that increase cGMP levels, imidazole was without effect, but carbamylcholine inhibited LT release. All agents that increase cAMP levels and carbamylcholine also prevented LT-induced cell damage, provided the cells were treated simultaneously with LT and the drugs (Prieur and Granger, 1975). The concentration of drugs required for inhibition of LT action was found to be higher than that required for blocking LT synthesis. The inhibition of LT production and action by some drugs that affect cAMP levels parallels the blocking effects of the same agents on lymphocyte-mediated cytotoxicity. The potent adenylate cyclase activator cholera toxin forms an exception, since it blocks lymphocyte cytotoxicity, but does not inhibit LT secretion (Henney *et al.*, 1974).

The only method of LT inactivation described as yet is based on the use of anti-LT antibodies. Seemingly specific antibodies were produced in several laboratories against human and guinea pig LT (Boulos *et al.*, 1974; Gately *et al.*, 1975). It was found that anti-LT antibody is species-specific, and within the same species, antibody prepared against LT induced by one stimulus will cross-react with LT induced by different stimuli. Anti-LT antibody does not react with MIF or mitogenic factor. An unexpected finding was the ability of antisera to human IgG, L-chain, and Fc fragment to react with LT. Antisera to guinea pig C2, C3, and C5 did not inactivate LT.

The ability of various drugs to inhibit LT action has been little investigated. Peter (1971) found that the lysosome-stabilizing antiinflammatory drugs chloroquine, triamcinolone, dexamethasone, and prednisolone prevent LT action. Two other antiinflammatory agents, sodium salicylate and phenylbutazone, did not modify LT activity. As mentioned above, elevation of the cAMP level in the target cells partially prevents the effect of LTs (Prieur and Granger, 1975). The systematic testing of drugs found to modify lymphocyte cytotoxicity for a possible effect on LT synthesis or action is indicated. These drugs include organophosphorus esterase inhibitors, heparin, insulin, and indomethacin.

7.3. Interferons

Interferons (IFs) are soluble materials released by a variety of cells in response to a variety of stimuli, and are characterized by the capacity to inhibit replication of a number of unrelated RNA and DNA viruses. IFs do not inactivate viruses directly and do not prevent virus absorption to cells, but prevent replication via a process requiring RNA and protein synthesis by the host cell. Evidence is accumulating in support of a more general biological role for IFs, as exemplified by their ability to inhibit the multiplication of tumor cells and normal cells, to enhance phagocytosis by macrophages, to block the growth of intracellular parasites other than viruses, to enhance lymphocyte cytotoxicity, and to inhibit both the sensitization stage and the expression of cell-mediated immunity. While it was originally thought that the production of IFs could be induced only by viruses, it soon became apparent that a number of nonviral agents are potent IF inducers. Among these agents are double-stranded RNA of normal cells, synthetic double-stranded RNA, intracellular microorganisms, lipopolysaccharides, a number of anionic polymers, and some cationic dyes. The subject was recently reviewed by M. Ho and Armstrong (1975). Spontaneous IF production by a variety of normal cells or cell lines has also been reported, but the presence of an unrecognized inducer should be suspected.

New perspectives in IF research were opened by the finding by Glasgow (1966) that peritoneal exudate cells from mice immunized to Chikungunya virus produced 2–10 times more IF than cells of normal mice. This result was reproduced in a number of experimental systems, including stimulation of blood lymphocytes from tuberculin-sensitive humans and of sensitized mouse peritoneal exudate cells with PPD (Green *et al.*, 1969; Milstone and Waksman, 1970), mixed lymphocyte cultures from mice with differences in histocompatibility antigens (Gifford *et al.*, 1971), and leukocytes from rabbits immunized with herpes simplex virus and incubated with ultraviolet-inactivated herpes virus (Lodmell and Notkins, 1974). A special case is represented by IF induction in lymphocytes by mitogens such as PHA (Wheelock, 1965), Con A (Wallen *et al.*, 1973), pokeweed mitogen (Friedman and Cooper, 1967), and antilymphocyte globulin or its bivalent $F(ab')_2$ fragment (Falcoff *et al.*, 1972).

IF production by antigen-stimulated sensitized lymphocytes is characterized by the unusual length of time (3 or 4 days) required for the accumulation of detectable amounts of mediator. On the other hand mitogen-induced IF is detected as early as 2 hr after stimulation, reaching a peak at 20 hr, and antilymphocyte-serum-induced IF is found after only 30 min of incubation. Addition of macrophages, but not of neutrophils, resulted in a considerable increase in IF production by both antigen- and mitogen-stimulated cells.

The cellular origin of antigen- and mitogen-induced lymphocyte-derived IFs has also been investigated. Treatment of mouse spleen cells with anti-θ serum and complement blocks IF production in response to PPD, PHA, and Con A, but not to pokeweed mitogen (Wallen *et al.*, 1973). It was also found that cells producing IF are distinct from those responding to the same stimuli by DNA synthesis. Stobo *et al.* (1974) also found that peripheral T cells were required for IF production after PHA stimulation in mice, while mature or immature thymocytes were unable to release IF. In both studies, it was not determined whether T cells actually release IF or are only required for IF production by another cell. Different results were obtained by Epstein *et al.* (1974), who found that in man, both T and B cells stimulated by PHA and pokeweed mitogen produce IF, but the B-cell response is delayed. Malignant plasma cells from the bone marrow of myeloma patients were found to produce IF spontaneously (Epstein and Salmon, 1974). Patients with thymic hypoplasia have a depressed T-cell IF response that is corrected by thymus grafting, while hypogammaglobulinemic patients have normal T-cell IF production (Epstein and Amman, 1974). The only exception to this is patients with IgA deficiency, who have an unexplained low IF response, while T-cell proliferation is normal.

The synthesis of IFs requires RNA and protein synthesis, but the situation is complicated by the fact that the inhibition of protein and RNA synthesis after induction enhances IF synthesis, possibly by blocking the formation of a protein that normally terminates production. Human IF synthesis is blocked by inhibitors of glycosylation (Havell *et al.*, 1975).

Youngner and Salvin (1973) found that IF produced by specific antigenic stimulation of mice is different in physicochemical properties from IF produced by nonspecific stimuli. They proposed the name "type I IF for the material produced by nonspecific stimuli and "type II IF" for the material induced by specific antigen. Type II IF is a trypsin-sensitive material with a molecular weight of 45,000–80,000, unstable at pH 2 (unlike type I IF), and stable at 56°C. IFs induced by PHA and antilymphocyte serum are also unstable at pH2 and 10, but PHA-induced IF is inactivated at 56°C. Not all antigen-induced IFs have properties identical to those of type II IF in mice. Human PPD-induced IF is stable at extremes of pH, and so are rabbit IF induced by PPD and mouse IF released in mixed lymphocyte cultures. Spontaneous IF is stable at pH 2 and relatively resistant to heating at 56°C. It is also of interest that in the mouse, type I and type II IFs are antigenically distinct. The close resemblance between the physicochemical characteristics of type II IF and MIF in the mouse is intriguing, and a possible identity of the two mediators has been suggested (Youngner and Salvin, 1973).

The biological importance of IFs induced by immunologic mechanisms is not clear. Cell-mediated immunity is definitely involved in host resistance against the herpes virus group and vaccinia virus, and it has been suggested that IF induced by specific immunologic mechanisms might block the spread of the virus (Lodmell and Notkins, 1974). A seemingly paradoxic situation is seen in herpes simplex infections in humans, where peak IF production occurs only 2–6 weeks after the onset of disease and could therefore have little influence on the evolution of the disease. It was suggested, however, that the delay in IF production by peripheral lymphocytes is due to localization of specifically responding cells at the sites of the viral attack (Rasmussen *et al.,* 1974).

In addition to this antiviral function, other less specific effects of IFs might be important. As mentioned before, IFs could enhance host defense by their reported phagocytosis-enhancing effect and by inhibiting tumor cell multiplication *in vitro* and the growth of transplanted tumors *in vivo*. Also, IFs have been reported to have a variety of stimulatory and inhibitory effects on the humoral and cell-mediated immune response. These effects include stimulation or inhibition of antibody formation against SRBC, inhibition of antigen-induced lymphocyte proliferation, enhancement of lymphocyte cytotoxicity, and prevention of the elicitation and induction of delayed-type hypersensitivity. A special place is occupied by type II IF released into the bloodstream of immunized mice 3–4 hr after specific antigenic stimulation *in vivo* (Stinebring and Absher, 1970). The phenomenon was studied in detail by Youngner and Salvin (1973), who found that intravenous BCG immunization followed by challenge with intravenous BCG elicits IF (and MIF) release into the circulation. It is probable that IF released into the blood is identical to IF induced *in vitro* by exposure of lymphocytes from animals sensitized to specific antigen. A strict correlation was found between the conditions of immunization that resulted in the *in vivo* release of IF and MIF and those that ensured protection against virulent *Mycobacterium tuberculosis*. It is therefore possible that antiviral mechanisms can be induced by the specific challenge of immunized animals with antigens unrelated to the virus. This induction would represent a parallel to the phenomenon of macrophage activation against bacterial attack which is also characterized by lack of specificity. The multiplicity of IF inducers available and the relative ease with which IFs can be produced in large amounts *in vitro* are promising conditions for their use in humans in situations other than viral infections (antitumor therapy, immunosuppression).

Little can be said about pharmacological modulation of IF production and action. It has been reported that treatment of cells with dibutyryl cAMP, or with drugs that elevate cAMP levels inhibits the production of IF induced by viruses or synthetic polynucleotide (Dianzani *et al.*, 1972). The inhibitory effect of cAMP was prevented by suppression of protein synthesis. On the other hand, cAMP and agents that increase cAMP concentrations were also found to potentiate the antiviral activity of IF. It is of interest that IF itself induced a moderate increase in cAMP levels 4 hr after addition to the cells, possibly by stimulation of adenylate cyclase (Weber and Stewart, 1975).

8. *In Vivo* Realities—Role of Lymphokines in Immunity and Nonimmunologic Processes

In this present review, I have repeatedly stressed that LKs are of relevance to immunology only if definite proof is available that they do indeed participate in immunologic processes in the intact animal. The term LK should be used in a broad but nevertheless circumscribed sense, as defining soluble materials of lymphocytic origin that are produced as the result of some form of stimulus-membrane interaction and that are distinct from immunoglobulins. Emphasis should not be placed solely on the fact that they have certain biological effects, unless such an effect can be defined in more precise molecular terms. Also, we have come lately to admit that both the cellular origin and the range of biological actions of LKs transcend the borders of classic immune phenomena. That they do could mean that the immunologically related manifestations of LKs might represent only the tip of the iceberg, and that we have been dealing merely with a particular manifestation of a wide class of soluble intercellular mediators produced by a variety of cells in response to certain stimuli, the nature of which is not yet understood. We must also consider, however, the possibility that we have been misled by an apparent similarity in the biological effects of materials of lymphoid and nonlymphoid origin, which does not reflect a true identity or even a close relationship. We should remember that the main biological activity detected in materials produced by nonlymphoid cells is inhibition of macrophage migration, which, as we have repeatedly said, can be the result of a number of cellular mechanisms. It is therefore possible that two unrelated materials, with two totally different *in vivo* functions, might have a similar effect on a target cell in an admittedly highly artifactual *in vitro* situation. Similarities in physicochemical characteristics between lymphoid and nonlymphoid materials are of doubtful significance, unless highly purified and rigorously characterized LKs become available. The strongest argument to date for a true identity of lymphoid and virus-induced MIF is the serologic cross-reaction among these substances found by Yoshida *et al.* (1975b).

A reasonable functional classification of LKs based on the mechanisms by which they bring about their effect would therefore be the following:*

1. *Inhibitory LKs,* which include LTs and materials such as proliferation-inhibitory factor and cloning-inhibitory factor (the relationship of which to LTs was discussed in Section 7.2). This category should probably also include materials recently described that have a direct toxic or multiplication-inhibitory action on bacteria and fungi and type II IF. The main biological phenomenon in which a function for such LKs is suspected is lymphocyte cytotoxicity (direct and antibody-dependent), with its possible relevance to allograft rejection, control of malignancy, and elimination of aberrant clones. This category should also include the recently recognized suppressor factors with a suspected role in the natural modulation of the immune response and in the maintenance of immunologic unresponsiveness.

2. *Stimulatory LKs,* which include the mitogenic factors that act on lymphocytes, the macrophage mitogenic factor (discussed in Chapter 5), hemopoietic colony-stimulating factors, and the recently recognized mediators of T–B and T–T cell cooperation. While a role for such LKs at the effector end of the immune response has been suggested (e.g., by inducing macrophage proliferation), their main function appears to be in the inductive phases of immunity. A fine equilibrium between stimulatory and inhibitory LKs is at least partly responsible for the quick responsiveness and self-limiting ability of the immune phenomena *in vivo.*

3. *Inflammatory LKs,* which form what is probably the biologically most significant category. The common denominator of this group is their property to recruit and activate a variety of circulatory cells that participate in inflammation. The group includes all chemotactic LKs and the MIFs, as well as mediators that influence vascular permeability and the clotting system via platelets or soluble clotting factors. The paramount importance of these factors lies in the fact that they are largely responsible for amplifying the specific interaction between sensitized lymphocyte and antigen. As an example, such interaction will result in the release of factors that increase vascular permeability (possibly via the activation of a cascade of immediate-type mediators), which is followed by the accumulation of inflammatory cells (neutrophils, macrophages, basophils, eosinophils) attracted to the site of

*Thanks are expressed to Dr. Stanley Cohen for suggesting such a classification in the course of a stimulating correspondence.

the immunologic event by a variety of chemotactic LKs. Once arrived, the cells are immobilized by exposure to MIF-like factors and subsequently activated. Some of the nonspecific cells recruited by this process will release secondary mediators (e.g., the release by macrophages of collagenase, other lysosomal enzymes, and plasminogen activator), which further accentuate the inflammatory process. It is probable that most of the defense mechanisms against infectious agents, for which cell-mediated immunity is responsible, are mediated via the inflammatory LKs. On the other hand, it would be dangerous to take the dogmatic view and identify inflammatory and other LKs exclusively with cell-mediated immunity. Induction of MIF release by soluble antigen-antibody complexes and the cooperation between complexes and lymphocytes in the release of eosinophil chemotactic LK are clear examples of the interrelationship of humoral and cell-mediated immunity.

Finally, the biological role of LKs might extend much beyond strictly immunologic phenomena. LKs might affect such other processes as tissue healing and regeneration, the removal of damaged or senescent tissue, the migration of tumor cells *in vivo,* clotting phenomena, and bone resorption. We should remember that the nonimmunologic function of LKs might turn out to be as important as the general physiologic role of immediate-type mediators, such as histamine and serotonin.

ACKNOWLEDGMENTS

The author's experimental work described in this chapter was supported by grant 5-RO1 AI-11194 from the National Institutes of Health, Bethesda, Md., by grant No. 480 from the U.S.-Israel Binational Science Foundation, and by a grant from F. Hoffman-La Roche & Co. Ltd., Basel, Switzerland.

References

Altman, L. C., and Kirchner, H., 1972, *J. Immunol.* **109**:1149–1151.
Altman, L. C., Chassy, B., and Mackler, B., 1975, *J. Immunol.* **115**:18–21.
Anderson, R., Glover, A., Koornhof, H. J., and Rabson, A. R., 1976, *J. Immunol.* **117**:428–432.
Andreis, M., Stastny, P., and Ziff, M., 1974, *Arthritis Rheum.* **17**:537–551.
Ashworth, L. A. E., Eckersley, B. J., and Ford, W. H., 1975, *Int. Arch. Allergy* **48**:143–155.
Balow, J. E., and Rosenthal, A. S., 1973, *J. Exp. Med.* **137**:1031–1041.
Bartfeld, H., and Atoynatan, T., 1969, *Proc. Soc. Exp. Biol. Med.* **130**:497–501.
Bartfeld, H., and Atoynatan, T., 1970, *Int. Arch. Allergy* **38**:549–553.
Bartfeld, H., and Atoynatan, T., 1971, *Nature (London) New Biol.* **231**:157–159.
Bennett, B., and Bloom, B. R., 1967, *Transplantation* **5**:996– 1000.
Bennett B., and Bloom, B. R., 1968, *Proc. Natl. Acad. Sci. U.S.A.* **59**:756–762.
Ben-Sasson, S. Z., and Rosenthal, A. S., 1975, *J. Immunol.* **115**:1140–1142.
Ben-Sasson, S. Z., Shevach, E., Green, I., and Paul, W. E., 1974, *J. Exp. Med.* **140**:383–395.
Berger, F. M., Fukui, G. M., Goldenbaum, E. G., De Angelo, M., and Chandlee, G. C., 1969, *J. Immunol.* **102**:1024–1031.
Bergstrand, H., and Kallen, B., 1973, *Scand J. Immunol.* **2**:173–187.
Bernstein, I. D., Thor, D. E., Zbar, B., and Rapp. H. J., 1971, *Science* **172**:729–731.
Bhisey, A. N., and Freed, J. J., 1971, *Exp. Cell. Res.* **64**:419–429.
Bloom, B. R., 1971, *Adv. Immunol.* **13**:101–208.
Bloom, B. R., and Bennett, B., 1966, *Science* **153**:80–82.
Bloom, B. R., and Bennett, B., 1970, *Ann. N.Y. Acad. Sci.* **169**:258–265.
Bloom, B. R., and Jimenez, L., 1970, *Am. J. Pathol.* **60**:453–465.
Bloom, B. R., Gaffney, J., and Jimenez, L. 1972, *J. Immunol.* **109**:1395–1398.

Bloom, B. R., Stoner, G., Gaffney, J., Shevach, E., and Green, I., 1975, *Eur. J. Immunol.* **5**:218–220.
Boetcher, D. A., and Leonard, E. J., 1973, *Immunol. Commun.* **2**:421–429.
Boros, D. L., Warren, K. S., and Pelley, R. P., 1973, *Nature (London)* **246**:224–226.
Boulos, G. N., Rosenau, W., and Goldberg, M. L., 1974, *J. Immunol.* **112**:1347–1353.
Bourne, H. R., Lehrer, R. I., Lichtenstein, L. M., Weissmann, G., and Zurier, R., 1973, *J. Clin. Invest.* **52**:698–708.
Braunstein, J. D., Hadden, E. M., Good, R. A., and Hadden, J. W., 1974, *Fed. Proc. Fed. Am. Soc. Exp. Biol.* **33**:650 (abstract).
Bremerskov, V., 1973, *Nature (London) New Biol.* **246**:174.
Bürk, R. R., 1973, *Proc. Natl. Acad. Sci. U.S.A.* **70**:369–372.
Caspary, E. A., 1972, *Clin. Exp. Immunol.* **11**:305–309.
Clinton, B. A., Magoc, T. J., and Aspinall, R. L., 1974, *J. Immunol.* **112**:1741–1746.
Cohen, S., and Ward, P. A., 1971, *J. Exp. Med.* **133**:133–146.
Cohen, S., Benacerraf, B., McCluskey, R., and Ovary, Z., 1967, *J. Immunol.* **98**:351–358.
Cohen, S., Ward, P. A., Yoshida, T., and Burek, C. L., 1973, *Cell. Immunol.* **9**:363–376.
Cohen, S., Fisher, B., Yoshida, T., and Bettigole, R. E., 1974, *N. Engl. J. Med.* **290**:882–886.
Daniels, J. C., Warren, K. S., and David, J. R., 1975, *J. Immunol.* **115**:1414–1421.
David, J. R., 1965, *J. Exp. Med.* **122**:1125–1134.
David, J. R., 1966, *Proc. Natl. Acad. Sci. U.S.A.* **56**:72–77.
David, J. R., and Becker, E. L., 1974, *Eur. J. Immunol.* **4**:287–289.
David, J. R., and David, R. A., 1972, *Prog. Allergy* **16**:300–449.
Davis, R. C., Cooperband, S. R., and Mannick, J., 1971, *J. Immunol.* **106**:755–760.
Daynes, R. A., and Granger, G. A., 1974, *Cell. Immunol.* **12**:252–262.
Dianzani, F., Neri, P., and Zucca, M., 1972, *Proc. Soc. Exp. Biol. Med.* **140**:1375–1378.
Dumonde, D. C., Wolstencroft, R. A., Panayi, G. S., Matthew, M., Morley, J., and Howson, W. T., 1969, *Nature (London)* **224**:38–42.
Dumonde, D. C., Page, D. A., Matthew, M., and Wolstencroft, R. A., 1972, *Clin. Exp. Immunol.* **10**:25–47.
Dvorak, A. M., Hammond, M. E., Dvorak, H. F., and Karnovsky, M. J., 1972, *Lab. Invest.* **27**:561–574.
Epstein, L. B., and Ammann, A. J., 1974, *J. Immunol.* **112**:617–626.
Epstein, L. B., and Salmon, S. E., 1974, *J. Immunol.* **112**:1131–1138.
Epstein, L. B., Kreth, H. W., and Herzenberg, L. A., 1974, *Cell. Immunol.* **12**:407–421.
Estensen, R. D., Hill, H. R., Quie, P. G., Hogan, N., and Goldberg, N. D., 1973, *Nature (London)* **245**:458–460.
Falcoff, R., Oriol, R., and Iscaki, S., 1972, *Eur. J. Immunol.* **2**:476–478.
Fauve, R. M., and Dekaris, D., 1968, *Science* **160**:795–796.
Fauve, R. M., Hevin, B., Jacob, H., Gaillard, J. A., and Jacob, F., 1974, *Proc. Natl Acad. Sci. U.S.A.* **71**:4052–4056.
Flanagan, T. D., Yoshida, T., and Cohen, S., 1973, *Infect. Immun.* **8**:145–150.
Fowles, R. E., Fajardo, I. M., Leibowitch, J. L., and David, J. R., 1973, *J. Exp. Med.* **138**:952–964.
Fox, R. A., and MacSween, J. M., 1974, *Immunol. Commun.* **3**:375–389.
Fox, R. A., Gregory, D. S., and Feldman, J. D., 1974, *J. Immunol.* **112**:1867–1872.
Friedman, R. M., and Cooper, H. L., 1967, *Proc. Soc. Exp. Biol. Med.* **125**:901–905.
Friedrich, W., Lazary, S., Geczy, C., and De Weck, A. L., 1975, *Int. Arch. Allergy* **49**:504–518.
Galindo, B., Lazdins, J., and Castillo, R., 1974, *Infect. Immun.* **9**:212–216.
Gately, M. K., Gately, C. L., Henney, C. S., and Mayer, M. M., 1975, *J. Immunol.* **115**:817–826.
Geczy, C. L., Friedrich, W., and De Weck, A. L., 1975, *Cell. Immunol.* **19**:65–77.
Gifford, G. E., Tibor, A., and Peavy, D. C., 1971, *Infect. Immun.* **3**:164–166.
Glasgow, L. A., 1966, *J. Bacteriol.* **91**:2185–2191.
Godal, T., Rees, R. J. W., and Lamvik, J. O., 1971, *Clin. Exp. Immunol.* **8**:625–637.
Goetzl, E. J., Wasserman, S. I., Gigli, I., and Austen, K. F., 1974, *J. Clin. Invest.* **53**:813–818.
Gorczynski, R. M., 1974, *J. Immunol.* **112**:1815–1825.
Granger, G. A., and Williams, T. W., 1968, *Nature (London)* **218**:1253–1254.
Granger, G. A., Moore, G. E., White, J. G., Matzinger, P., Sundsmo, J. S., Shupe, S., Kolb, W. P., Kramer, J., and Glade, P. R., 1970, *J. Immunol.* **104**:1476–1485.
Green, J. A., Cooperband, S. R., and Kibrick, S., 1969, *Science* **164**:1415–1417.

Hadden, J. W., Leu, R., Goldberg, N. D., and Hadden, E. M., 1974a, *Fed. Proc. Fed. Am. Soc. Exp. Biol.* **33**:745 (abstract).
Hadden, J. W., Hadden, E. M., and Goldberg, N. D., 1974b, in: *Cyclic AMP, Cell Growth, and the Immune Response* (W. Braun, L. D. Lichtenstein, and C. W. Parker, eds.), pp. 237–246, Springer-Verlag, New York.
Hadden, J. W., Sadlick, J. R., and Hadden, E. M., 1975, *Nature (London)* **257**:483–485.
Halliday, W. J., and Miller, S., 1972, *Int. J. Cancer* **9**:477–483.
Hammond, M. E., Roblin, R. O., Dvorak, A. M., Selvaggio, S. S., Black, P. H., and Dvorak, H. F., 1974, *Science* **185**:955–957.
Hammond, M. E., Selvaggio, S. S., and Dvorak, H. F., 1975, *J. Immunol.* **115**:914–921.
Haslam, R. J., and Lynham, J. A., 1972, *Life Sci.* **11**:1143–1154.
Hattler, B. G., Rocklin, R., Ward, P. A., and Rickles, F. R., 1973, *Cell. Immunol.* **9**:289–296.
Havell, E. A., Vilcek, J., Falcoff, E., and Berman, B., 1975, *Virology* **63**:475–483.
Havemann, K., Horvat, M., Sodomann, C. P., Havemann, K., and Burger, S., 1972, *Eur. J. Immunol.* **2**:97–99.
Hay, J. B., Lachmann, P. J., and Trnka, Z., 1973, *Eur. J. Immunol.* **3**:127–131.
Henney, C. S., Gaffney, J., and Bloom, B. R., 1974, *J. Exp. Med.* **140**:837–852.
Higgins, T. J., Winston, C. T., and David, J. R., 1973, *Fed. Proc. Fed. Am. Soc. Exp. Biol.* **32**:878 (abstract).
Ho, M., and Armstrong, J. A., 1975, Interferon, *Annu. Rev. Microbiol.* **29**:131–161.
Ho, R. J., and Sutherland, E. W., 1971, *J. Biol. Chem.* **246**:6822–6827.
Houck, J. C., and Chang, C. M., 1975, *Proc. Soc. Exp. Biol. Med.* **148**:104–106.
Houck, J. C., Attallah, A. M., and Lilly, J. R., 1973, *Nature (London)* **245**:148–150.
Jeffes, E. W. B., and Granger, G. A., 1975, *J. Immunol.* **114**:64–69.
Johnson, G. S., and Pastan, I., 1972, *Nature (London) New Biol.* **236**:247–249.
Johnson, G. S., Morgan, W. D., and Pastan, I., 1972, *Nature (London)* **235**:54–56.
Kleinerman, E. S., Snyderman, R., and Daniels, C. A., 1974, *J. Immunol.* **113**:1562–1567.
Koopman, W. J., Gillis, M. H., and David, J. R., 1973, *J. Immunol.* **110**:1609–1614.
Kotkes, P., and Pick, E., 1975a, in: *The Immunological Basis of Connective Tissue Disorders* (L. G. Silvestri, ed.), pp. 141–153, North-Holland Publishing Co., Amsterdam and Oxford.
Kotkes, P., and Pick, E., 1975b, *Clin. Exp. Immunol.* **19**:105–120.
Kotkes, P., and Pick, E., 1976, *Cell. Immunol.* **27**:353–354 (abstract).
Kramer, S., and Granger, G. A., 1975, *Cell. Immunol.* **15**:57–68.
Krejci, J., Svejcar, J., Pekarek, J., and Johanovsky, J., 1968, *Z. Immunitaetsforsch.* **136**:259–267.
Krug, F., Parikh, I., Illiano, G., and Cuatrecasas, P., 1973, *Biochem. Biophys. Res. Commun.* **50**:985–991.
Kuhner, A. L., Remold, H. G., and David, J. R., 1975, *Fed. Proc. Fed. Am. Soc. Exp. Biol.* **34**:977 (abstract).
Leu, R. W., Eddleston, A. L. W. F., Hadden, J. W., and Good, R. A., 1972, *J. Exp. Med.* **136**:589–603.
Leu, R. W., Eddleston, A. W. L. F., Good, R. A., and Hadden, J. W., 1973, *Exp. Cell. Res.* **76**:458–461.
Lies, R. B., and Peter, J. B., 1973, *Cell. Immunol.* **8**:332–335.
Lipton, A., Klinger, I., Paul, D., and Holley, R. W., 1971, *Proc. Natl. Acad. Sci. U.S.A.* **68**:2799–2801.
Lodmell, D. L., and Notkins, A. L., 1974, *J. Exp. Med.* **140**:764–778.
Lolekha, S., and Gotoff, S., 1971, *Cell. Immunol.* **2**:386–398.
Lolekha, S., Dray, S., and Gotoff, S. P., 1970, *J. Immunol.* **104**:296–304.
Lomnitzer, R., Rabson, A. R., and Koornhof, H. J., 1976a, *Clin. Exp. Immunol.* **24**:42–48.
Lomnitzer, R., Rabson, A. R., and Koornhof, H. J., 1976b, *Clin. Exp. Immunol.* **25**:303–310.
Mahmoud, A. A. F., Mandel, M. A., Warren, K. S., and Webster, L. T., 1975, *J. Immunol.* **114**:279–283.
Maillard, J. L., Pick, E., and Turk, J. L., 1972, *Int. Arch. Allergy* **42**:50–68.
Malley, A., and Baecher, L., 1971, *J. Immunol.* **107**:586–588.
Manheimer, S., and Pick, E., 1973, *Immunology* **24**:1027–1034.
May-Levin, F., Graffte, G., and Brule, G., 1972, *Schweiz. Med. Wochenschr.* **102**:1188–1190.
Meade, C. J., Lachmann, P. J., and Brenner, S., 1974, *Immunology* **27**:227–240.
Milstone, L. M., and Waksman, B. H., 1970, *J. Immunol.* **105**:1068–1071.
Mizoguchi, Y., Yamamoto, S., and Morisawa, S., 1973, *J. Biochem.* **73**:467–474.

Morita, C., and Soekawa, M., 1972, *Poult. Sci.* **51**:1133–1136.
Morley, J., 1974, *Acta Allergol.* **29**:185–208.
Morley, J., Bray, M. A., Gordon, D., and Paul, W., 1975, in: *The Immunological Basis of Connective Tissue Disorders* (L. Silvestri, ed.), pp. 129–140, North-Holland Publishing Co., Amsterdam and Oxford.
Namba, Y., and Waksman, B. H., 1975, *J. Immunol.* **115**:1018–1022.
Nath, I., Poulter, L. W., and Turk, J. L., 1973, *Clin. Exp. Immunol.* **13**:455–466.
Nathan, C. F., Karnovsky, M. L., and David, J. R., 1971, *J. Exp. Med.* **133**:1356–1376.
Nelson, R. D., and Leu, R. W., 1975, *J. Immunol.* **114**:606–609.
Ohishi, M., and Onoue, K., 1975, *Cell. Immunol.* **18**:220–232.
Pantalone, R. M., and Page, R., 1975, *Proc. Natl. Acad. Sci. U.S.A.* **72**:2091–2094.
Papageorgiou, P. S., and Glade, P. R., 1974, *Cell. Immunol.* **12**:326–330.
Papageorgiou, P. S., Henley, W. L., and Glade, P. R., 1972, *J. Immunol.* **108**:494–504.
Papermaster, B. W., Holtermann, O. A., Rosner, D., Klein, E., and Dao, T., 1974, *Res. Commun. Chem. Pathol. Pharmacol.* **8**:413–416.
Pekarek, J., and Krejci, J., 1974, *J. Immunol. Methods* **6**:1–22.
Pekarek, J., Svejcar, J., and Johanovsky, J., 1971, *Immunology* **20**:895–900.
Peter, J. B., 1971, *Cell. Immunol.* **2**:199–202.
Peter, J. B., Stratton, J. A., Stempel, K. E., Yu, D., and Cardin, C., 1973, *J. Immunol.* **111**:770–782.
Pick, E., 1972a, *Nature (London)* **238**:176–177.
Pick, E., 1972b, *Isr. J. Med. Sci.* **8**:654 (abstract).
Pick, E., 1973, *Eur. J. Immunol.* **3**:317–319.
Pick, E., 1974, *Immunology* **26**:649–658.
Pick, E., and Abrahamer, H., 1973, *Int. Arch. Allergy* **44**:215–220.
Pick, E., and Manheimer, S., 1973, *Int. Arch. Allergy* **45**:295–298.
Pick, E., and Manheimer, S., 1974, *Cell. Immunol.* **11**:30–46.
Pick, E., and Turk, J. L., 1972a, *Clin. Exp. Immunol.* **10**:1–23.
Pick, E., and Turk, J. L., 1972b, *Immunology* **22**:39–49.
Pick, E., Krejci, J., Cech, K., and Turk, J. L., 1969, *Immunology* **17**:741–767.
Pick, E., Brostoff, J., Krejci, J., and Turk, J. L., 1970, *Cell. Immunol.* **1**:92–109.
Pick, E., Godny, Y., and Gold, E. F., 1975a, *Eur. J. Immunol* **5**:584–587.
Pick, E., Abrahamer, H., and Kotkes, P., 1975b, *Isr. J. Med. Sci.* **11**:1379 (abstract).
Piessens, W. F., Churchill, W. H., and David, J. R., 1975, *J. Immunol.* **114**:293–299.
Plaut, M., Lichtenstein, L. M., and Henney, C. S., 1973, *J. Immunol.* **110**:771–780.
Pollock, E. M., and Vazquez, J. J., 1971, *J. Reticuloendothel. Soc.* **10**:205–211.
Pollock, E. M., Pegram, C. N., and Vazquez, J. J., 1971, *J. Reticuloendothel. Soc.* **9**:383–391.
Poste, G., 1975a, *Cancer Res.* **35**:2558–2566.
Poste, G., 1975b, *Exp. Cell Res.* **92**:283–290.
Postlethwaite, A. E., and Snyderman, R., 1975, *J. Immunol.* **114**:274–278.
Prieur, A., and Granger, G. A., 1975, *Transplantation* **20**:331–337.
Prystowsky, M. B., Sorokin, C. F., Ceglowski, W. S., Hirschhorn, K., and Glade, P., 1975, *Int. Arch. Allergy* **48**:225–235.
Ramseier, H., 1967, *Science* **157**:554–556.
Ranlov, P., and Hardt, F., 1970, *Transplantation* **10**:438–442.
Rasmussen, L. E., Jordan, G. W., Stevens, D. A., and Merigan, T. C., 1974, *J. Immunol.* **112**:728–736.
Reaven, E. P., and Axline, S. G., 1973, *J. Cell. Biol.* **59**:12–27.
Remold, H. G., 1973, *J. Exp. Med.* **138**:1065–1076.
Remold, H. G., 1974, *J. Immunol.* **112**:1571–1577.
Remold, H. G., and David, J. R., 1971, *J. Immunol.* **107**:1090–1098.
Remold, H. G., and Mednis, A., 1972, *Fed. Proc. Fed. Amer. Soc. Exp. Biol.* **31**:753 (abstract).
Remold, H. G., and Rosenberg, R. G., 1975, *J. Biol. Chem.* **250**:6608–6613.
Remold, H. G., Katz, A. B., Haber, E., and David, J. R., 1970, *Cell. Immunol.* **1**:133–145.
Remold, H. G., David, R. A., and David, J. R., 1972, *J. Immunol.* **109**:578–586.
Remold-O'Donnell, E., and Remold, H. G., 1974, *J. Biol. Chem.* **249**:3622–3627.
Rivkin, I., Rosenblatt, J., and Becker, E., 1975, *J. Immunol.* **115**:1126–1134.
Rocklin, R. E., 1975, *Fed. Proc. Fed. Am. Soc. Exp. Biol.* **34**:977 (abstract).
Rocklin, R. E., Remold, H. G., and David, J. R., 1972, *Cell. Immunol.* **5**:436–445.

Rocklin, R. E., MacDermott, R. P., Chess, L., Schlossman, S. F., and David, J. R., 1974, *J. Exp. Med.* **140**:1303–1316.
Rosenstreich, D. L., Blake, T., and Rosenthal, A. S., 1971, *J. Exp. Med.* **134**:1170–1186.
Ruddle, N. H., and Waksman, B. H., 1968, *J. Exp. Med.* **128**:1267–1279.
Rühl, H., Vogt, W., Bochert, G., Schmidt, S., Moelle, R., and Schaoua, H., 1974, *Immunology* **26**:989–994.
Salvin, S. B., and Nishio, J., 1972, *J. Exp. Med.* **135**:985–995.
Salvin, S. B., Sell, S., and Nishio, J., 1971, *J. Immunol.* **107**:655–662.
Salvin, S., Youngner, J. S., and Lederer, W. H., 1973, *Infect. Immun.* **7**:68–75.
Sandler, J. A., Gallin, J. I., and Vaughan, M., 1975, *J. Cell Biol.* **67**:480–484.
Schlag, W., 1971, *Klin. Wochenschr.* **49**:1030–1031.
Schmidt, M. E., Douglas, S. D., and Rubin, A., 1973, *Cell. Immunol.* **9**:45–59.
Schreiner, G. F., and Unanue, E. R., 1975, *J. Immunol.* **114**:802–808.
Shacks, S. J., Chiller, J., and Granger, G. A., 1973, *Cell. Immunol.* **7**:313–321.
Smyth, A. C., and Weiss, L., 1970, *J. Immunol.* **105**:1360–1374.
Snyderman, R., Shin, H. S., and Dannenberg, A. M., 1972, *J. Immunol.* **109**:896–898.
Sonozaki, H., and Cohen, S., 1971, *Cell. Immunol.* **2**:341–352.
Sorg, C., and Bloom, B. R., 1973, *J. Exp. Med.* **137**:148–170.
Sorg, C., and Hämmerling, G., 1975, *Z. Immunitaetsforsch.* **150**:243–244 (abstract).
Soriano, R. B., South, M. A., Goldman, A. S., and Smith, O. W., 1973, *J. Pediatr.* **83**:951–958.
Stastny, P., Rosenthal, M., Andreis, M., and Ziff, M., 1973, *Arthritis Rheum.* **16**:572 (abstract).
Stevenson, R. D., 1973, *Clin. Exp. Immunol.* **14**:417–426.
Stinebring, W. R., and Absher, P. M., 1970, *Ann. N.Y. Acad. Sci.* **173**:714–718.
Stobo, J., Green, I., Jackson, L., and Baron, S., 1974, *J. Immuol.* **112**:1589–1593.
Sugane, K., Kasahara, T., and Shioiri-Nakana, K., 1975, *Jpn. J. Exp. Med.* **45**:19–24.
Sultzer, B. M., and Craig, J. P., 1973, *Nature (London) New Biol.* **244**:178–180.
Svejcar, J. and Johanovsky, J., 1961, *Z. Immunitaetsforsch.* **56**:398–419.
Svejcar, J., Pekarek, J., and Johanovsky, J., 1968, *Immunology* **15**:1–11.
Svejcar, J., Pekarek, J., and Johanovsky, J., 1971, *Z. Immunitaetsforsch.* **141**:119–128.
Thomas, D. B., 1972, *Eur. J. Immunol.* **2**:478–481.
Till, G., and Ward, P. A., 1975, *J. Immunol.* **114**:843–847.
Tubergen, D. B., Feldman, J. D., Pollock, E. M., and Lerner, R. A., 1972, *J. Exp. Med.* **135**:255–261.
Wahl, L. M., Wahl, S. M., Mergenhagen, S. E., and Martin, G. R., 1975, *Science* **187**:261–263.
Wahl, S. M., 1975, *Ann. N.Y. Acad. Sci.* **256**:375–385.
Wahl, S. M., Altman, L. C., Oppenheim, J. J., and Mergenhagen, S. F., 1974a, *Int. Arch. Allergy* **46**:768–784.
Wahl, S., Iverson, G. M., and Oppenheim, J. J., 1974b, *J. Exp. Med.* **140**:1631–1645.
Wahl, S. M., Altman, L. C., and Rosenstreich, D. L., 1975, *J. Immunol.* **115**:476–481.
Walker, S. M., and Lucas, Z. J., 1974, *J. Immunol.* **113**:813–823.
Wallen, W. C., Dean, J. H., and Lucas, D., 1973, *Cell. Immunol.* **6**:110–122.
Ward, P. A., 1971, *Am. J. Pathol.* **64**:521–530.
Ward, P. A., and Rocklin, R. E., 1975, *J. Immunol.* **115**:309–311.
Ward, P. A., and Volkman, A., 1975, *J. Immunol* **115**:1394–1399.
Ward, P. A., Remold, H. G., and David, J. R., 1970, *Cell. Immunol.* **1**:162–174.
Ward, P. A., Dvorak, H. F., Cohen, S., Yoshida, T., Data, R., and Selvaggio, S. S., 1975, *J. Immunol.* **114**:1523–1531.
Warren, K. S., Mahmoud, A. A. F., Boros, D. L., Rall, T. W., Mandel, M. A., and Carpenter, C. C. J., 1974, *J. Immunol.* **112**:996–1007.
Weber, J. M., and Stewart, R. B., 1975, *J. Gen. Virol.* **28**:363–372.
Weiss, L. and Glaves, D., 1975, *J. Immunol.* **115**:1362–1365.
Weston, W. L., Claman, H. N., and Krueger, G. G., 1973, *J. Immunol.* **110**:880–883.
Wheelock, E. F., 1965, *Science* **149**:310, 311.
Wilkinson, P. C., 1975, *Nature (London)* **255**:485–487.
Williams, T. J., Morley, J., and Wolstencroft, R. A., 1972, *J. Immunol. Methods* **2**:137–143.
Williams, T. W., and Granger, G. A., 1969a, *J. Immunol.* **102**:911–918.
Williams, T. W., and Granger, G. A., 1969b, *J. Immunol.* **103**:170–178.
Willingham, M. C., and Pastan, I., 1975a, *Proc. Natl. Acad. Sci. U.S.A.* **72**:1263–1267.

Willingham, M. C. and Pastan, I., 1975b, *J. Cell Biol.* **67**:146–159.

Wright, D. G. Kirkpatrick, I. C. H., and Gallin, J. I., 1976, in: *Modulation of Host Immune Resistance in the Prevention or Treatment of Induced Neoplasia* (M. Chirigos, ed.), Fogarty International Center Proceedings No. 28, U.S. Government Printing Office, Washington, D.C., in press.

Yamamoto, K., and Takahashi, Y., 1971, *Nature (London) New Biol.* **233**:261, 262.

Yoshida, T., and Cohen, S., 1974, *J. Immunol.* **112**:1540–1547.

Yoshida, T., and Reisfeld, R. A., 1970, *Nature (London)* **226**:856, 857.

Yoshida, T., Janeway, C. A., and Paul, W. E., 1972, *J. Immunol.* **109**:201–206.

Yoshida, T., Sonozaki, H., and Cohen, S., 1973, *J. Exp. Med.* **138**:784–797.

Yoshida, T., Bigazzi, P. E., and Cohen, S., 1975a, *J. Immunol.* **114**:688–691.

Yoshida, T., Bigazzi, P. E., and Cohen, S., 1975b, *Proc. Natl. Acad. Sci. U.S.A.* **72**:1641–1644.

Yoshinaga, M., Waksman, B. H., and Malawista, S. E., 1972, *Science* **176**:1147–1149.

Youngner, J. S., and Salvin, S. B., 1973, *J. Immunol.* **111**:1914–1922.

11

Mechanism of Action of Antiallergic Drugs and Relationship of Cyclic Nucleotides to Allergy

RONALD G. COFFEY and ELLIOTT MIDDLETON, JR.

1. Introduction

In the last two decades, diverse medical and scientific disciplines including pharmacology, endocrinology, immunology, and biochemistry have found common ground, both theoretically and in the design of experiments, due to the discovery of the second messenger system by Sutherland and colleagues (Sutherland and Rall, 1960; Robison *et al.,* 1971). Nearly all hormones, a growing list of other cell–cell mediators or effector substances, and a large number of drugs have found their mechanism of action at the level of cyclic adenosine 3′,5′-monophosphate (cAMP) or cyclic guanosine 3′,5′-monophosphate (cGMP). It is therefore not surprising that nearly all antiallergic agents can now be classified under either of two categories of biochemical mechanisms: (1) effects mediated by changes in cAMP levels or (2) effects mediated by changes in cGMP levels.

Allergy of the immediate-hypersensitivity type includes, by definition, all pathophysiologic conditions that result when specific antigen interacts with immunoglobulin E (IgE, reagin; Ishizaka and Ishizaka, 1973) bound to tissue mast cells or circulating basophils: allergic asthma, allergic rhinitis, anaphylaxis, and certain cases of urticaria, angioedema, atopic dermatitis (eczema), drug, food, and insect sting hypersensitivities. The intent of this chapter is to describe briefly each class of antiallergic agent in terms of known or suspected effects on cyclic nucleotide levels and to relate these effects to clinical response. The discussion is restricted to asthma

RONALD G. COFFEY • Laboratory of Immunopharmacology, Memorial Sloan-Kettering Cancer Center, New York, New York 10021. ELLIOTT MIDDLETON, JR. • Allergy Laboratories, Buffalo General Hospital, State University of New York at Buffalo, Buffalo, New York 14214.

because of its predominant position, both in terms of morbidity and mortality and in terms of the extensive research focused on this disorder. Some new ideas are put forward in the hope that they might provoke new experimentation to increase our understanding of the biochemical and pharmacological abnormalities that underlie the common allergic disorders.

2. Cyclic Nucleotide Metabolism and Actions

Since most of the mechanisms of action of antiallergic agents are now understood in terms of cyclic nucleotide metabolism, a brief review of this subject follows. The reviews by Sutherland and Rall (1960), Robison *et al.* (1971), and Goldberg *et al.* (1973a) should be consulted for more thorough discussions.

cAMP is formed from ATP due to the action of the plasma membrane enzyme adenylate cyclase, as shown in Figure 1. Catecholamines and many other hormones stimulate this reaction, depending in part on the presence of specific hormone receptors on the cell surface. The stimulation may require intracellular GTP acting at an allosteric site on the enzyme to produce the activated state (Schramm and Rodbell, 1975). Many hormones that do not stimulate adenylate cyclase have recently been found to stimulate the formation of cGMP from GTP by an analogous reaction catalyzed by guanylate cyclase, an enzyme found in both plasma mem-

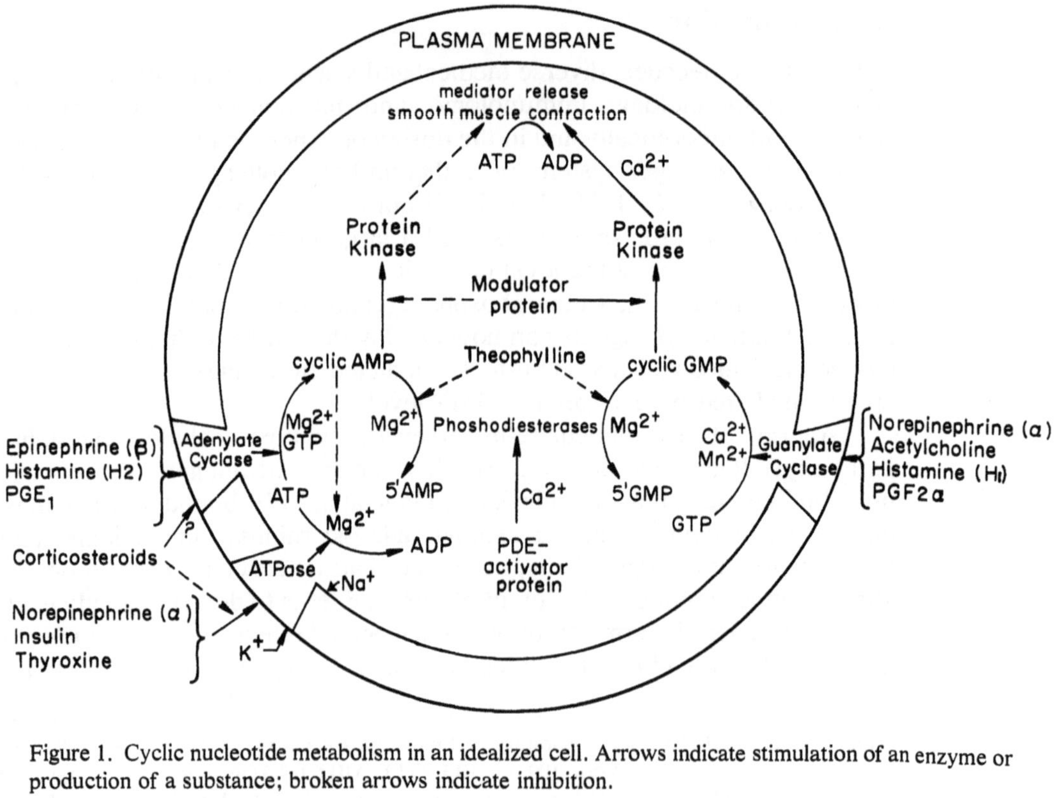

Figure 1. Cyclic nucleotide metabolism in an idealized cell. Arrows indicate stimulation of an enzyme or production of a substance; broken arrows indicate inhibition.

TABLE 1. Agents That Alter Cyclic Nucleotide Levels[a]

Agent	Cell: Mast cell cGMP	Mast cell cAMP	Lymphocyte cGMP	Lymphocyte cAMP	Lung tissue cGMP	Lung tissue cAMP	Other smooth muscle cGMP	Other smooth muscle cAMP
α-Adrenergic		↓ (2)				↓ (12)	↑ (20,21)	0 (20,21)
β-Adrenergic		↑ (2)		↑ (4,16,17)	↓ (14)	↑ (12,14)	↓ (3)	↑ (3,21)
Bradykinin					↑ (22)	↑ (22)[b]		
Cholinergic[c]			↑ (6,10,11)	0 (1)	↑ (6,14,18,22)	0 (12,14,18)	↑ (6,20,21)	0 (6,20)
Corticosteroid		↑ (2)		↑ (16,17)	↓ (5,6)			
Estrogen							↑ (13)	
Histamine (*H-1*)[d]					↑ (18)	0 (18)	↑ (20)	
Histamine (*H-2*)[d]				↑ (4,15)		↑ (22)		
Ionophore + Ca^{2+}	↑ (1)		↑ (10)	0 (10)				
Ionophore + Mg^{2+}			0 (10)	↑ (10)				
Insulin			↑ (11)	0 (11)				
Mitogen			↑ (8–10)	0 (8–10)				
$PGF_{2\alpha}$						0 or ↑ (12)	↑ (3,7,21)	0 (3,7)
PGE_1 or E_2				↑ (17)		↑ (12)	↓ (3)	↑ (3)
Oxytocin							↑ (6,7,21)	0 (7)
Secretin					↑ (23)			
Serotonin			↑ (19)				↑ (6,7,21)	0 (7)

[a]Symbols: (↑) Increase in cAMP or cGMP; (↓) decrease; (0) no change. The numbers in parentheses denote the following references: **(1)** Coffey and Hadden (unpublished data); **(2)** Coffey and Middleton (1973); **(3)** Dunham *et al.* (1974); **(4)** Gillespie *et al.* (1974); **(5)** Goldberg *et al.* (1973a); **(6)** Goldberg *et al.* (1973b); **(7)** Goldberg *et al.* (1974); **(8)** Hadden *et al.* (1972b); **(9)** Hadden *et al.* (1974); **(10)** Hadden *et al.* (1975); **(11)** Illiano *et al.* (1973); **(12)** Kaliner *et al.* (1972); **(13)** Kuehl *et al.* (1974); **(14)** Kuo and Kuo (1973); **(15)** Lichtenstein (1973); **(16)** Logsdon *et al.* (1972); **(17)** Parker (1973); **(18)** Polson *et al.* (1976); **(19)** Sandler *et al.* (1975); **(20)** Schultz *et al.* (1973); **(21)** Schultz *et al.* (1975); **(22)** Stoner *et al.* (1974); **(23)** Thompson *et al.* (1974).
[b]The action to increase cAMP is indirect, probably due to PG release.
[c]Muscarinic cholinergic action, blocked by atropine, is indicated.
[d]*H-1* and *H-2* receptor activation is assumed in accordance with the developing literature for some cases in which selective blockade was not employed.

brane and cytosol fractions of cells. Hormones and other agents capable of stimulating accumulation of cAMP or cGMP in lymphocytes, mast cells, lung, and other smooth-muscle-containing tissues are listed in Table 1. In working with broken cell preparations, adenylate cyclase was found to require Mg^{2+} and to be inhibited by Ca^{2+} (Steer and Levitzki, 1975), while guanylate cyclase requires Mn^{2+}, and at suboptimal levels of the latter, it is further stimulated by Ca^{2+} (G. Schultz *et al.*, 1973). Furthermore, Ca^{2+} is necessary for maintenance of basal cGMP levels, for the stimulation of guanylate cyclase by many agents, and also for the expression of most cGMP-mediated events (Goldberg *et al.*, 1973a,b; Schultz *et al.*, 1973).

cAMP mediates the hormonal message by increasing the activity of intracellular protein kinases (cf. Langan, 1973), which catalyze the phosphorylation of a variety of enzymes and other proteins in the plasma membrane, cytoplasm and nucleus. Among the many and diverse biochemical changes in differentiated tissues caused by this cascade of reactions, of which enhanced glycogenolysis was the first to be discovered (Sutherland and Rall, 1960), those listed in Table 2 are the most relevant for the topic of this section. cAMP stimulates phosphorylation of smooth muscle membrane proteins, and this stimulation is thought to be related to increased Ca^{2+} binding and subsequent muscle relaxation (G. Schultz *et al.*, 1973). Inhibition of glucose and cation transport (Hadden *et al.*, 1971a,b) may also contribute to the effects of cAMP. The mechanisms by which cAMP inhibits a variety of immunologic responses—including inhibition of mediator release from mast cells (Assem, 1971; Kaliner *et al.*, 1972; Austen, 1973) (see also Chapter 7) and basophils (Lichtenstein, 1973), prevention of leukotaxis (Hill *et al.*, 1975), prevention of neutrophil lysosomal enzyme discharge (Ignarro and George, 1974; R. J. Smith and Ignarro, 1975), and inhibition of lymphocyte-mediated cytotoxicity (Strom *et al.*, 1973) and lymphocyte clonal proliferation (Hadden *et al.*, 1972b, 1974, 1975)—as they relate to allergy as well as to other immunologic disorders are under active investigation.

In every instance, an effect opposing that of cAMP has been documented for cGMP or agents that increase cGMP levels in cells, and these observations prompted the formulation by Goldberg, Hadden, and colleagues of the dualism or Yin–Yang theory of biological regulation (Goldberg *et al.*, 1973b, 1974, 1975; Hadden *et al.*, 1972b, 1974, 1975). Demonstrations of intracellular mechanisms for

TABLE 2. Relationship of Cell Functions to Cyclic AMP

Cell type	Effect of increasing cyclic AMP
Tracheobronchial smooth muscle	Relaxation
Bronchial and pulmonary vessels	Vasodilation
Adrenal cortex	Stimulation of cortisol synthesis, and secretion
Mast cell, basophil	Inhibition of mediator release
Lymphocyte	Inhibition of clonal proliferation; inhibition of lymphokine production
Eosinophil	Decrease in eosinophilia; inhibition of leukotaxis

cGMP effects have taken a discouraging amount of time and effort, but four now appear to be related to some effects: stimulation of RNA polymerase I (L. D. Johnson and Hadden, 1975), stimulation of specific nuclear acidic protein phosphorylation (E. M. Johnson and Hadden, 1975), increased activity of phosphoribosyl pyrophosphate synthetase (Chambers *et al.*, 1974), and stimulation of specific cGMP-dependent protein kinases (Kuo, 1975), which may stimulate phosphorylation of selective proteins (Casnellie and Greengard, 1974).

Following the intracellular changes exerted by the increased levels of the cyclic nucleotides, their levels must be restored to resting or baseline values for the maintenance of homeostasis. This restoration is accomplished by the degradative action of phosphodiesterase (PDE) enzymes. Most tissues possess at least three molecular forms of PDE, one that specifically catalyzes conversion of cAMP to 5′-AMP, one that converts cGMP to 5′-GMP, and one or more that act on both nucleotides (cf. Appleman *et al.*, 1973, for a review). Kinetic analysis of the cAMP-PDE enzymes usually shows that stimulated nucleotide levels return slowly to baseline (negative cooperativity). Other interesting features of PDEs are: (1) stimulation of one cAMP-PDE by physiologic levels of cGMP; (2) inhibition of a cGMP-PDE by high levels of cAMP; (3) activation by cAMP of new synthesis of cAMP-PDE molecules; and (4) the presence of low K_m (high-affinity) PDEs in association with the plasma membrane. The latter are suspected of being important with regard to rapid adjustment of the levels of cyclic nucleotides associated with the plasma membrane following hormone or drug stimulation of the cyclases, and also with regard to effects of certain drugs and perhaps hormones such as insulin and growth hormone (Zinman and Hollenberg, 1974; Van Inwegen *et al.*, 1975) on PDE activities.

To summarize briefly, cells possess several mechanisms by which drugs and hormones (first messengers) influence the expression of specialized functions. cAMP has a negative influence on allergic and inflammatory processes, while cGMP (together with its partner, Ca^{2+}) exerts actions opposite to those of cAMP and promotes or enhances such processes as mediator release, smooth muscle contraction, and leukotaxis. The activities of the three types of enzymes—the cyclases, the PDEs, and the protein kinases—together with Ca^{2+}, form the basic elements of biological regulatory mechanisms to be considered in the following sections.

3. Pathophysiology of Asthma

3.1. Background

Asthma, or reversible obstructive airway disease, is the most serious allergic disorder known, afflicting an estimated 9 million Americans and responsible for about 2000 deaths annually. The pathophysiology has been reviewed extensively (Middleton, 1965, 1972; Rose and Radermecker, 1971; Vaughan *et al.*, 1973; Levinson *et al.*, 1974). Briefly, asthma is characterized by episodic bronchial obstruction caused by edema of the bronchial mucosa and submucosa, viscous mucus plugs in the bronchi and bronchioles, and bronchial smooth muscle contraction. Other pathologic features include peripheral blood eosinophilia, infiltration of eosinophils in the bronchial wall and shedding of superficial columnar epithelial cells and eosinophils into the bronchial lumen, dilation of submucosal capillaries, mast cell degranulation, and thickening of the mucosal basement membrane. These features occur in both extrinsic asthma, for which the provoking allergen can be identified, and intrinsic asthma, the causal mechanisms of which are poorly understood. Increased serum IgE levels are seen in many but not all cases of extrinsic asthma. In the case of immunologically mediated tissue injury, each of these changes can be accounted for by the chemical mediators of immediate-type allergic inflammation discussed in Section 3.2. Such diverse agents as cold air, dust, fumes, exercise, infection, and emotional stress may also trigger an asthmatic attack in susceptible patients. Irritation of the respiratory tract by some of these factors, e.g., histamine, can produce in the asthmatic patient an excessive stimulation of the subepithelial irritant receptors and excessive reflex output by efferent parasympathetic (vagal) nerves that innervate the smooth muscle, glands, blood vessels, and mucous membranes (Nadel, 1973; Gold, 1973), culminating in a narrowing of the airways. Especially important is the narrowing of the smaller airways, which may be chronically constricted to some degree even in symptom-free asthmatic patients (Levinson *et al.*, 1974).

3.2. Chemical Mediators

The chemical mediators of immediate-type allergic inflammation which are discussed thoroughly in this volume by Gillespie (Chapter 6) and Goetzl and Austen (Chapter 7), now include histamine, slow-reacting substance of anaphylaxis (SRS-A), eosinophil chemotactic factor of anaphylaxis (ECF-A), basophil kallikrein of anaphylaxis (BK-A), platelet-activating factor (PAF) and possibly kinins and prostaglandins of the F series. These substances are released from blood basophils and tissue mast cells following a multistep sequence of reactions that begins with antigen combining with IgE molecules on the surfaces of the cells. Although all the steps have not been elucidated, they include activation of a cellular serine esterase, Ca^{2+} uptake, and an energy-dependent exocytosis involving microtubule function (Austen, 1973; Lichtenstein, 1975). The Ca^{2+} requirement for basophil degranulation has long been appreciated, but only recently was it unequivocally demonstrated in isolated mast cells (Diamant and Patkar, 1975).

The biological regulation of mediator release by cyclic nucleotides is a good example of the dualism theory. cAMP inhibits release, possibly by interfering with microtubule function (Lichtenstein, 1975), while cGMP augments release (Kaliner *et al.*, 1972). Consequently, β-adrenergic agonists and other agents that increase intracellular levels of cAMP will inhibit, while α-adrenergic and cholinergic agonists, and other agents that increase levels of cGMP, will augment, mediator release. Histamine may regulate its own release, since it can act on H_2 receptors to increase leukocyte cAMP levels at concentrations normally encountered in allergic reactions (Lichtenstein, 1975). Since ATP is utilized during the release reaction (Diamant, 1975), α-adrenergic stimulation and β-adrenergic inhibition of ATPase (Coffey and Middleton, 1973) may represent other regulatory mechanisms.

Entry of Ca^{2+} into or translocation to appropriate sites is now thought to represent the intracellular trigger for the antigen-activated cell to undergo the degranulation and release reaction (Diamant and Patkar, 1975). Others (Lichtenstein, 1975) believe that a reduction in cAMP represents the release signal, but since the reaction occurs so quickly (at least in rat mast cells, in which reaction is complete in 10–30 sec), one may wonder whether a decrease in cAMP can be followed sufficiently rapidly by inactivation of protein kinases and subsequent dephosphorylation of their substrates to effect such a concerted process. Alternatively, cGMP, together with Ca^{2+}, may constitute components of the release signal (Coffey and Middleton, 1973; Taylor and Sheldon, 1974). This possibility is supported by the observation that two mast-cell-degranulating agents, phorbol myristate acetate and the ionophore A23187 (E. I. Lilly and Co.) cause cGMP accumulation in other cells (Goldberg *et al.*, 1974; Hadden *et al.*, 1975; R. J. Smith and Ignarro, 1975).

All the possibilities discussed above are under active investigation in several laboratories. The application of experimental findings with several drugs such as cromolyn that inhibit release by mechanisms not fully understood holds much promise for asthmatic patients who are exquisitely sensitive to the mediators. Heightened sensitivity to histamine and other mediators can also be obtained experimentally by use of β-adrenergic blocking drugs (Szentivanyi, 1968), and this finding became the cornerstone of the theory to be discussed in the next section.

3.3. β-Adrenergic Blockade Theory

Several metabolic studies in humans and in pharmacologically manipulated animals supported the notion of inadequate adrenergic responsiveness in asthmatics, and led to the β-adrenergic blockade theory of asthma (Reed, 1965; Szentivanyi, 1968). The evidence for and against this theory has been frequently reviewed (Middleton, 1972, 1975a; Middleton and Coffey, 1973; Parker, 1973; Reed, 1974; Nelson, 1975), and a discussion of the most recent experimental evidence is given after the following brief review of adrenergic pharmacology.

The naturally occurring catecholamines are epinephrine, which is formed from norepinephrine and secreted by the adrenal medulla, and norepinephrine, which is stored in and secreted from sympathetic postganglionic nerves. Catecholamines elicit two pharmacologically opposing responses termed *α-adrenergic* and *β-adrenergic* (Ahlquist, 1948). Each tissue is thought to respond in predominantly an α or a β fashion, depending on which type of adrenergic receptor predominates. α-Receptor stimulation in smooth muscle is associated with contraction (except in the gut), and β-receptor stimulation causes smooth muscle relaxation. The rank order of potency of catecholamines and effectiveness of selective antagonists in blocking their effects led A. M. Lands *et al.* (1967) to subdivide β-adrenergic responses into β-1 and β-2 classes. The smooth muscle of respiratory tract is characterized as a β-2-responsive tissue, although there is now strong evidence that it also possesses α-adrenergic receptors (Fleisch *et al.*, 1973). Smooth muscles of blood vessels, uterus, and vas deferens are also classed as β-2, while those of coronary artery, alimentary tract, and cardiac tissue are classed as β-1.

β-Adrenergic responses are well known to be mediated by cAMP (Robison *et al.*, 1971), and the effects of catecholamines in relieving the asthmatic condition are believed to result from β-adrenergic stimulation of adenylate cyclase (see Table 2). The α-adrenergic responses to epinephrine are opposed to those listed in Table 2, but the mechanisms by which they occur are not completely understood. The first proposal involved a reduction in cAMP levels (Robison *et al.*, 1971), and this reduction was documented in human lung tissue (Kaliner *et al.*, 1972). The second proposal involved stimulation of membrane-bound ATPase, and this stimulation was demonstrated in a few cell types, including lymphocytes (Coffey *et al.*, 1975), mast cells (Coffey and Middleton, 1973), and neutrophils and macrophages (Coffey *et al.*, 1971). Such stimulation has been tentatively related to α-adrenergic augmentation of cation and nutrient transport (Hadden *et al.*, 1971a,b) and secretory (Coffey and Middleton, 1973), motile, contractile, and other energy-requiring processes coupled to ATP hydrolysis (Coffey *et al.*, 1974). The third proposal regarding the mechanism of α-stimulation involved stimulation of guanylate cyclase either directly (Goldberg *et al.*, 1974; G. Schultz *et al.*, 1975) or indirectly through release of acetylcholine (ACh) (Ball *et al.*, 1972).

Applying these concepts of adrenergic pharmacology to studies in asthma, most experimentors concluded that there is a variable degree of β-adrenergic blockade in most symptomatic and some asymptomatic patients, but all do not agree that the blockade is the first cause of or the final common pathway for the disorder. In support of the theory, Bernstein *et al.*, (1972) demonstrated reduced responses of urinary cAMP following administration of epinephrine, but normal increases following glucagon. Studies with isolated human leukocytes or purified lymphocytes (Falliers *et al.*, 1971; Logsdon *et al.*, 1972; Parker and Smith, 1973; Gillespie *et al.*, 1974; Alston *et al.*, 1974) also showed reduced β-adrenergic stimulation of adenylate cyclase, especially during symptomatic periods (Parker and Smith, 1973), and in some studies (Logsdon *et al.*, 1973; Parker *et al.*, 1973a,b; Gillespie *et al.*, 1974), the basal cAMP levels were reduced as well.

The possibility that sympathomimetic therapy produces reduced responsiveness of β-adrenergic receptors is suggested by the animal studies of Mukherjee and Lefkowitz (1976). Interestingly, addition of GTP rapidly restored responsiveness. In the human metabolic studies of Nelson *et al.* (1975), ephedrine therapy resulted in diminished blood glucose responses to ephinephrine. Also, in studies of receptor desensitization to isoproterenol and other agonists in peripheral blood adherent mononuclear cells, Kalisker and Middleton (in preparation) found that cAMP responses were reduced in both normals and asthmatics taking the β-agonists, and were higher and comparable when the drugs were not being taken. In most of the studies cited, however, the cells of normal subjects, also given a regimen of ephedrine and other antiasthmatic drugs for periods ranging from 5 to 15 days, showed normal responses to epinephrine or isoproterenol. Similar results for blood glucose were obtained by Fireman *et al.* (1970) after 30 days of oral ephedrine therapy, and recent experiments by Svedmyr *et al.* (1976) revealed no drug-related reduction in lung function responses to catecholamines. In addition, recent studies of β-adrenergic responses of lymphocytes (Lee *et al.*, 1975) and polymorphonuclear leukocytes (Busse, 1975) in asthmatic patients not receiving sympathomimetic therapy support the hypothesis of β-adrenergic blockade. It is apparent that a need exists for more studies with isolated cell types before this controversy can be satisfactorily resolved.

Assuming the validity of the many reports supporting β-adrenergic blockade in asthma, many questions remain regarding its molecular nature: (1) Are the numbers of β-receptors diminished in cells of allergic patients? Two types of studies suggest that they are not: (a) Isolated asthmatics' leukocytes bind as much labeled epinephrine as normal cells (Sokol and Beall, 1975), although recently developed methodology (Mukherjee and Lefkowitz, 1976) for distinguishing specific β-receptor binding from α- and nonspecific binding must be employed in corroborative experiments. (b) The β-blockade, defined by subsensitivity of adenylate cyclase to stimulation by isoproterenol, was effectively removed by incubating leukocytes of asthmatics with the α-adrenergic blockers phentolamine (Logsdon *et al.*, 1973) and thymoxamine (Alston *et al.*, 1974), suggesting either that the cells possessed a normal number of β-receptors that were "unblocked" by the pharmacological manipulation or that blockade of unusually responsive α-receptors permitted normal stimulation of β-receptors. (2) Are the numbers or responsiveness of α-receptors increased in cells of allergic patients? ATPase activities are linked to α-stimulation, and are significantly elevated in both leukocytes (Coffey *et al.*, 1974) and platelets (Coffey and Middleton, 1975) of asthmatics. Specific inhibition of Mg^2-dependent, Na^+, K^+-stimulated ATPase by ouabain resulted in normal responsiveness of asthmatic leukocyte adenylate cyclase to isoproterenol (Alston *et al.*, 1974), suggesting again that the β-blockade is not the result of a reduced number of β-receptors, but rather an expression of imbalance between activities of two competing catecholamine-responsive enzyme systems. (3) If the receptors are indeed blocked, does the block occur at the level of the β-receptor itself (now known to be a protein; Lefkowitz *et al.*, 1976), at the level of a phospholipid component (Lefkowitz *et al.*, 1976) of the receptor or "transducer," or even nearer the catalytic site of adenylate cyclase? The latter situation could be produced by excessive guanylate cyclase activity, which might reduce the amount of GTP below the level required for activation of adenylate cyclase. Data have not yet arrived for tissues of patients with asthma or other allergic disorders. (4) Another possibility could involve increased cellular Ca^{2+}, which stimulates guanylate cyclase, inhibits adenylate cyclase, and may be involved in catecholamine tachyphylaxis, possibly produced by Ca^{2+} activation of a PDE activator protein (J. Schultz, 1975). In support of this notion is the fact that aminophylline (a PDE inhibitor) prevented isoproterenol desensitization in rat aorta (Fleisch *et al.*, 1973). Of possible relevance is the finding (Coffey *et al.*, 1972) of greatly elevated divalent-cation-dependent ATPase activity in membranes of leukocytes of asthmatics, measured in the absence of divalent cations. This activity could be reduced to normal negligible levels with EGTA, suggesting that the elevated activity was due to increased Ca^{2+} binding in the membranes. (5) Last, the question of an abnormality in endogenous catecholamine production in asthmatics was raised by Mathé and Knapp (1969), who found evidence of decreased epinephrine in the urine of asthmatics subjected to psychological stress. Also, Griffiths *et al.* (1972) measured an abnormally high increase in plasma norepinephrine in asthmatics following exercise. Morris *et al.*, (1972) found elevated levels of epinephrine in the urine of asthmatics at rest, but subnormal increases in epinephrine in response to the stress of asthmatic attacks.

In summary, an abundance of literature exists that not only supports β-adrenergic blockade in several tissues of asthmatic patients, but also suggests a relative increase in α-adrenergic response that may be related to enhanced ATPase and guanylate cyclase activities. Balance in adrenergic responsiveness can apparently be restored by pharmacological manipulation. The defective aspect(s) of the receptor mechanisms that regulate responses to hormones and mediators may involve subtle abnormalities in membrane structure.

4. Drugs Used in Treatment of Asthma

4.1. Sympathomimetic Amines and Antagonists

Sympathomimetic amines are commonly used to control hypersensitivity states, especially asthma, anaphylaxis, rhinitis, urticaria, angioedema, and insect sting reactions. Examples are epinephrine, isoproterenol, and ephedrine. The latter has been used the longest of any, but Furchgott (1970) stated that it has no β-agonistic properties. It has an indirect effect in releasing norepinephrine from nerve storage pools. The released norepinephrine may then exert beneficial β-adrenergic effects, but may also activate α-receptors. Epinephrine also has both α- and β-agonistic effects, while isoproterenol (in the absence of β-blockade) acts almost exclusively on the β-receptors. More selective β-2 stimulators are discussed in recent reviews by Avner (1975), Leifer and Wittig (1975), and van As (1975): isoetharine, metaproterenol (orciprenaline), albuterol (salbutamol), terbutaline, fenoterenol, salmefamol, trimetoquinol, hexoprenaline, rimiterol, and carbuterol are examples. These agents are probably also the best activators of adenylate cyclase in lung, and have a duration of action of 3–6 hr. This duration is considerably longer than that of isoproterenol, the agonist most often used at present. One disadvantage of isoproterenol is its metabolism to 3-methoxy-isoproterenol, a β-blocking compound thought by some workers to be partially responsible for deaths involving isoproterenol overusage. Of the β-agonists, only four are at present available as aerosols in the United States: epinephrine, isoproterenol, isoetharine, and metaproterenol.

The combined use of sympathomimetic amines and a specific β-1-receptor-blocking compound such as sotalol, in patients with certain cardiovascular diseases, was suggested to obviate side effects on cardiac force and rate of contraction, but use of this drug involves a slight risk of aggravating asthma in some patients (Powles *et al.*, 1969).

Combining sympathomimetic amines with α-adrenergic antagonists may also be useful in the management of asthma, as suggested by the leukocyte enzyme studies cited above and by clinically improved airway conductance following administration of dibenamine (Klotz and Bernstein, 1950), thymoxamine (Griffin *et al.*, 1972), and phentolamine (Marcelle, 1969; Gross *et al.*, 1974). Some α-blocking compounds such as phentolamine and phenoxybenzamine also have antihistaminic properties, and these agents as well as thymoxamine inhibit histamine-induced airway narrowing (Bianco *et al.*, 1972; Gaddie *et al.*, 1972; Kerr *et al.*, 1970). Another new α-blocking agent, indoramin, has been shown to inhibit exercise-induced asthma (Bianco *et al.*, 1974). At least two possible mechanisms for the effects described above are: (1) prevention of α-adrenergic increases in cGMP and (2) independent effects of α-blocking compounds in increasing cAMP levels (Logsdon *et al.*, 1973; Middleton, 1974).

In conclusion, catecholamines and especially the newer β-2 sympathomimetic amines represent an important part of asthma therapy. Presumably by increasing cAMP levels they inhibit mediator release and bronchial smooth muscle contraction. In many patients, however, therapy with sympathomimetics may not provide complete relief, indicating the need for other agents such as cAMP-PDE inhibitors, which may increase cAMP levels by a mechanism that is not suppressed by β-adrenergic blockade.

4.2. Phosphodiesterase Inhibitors

The most-studied inhibitors of PDEs are methyl xanthines such as theophylline and caffeine. They inhibit breakdown of both cAMP and cGMP *in vitro,* usually by a competitive mechanism, but usually mimic effects of cAMP on tissues and often cause effects synergistic with agents that stimulate adenylate cyclase (Goldberg *et al.,* 1973a). Thus, it is suspected but not yet proved that the predominant effect of methyl xanthines *in vivo* is on cAMP-PDE, and this effect might explain their efficacy in the management of asthma. A disturbing fact observed by ourselves and others is that theophylline does not effectively inhibit cAMP-PDE *in vitro* at the concentrations (10^{-6}–10^{-5} M) found effective *in vivo.* It may therefore influence other mechanisms such as the Ca^{2+}-dependent regulator protein of PDE (J. Schultz, 1975) or affect levels of membrane-bound Ca^{2+} by an action independent of PDE inhibition (Schwabe and Ebert, 1972). To date, attempts to demonstrate abnormalities in cAMP-PDE in leukocytes of asthmatics have been unsuccessful (Parker, 1973; Coffey and Middleton, unpublished results), but the cGMP-PDE enzymes have not yet been investigated.

The only PDE inhibitor now in use for the treatment of asthma is theophylline or its more water-soluble form, aminophylline (ethylenediamine·2 theophylline). Different patients exhibit different rates of theophylline metabolism, so individualization of dosage becomes very important (Weinberger and Riegelman, 1974). Theophylline may not be as potent or as selective for cAMP-PDE as other compounds now being tested. For example, 1-methyl-3-isobutylxanthine is much more potent and appears to have a greater selectivity for cGMP-PDE (G. Schultz *et al.,* 1973), but has not been tested clinically. Among the more potent PDE inhibitors now under study are the imidazolidinones, especially RO 20-1724, which has up to 1000 times the potency of theophylline (Sheppard, 1973) and seems to have no lipolytic or cardiac effects, and papaverine, which is 10–100 times as potent as theophylline (Goldberg *et al.,* 1970). Other drugs in current use for other disorders have been reported to inhibit cAMP-PDE, including the phenothiazine-type tranquilizers and reserpine derivatives, the antidepressant imipramine, diuretics such as furosemide, hypoglycemic agents such as chloropropamide and tolbutamide, and α-adrenergic antagonists, including dihydroergotamine and phentolamine (Appleman *et al.,* 1973; Kuehl, 1974). Interestingly, most of these compounds also inhibit ATPase activity (Roufogalis, 1975). An ideal compound for the treatment of asthma would inhibit cAMP-PDE while stimulating cGMP-PDE. Such properties are not inconceivable, since they represent the exact opposite of those postulated for imidazole (Goldberg *et al.,* 1970).

4.3. Corticosteroids

In addition to the sympathomimetic amines and PDE inhibitors that act directly on the cAMP system, corticosteroids are used widely in the management of allergic states, and also affect the cyclic nucleotide system by mechanisms not well understood.

At the tissue level, corticosteroids exert a wide range of antiallergic and antiinflammatory actions, including lymphopenia and relatively greater loss of T than B cells from the circulation (a result of redistribution to the bone marrow; Fauci, 1975), inhibition of release of lysosomal enzymes (Weissmann, 1973) and histamine (Coffey and Middleton, 1973; Greaves and Plummer, 1974), and inhibition of several other processes, including leukotaxis and eosinophilia, effects that were recently reviewed by Baxter and Harris (1975), Leung and Munck (1975), and Middleton (1975b). It is also claimed that corticosteroids inhibit endogenous histamine formation (Aviado and Carillo, 1970), and more recently, it was proposed (Hong and Levine, 1976) that corticosteroids act by inhibiting release of arachidonic acid, the precursor of prostaglandins, with profound effects, which are discussed in Section 4.6.

Regarding well-known molecular mechanisms, steroids combine with specific cytoplasmic receptors that enter the nucleus to act on nuclear receptors, stimulating selective mRNA synthesis (O'Malley, 1971). This scheme was first established for estrogen, but now appears valid for all steroids including the glucocorticosteroids in lung (Toft and Chytil, 1973). Since about 6–10 hr is required for corticosteroids to exert clinical improvement in asthma, most of the effects are probably mediated by nuclear mechanisms, the predominant one being a general suppression of tissue protein synthesis and cell proliferation. However, corticosteroids selectively stimulate synthesis of several proteins, including tyrosine aminotransferase, tryptophan oxygenase, tryptophan hydroxylase, phosphoenolpyruvate carboxykinase, glycerophosphate dehydrogenase, and glutamine synthetase (Leung and Munck, 1975; Wicks *et al.*, 1974). Many of these effects are also produced by cAMP, but different nuclear mechanisms are involved (Krone *et al.*, 1975). It is not readily apparent how increased activities of the enzymes listed to date can elicit any of the antiallergic or antiinflammatory responses to corticosteroids, while inhibition by corticosteroids of synthesis of a protein involved in glucose utilization (Leung and Munck, 1975) could be an important mechanism, since mediator release requires glucose.

Of undetermined mechanism but unquestionable importance is the old observation that corticosteroids exert a "sparing action" on or a "permissive effect" for the stimulation by catecholamines of β-receptors (Brodie *et al.*, 1966). Townley *et al.* (1970) proposed this mechanism to account for corticosteroid-induced reduction of the glycemic abnormality of asthma. In a recent discussion of this effect, Geddes *et al.* (1974) concluded that corticosteroid inhibition of norepinephrine uptake into extraneuronal tissue is the most plausible mechanism. We observed that a single injection of 40 mg methyl prednisolone restored normal levels as well as circadian rhythm of cAMP excretion in asthmatic children (Coffey and Middleton, 1974). This effect lasted 2–3 days, and may relate to the restoration of β-adrenergic responsiveness in the subjects. Similarly, in leukocytes of asthmatic patients, corticosteroid therapy restores responsiveness of adenylate cyclase to isoproterenol stimulation (Logsdon *et al.*, 1972; Parker *et al.*, 1973a,b) and reduces ATPase activities to normal levels (Coffey *et al.*, 1974; Coffey and Middleton, 1975). Direct stimulation of adenylate cyclase by corticosteroids has not been documented in membrane preparations, although cAMP levels are increased, possibly due to decreases in cAMP-PDE, after several hours of exposure of cells in culture (Manganiello and Vaughan, 1972). On the other hand, Logsdon *et al.* (1972) and Parker *et al.* (1973a) observed stimulation of cAMP accumulation in human leukocytes and lymphocytes within 2–5 min after addition of physiologic levels of corticosteroids *in vitro*. These results suggest that steroids may also act on receptors at the cell surface (Suyemitsu and Terayama, 1975) to modulate metabolism. In other experiments, we found progressive inhibition in broken cell membrane preparations of leukocyte ATPase (Coffey *et al.*, 1974) and cytoplasmic cAMP-PDE (Logsdon *et al.*, 1972) activities by corticosteroids, and others (Lavin *et al.*, 1975) confirmed the latter effect for both low- and high-K_m types of cAMP-PDE in human lymphocytes. It therefore seems reasonable to propose that some of the beneficial effects of corticosteroids may be mediated by stimulation of cAMP accumulation and inhibition of ATPase activities by mechanisms involving only plasma membrane and cytoplasmic receptors.

Detailed studies on cGMP modulation by corticosteroids should also be performed, since mediator release in the lung is augmented by cGMP (Kaliner *et al.*, 1972), and smooth muscle contraction may be mediated by this nucleotide (Goldberg *et al.*, 1973a,b; G. Schultz *et al.*, 1973, 1975). The observation that hydrocortisone treatment reduces lung cGMP levels (Goldberg *et al.*, 1973b) may be of extreme importance. It will be of great interest to examine whether corticosteroids actually fulfill the role for the ideal PDE modulator, activating cGMP-PDE while inhibiting cAMP-PDE.

It is not known whether any of the actions of corticosteroids discussed above are abnormal in asthmatics, but since R. S. Smith *et al.* (1973) reported abnormal responses of lymphocyte immunoglobulin synthesis following exposure to hydrocortisone, and Schwartz *et al.* (1968) found reduced eosinopenic responses to corticosteroids in asthma, it appears important to investigate steroid receptor functions.

Corticosteroids widely used by oral or intravenous administration to treat asthma and various allergic states include prednisone, methylprednisolone, and hydrocortisone. Side effects are minimal if the drugs are used briefly and infrequently. When used at high dosage over long periods of time, the steroids can cause serious side effects such as hypothalamic–pituitary suppression of ACTH release, Cushingoid changes, and retardation of growth. Alternate-day steroid therapy given in the morning is therapeutically effective and seems to cause far fewer side effects (Morris, 1973, 1975). Aerosolized beclomethasone dipropionate has been found extremely effective in recent clinical tests, and does not appear to confer unwanted side effects seen with other systemically active steroids (Kreus *et al.*, 1975; Godfrey, 1975).

4.4. Atropine

Asthma has long been considered a disorder of autonomic imbalance with parasympathetic (cholinergic) predominance, and evidence of the hyperirritability of the airways supports this contention (Nadel, 1973; Gold, 1973). Stimulation of the subepithelial receptors of the tracheobronchial tree by cold air, dust, SO_2 or mediators released by antigen in sensitized subjects initiates a vagal reflex that induces bronchoconstriction. In the asthmatic patient this mechanism could provide a positive feedback loop (Gold, 1973): histamine released following IgE–antigen reactions stimulates afferent parasympathetic nerves, which could result reflexly in greater release of ACh from efferent vagal fibers, augmenting smooth muscle contraction (G. Schultz *et al.*, 1973) and mediator release (Kaliner *et al.*, 1972; Austen, 1973), assuming apposition of cholinergic nerves and mast cells. In experimental animals, it was shown that the increase in airway resistance could be abolished by interrupting either the afferent or efferent limbs of the vagus or by atropine sulfate, which blocks the muscarinic cholinergic receptors. Since ACh and its analogues carbachol and mecholyl act on these receptors to increase levels of cGMP (George *et al.*, 1970; Goldberg *et al.*, 1973a; G. Schultz *et al.*, 1973) with the associated augmentation of smooth muscle contraction and mediator release, atropine would be expected to inhibit these responses.

The supposed disadvantage of atropine is its drying effect, which could enhance mucus plug formation, but recent clinical trials with atropine (cf. Cropp, 1975; Gold, 1973) and ipatropium bromide, a quaternary atropine salt (Simonsson *et al.*, 1975), indicate that the renewed interest in this type of treatment is justified. Interestingly, Patel (1975) found that 1.2 mg aerosolized atropine sulfate produced significant increases in forced expiratory volume (FEV_1) and specific airway conductance following $PGF_{2\alpha}$-induced bronchoconstriction in asthmatics. These results prompted the suggestion that $PGF_{2\alpha}$ may activate cholinergic receptors, but our interpretation would be that $PGF_{2\alpha}$ stimulates the afferent limb of the bronchoconstrictor reflex, resulting in the reflex discharge from the efferent nerve endings of ACh. The action of ACh on cholinergic receptors is then blocked by atropine. A mechanistic distinction between these possibilities could be made using isolated cells.

4.5. Antihistamines

Histamine, like the catecholamines, acts on two sets of receptors termed H_1 and H_2 (Black *et al.*, 1972; Fleisch *et al.*, 1973). Activation of the H_2 receptors is associated with increased cAMP levels, and may provide a feedback inhibition of histamine release (Lichtenstein, 1973). This is a potentially valuable homeostatic mechanism that conceivably may not operate correctly in allergic patients. Several new compounds, including burimamide, metiamide and cimetidine, block H_2 receptors and would prevent histamine-induced increases in cAMP, so we do not expect these compounds to be useful for allergic therapy. Activation of H_1 receptors is now thought to be associated with increased cGMP levels in lung (Goldberg *et al.*, 1973b; Stoner *et al.*, 1974; Polson *et al.*, 1976). Blockade of this interaction by promethazine, diphenhydramine, mepyramine, or other antihistamines (many of which also possess α-adrenergic antagonistic properties) may be of some benefit to certain patients with asthma. The older literature suggests that they are not, although they have been used for many years in the management of allergic rhinitis, urticaria, and other allergic disorders. Recent clinical experiments (Karlin, 1975), however, showed beneficial effects of chlorpheniramine in some asthmatics, and a report (Lichtenstein, 1973) that some antihistamines at low concentrations inhibit immunologic histamine release indicate that further study of these agents is warranted.

4.6. Prostaglandins

Prostaglandins (PGs) have been considered both as possible mediators of the pathogenesis of asthma and as therapeutic agents. Human lung contains several

PGs, PGE_2 and $F_{2\alpha}$ being the most abundant (Karim *et al.*, 1967). Predictions that endogenous $PGF_{2\alpha}$ may play an important role in the pathogenesis of asthma (Karim *et al.*, 1967; Mathé *et al.*, 1973; Paterson *et al.*, 1973) are supported by the facts that asthmatics are exquisitely sensitive to the bronchoconstrictor effects of aerosolized $PGF_{2\alpha}$ (Mathé *et al.*, 1973; Patel, 1975), and that an 8-fold increase in plasma levels of the primary metabolite of $PGF_{2\alpha}$ were found in the plasma of asthmatic patients following allergen challenge (Green *et al.*, 1974). In contrast, PGE_1 and PGE_2 cause relaxation of tracheobronchial smooth muscle (Sweatman and Collier, 1968; A. P. Smith, 1973) and inhibit immunologic release of histamine from human leukocytes (Lichtenstein and Henney, 1972) and lung fragments (Tauber *et al.*, 1973).

PGE_1 and E_2 stimulate adenylate cyclase in most tissues (Kuehl, 1974; Butcher and Baird, 1968), while $PGF_{2\alpha}$ stimulates cGMP accumulation (Dunham *et al.*, 1974). The effects of PGE_1, unlike those of isoproterenol, are not diminished in leukocytes of asthmatics (Parker *et al.*, 1973b; Coffey and Middleton, unpublished observations). It is therefore reasonable to expect that aerosolized PGE_1 or PGE_2 would be of great benefit to asthmatics, stimulating cAMP production through receptors that are not blocked, and overcoming an imbalance, if any, in the PGE_2/$PGF_{2\alpha}$ ratio. In the experiments of A, P. Smith (1973), however, the bronchodilator potency of PGE_2 was about one-tenth that of isoproterenol on a weight basis, the peak effect of PGE_2 was delayed by a few minutes, and its duration of action was only about 1 hr, which is less than that of the β-2 agonists. In addition, serious side effects including upper airway irritation, cough, expectoration, and even aggravation of asthma (which could be relieved by isoproterenol) may occur in some patients (A. P. Smith, 1973), indicating that experimental use of PGE_1 or PGE_2 in asthma requires further study. A possibly insurmountable problem involves the metabolism of PGE_2 (as well as $PGF_{2\alpha}$) to the 15-keto derivative, which is a more potent bronchoconstrictor than $PGF_{2\alpha}$ (Dawson and Sweatman, 1975).

The pharmacological manipulation of PG levels through inhibition of synthesis represents another possible approach. Nonsteroidal analgesic antiinflammatory compounds such as aspirin, indomethacin, and the fenamate drugs (flufenamic acid, meclofenamic acid, ibuprofen) inhibit synthesis of all PGs (Vane, 1971) by inhibition of the oxygenase that catalyzes conversion of arachidonic acid hydroperoxide to the cyclic endoperoxide precursor of both PGE_2 and $PGF_{2\alpha}$ (W. E. M. Lands *et al.*, 1974). Interestingly, indomethacin and the fenamates are also potent cAMP-PDE inhibitors (Kuehl, 1974). Aspirin does inhibit SRS-A- and $PGF_{2\alpha}$-induced bronchoconstriction in isolated human tissue, but is contraindicated for aspirin-sensitive asthmatics. Clinical trials with the fenamates have proved disappointing (Fleisch *et al.*, 1973). Pyrazalones such as phenylbutazone appear to inhibit both the cyclic endoperoxide reductase (which catalyzes the formation of $PGF_{2\alpha}$) and the isomerase (which catalyzes the formation of PGE_2) (Flower and Vane, 1974). Such drugs would probably not produce a more favorable PGE/PGF ratio in asthmatics, but the prospect of new drugs selectively inhibiting only the reductase offers hope. Other prospects include manipulation of the PG synthesis system at the level of endoperoxides. Some workers (Gorman, 1975) now believe that these intermediates may possess far greater biological activity than the final PG molecules, and that their effects mimic those of $PGF_{2\alpha}$, rather than those of the PGEs. The possibility that these labile but very powerful bronchoconstrictors are released prematurely in response to bronchial irritation should be investigated, since they have up to 15 times the effect of $PGF_{2\alpha}$ (Gorman, 1975). Inhibition of the formation of PG molecules and their precursors (possibly by corticosteroids, as mentioned in Section 4.3) therefore merits further study.

Last, pharmacological inhibition of $PGF_{2\alpha}$-induced bronchoconstriction may prove therapeutically useful. Polyphloretin phosphate inhibited human bronchial smooth muscle contraction induced *in vitro* by $PGF_{2\alpha}$ (Mathé *et al.*, 1971) as well as by SRS-A (Mathé and Strandberg, 1971). This inhibition may be a selective effect on a cGMP-mediated step, since the compound did not inhibit the relaxant effects of PGE_2 in experimental animals (A. P. Smith, 1973), and since Kuehl *et al.* (1971) found that it acts not at the PG receptor level, but rather at a protein kinase step. Preliminary studies with polyphloretin phosphate showed no improvement on airways of asthmatics (A. P. Smith, 1973). Some of the bronchoconstrictive effects of $PGF_{2\alpha}$ may be indirect, mediated by the cholinergic system as suggested by Patel (1975), who found that inhaled atropine but not sodium cromoglycate or thymoxamine prevented the bronchoconstriction. A combination therapy consisting of drugs aimed at inhibiting the synthesis, secretion, and cellular actions of $PGF_{2\alpha}$ can therefore be envisioned in future clinical trials.

4.7. Cromolyn, Hetrazan, and Chlorphenesin

Drugs that cannot be classified according to molecular mechanisms of action include disodium cromoglycate (Cromolyn, Intal, Aarane), diethylcarbamazine (Hetrazan), and chlorphenesin.

Cromolyn now has an established reputation as an effective adjunct in managing asthma, and possibly also Type III immunologic lung injury, allergic rhinitis, and vernal keratoconjunctivitis (Pepys, 1973). Its mechanism of action is unknown, although it has been suggested that it involves changes in Ca^{2+} flux (Kerr *et al.*, 1970; H. G. Johnson and Bach, 1975), and possibly inhibition of cAMP-PDE (Rachelevsky *et al.*, 1975). Another possibility is suggested by the close similarity of its structure and that of a recently developed antagonist of SRS-A (Augustein *et al.*, 1973). Comparing the effect of cromolyn on histamine-induced bronchoconstriction in asthmatics with the effects of phentolamine and phenoxybenzamine, Kerr *et al.* (1970) postulated that cromolyn may have partial α-blocking action. The principal effect is the inhibition of mediator release at a step following the antigen–antibody reaction, and this inhibition may be due to a stabilization of mast cell membranes (Altounyan *et al.*, 1971). It exhibits a limited dose–response relationship *in vitro,* inhibiting mediator release from human lung only at 0.1–10 μg/ml (Orange and Austen, 1971). The clinical effectiveness of cromolyn is not limited to reagin-mediated asthma; it is also effective in some patients with intrinsic asthma, and can partially prevent exercise-induced asthma in many patients. Cromolyn therapy frequently allows a reduction in steroid requirements (Pepys, 1973). Similar effects may be obtained with a new compound, 2-*o*-propoxyphenyl-8-azapurin-6-one, which was recently developed and found to be at least 10 times more effective than cromolyn in preventing mediator release and anaphylactic bronchospasm in guinea pigs and in isolated human bronchial muscle (Broughton *et al.*, 1974). Its mechanism of action is also undetermined. Other drugs with cromolyn-like activity are under development (Assem *et al.*, 1974).

Like cromolyn, Hetrazan inhibits release of mediators from lung (Orange *et al.*, 1970) by an unknown mechanism, but unlike cromolyn, Hetrazan has had only limited clinical testing. This antifilarial drug appeared to have a beneficial effect on asthma when it was given for concurrent infestation of filaria (Mallen, 1965).

Chlorphenesin carbamate is used as a muscle relaxant, and also inhibits mediator release from lung (Malley and Baecher, 1971) by an unknown mechanism. We are not aware of any clinical studies involving its use in allergy therapy.

4.8. Cyclic AMP and Analogues

It might seem reasonable to consider the use of cAMP or its more lipophilic mono- and dibutyryl-substituted derivatives in asthma, but we are not aware of any clinical studies. Paradoxically, when these compounds are added to *in vitro* systems, they frequently cause effects opposite to those obtained by stimulating intracellular increases in cAMP (Goldberg *et al.*, 1973b). Exogenous dibutyryl cAMP was shown to produce smooth muscle relaxation (Sheppard, 1973), and the 8-benzylthio derivative was 7 times as potent in guinea pig tracheal strips (Rubin *et al.*, 1971), while cAMP produced no effect unless theophylline was also added (Middleton and Fink, 1968), or caused contraction in several experiments (cf. Fleisch *et al.*, 1973). Nevertheless, cAMP was found to inhibit mediator release from lung tissue *in vitro* (Kaliner *et al.*, 1972). The possible clinical usefulness of cAMP or its analogues must await further investigation.

5. Summary and Speculation

It is apparent from the foregoing discussion that asthma is characterized by an imbalance in both α- and β-adrenergic receptor responsiveness as well as cholinergic hyperresponsiveness. Nearly all agents used in the treatment of allergic diseases may be associated with increased cAMP levels or decreased cGMP levels. The origin and identity of the factor, agent, or condition that causes receptor imbalance is completely unknown. Two animal studies (Fink and Schlueter, 1969; Busse and Reed, 1974) and one human platelet study (Solinger *et al.*, 1973) suggest that there may be a causative factor in the plasma of hypersensitive animals and asthmatic patients that confers cellular abnormalities on cells of normal subjects. However, these observations were not confirmed in human leukocyte cAMP studies (Gillespie *et al.*, 1974). The production of β-adrenergic blockade with products isolated from *Bordetella pertussis* (Parker and Morse, 1973) raises the possibility that the origin of the factor(s) may be viral or bacterial, as proposed by Szentivanyi (1968). Reports of endotoxin-induced enhancement of α-adrenergic responses in human bronchial smooth muscle (Simonsson *et al.*, 1972) suggest the importance of bacterial products in the development of adrenergic imbalance.

The demonstration of receptor imbalance in nonpulmonary cells of patients with asthma argues against a specific defect restricted to the target organ. The abnormalities discovered in leukocytes may reflect a more exaggerated form in receptor imbalances thought to exist in the lungs of asthmatic patients. Further experiments with *in vitro* systems may provide insights into the molecular details of abnormal receptor function. These receptor imbalances are characterized by subresponsive β-adrenergic and overly responsive α-adrenergic and muscarinic cholinergic receptor interactions with cellular enzymes, resulting in depressed adenylate cyclase, elevated ATPase, and possibly elevated guanylate cyclase activities. These elevated activities could result in reduced cAMP levels in two ways: (1) If a restricted membrane pool of ATP serves as substrate for both ATPase and adenylate cyclase, stimulation of the former would reduce availability of ATP for the latter enzyme and result in a lowering of cAMP levels. Conversely, cAMP acts to reduce ATPase activities (Mózsik, 1970; Luly *et al.*, 1972; Coffey *et al.*, 1975). (2) The elevated levels of cGMP could reduce cAMP by activating a specific PDE (Franks and MacManus, 1971). Stimulation of guanylate cyclase could also reduce β-adrenergic activation of adenylate cyclase by lowering the level of membrane-associated GTP, which may be a necessary component of the receptor–adenylate cyclase system (Schramm and Rodbell, 1975). In any event, stimulation of guanylate cyclase by ACh results in catecholamine-subsensitive adenylate cyclase (Kuo and Kuo, 1973).

Elevated ATPase activities may be a result of an imbalance in cellular receptors for hormones other than epinephrine. Mg^{2+}-dependent ATPases are also stimulated directly by insulin (Hadden *et al.*, 1972a; Jarett and Smith, 1974), growth hormone (Aizono *et al.*, 1974), carbachol, and histamine (Narumi and Kanno, 1973), while Mg^{2+}- and Na^+,K^+-ATPases are stimulated indirectly by thyroxine (Ismael-Beigi and Edelman, 1974). The latter is noteworthy in that thyroxine is required for optimum β-adrenergic responsiveness (Van Inwegen *et al.*, 1975). An imbalance in membrane phospholipid constituents could also produce altered ATPase and adenylate cyclase activities, since phospholipids (particularly phosphatidyl serine) are required for Na^+,K^+-ATPases (Whittam and Wheeler, 1970), while phosphatidyl inositol is required for β-adrenergic stimulation of adenylate cyclase (Levey, 1971). Phospholipids also determine temperature transition points for activation energies (Wisnieski *et al.*, 1974), and a phospholipid imbalance that produces an altered transition point could predispose a tissue to α-adrenergic responses (Fleisch *et al.*, 1973; Kunos *et al.*, 1974) and increase the guanylate cyclase/adenylate cyclase activity ratio (Amer and Byrne, 1975). A similar shift could account for the temperature-dependent interconversion of histamine receptor responses (Kenakin *et al.*, 1974).

In speculating about metabolic defects distal to the hormone receptors, it should be noted that the lung contains not only the highest level of cGMP and guanylate cyclase activity among mammalian tissues (Goldberg *et al.*, 1973a), but also the highest level of the protein kinase modulator protein that activates cGMP-dependent protein kinase (Kuo, 1975). Abnormalities in the levels of the protein kinases or the modulator protein could predispose a tissue to imbalanced responses to the cyclic nucleotides. It is of interest that the level of the cGMP-dependent protein kinase in lung decreases, while that of the cAMP-dependent protein kinase increases, with age (Kuo, 1975). It will be interesting to learn whether these changes are related to the observation that α-receptors decrease more rapidly than β-receptors in tissues of aging animals (Fleisch *et al.*, 1973).

In conclusion, we now understand how many, but certainly not all, antiallergic drugs exert their effects at the molecular level. Yet only the first stage of a biochemical understanding of allergic diseases has been achieved to date. In addition to immunologic studies, urgently needed biochemical studies include the quantitation of membrane phospholipids, divalent cations, and guanylate cyclase activities, and the extent to which the latter can be stimulated by cholinergic agents and mediators liberated from mast cells. Of equal importance but more difficult may be the isolation and quantitation of β-, α-, and muscarinic cholinergic receptors. In the light of rapidly expanding knowledge on how receptors are linked to enzymic activation, such information should eventually permit theoretical calculations of functional receptor imbalance and suggest pharmacological manipulations to restore balance.

References

Ahlquist, R. P., 1948, *Am. J. Physiol.* **153**:586–600.

Aizono, Y., Roberts, J. E., Sonenberg, M., and Swislocki, N. I., 1974, *Arch. Biochem. Biophys.* **163**:634–643.

Alston, W. C., Patel, K. R., and Kerr, J. W., 1974, *Brit. Med. J.* **1**:90–93.

Altounyan, R. E., Cox, J. S. G., and Orr, T. S. C., 1971, in: *New Concepts in Allergy and Clinical Immunology* (U. Serafini, A. W. Frankland, C. Mesala, and J. M. Jamar, eds.), pp. 377–384, Excerpta Medica, Amsterdam.

Amer, M. S., and Byrne, J. E., 1975, *Nature (London)* **256**:421–424.

Appleman, M. M., Thompson, W. J., and Russell, T. R., 1973, *Adv. Cyclic Nucleotide Res.* **3**:65–98.

Assem, E. S. K., 1971, *Postgrad. Med. J. Suppl.* **47**:31–34.

Assem, E. S. K., Evans, J. A., and McAllen, M., 1974, *Br. Med. J.* **2**:93–95.

Augustein, J., Farmer, J. B., Lee, T. B., Sheard, P., and Tattersall, M. L., 1973, *Nature (London) New Biol.* **245**:215.

Austen, K. F., 1973, in: *Asthma: Physiology, Immunopharmacology and Treatment* (K. F. Austen and L. M. Lichtenstein, eds.), pp. 111–119, Academic Press, New York.

Aviado, T. M., and Carillo, L. R., 1970, *Clin. Pharmacol.* **10**:3–11.

Avner, S. E., 1975, *Pediatr. Clin. North Am.* **22**:129–139.

Ball, J. H., Kaminsky, N. I., Hardman, J. G., Broadus, A. E., Sutherland, E. W., and Liddle, G. W., 1972, *J. Clin. Invest.* **51**:2124–2129.

Baxter, J. D., and Harris, A. W., 1975, *Transplant. Proc.* **7**:55–65.

Bernstein, R. A., Linarelli, L., Facktor, M. A., Friday, G. A., Drash, A., and Fireman, P., 1972, *J. Lab. Clin. Med.* **80**:772–779.

Bianco, S., Griffin, J. P., Kamburoff, P. L., and Prime, F. J., 1972, *Br. J. Dis. Chest* **66**:27–32.

Bianco, S., Griffin, J. P., Kamburoff, P. L., and Prime, F. J., 1974, *Br. Med. J.* **4**:18–20.

Black, J. W., Duncan, W. A. M., Durant, C. J., Ganellin, C. R., and Parsons, E. M., 1972, *Nature (London)* **236**:385–390.

Brodie, B. B., Davies, J. I., Hynie, S., Krishna, G., and Weiss, B., 1966, *Pharmacol. Rev.* **18**:273–289.

Broughton, B. J., Chaplen, P., Knowles, P., Lunt, E., Pain, D. L., Wooldridge, K. R. H., Ford, R., Marshall, S., Walker, J. L., and Maxwell, D. R., 1974, *Nature (London)* **251**:650–652.

Busse, W. W., 1975, *Clin. Res.* **23**:502A.

Busse, W. W., and Reed, C. E., 1974, *J. Allergy Clin. Immunol.* **53**:271–277.

Butcher, R. W., and Baird, C. E., 1968, *J. Biol. Chem.* **243**:1713–1717.

Casnellie, J. E., and Greengard, P., 1974, *Proc. Natl. Acad. Sci. U.S.A.* **71**:1891–1895.

Chambers, D. A., Martin, D. W., Jr., and Weinstein, Y., 1974, *Cell* **3**:375–380.

Coffey, R. G., and Middleton, E., Jr., 1973, *Int. Arch. Allergy Appl. Immunol.* **45**:593–611.

Coffey, R. G., and Middleton, E., Jr., 1974, *J. Allergy Clin. Immunol.* **54**:41–53.

Coffey, R. G., and Middleton, E., Jr., 1975, *Int. Arch. Allergy Appl. Immunol.* **48**:171–181.

Coffey, R. G., Hadden, J. W., Hadden, E. M., and Middleton, E., Jr., 1971, *Fed. Proc. Fed. Am. Soc. Exp. Biol.* **30**:497.

Coffey, R. G., Logsdon, P. J., and Middleton, E., Jr., 1972, *J. Allergy Clin. Immunol.* **49**:87–88.

Coffey, R. G., Hadden, J. W., and Middleton, E., Jr., 1974, *J. Clin. Invest.* **54**:138–146.

Coffey, R. G., Hadden, E. M., and Hadden, J. W., 1975, *Endocrine Res. Commun.* **2**:179–198.

Cropp, G. J. A., 1975, *Am. Rev. Respir. Dis.* **112**:599–606.

Dawson, W., and Sweatman, W. J. F., 1975, *Int. Arch. Allergy* **49**:213–216.

Diamant, B., 1975, *Int. Arch. Allergy* **49**:155–171.

Diamant, B., and Patkar, S. A., 1975, *Int. Arch. Allergy* **49**:183–207.

Dunham, E. W., Haddox, M. K., and Goldberg, N. D., 1974, *Proc. Natl. Acad. Sci. U.S.A.* **71**:815–819.

Falliers, C. J., de A., Cardoso, R. R., Bane, H. N., Coffey, R., and Middleton, E., Jr., 1971, *J. Allergy* **47**:207–219.

Fauci, A. S., 1975, *Immunology* **28**:669–680.
Fink, J. N., and Schlueter, D. P., 1969, *J. Allergy* **43**:167–168.
Fireman, P., Palm, C. R., Friday, G. A., and Drash, A. L., 1970, *J. Allergy* **45**:117.
Fleisch, J. H., Kent, K. M., and Cooper, T., 1973, in: *Asthma: Physiology, Immunopharmacology and Treatment* (K. F. Austen and L. M. Lichtenstein, eds.), pp. 139–164, Academic Press, New York.
Flower, R. J., and Vane, J. R., 1974, in: *Prostaglandin Synthetase Inhibitors—Their Effects on Physiological Functions and Pathological States* (H. R. Robinson and J. R. Vane, eds.), pp. 9–18, Raven Press, New York.
Franks, D. J., and MacManus, J. P., 1971, *Biochem. Biophys. Res. Commun.* **42**:844–849.
Furchgott, R. F., 1970, *Fed. Proc. Fed. Am. Soc. Exp. Biol.* **29**:1352–1361.
Gaddie, J., Legge, J. S., Petrie, G., and Palmer, K. N. V., 1972, *Br. J. Dis. Chest* **66**:141–146.
Geddes, B. A., Jones, T. R., Dvorsky, R. J., and Lefcoe, N. M., 1974, *Am. Rev. Respir. Dis.* **110**:420–427.
George, W., Polson, J. B., O'Toole, A. G., and Goldberg, N., 1970, *Proc. Natl. Acad. Sci. U.S.A.* **66**:398–403.
Gillespie, E., Valentine, M., and Lichtenstein, L. M., 1974, *J. Allergy Clin. Immunol.* **53**:27–33.
Godfrey, S., 1975, *Pediatr. Clin. North Am.* **22**:147–155.
Gold, W. M., 1973, in: *Asthma: Physiology, Immunopharmacology and Treatment* (K. F. Austen and L. M. Lichtenstein, eds.), pp. 169–182, Academic Press, New York.
Goldberg, N. D., Lust, W. D., O'Dea, R. F., Wei, S., and O'Toole, A. G., 1970, *Adv. Biochem. Psychopharmacol.* **3**:67–87.
Goldberg, N. D., O'Dea, R. F., and Haddox, M. K., 1973a, *Adv. Cyclic Nucleotide Res.* **3**:155–223.
Goldberg, N. D., Haddox, M. K., Hartle, D. K., and Hadden, J. W., 1973b, in: *Pharmacology and the Future of Man, Proceedings of the Fifth International Congress of Pharmacology:* Vol. 5, pp. 146–169, S. Karger, Basel.
Goldberg, N. D., Haddox, M. K., Dunham, E., Lopez, C., and Hadden, J. W., 1974, in: *Control of Proliferation in Animal Cells* (B. Clarkson and R. Baserga, eds.), Vol. 1, pp. 609–626, *Cold Spring Harbor Conferences on Cell Proliferation,* Cold Spring Harbor Press, New York.
Goldberg, N. D., Haddox, M. K., Nicol, S. E., Glass, D. B., Sanford, C. H., Kuehl, F. A., and Estensen, R., 1975, *Adv. Cyclic Nucleotide Res.* **5**:307–330.
Gorman, R. R., 1975, *J. Cyclic Nucleotide Res.* **1**:1–10.
Greaves, M. W., and Plummer, V. M., 1974, *Immunology* **27**:359–364.
Green, K., Hedquist, P., and Svanborg, N., 1974, *Lancet* **2**:1419–1421.
Griffin, J. P., Kamburoff, P. L., Prime, F. J., and Arbab, A. G., 1972, *Lancet* **1**:1288.
Griffiths, J., Leung, F. Y., Grzybowski, S., and Chan-Yeung, M. M. W., 1972, *Chest* **62**:527–533.
Gross, G. N., Souhrada, J. F., and Farr, R. S., 1974, *Chest* **66**:397–401.
Hadden, J. W., Hadden, E. M., and Good, R. A., 1971a, *Biochim. Biophys. Acta* **237**:339–347.
Hadden, J. W., Hadden, E. M., and Good, R. A., 1971b, *Exp. Cell Res.* **68**:217–219.
Hadden, J. W., Hadden, E. M., Wilson, E. E., Good, R. A., and Coffey, R. G., 1972a, *Nature (London) New Biol.* **235**:174–176.
Hadden, J. W., Hadden, E., Haddox, M., and Goldberg, N., 1972b, *Proc. Natl. Acad. Sci. U.S.A.* **69**:3024–3027.
Hadden, J. W., Hadden, E. M., and Goldberg, N. D., 1974, in: *Cyclic AMP, the Immune Response, and Tumor Growth* (W. Braun, L. M. Lichtenstein, and C. W. Parker, eds.), pp. 237–246, Springer-Verlag, New York.
Hadden, J. W., Johnson, E. M., Hadden, E. M., Coffey, R. G., and Johnson, L. D., 1975, in: *Immune Recognition, Proceedings of the Ninth Leukocyte Culture Conference (1974),* (A. S. Rosenthal, ed.), pp. 359–389, Academic Press, New York.
Hill, H. R., Estensen, R. D., Quie, P. G., Hogan, N. A., and Goldberg, N. D., 1975, *Metabolism* **24**:447–456.
Hong, S.-C. L., and Levine, L., 1976, *Proc. Natl. Acad. Sci. U.S.A.* **73**:1730–1734.
Ignarro, L. J., and George, W. J., 1974, *Proc. Natl. Acad. Sci. U.S.A.* **71**:2027–2031.
Illiano, G., Tell, G. P. E., Siegel, M. I., and Cuatrecasas, P., 1973, *Proc. Natl. Acad. Sci. U.S.A.* **70**:2443–2447.
Ishizaka, K., and Ishizaka, T., 1973, in: *Asthma: Physiology, Immunopharmacology and Treatment* (K. F. Austen and L. M. Lichtenstein, eds.), pp. 55–68, Academic Press, New York.
Ismail-Beigi, F., and Edelman, I. S., 1974, *Proc. Soc. Exp. Biol. Med.* **146**:983–988.

Jarett, L., and Smith, R. M., 1974, *J. Biol. Chem.* **249**:5195–5199.
Johnson, E. M., and Hadden, J. W., 1975, *Science* **187**:1198–1200.
Johnson, H. G., and Bach, M. K., 1975, *J. Immunol.* **114**:514–516.
Johnson, L. D., and Hadden, J. W., 1975, *Biochem. Biophys. Res. Commun.* **66**:1498–1505.
Kaliner, M., Orange, R. P., and Austen, K. F., 1972, *J. Exp. Med.* **136**:556–567.
Karim, S. M. M., Sandler, M., and Williams, C., 1967, *Br. J. Pharmacol. Chemother.* **31**:340–344.
Karlin, J. M., 1975, *Pediatr. Clin. North Am.* **22**:157–162.
Kenakin, T. P., Krueger, C. A., and Cook, D. A., 1974, *Nature (London)* **252**:54–55.
Kerr, J. W., Govindaraj, M., and Patel, K. R., 1970, *Brit. Med. J.* **2**:139–141.
Klotz, S. D., and Bernstein, C., 1950, *Ann. Allergy* **8**:767–771.
Kreus, K.-E., Viljanen, A. A., Kujala, E., and Kreus, R., 1975, *Scand. J. Respir. Dis.* **56**:47–57.
Krone, W., Huttner, W. B., Seitz, H. J., and Tarnowski, W., 1975, *FEBS Lett.* **52**:85–89.
Kuehl, F. A., Jr., 1974, *Prostaglandins* **5**:325–340.
Kuehl, F. A., Jr., Humes, J. L., Mandel, L. R., Cirillo, V. J., Zanetti, M. E., and Ham, E. A., 1971, *Biochem. Biophys. Res. Commun.* **44**:1464–1470.
Kuehl, F. A., Jr., Ham, E. A., Zanetti, M. E., Sanford, C. H., Nicol, S. E., and Goldberg, N. D., 1974, *Proc. Natl. Acad. Sci. U.S.A.* **71**:1866–1870.
Kunos, G., Vermes-Kunos, I., and Nickerson, M., 1974, *Nature (London)* **250**:779–781.
Kuo, J. F., 1975, *Proc. Natl. Acad. Sci. U.S.A.* **72**:2256–2259.
Kuo, J. F., and Kuo, W.-N., 1973, *Biochem. Biophys. Res. Commun.* **55**:660–665.
Lands, A. M., Arnold, A., McAuliff, J. P., Ludena, F. P., and Brown, T. G., Jr., 1967, *Nature (London)* **214**:597–598.
Lands, W. E. M., LeTellier, P. R., Rome, L., and Vanderhoek, J. Y., 1974, in: *Prostaglandin Synthetase Inhibitors—Their Effects on Physiological Functions and Pathological States* (H. R. Robinson and J. R. Vane, eds.), pp. 1–7, Raven Press, New York.
Langan, T. A., 1973, *Adv. Cyclic Nucleotide Res.* **3**:99–153.
Lavin, N., Rachelefsky, G., and Kaplan, S. A., 1975, *Horm. Metab. Res.* **7**:253–258.
Lee, T. P., Busse, W. W., and Reed, C. E., 1975, *Clin. Res.* **23**:503A.
Lefkowitz, R. J., Limbird, L. E., Mukherjee, C., and Caron, M. G., 1976, *Biochim. Biophys. Acta* **457**:1–39.
Leifer, K. N., and Wittig, H. J., 1975, *Ann. Allergy* **35**:69–80.
Leung, K., and Munck, A., 1975, *Annu. Rev. Physiol.* **37**:245–272.
Levey, G. S., 1971, *J. Biol. Chem.* **246**:7405–7407.
Levinson, H., Collins-Williams, C., Bryan, A. C., Reilly, B. J., and Orange, R. P., 1974, *Pediatr. Clin. North Am.* **21**:951–965.
Lichtenstein, L. M., 1973, in: *Asthma: Physiology, Immunopharmacology, and Treatment* (K. F. Austen and L. M. Lichtenstein, eds.), pp. 91–104, Academic Press, New York.
Lichenstein, L. M., 1975, *Int. Arch. Allergy* **49**:143–154.
Lichenstein, L. M., and Henney, C. S., 1972, in: *Prostaglandins in Cellular Biology* (P. W. Ramwell and B. B. Pharriss, eds.), pp. 293–308, Plenum Press, New York.
Logsdon, P. J., Middleton, E., Jr., and Coffey, R. G., 1972, *J. Allergy Clin. Immunol.* **50**:45–56.
Logsdon, P. J., Carnright, D. V., Middleton, E., Jr., and Coffey, R. G., 1973, *J. Allergy Clin. Immunol.* **52**:148–157.
Luly, P., Barnabei, O., and Tria, E., 1972, *Biochim. Biophys. Acta* **282**:447–452.
Mallen, M. S., 1965, *Ann. Allergy* **23**:534–537.
Malley, A., and Baecher, L., 1971, *J. Immunol.* **107**:586–588.
Manganiello, V., and Vaughan, M., 1972, *J. Clin. Invest.* **51**:2763–2767.
Marcelle, R., 1969, *Acta Allergol.* **24**:432–436.
Mathé, A. A., and Knapp, P. H., 1969, *N. Engl. J. Med.* **281**:234–238.
Mathé, A. A., and Strandberg, K., 1971, *Acta Physiol. Scand.* **82**:460–465.
Mathé, A. A., Strandberg, K., and Astrom, A., 1971, *Nature (London) New Biol.* **230**:215–216.
Mathé, A. A., Hedqvist, P., Holmgren, A., and Svanborg, N., 1973, *Brit. Med. J.* **1**:193–196.
Middleton, E., Jr., 1965, in: *Immunological Diseases* (M. Samter, ed.), pp. 578–599, Little, Brown and Co., Boston.
Middleton, E., Jr., 1972, *Adv. Intern. Med.* **18**:177–197.
Middleton, E., Jr., 1974, in: *Allergology, Proceedings of the Eighth International Congress of Allergology* (Y. Yamamura, ed.), pp. 317–324, Excerpta Medica, Amsterdam.

Middleton, E., Jr., 1975a, *Pediatr. Clin. North Am.* **22**:111–119.
Middleton, E., Jr., 1975b, in: *New Directions in Asthma* (M. Stein, ed.), pp. 433–446, American College of Chest Physicians, Park Ridge, Illinois.
Middleton, E., Jr., and Coffey, R. G., 1973, *Annu. Rep. Med. Chem.* **8**:273–283.
Middleton, E., Jr., and Fink, S. R., 1968, *J. Clin. Invest.* **47**:69a.
Morris, H. G., 1973, in: *Annual Review of Allergy of 1972*, Vol. 1 (C. Frazier, ed.), p. 105, Medical Examination Publishing Co., New York.
Morris, H. G., 1975, *Pediatr. Res.* **9**:579–583.
Morris, H. G., DeRoche, G., and Earle, M., 1972, *J. Allergy Clin. Immunol.* **50**:138–145.
Mózsik, G. Y., 1970, *Eur. J. Pharmacol.* **9**:207–210.
Mukherjee, C., and Lefkowitz, R. J., 1976, *Proc. Natl. Acad. Sci. U.S.A.* **73**:1494–1498.
Nadel, J. A., 1973, in: *Asthma: Physiology, Immunopharmacology and Treatment* (K. F. Austen and L. M. Lichtenstein, eds.). pp. 29–37, Academic Press, New York.
Narumi, S., and Kanno, M., 1973, *Biochem. Biophys. Acta* **311**:80–89.
Nelson, H. S., 1975, *Pediatr. Clin. North Am.* **22**:53–61.
Nelson, H. S., Black, J. W., Branch, L. B., Pfuetze, B., Spaulding, H., Summers, R., and Wood, D., 1975, *J. Allergy Clin. Immunol.* **55**:299–309.
O'Malley, B. W., 1971, *N. Engl. J. Med.* **284**:370–377.
Orange, R. P., and Austen, K. F., 1971, in: *Progress in Immunology* (B. Amos, ed.), pp. 173–186, Academic Press, New York.
Orange, R. P., Stechschulte, D. J., and Austen, K. F., 1970, *J. Immunol.* **105**:1087–1095.
Parker, C. W., 1973, in: *Asthma: Physiology, Immunopharmacology and Treatment* (K. F. Austen and L. M. Lichtenstein, eds.), pp. 185–206, Academic Press, New York.
Parker, C. W., and Morse, S. I., 1973, *J. Exp. Med.* **137**:1078–1091.
Parker, C. W., and Smith, J. W., 1973, *J. Clin. Invest.* **52**:48–59.
Parker, C. W., Baumann, M. L., and Huber, M. G., 1973a, *J. Clin. Invest.* **52**:1336–1341.
Parker, C. W., Huber, M. G., and Baumann, M. L., 1973b, *J. Clin. Invest.* **52**:1342–1348.
Patel, K. R., 1975, *Br. Med. J.* **2**:360–362.
Paterson, N. A. M., Ahmad, D., and Lefcoe, N. M., 1973, *Br. J. Dis. Chest* **67**:197–207.
Pepys, J., 1973, in: *Asthma: Physiology, Immunopharmacolocy and Treatment* (K. F. Austen and L. M. Lichtenstein, eds.), pp. 280–292, Academic Press, New York.
Polson, J. B., Krzanowski, J. J., and Szentivanyi, A., 1976, *Naunyn-Schmiedebergs Arch. Pharmacol.* **295**:27–32.
Powles, R., Shinebourne, E., and Homer, J. A., 1969, *Thorax* **24**:616–618.
Rachelevsky, G. S., Lavin, N., and Kaplan, S. A., 1975, *J. Allergy Clin. Immunol.* **55**:117–118.
Reed, C. E., 1965, *Rec. Prog. Horm. Res.* **21**:402–415.
Reed, C. E., 1974, *J. Allergy Clin. Immunol.* **53**:34–41.
Robison, G. A., Butcher, R. W., and Sutherland, E. W., 1971, in: *Cyclic AMP*, pp. 223–228, Academic Press, New York.
Rose, B., and Radermecker, M., 1971, in: *Immunological Diseases* (M. Samter, ed.), pp. 859–877, Little, Brown and Co., Boston.
Roufogalis, B. D., 1975, *J. Neurochem.* **24**:51–62.
Rubin, B., O'Keefe, E. H., Waugh, M. H., Kotler, D. G., DeMaio, D. A., and Horovitz, Z. P., 1971, *Proc. Soc. Exp. Biol. Med.* **137**:1244–1248.
Sandler, J. A., Clyman, R. I., Manganiello, V. C., and Vaughan, M., 1975, *J. Clin. Invest.* **55**:431–435.
Schramm, M., and Rodbell, M., 1975, *J. Biol. Chem.* **250**:2232–2237.
Schultz, G., Hardman, J. G., and Sutherland, E. W., 1973, in: *Asthma: Physiology, Immunopharmacology and Treatment* (K. F. Austen and L. M. Lichtenstein, eds.), pp. 123–138, Academic Press, New York.
Schultz, G., Schultz, K., and Hardman, J. G., 1975, *Metabolism* **24**:429–437.
Schultz, J., 1975, *J. Neurochem.* **24**:495–502.
Schwabe, U., and Ebert, R., 1972, *Naunyn-Schmiedebergs Arch. Pharmacol.* **274**:287–298.
Schwartz, H. J., Lowell, F. C., and Melby, J. C., 1968, *Ann. Intern. Med.* **69**:493–499.
Sheppard, H., 1973, in: *Asthma: Physiology, Immunopharmacology and Treatment* (K. F. Austen and L. M. Lichtenstein, eds.), pp. 235–248, Academic Press, New York.
Simonsson, B. G., Svedmyr, N., Skoogh, B. E., Anderson, R., and Bergh, N. B., 1972, *Scand. J. Respir. Dis.* **53**:227–236.

Simonsson, B. G., Jonson, B., and Ström, B., 1975, *Scand. J. Respir. Dis.* **56**:138–149.
Smith, A. P., 1973, in: *Asthma: Physiology, Immunopharmacology and Treatment* (K. F. Austen and L. M. Lichtenstein, eds.), pp. 267–275, Academic Press, New York.
Smith, R. J., and Ignarro, L. J., 1975, *Proc. Natl. Acad. Sci. U.S.A.* **72**:108–112.
Smith, R. S., Sherman, N. A., and Middleton, E., Jr., 1973, *J. Allergy Clin. Immunol.* **51**:328–334.
Solinger, A., Bernstein, L., and Glueck, H. I., 1973, *J. Allergy Clin. Immunol.* **51**:29–34.
Sokol, W. N., and Beall, G. N., 1975, *J. Allergy Clin. Immunol.* **55**:310–324.
Steer, M. L., and Levitzki, A., 1975, *J. Biol. Chem.* **250**:2080–2084.
Stoner, J., Manganiello, V. C., and Vaughan, M., 1974, *Mol. Pharmacol.* **10**:155–161.
Strom, T. B., Carpenter, C. B., Garovoy, M. R., Austen, K. F., Merrill, J. P., and Kaliner, M., 1973, *J. Exp. Med.* **138**:381–393.
Sutherland, E. W., and Rall, T. W., 1960, *Pharmacol. Rev.* **12**:265–299.
Suyemitsu, T., and Terayama, H., 1975, *Endocrinology* **96**:1499–1508.
Svedmyr, N., Larsson, S., and Thiringer, G., 1976, *Chest* **69**:479–483.
Sweatman, W. J. F., and Collier, H. O. J., 1968, *Nature (London)* **217**:69.
Szentivanyi, A., 1968, *J. Allergy* **42**:203–232.
Tauber, A. I., Kaliner, M., Stechschulte, D. J., and Austen, K. F., 1973, *J. Allergy Clin. Immunol.* **51**:106.
Taylor, W. A., and Sheldon, D., 1974, *Int. Arch. Allergy* **47**:696–707.
Thompson, W. J., Johnson, D. G., Lavis, V. R., and Williams, R. H., 1974, *Endocrinology* **94**:276–278.
Toft, D., Chytil, F., 1973, *Arch. Biochem. Biophys.* **157**:464–469.
Townley, R. G., Daley, D., and Selenke, W., 1970, *J. Allergy* **45**:71–86.
van As, A., 1975, in: *New Directions in Asthma* (M. Stein, ed.), pp. 415–432, American College of Chest Physicians, Park Ridge, Illinois.
Vane, J. R., 1971, *Nature (London) New Biol.* **231**:232–235.
Van Inwegen, R. G., Robison, G. A., Thompson, W. J., Armstrong, K. J., and Stouffer, J. E., 1975, *J. Biol. Chem.* **250**:2452–2456.
Vaughan, J. H., Tan, E. M., Mathison, D. A., Stevenson, D. D., Berman, S. Z., and Braude, A. I., 1973, in: *Asthma: Physiology, Immunopharmacology and Treatment* (K. F. Austen and L. M. Lichtenstein, eds.), pp. 1–10, Academic Press, New York.
Weinberger, M. M., and Riegelman, S., 1974, *N. Engl. J. Med.* **291**:151–153.
Weissman, G., 1973, in: *Asthma: Physiology, Immunopharmacology and Treatment* (K. F. Austen and L. M., Lichtenstein, eds.), pp. 221–230, Academic Press, New York.
Whittam, R., and Wheeler, K. P., 1970, *Annu. Rev. Physiol.* **32**:21–60.
Wicks, W. D., Barnett, C. A., and McKibbin, J. B., 1974, *Fed. Proc. Fed. Am. Soc. Exp. Biol.* **33**:1105–1111.
Wisniewski, B. J., Parkes, J. G., Huang, Y. O., and Fox, C. F., 1974, *Proc. Natl. Acad. Sci. U.S.A.* **71**:4381–4385.
Zinman, B., and Hollenberg, C. H., 1974, *J. Biol. Chem.* **249**:2182–2187.

12

Modulation of the Expression of the Immune Response by Antiinflammatory Drugs

ROBERT J. PERPER and PHILIP DAVIES

1. Introduction

The cellular and humoral processes that mediate diseases manifested by acute and chronic inflammation are complex and as yet incompletely understood. The mediation of tissue damage, destruction, and repair probably involves a series of consecutive events involving both cells and humoral mediators. Some of these pathways are depicted schematically in Figure 1. In view of the complexity of the inflammatory process in its various forms, it is not surprising that the mode of action of antiinflammatory agents is poorly understood, especially since in most instances available drugs provide palliation in clinical diseases, rather than prevention or reversal of disease progression.

The initiation of immune responses involves at least three major cell types, namely, T and B lymphocytes and macrophages, while expression of the response involves several others, including neutrophils, platelets, eosinophils, and basophils. In addition, the inflammatory sequelae secondary to the expression of cellular immunity, or the interaction of antibody with specific antigen, or both, can activate many humoral systems to generate mediators that cause acute inflammation. These include the complement, clotting, and kinin systems, as well as soluble mediators released from mast cells, basophils, eosinophils, and platelets. It is therefore apparent that the elucidation of the mechanisms by which steroidal and nonsteroidal antiinflammatory drugs modulate the initiation and the expression of the immune response is a formidable undertaking. Because of the complexity of the problem, a

ROBERT J. PERPER and PHILIP DAVIES • Merck Institute for Therapeutic Research, Rahway, New Jersey 07065.

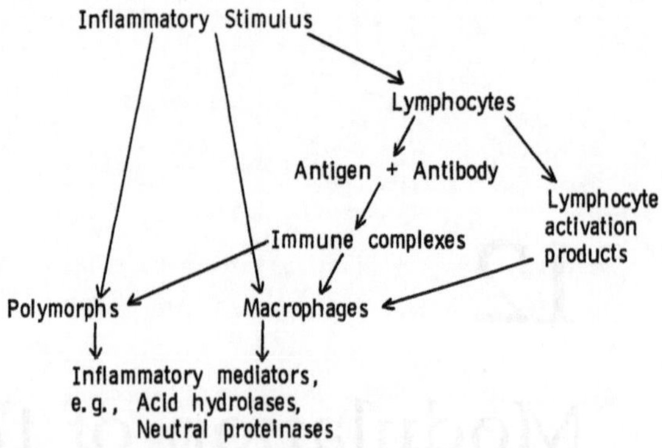

Figure 1. Schematic representation of the release of inflammatory mediators from polymorphs and macrophages by immunologic and nonimmunologic stimuli.

clear understanding of how these drugs affect the overall response is not possible at present. Information is available on the influence of antiinflammatory drugs on individual components of the reaction, and these drugs will be reviewed. We will not attempt to survey all the published literature on the subject, but will restrict ourselves to some of those cellular and humoral events that appear relevant to the initiation of immune response and its expression as immune-based inflammatory processes.

The term *antiinflammatory drugs* is a nonspecific one that encompasses a vast array of pharmacologically active agents. These agents include specific antagonists of mediators, which are exemplified by the antihistamines; immunosuppressive agents that act on cells participating in the inflammatory response, such as macrophages and lymphocytes; glucocorticosteroids, which have multiple actions; antirheumatic agents such as gold salts, penicillamine, and chloroquine, which show activity only after a considerable period of therapy; and finally, the nonsteroidal antiinflammatory drugs, which are exemplified by indomethacin, phenylbutazone, and aspirin. In this review, we will not consider antagonists of specific mediators of inflammation, which are covered elsewhere in this volume, but will limit ourselves to the other agents that have been shown to modulate one stage or another of the immune response, emphasizing those studies in which the drug effect can be related to effects on the overall immune response indicated by modification of immune-based inflammatory processes. It is our opinion that agents characterized in this way offer the best possibility of controlling immune-based inflammatory processes without compromising other immunologically based host defense processes in an unacceptable way.

2. Effect of Antiinflammatory Agents on Lymphocytes and the Immune Response

2.1. Corticosteroids

Glucocorticoids are transported to their target cells by a specific plasma α-globulin named *transcortin* [corticosteroid-binding globulin (CBG)] (Sandberg and Slaunwhite, 1963). Steroids bind to a cytoplasmic receptor protein, undergo modification, and enter the cell nucleus, thus gaining access to DNA. The sequela of this interaction is an altered rate of ribosomal and tRNA synthesis as well as an alteration in the rate of mRNA synthesis. The net result is an altered rate of the synthesis of specific proteins either stimulatory to RNA synthesis in some tissues, i.e., liver, or suppressive in others (lymphoid tissues). For reviews, see Kornel (1973) and E. B. Thompson and Lippman (1974).

Since the discovery (Ingle, 1938; White, 1948) that cortisol causes a loss of mass in all lymphatic tissue and a lymphopenia, the biochemical basis for this effect has been extensively investigated, but remains unclear. Biochemical changes include the inhibition of the synthesis of nucleic acids and proteins, the inhibition of transport of hexoses, and the incorporation of orthophosphate into ATP of thymocytes (which are effects that require RNA and protein synthesis according to Makman *et al.*, 1970). Also, there occurs an inhibitory action on amino acid transport with an increased rate of release of amino acids (Makman *et al.*, 1970). The marked inhibitory effect of cortisol on thymocyte metabolic activity contrasts with its stimulatory effect in some other cell types. This paradox might be a function of the measurements made; however, it has been shown that cortisol can induce the synthesis of a protein inhibitor of transport and phosphorylation processes in rat thymocytes (Makman *et al.*, 1971). Thus, the main action of cortisol might be to stimulate the production of an inhibitor, rather than to inhibit metabolic processes directly.

The lymphoid tissues of all species are not equally susceptible to the action of corticosteroids. The rat, mouse, and rabbit are relatively sensitive, whereas man, the monkey, and the guinea pig are resistant (Claman, 1972). When corticosteroids are administered systemically, the lymphoid tissues most sensitive are the cortical zone of the thymus, the periarticular sheaths of the spleen, and the paracortical area of the lymph nodes (Dukor *et al.*, 1968; Raff and Owen, 1971). The precursors of antibody-forming cells in mouse bone marrow are resistant to high doses of cortisone *in vivo*, as evidenced by their ability to cooperate with thymus cells after adoptive transfer to irradiated recipients (Levine and Claman, 1970). The small population of thymocytes that remains after steroid treatment produces a greater graft-vs.-host (GVH) reaction than do untreated thymus or spleen cells (Blomgren and Anderson, 1969; Cohen *et al.*, 1970), and bone marrow cells from similarly treated animals also have an enhanced ability to mount GVH reactions. The changes in GVH reactivity are paralleled by increases in phytohemagglutinin (PHA) responsiveness (both are T-cell functions), and have been shown to result from PHA-responsive cells entering the bone marrow from the periphery, in particular from the spleen (Moorhead and Claman, 1972). Thus, after steroid administration, there is a shift in populations of lymphoid cells from one lymphoid organ to another. Aside from species, organ, and interorgan sensitivity of various lymphocytes to steroids, there are recent reports indicating that certain subclasses, i.e., suppressor T lymphocytes, are differentially susceptible to steroid effects (Ha *et al.*, 1974); however, the final analysis of this subclass susceptibility to steroids remains incomplete.

The selectivity of corticosteroids for the various lymphoid tissues mentioned above makes it extremely difficult to analyze the effect of these agents in an intact immune response. The issue becomes even more complicated because of the profound inhibitory effect that corticosteroids have on macrophage function (Weston *et al.*, 1972; J. Thompson and Van Furth, 1973). Thus, the effect of corticosteroids on the immune response is one in which multiple loci can be affected. *In vitro* immune response to antigen (Seeger and Oppenheim, 1970; Nelson and Leu, 1975; Lipsky *et al.*, 1976) as well as mitogen responses are dependent on macrophage participation as well as T and B lymphocytes. Steroids inhibit reproducibly both the primary immune response and mitogen responses. Some reports implicate the B cell as a target for steroids (Cohen and Claman, 1971), whereas others attribute the inhibitory effect on the primary *in vitro* response of spleen cells, or those obtained from treated animals, to the T-cell population (Segal *et al.*, 1972; Vann, 1974). Finally, it was shown that the inhibitory effect of corticosteroids on the *in vitro* response of human lymphocytes to various mitogens is at the level of the macrophage (Blomgren, 1974). Other results indicate, however, that with certain mitogens, such as pokeweed, no effect is seen after corticosteroid therapy (Heilman, 1972, 1973). Such conflicting results are not unexpected, since three factors must be considered: differential susceptibility to the steroids of the several cell types involved in the immune response, source of cells as regards different localization patterns after steroid administration, and specificity of steroids for subclasses of lymphocytes with immunoregulatory potential.

In vivo, corticosteroids have a profound effect on both primary and secondary humoral antibody formation in steroid-sensitive species. The primary response is more sensitive than is the secondary response, and treatment before antigen is more effective than treatment started after the induction of the response (Makinodan *et al.*, 1970; Berglund, 1956; Dukor and Dietrich, 1968). In steroid-resistant species, such as man, steroids have little (Butler and Rossen, 1973) if any (Tuchinda *et al.*, 1972) effect on the humoral immune response.

Corticosteroids have a marked inhibitory effect on the expression of cell-mediated immunity. Since corticosteroids have potential activity in multiple pathways connected with the generalized inflammatory reaction, it has been difficult to determine whether the agent has a fundamental effect on cell-mediated immunity at the level of antigen recognition. Cell-mediated immunity to defined antigens, in transplantation or in autoimmune diseases, is expressed by inflammatory reactions, which consist of a characteristic mononuclear cell infiltration composed of lymphocytes and macrophages. Since steroids are lympholytic and cause a monocytopenia and a lymphopenia, as well as inhibiting lymphocyte proliferation, it is understandable that the expression of delayed hypersensitivity would be inhibited by this class of drugs. The events by which these cell types accumulate at the site of inflammation are dependent on chemotaxis, production of soluble mediators from lymphocytes (lymphokines) that expand the inflammatory reaction, and finally cell division. Corticosteroids prevent emigration of monocytes through vascular endothelium (J. Thompson and Van Furth, 1970; Perper *et al.*, 1974). An earlier report that lymphocytes are responsive to chemotactic factors (Ward *et al.*, 1971) was not confirmed by others (Keller and Sorkin, 1967; Perper *et al.*, 1975). Thus, a direct effect on lymphocyte emigration from the blood to the site of a delayed hypersensitivity reaction cannot be assumed at this time. It should be noted, however, that lymphopenia induced by steroid treatment would be expected to reduce the number of lymphocytes entering the lesion, since the number of cells emigrating is related to the number of circulating cells (Perper *et al.*, 1974). Steroids, however, do have an effect on the expression of the cellular reactions, since they have been reported to inhibit the effect of two lymphokines, cytotoxic and macrophage migration inhibitory factor (MIF), on their respective target cells (Weston *et al.*, 1973; Balow and Rosenthal, 1973; Peter, 1971), even though they do not prevent the synthesis or release of these lymphokines. Finally, steroids interfere with lymphocyte proliferation, as noted above. A combination of these three factors (recruitment, expansion, and proliferation) would result in a reduction of lymphocyte and macrophage accumulation at the site of a delayed hypersensitivity reaction. Treatment of man and animals with steroids results in inhibition of the expression of delayed hypersensitivity reactions, allograft rejection, and many autoimmune diseases.

In summary, the effect of corticosteroids on the lymphocyte in both humoral and cellular immune responses results from an indirect rather than a direct effect on the immune response. In the case of humoral antibody production, lymphocyte redistribution and a direct effect on lymphocyte metabolism result in a functional depletion of the pool of potentially available antibody-secreting cells. A similar effect occurs during the expression of cellular immunity, and in addition, the target organs of lymphocyte activation are somehow protected. Finally, the effect of steroids on lymphocytes is dependent on species, organ, and subclass of lymphocyte.

2.2. Nonsteroid Antiinflammatory Drugs

The prototypes for this class of agents are indomethacin, phenylbutazone, and aspirin. There are between 10 and 20 new agents with similar biological profiles (inhibition of PG synthetase activity), they are covered in detail in other chapters, and therefore will not be discussed in this review. The effect of such agents on immune responses has not been studied in great detail, undoubtedly because of the marginal effects on the intact immune response, both *in vivo* and *in vitro*.

There have been a number of papers concerning the effect of these various drugs on mitogen-induced lymphocyte transformation *in vitro*. Forbes and Smith (1967) first reported that pharmacological concentrations of phenylbutazone, oxyphenbutazone, mefenamic acid, salicylate, indomethacin, and chloroquine all inhibit protein synthesis of resting human peripheral blood, lymph node, or thymus lymphocytes. Pachman *et al.* (1971) confirmed and extended the aspirin studies, and found that DNA, RNA, and protein synthesis in resting lymphocytes or those stimulated with PHA or antigen were reversibly inhibited. In addition, they noted an uncoupling of oxidative phosphorylation, as evidenced by increased glucose consumption, lactic acid production, and enhanced oxygen consumption. There are conflicting reports relative to the blastogenic response of patients receiving aspirin *in vivo*. Smith *et al.* (1975) found no effect of aspirin treatment on the response of patients' lymphocytes to PHA or allogeneic lymphocytes using 60 mg 5 times daily for 14 days. Measurements were made 10 days after the last dose. In contrast, Crout *et al.* (1975) found significant inhibition of lymphocyte responses to PHA and pokeweed mitogen in patients receiving 900 mg aspirin p.o. 5 times a day for 4 days. Lymphocytes showed maximum inhibition of response to mitogen 12 hr after the last dose, and the inhibition was not correlated with the plasma levels of salicylate. No change in the proportion of T or B cells was noted.

The significance of inhibition of lymphocyte transformation by nonsteroid antiinflammatory drugs is obscure, since no marked effect on the expression of cellular immunity has been observed *in vivo*. There is one report in which prolongation of guinea pig skin allograft rejection occurred following treatment with indomethacin given at an extraordinarily high dose of 50 mg/kg (Coppola *et al.*, 1967). The relevance of this finding remains unclear.

Even though the nonsteroidal antiinflammatory drugs have not been reported to inhibit classic delayed hypersensitivity reactions or humoral antibody formation, they do have substantial therapeutic and prophylactic effects in immunologically induced inflammatory diseases in animals, such as experimental allergic encephalomyelitis in guinea pigs (Rosenthale and Nagra, 1967) and adjuvant-induced polyarthritis in rats (Winder *et al.*, 1969; Walz *et al.*, 1971). In these latter cases, the effect is undoubtedly on the inflammatory response and not due to any central influence on immune reactivity, since by appropriate timing schedules, these two reactions can be analyzed separately (Perper *et al.*, 1971). Thus, the nonsteroidal antiinflammatory agents do not seem to have any central effect on the immune system *in vivo*, even though they do inhibit lymphocyte transformation *in vitro*.

2.3. Miscellaneous Antiinflammatory Agents

We will not attempt to review all the literature concerning various new agents that have been reported to modify the immune response in one way or another, since it is difficult to determine which of these agents can be classified as antiinflammatory in the classic sense of suppressing rubor, tumor, calor, and dolor. Several agents have been reported to be active in rheumatoid arthritis in man in alleviating the inflammatory component of the disease, so that mention should be made of some of these agents, since they do have antiinflammatory activity *in vivo*.

Penicillamine was first described to have antiarthritic activity in 1963 (Jaffe, 1963). This observation was confirmed by several other investigators, culminating in a multicenter trial in England (Multicenter Trial Group, 1973) in which the beneficial effect of this agent in rheumatoid arthritis was established. Although the agent is proved effective in man, it is inactive in models of chronic inflammation in animals (Liyanage and Currey, 1972), and its mechanism of action remains unknown. It does, however, influence several aspects of the immune response in treated patients. Patients with rheumatoid arthritis have present in their circulation immune complexes composed of IgM and IgG antibodies (rheumatoid factor) directed against their own immunoglobulins (Winchester, 1975). After several months' treatment with penicillamine, there occurs a fall in the amount of circulating immune complexes, as measured by ultracentrifugal analysis, precipitation with monoclonal IgM rheumatoid factor, or latex fixation (Jaffe, 1975; Zucker *et al.*, 1970). There is also a lowering of the serum IgG and IgM but not IgA levels (Bluestone and Goldberg, 1973). There is no effect on PHA-induced lymphocyte transformation (Zucker *et al.*, 1970). With the exception of a single report (Schumacher *et al.*, 1975), there is no experimental model in which penicillamine has been shown to effect immunoglobulin levels, circulating immune complexes, or lymphocyte functions. The mechanisms by which circulating complexes and immunoglobulin levels are reduced are unknown. *In vitro,* the drug reduces disulfide bonds of macroglobulins; however, very high concentrations of drug are required. It is therefore unlikely that it is this effect that results in the lowering of immunoglobulin levels *in vivo*. From the clinical observations, the drug apparently has a central effect on only a selected subpopulation of lymphocytes that are capable of producing certain immunoglobulin heavy chains, since it does not affect IgA levels. Penicillamine influences various parameters, including serum copper levels (Jaffe, 1965), sulfhydryl levels (Lorber *et al.*, 1964), pyridoxine metabolism (Jaffe *et al.*, 1964), and collagen cross-linking (Nimni and Bavetta, 1965); however, none of these effects can be directly related to its antiarthritic effects in patients. Thus, the agent affects the immune response in an as yet undetermined manner that results in antiinflammatory activity in human beings *in vivo*.

Levamisole [1,2,3,5,6-tetrahydro-6-phenylimidazo(2,1-β)-thiazol, monohydrochloride], an effective anthelmintic, is currently being tested in man for antiarthritic activity with as yet undetermined efficacy. In one open study in patients with rheumatoid arthritis, it was found that levamisole was as active as D-penicillamine in reducing rheumatoid factor levels and alleviating symptoms (Huskisson *et al.*, 1976). This result is similar to that of another trial (Schuermans, 1975), but was not confirmed in a recently reported double-blind trial (Diani and Pras, 1975). The effect of this agent on lymphocytes is somewhat controversial. The overall impression is that by using appropriate, somewhat specialized protocols, immunoenhancement can be observed. Enhancement of *in vitro* transformation was observed in several laboratories (Hokama *et al.*, 1974; Lichtenfeld *et al.*, 1974; Pabst and Crawford, 1974; Hadden *et al.*, 1975; Sampson and Lui, 1976). Treatment with this agent *in vivo* results in enhanced delayed hypersensitivity reaction (Tripodi *et al.*, 1973) and humoral immune responses (Renoux and Renoux, 1973). Thus, although this agent has effects *in vivo* and *in vitro* on immune responsiveness, we will have to await more double-blind clinical trials to determine whether it has antiarthritic activity either in experimental animals or in man (see Chapter 14 for further discussion).

Sheep lymphocytes exposed to gold as sodium aurothiomalate develop abnormal multivesicular bodies (Cahill, 1971a) and show a diminished blastogenic response to PHA (Cahill, 1971b). Gold has a similar effect on blastogenesis induced by streptolysin S (Fikrig and Smithwick, 1965). The effects of gold on immune parameters in rheumatoid arthritis were surveyed (Freyberg *et al.*, 1972), but no insight into its mechanism of action is available at present.

3. Neutrophils

Human and animal neutrophils secrete both acid hydrolases (Weissman *et al.*, 1975) and neutral proteinases (Oronsky *et al.*, 1973a) after exposure to certain kinds of antigen–antibody complexes. The cells remain viable during the release of these enzyme systems. Corticosteroids and certain nonsteroidal antiinflammatory drugs were shown to inhibit the release of neutral proteinases (Perper and Oronsky, 1974). Cyclic nucleotides were shown to modulate the secretion of acid hydrolases in a positive or negative way (Weissman *et al.*, 1975) (see Chapter 4). The neutral proteinases are capable of causing the degradation of connective tissue components (Oronsky *et al.*, 1973b), as well as activating both the complement (I. M. Goldstein and Weissman, 1974) and kinin systems (Movat *et al.*, 1972). These data indicate that under certain conditions *in vitro*, some antiinflammatory agents can inhibit the inflammatory as well as the destructive events secondary to immunologic reactions. Whether these agents are active in these systems under *in vivo* conditions is not known; however, the *in vitro* observations should serve as a basis for the future design of specific agents that interfere with the expression of certain types of immunologically induced inflammatory reactions.

4. Macrophages

Macrophages are distributed widely throughout the body and assume a variety of morphological guises dependent on their stage of maturation and tissue of localization. These various forms were collectively designated the *mononuclear phagocyte system* by Van Furth *et al.* (1972), and readers are referred to this article for further morphological and functional definition of this cell type.

Mononuclear phagocytes are derived from bone marrow (Volkman and Gowans, 1965; Virolainen, 1968; Van Furth and Cohn, 1968), where they differentiate from a primitive precursor stem cell (Metcalf and Moore, 1971). The most immature recognizable form of bone marrow mononuclear phagocyte is the monoblast (Goud *et al.*, 1975), which matures into the promonocyte and finally into the monocyte; monocytes then form a nondividing pool of cells that are recruited into the circulation and finally into various tissues, where they differentiate further into macrophages. Macrophages are thought to play an important role in both the afferent and efferent limbs of immune responses. The role of macrophages in the presentation of antigen to immunocompetent cells has been widely documented (Unanue, 1972), although the mechanisms of this presentation remain unclear. The macrophage is also a target for the products of stimulated lymphocytes, responding in a variety of ways. These responses include the production or release or both of several types of mediators of the inflammatory response (Table 1). It is clear from Table 1 that the macrophage is a source of several classes of inflammatory mediators. At present, it is not clear whether the secretion of all these classes is modulated by products of stimulated lymphocytes. This is an important area of further investigation, as is the effect of various drugs on these secretory processes.

4.1. Effects of Drugs on Promonocytes and Monocytes in the Bone Marrow

Van Furth and his colleagues showed that the proliferation of promonocytes and monocytes in bone marrow of mice is extremely susceptible to certain drugs (J. Thompson and Van Furth, 1970, 1973). A single subcutaneous injection of 25 μg dexamethasone into mice caused a rapid decrease in the number of peripheral blood monocytes. Maximum depression was observed after 6 hr, with a return to normal within 12 hr and a significant increase above normal values by 24 hr after injection of dexamethasone. Repeated injections of dexamethasone prolonged the monocytopenia. A much more prolonged depression of peripheral blood monocyte counts was observed after a single injection of 15 mg hydrocortisone given in the form of a subcutaneous depot. Monocyte levels were profoundly depressed for at least 7 days, with a slow increase toward normal being seen in the subsequent 7 days, but during this period many animals succumbed in a cachectic state.

In marked contrast to its effects on peripheral blood monocyte levels, hydrocortisone reduces the number of peritoneal macrophages (monocytes that have emigrated from peripheral blood and differentiated) by a maximum of only 30% during a 1-week period. When dividing monocyte precursors in bone marrow were

TABLE 1. Secretion of Inflammatory Mediators by Macrophages

Mediator	Stimulus	Source	References
Neutral proteinases			
Plasminogen activator	None Endotoxin Phagocytizable particle	Murine peritoneal cells induced by thioglycollate broth	Unkeless *et al.* (1974), Gordon *et al.* (1974)
Collagenase	None Phagocytizable particle Endotoxin	Murine peritoneal cells induced by thioglycollate broth	Werb and Gordon (1975a), Wahl *et al* (1974)
	Lymphocyte activation products	Oil-induced guinea pig peritoneal cells	Wahl *et al.* (1975)
Elastase	None Phagocytizable particles	Murine peritoneal cells induced by thioglycollate broth	Werb and Gordon (1975b)
Acid hydrolases	Lymphocyte activation products	Unstimulated murine peritoneal cells	Pantalone and Page (1975)
	Antigen–antibody complexes	Unstimulated murine peritoneal cells	Cardella *et al.* (1974)
	Nonimmunogenic inflammatory materials	Murine peritoneal cells	P. Davies and Allison (1976)
Prostaglandins	Lymphocyte activation products	Guinea pig peritoneal cells	Bray *et al.* (1974)
	None	Rheumatoid synovium	Dayer *et al.* (1976)
Complement components			
C3, C4	None	Human peritoneal cells	Stecher *et al.* (1967)
C2, C3, C4	None		
C3, Factor B	None	Human monocytes	Einstein *et al.* (1976)
		Murine peritoneal cells	Hadding *et al.* (1976)
Pyrogen	Endotoxin	Human peripheral blood monocytes	Bodell (1974)
	Phagocytosis	Human peripheral blood monocytes	Dinarello *et al.* (1974)
Factors that influence lymphocyte proliferation	Various	Various	Waksman and Namba (1976), Wood *et al.* (1976)

labeled with tritiated thymidine, the highest percentage of labeled mononuclear phagocytes in the peritoneal cavity was observed to be 15% 60 hr later. This result is consonant with the observation of Van Furth and Cohn (1968) that peritoneal macrophages have a turnover period of 40 days. In hydrocortisone-treated mice, the maximum percentage of thymidine-labeled macrophages did not exceed 5% at any time. When mice were injected intraperitoneally with fetal calf serum to provoke a sterile inflammatory response, there was an increase in both peripheral blood and peritoneal cavity mononuclear phagocyte count, with a maximum being seen after

72 hr. This increase was effectively prevented by hydrocortisone administered before or after the inflammatory stimulus. A marked increase in the number of thymidine-labeled peritoneal mononuclear phagocytes was observed in animals injected intraperitoneally with fetal calf serum, reaching close to 70% 72 hr after injection of calf serum. Treatment of animals with intraperitoneal sterile inflammation with hydrocortisone caused a marked diminution in both the number and percentage of thymidine-labeled mononuclear phagocytes.

These observations have been interpreted to indicate an inhibitory effect of steroids on the transit of monocytes from peripheral blood into the peritoneal cavity. The rate of disappearance of monocytes from peripheral blood exceeds that to be expected due to their normal transit time through peripheral blood, and J. Thompson and Van Furth (1970) postulate that they are sequestered in an extravascular pool of unknown location.

In a subsequent study, J. Thompson and Van Furth (1973) demonstrated a direct effect of steroids on the number of promonocytes and monocytes in bone marrow in mice. Hydrocortisone caused a slight decrease in the number of bone marrow monocytes and promonocytes. There was little effect of thymidine incorporation by promonocytes, with some inhibition of monocyte release from bone marrow, but not of sufficient extent to account for steroid-induced monocytopenia in peripheral blood.

Both 6-mercaptopurine and its derivative azathioprine possess antiinflammatory activity, and they have been shown to reduce cellular infiltration at sites of inflammation (A. R. Page *et al.*, 1962; Hurd and Ziff, 1968; Arinoviche and Loewi, 1970; Phillips and Zweiman, 1973).

In mice, 200 mg azathioprine/kg causes a gradual decrease in the number of peripheral blood leukocytes, with monocytes falling to 10% of their initial level after 4 days (Gassmann and Van Furth, 1975). A lower dose of azathioprine, 3 mg/kg, equivalent to a nontoxic, antiinflammatory dose in man, causes a fall of peripheral blood monocyte counts to 50% of normal. Prolonged administration of azathioprine at a dose of 200 mg/kg was required to cause a decrease in the number of peritoneal macrophages. Azathioprine caused a marked fall in the number of peritoneal macrophages and peripheral blood monocytes in mice in which an inflammatory response was provoked by an intraperitoneal injection of fetal calf serum. Labeling of macrophage precursors with tritiated thymidine showed that azathioprine was effective in preventing the recruitment of labeled macrophages into sites of sterile inflammation, as described here.

Taking into consideration the known time that monocytes spend in the bloodstream (Van Furth, 1970), azathioprine prevents the release of any new monocytes from bone marrow. It is not clear how this information relates to azathioprine-induced changes in mononuclear phagocyte kinetics in man, since Gassmann and Van Furth (1975) point out that humans are much more sensitive to the effects of this immunosuppressant.

Van Furth *et al.* (1975) studied the effect of azathioprine on the mitotic activity of mouse promonocytes both *in vivo* and *in vitro*. High doses of azathioprine gave a 70% decrease in the number of bone marrow monocytes within 96 hr. When bone marrow cells from azathioprine-treated mice were exposed to [^{3}H]thymidine for a short time *in vitro*, an unexpected increase in the number of labeled promonocytes from a control value of approximately 50% to over 90% was observed. Since azathioprine did not lower the number of bone marrow promonocytes and the total number of promonocytes synthesizing DNA was not reduced, the data suggest an effect on the cell cycle of these cells. Determination of DNA synthesis and cell cycle times showed that the former was significantly prolonged and the latter was increased by approximately 6 hr. Cytophotometric determination of the DNA content of nuclei showed significant increases in cells from azathioprine-treated animals, suggesting that cells do not proceed through the G_2 phase of the cell cycle to mitosis.

4.2. Effects of Glucocorticoids on the Response of Mononuclear Phagocytes to Lymphocyte Activation Products

Since corticosteroids have been shown to inhibit delayed hypersensitivity responses in certain situations (Claman, 1972), *in vitro* studies demonstrating that corticosteroids reverse the inhibition of macrophage migration caused by soluble mediators from lymphocytes stimulated with specific antigen may represent a mechanism of the *in vivo* effect. Lockshin (1972) showed that dexamethasone given *in vivo* to guinea pigs did not influence the subsequent capacity of lymphocytes from these animals to produce migration inhibitory factor. However, addition of dexamethasone to macrophages responding to supernatants of stimulated lymphocytes *in vitro* resulted in complete suppression of the response. These experiments did not distinguish between an effect on the MIF or on the responding cells, but a subsequent investigation by Balow and Rosenthal (1973) showed that steroids inhibited the interaction of the lymphocyte products with responding macrophages. Activity of steroids was detected whether assayed in a mixture of sensitized lymphocytes and macrophages or macrophages exposed to the supernatants of stimulated lymphocytes. Both hydrocortisone and dexamethasone reversed the inhibition of macrophage migration at pharmacological levels of 10 μg/ml. Other steroids such as deoxycorticosterone, estrogens, testosterone, and progesterone were found to be inactive. None of the steroids examined affected macrophage migration in the absence of products of stimulated lymphocytes. The activity of the steroids was found to depend on their dose and also that of stimulating antigen, being less effective in the presence of higher antigen concentrations. Steroids were found not to have any effect on the processing of antigen, nor did they suppress the production of MIF by sensitized lymphocytes. That they did not was shown by dialysis of supernatants from immune lymphocytes exposed to antigen in the presence of hydrocortisone. These supernatants displayed the same inhibitory activity as those from immune cells exposed to antigen in the absence of steroid. Readdition of steroid to dialyzed supernatants depleted their inhibitory capacity to their previous levels. Weston *et al.* (1973) showed that a macrophage-aggregating factor or factors released from sensitized guinea pig lymphocytes exposed to specific antigen (purified protein derivative) was rendered inactive in the presence of hydrocortisone. Once again, it was shown that the steroid interfered with the interaction of the lymphocyte product with macrophages, rather than with its production by lymphocytes.

A further example of steroid-induced inhibition of the interaction of lymphocyte activation products with macrophages was provided by Dimitriu (1976). A so-called "macrophage arming factor" is produced by a mixed lymphocyte reaction between cells from a skin graft recipient and the donor's splenocytes. This factor confers on macrophages cytotoxic activity against tumor cells maintained in culture. Macrophages obtained from steroid-treated mice or from mice treated with 0.001–0.1 μg hydrocortisone or methylprednisolone/ml *in vitro* were not able to interact with the lymphocyte product to render themselves "armed" against the tumor cell line. Corticosteroids did not influence the production of the "arming" factor by lymphocytes from steroid-treated animals or when added to lymphocytes *in vitro*.

4.3. Direct Effects of Corticosteroids on Macrophages

In vitro studies have shown that corticosteroids influence various functions of monocytes and macrophages. Wiener and Marmary (1969) showed that hydrocortisone at concentrations ranging from 1×10^{-7} to 1×10^{-4} M caused decreases in cellular levels of acid phosphatase and acid proteinase in mouse peritoneal macrophages. Cells treated with 1×10^{-4} M hydrocortisone were smaller and displayed fewer cytoplasmic processes, but there was no change in their pinocytic activity as determined by uptake of radioactive inulin. Hydrocortisone did not influence the digestion of heat-aggregated human serum albumin or *Salmonella typhimurium* (Weiner *et al.*, 1972). Phagocytosis of these two stimuli was inhibited by hydrocortisone, but only at extremely high concentrations of 1×10^{-4} M.

Rinehart *et al.* (1974) examined the effect of hydrocortisone on several aspects of human peripheral blood monocyte functions. Both random movement and chemotaxis of monocytes in response to *Escherichia coli* culture filtrate were found to be inhibited by hydrocortisone at doses 16 μg/ml(10^{-7} M) or greater. Similar doses of steroids also impaired the killing of *Staphylococcus aureus*. However, no marked effects were seen on the phagocytosis of *Cryptococcus neoformans* or the binding of IgG coating erythrocytes nor was there any stimulation of the hexose monophosphate shunt in phagocytizing cells.

Schreiber *et al.* (1975) showed that extremely high concentrations of corticosteriods (10^{-4}–10^{-3} M hydrocortisone) dispersed in cholesterol–phospholipid sonicates inhibit the complement and IgG receptor activity in a dose-dependent and a rapid time-dependent manner (maximum effects were seen within 15 min of adding the corticosteroid dispersion). The cells were able to exclude trypan blue and ingest latex, indicating their viability over a short period of time. It would be useful, however, to confirm the lack of toxicity of the steroids by examining parameters of viability some time (say 24 hr) after the removal of the steroids to exclude toxic effects that are either delayed or are of such a subtle nature that they are not immediately detectable by the trypan blue dye exclusion test or latex ingestion assay.

Van Zwet *et al.* (1975) concluded that hydrocortisone causes only slight decreases in the capacity of murine peritoneal macrophages to phagocytize several types of bacteria *in vitro*. Peritoneal macrophages from hydrocortisone-treated mice showed normal phagocytic activity in response to these stimuli. Of several organisms tested, only the killing of *Salmonella typhimurium* was diminished when macrophages were obtained from hydrocortisone-treated mice. These findings are supported by the observations of Van Furth and Jones (1975) that glucocorticosteroids have no effect on the fusion of lysosomes with phagosomes containing dead microorganisms, nor do they influence the metabolic events accompanying phagocytosis by macrophages (McCall *et al.*, 1971; Wang *et al.*, 1972). It must be borne in mind that these studies were carried out with nonstimulated cells, and that since lymphocyte activation products increase macrophage bactericidal activity (Fowles *et al.*, 1973; Nathan *et al.*, 1973), glucocorticoids would diminish the bactericidal activity of these cells in view of their inhibitory effects on lymphocyte activation product–macrophage interaction.

4.4. Effects of Antiinflammatory Drugs on the Secretory Activity in Macrophages

It is now clear that macrophages secrete a variety of products, many of them relevant to inflammatory processes (P. Davies and Allison, 1976; Waksman and Namba, 1976). There are indications that the release of some of these products is susceptible to inhibition by antiinflammatory drugs.

It was recently shown that macrophages secrete neutral proteinases such as plasminogen activator, collagenase, and elastase under certain conditions (Unkeless *et al.*, 1974; Gordon *et al.*, 1974; Wahl *et al.*, 1974, 1975; Werb and Gordon, 1975a,b). Reich (1975) and his colleagues showed that the secretion of plasminogen activator by macrophages is sensitive to physiologic amounts of hydrocortisone and very small amounts of glucocorticoids such as dexamethasone. On the other hand, nonsteroidal antiinflammatory compounds, such as aspirin and indomethacin, do not have any effect on plasminogen activator secretion by macrophages. The effect of corticosteroids is dependent on inhibition of RNA synthesis.

There are reports indicating that antiinflammatory drugs can inhibit the release of acid hydrolases from mouse peritoneal macrophages. Ringrose *et al.* (1975) showed that corticosteroids such as dexamethasone, prednisolone, and hydrocortisone reduce the selective release of lysosomal enzymes from macrophages induced by zymosan particles. The effect is dose-dependent in a biphasic manner, with a maximum inhibitory effect being seen between 3×10^{-6} and 3×10^{-7} M. These workers also showed that pharmacological concentrations of indomethacin gave a slight inhibition of lysosomal enzyme release from immune peritoneal macrophages induced by zymosan.

Finlay *et al.* (1975) showed that indomethacin increases lysosomal enzyme levels in cultured mouse macrophages, and, as well, inhibits their release by inflammatory stimuli. Increases in the cellular levels of lysosomal enzymes were observed with doses of indomethacin as low as 5×10^{-8} M when the cells were exposed to the drug for 72 hr. Maximum effects were seen with doses of indomethacin between 1×10^{-6} and 1×10^{-5} M. In cultures exposed to high doses of indomethacin, above 5×10^{-4} M, toxic effects were seen, with decreases in cellular levels of acid hydrolases and detachment of macrophages. The effects of indomethacin appear to be dependent on an intact protein synthesis mechanism, since low doses of puromycin inhibited the increases in acid hydrolase levels induced by indomethacin.

Macrophages pretreated with 1×10^{-5} M indomethacin release significantly less acid hydrolases when exposed to the type C mucopolysaccharide–peptidoglycan component of the cell walls of Group A streptocci. This material is inflammatory, causing a chronic inflammatory lesion when injected intradermally (R. C. Page *et al.*, 1974) or at other sites (Schwab *et al.*, 1959), and induces the selective release of a major proportion of macrophage lysosomal enzymes (P. Davies *et al.*, 1974). Although it is clear that there is a close relationship between the capacity of substances to induce the selective release of acid hydrolases from macrophages and to cause chronic inflammation (P. Davies and Allison, 1976), further investigations with other inflammatory stimuli are required to determine whether the inhibition of acid hydrolase release from macrophages represents a site of action for indomethacin.

Both chloroquine and gold salts are characterized by a latent period before their clinical effectiveness in rheumatoid arthritis is manifested. A common feature of these two classes of compounds is their accumulation within lysosomes of various cells (P. Davies and Allison, 1972; De Duve *et al.*, 1974), which allows them to be classified as lysosomotropic compounds (De Duve *et al.*, 1974). Fedorko *et al.* (1968a,b) described the changes that occur in macrophages exposed to chloroquine (30 μg/ml). Within 1 hr, cells were seen to develop phase-lucent vacuoles that grew larger with time and gave a positive reaction for acid phosphatase. Electron microscopy showed these vacuoles to be autophagic. Subsequent studies showed chloroquine to be a potent inhibitor of protein degradation in a variety of cells (Wibo and Poole, 1974; J. L. Goldstein *et al.*, 1975), and this finding suggests a mechanism by which the drug induced autophagocytosis as a consequence of the derangement of intracellular protein catabolism.

The accumulation of gold within synovial lining cells during chrysotherapy of rheumatoid arthritis was shown by Lewis and Ziff (1968). The revelance of this accumulation to the usefulness of this type of therapy in rheumatoid arthritis (Hill, 1968) is not clear, especially in view of the finding that thiomalic acid, as well as gold thiomalate, accumulates at such sites (Norton *et al.*, 1968) during treatment of patients with rheumatoid arthritis. *In vitro* studies have shown that colloidal gold accumulates in lysosomes of cultured macrophages in a time- and temperature-dependent fashion. That it does was demonstrated both morphologically (Cohn and Fedorko, 1969; Wills *et al.*, 1972) and with the use of radioactive colloidal gold (P. Davies *et al.*, 1973a). Cells accumulating colloidal gold *in vitro* retain over 95% of the endocytosed material for at least 3 days (P. Davies *et al.*, 1973b). Gold is a potent inhibitor of certain hydrolytic enzymes at 0.01–5.0 mg/ml, concentrations that may well be attained with secondary lysosomes. Indeed, it was shown that rats pretreated with sodium aurothiomalate have a markedly decreased capacity to degrade intravenously administered ^{125}I-labeled albumin, which accumulates within secondary lysosomes in the liver (M. Davies *et al.*, 1971).

5. Conclusions

Studies on the effects of antiinflammatory drugs on the immune response have been centered on the expression of immunologic reactions, with particular emphasis directed at the level of the macrophage and the neutrophil. The interaction of immune complexes with macrophages and neutrophils and of lymphokines with the macrophage results in the secretion of mediators of tissue damage as well as the induction of acute inflammatory reactions, predominantly by conversion of zymogens into pharmacologically active mediators. Antiinflammatory drugs have been shown to have few well-defined effects on the early events of the immune response.

They have been shown, in certain instances, to inhibit the activity of mediators of its expression, either at the level of interaction of immune complexes and lymphokines with target cells or by inhibiting the formation or the activity of the mediators of the acute and chronic phases of inflammatory responses. The development of new agents that can modulate responses of lymphocytes and their accesory target cells that result in release of the mediators of immunologic reactivity offers a valid therapeutic goal, since it offers a means for inhibiting the pathologic sequelae of immune reactions without compromising host defense mechanisms in an unacceptable fashion.

References

Arinoviche, R., and Loewie, G., 1970, *Ann. Rheum. Dis.* **29**:32–39.
Balow, J. E., and Rosenthal, A. S., 1973, *J. Exp. Med.* **137**:1031–1041.
Berglund, K., 1956, *Acta. Pathol. Microbiol. Scand.* **38**:311–328.
Blomgren, H., 1974, *Scand. J. Immunol.* **3**:655–664.
Blomgren, H., and Anderson, B., 1969, *Exp. Cell Res.* **57**:185–192.
Bluestone, R., and Goldberg, L. S., 1973, *Ann. Rheum. Dis.* **32**:50–52.
Bodell, P., 1974, *J. Exp. Med.* **140**:954–965.
Bray, M. A., Gordon, D., and Morley, J., 1974, *Br. J. Pharmacol.* **52**:435P.
Butler, W. T., and Rossen, R. D., 1973, *J. Clin. Invest.* **52**:2629–2640.
Cahill, R. N. P., 1971b, *Experientia* **27**:913–914.
Cardella, C. J., Davies, P., and Allison, A. C., 1974, *Nature (London)* **247**:46–48.
Claman, H. N., 1972, *N. Engl. J. Med.* **287**:388–397.
Cohen, J. J., and Claman, H. N., 1971, *J. Exp. Med.* **133**:1026–1034.
Cohen, J. J., Fischbach, M., and Claman, H. M., 1970, *J. Immunol.* **105**:1146–1150.
Cohn, Z. A., and Fedorko, M. E., 1969, in: *Lysosomes in Biology and Pathology* (J. T. Dingle and H. B. Fell, eds.), Vol. 1, pp. 43–63, North-Holland Publishing Co., Amsterdam.
Coppola, E. O., Hemstreet, G. P., and Villegar, G. R., 1967, in: *Pharmacological Treatment in Organ and Tissue Transplantation* (A. Bertelli and A. P. Monaco, eds.), pp. 79–84, Excerpta Medica Foundation, Amsterdam.
Crout, J. E., Hepburn, B., and Ritts, R. E., 1975, *N. Engl. J. Med.* **292**:221.
Davies, M., Lloyd, J. B., and Beck, F., 1971, *Biochem. J.* **121**:21–26.
Davies, P., and Allison, A., 1972, *Crit. Rev. Toxicol.* **2**:283–323.
Davies, P., and Allison, A. C., 1976, in: *Immunobiology of the Macrophage* (D. S. Nelson, ed.), pp. 427–461, Academic Press, New York.
Davies, P., Allison, A. C., and Haswell, A. D., 1973a, *Biochem. Biophys. Res. Commun.* **52**:627–634.
Davies, P., Allison, A. C., and Haswell, A. D., 1973b, *Biochem. J.* **134**:33–41.
Davies, P., Page, R. C., and Allison, A. C., 1974, *J. Exp. Med.* **139**:1262–1282.
Dayer, J. M., Drane, S. M., Russell, R. G. M., and Robinson, D. R., 1976, *Proc. Natl. Acad. Sci. U.S.A.* **73**:945–949.
De Duve, C., De Barsy, T., Poole, B., Trouet, A., Fulkens, P., and Van Hoff, F., 1974, *Biochem. Pharmacol.* **23**:2495–2531.
Diani, Y., and Pras, M., 1975, *Lancet* **2**:556.
Dimitriu, A., 1976, *Cell. Immunol.* **21**:79–87.
Dinarello, C. A., Goldin, N. P., and Wolff, S. M., 1974, *J. Exp. Med.* **139**:1369–1381.
Dukor, P., and Dietrich, F. M., 1968, *Int. Arch. Allergy Appl. Immunol.* **34**:32–48.
Dukor, P., Miller, J. F. A. P., and Sacquet, E., 1968, *Clin. Exp. Immunol.* **3**:191–212.
Einstein, L. P., Schneeberger, E. E., and Colten, H. R., 1976, *J. Exp. Med.* **143**:114–126.
Fedorko, M. E., Hirsch, J. G., and Cohn, Z. A., 1968a, *J. Cell Biol.* **38**:377–391.
Fedorko, M. E., Hirsch, J. G., and Cohn, Z. A., 1968b, *J. Cell Biol.* **38**:392–402.
Fikrig, S. M., and Smithwick, E. M., 1965, *Arthritis Rheum.* **11**:478–479.
Finlay, C., Davies, P., and Allison, A. C., 1975, *Agents Actions* **5**:345–353.
Forbes, I. J., and Smith, J. L., 1967, *Lancet* **2**:334–337.
Fowles, R. E., Fajardo, I. M., Leibowitch, J. L., and David, J. R., 1973, *J. Exp. Med.* **138**:952–964.

Freyberg, R. H., Ziff, M., and Baum, J., 1972, in: *Arthritis and Allied Conditions* (J. L. Hollander and D. J. McCarty, Jr., eds.), pp. 455–482, Lea & Febiger, Philadelphia.
Gassman, A. E., and Van Furth, R., 1975, *Blood* **46**:51–64.
Goldstein, I. M., and Weissman, G., 1974, *J. Immunol.* **113**:1583–1588.
Goldstein, J. L., Brunschede, G. Y., and Brown, M. S., 1975, *J. Biol. Chem.* **250**:7854–7862.
Gordon, S., Unkeless, J. C., and Cohn, Z. A., 1974, *J. Exp. Med.* **140**:995–1010.
Goud, T. J. L. M., Schotte, C., and Van Furth, R., 1975, *J. Exp. Med.* **142**:1180–1199.
Ha, T. Y., Waxman, B. H., and Treffers, H. P., 1974, *J. Exp. Med.* **139**:13–23.
Hadden, J. W., Coffey, R. G., Hadden, E. M., Lopez-Corrales, E., and Sunshine, G. H., 1975, *Cell Immunol.* **20**:98–103.
Hadding, U., Bentley, C., Bitter-Suermann, D., Brade, V., 1976, *Fed. Proc. Fed. Am. Soc. Exp. Biol.* **35**:654.
Heilman, D. H., 1972, *Clin. Exp. Immunol.* **11**:393–403.
Heilman, D. H., 1973, *Clin. Exp. Immunol.* **15**:203–212.
Hill, D. F., 1968, *Med. Clin. North Am.* **52**:733–738.
Hokama, Y., Kimura, L., Perreira, S., and Palumbo, N., 1974, *Fed. Proc. Fed. Am. Soc. Exp. Biol.* **33**:650.
Hurd, E. R., and Ziff, M., 1968, *J. Exp. Med.* **128**:780–785.
Huskisson, E. C., Dieppe, P. A., Scott, J., Trapnell, J., Balme, H. W., and Willoughby, D. A., 1976, *Lancet* **1**:393.
Ingle, D. J., 1938, *Proc. Soc. Exp. Biol. Med.* **38**:443–444.
Jaffe, I. A., 1963, *Ann. Rheum. Dis.* **22**:71–76.
Jaffe, I. A., 1965, *Arthritis Rheum.* **8**:1064–1079.
Jaffe, I. A., 1975, *Ann. N. Y. Acad. Sci.* **256**:330–337.
Jaffe, I. A., Altman, K., and Merryman, P., 1964, *J. Clin. Invest.* **43**:1869–1873.
Keller, H. V., and Sorkin, E., 1967, *Int. Arch. Allergy Appl. Immunol.* **31**:575–586.
Kornel, L., 1973, *Acta Endocrinol. Suppl.* 178, p. 74.
Levine, M. A., and Claman, H., 1970, *Science* **167**:1515–1517.
Lewis, D. C., and Ziff, M., 1968, *Arthritis Rheum.* **9**:682–692.
Lichtenfeld, J. L., Desner, M., Mardiney, M. R., and Wiernik, P. H., 1974, *Fed. Proc. Fed. Am. Soc. Exp. Biol.* **33**:790.
Lipsky, P. E., Ellner, J. J., and Rosenthal, A. S., 1976, *J. Immunol.* **116**:868–875.
Liyanage, S. P., and Currey, H. L. F., 1972, *Ann. Rheum. Dis.* **31**:521.
Lockshin, M. D., 1972, *Experientia* **28**:571–572.
Lorber, A., Pearson, C. M., Meredith, W. L., and Gnatz-Mandell, L. E., 1964, *Ann. Intern. Med.* **61**:423–434.
Makinodan, T., Santos, G. W., and Quinn, R. P., 1970, *Pharmacol. Rev.* **22**:189–247.
Makman, M. H., Nakagawa, S., Dvorkin, B., and White, A., 1970, *J. Biol. Chem.* **245**:2556–2563.
Makman, M. H., Dvorkin, B., and White, A., 1971, *Proc. Natl. Acad. Sci. U.S.A.* **68**:1269–1273.
McCall, C. E., Volk, J. V., Cooper, M. R., and DeChatelet, L. R., 1971, *Infect. Immun.* **4**:315–317.
Metcalf, D., and Moore, M. A. S., 1971, *Haemopoietic Cells,* North-Holland Publishing Co., Amsterdam.
Moorhead, J. W., and Claman, H. M., 1972, *Cell. Immunol.* **5**:74–86.
Movat, H. Z., Steinberg, S. G., Habal, F. M., and Ranadive, N. S., 1972, *Lab. Invest.* **29**:669–684.
Multicenter Trial Group, 1973, *Lancet* **1**:275–280.
Nathan, C. F., Remold, H. G., and David, J. R., 1973, *J. Exp. Med.* **137**:275–290.
Nelson, R., and Leu, R. W., 1975, *J. Immunol.* **114**:606–609.
Nimni, M. E., and Bavetta, L. A., 1965, *Science* **150**:905–907.
Norton, W. L., Lewis, D. C., and Ziff, M., 1968, *Arthritis Rheum.* **11**:436–443.
Oronsky, A. L., Perper, R. J., and Schroder, H. C., 1973a, *Nature (London)* **246**:417–419.
Oronsky, A. L., Ignarro, L. J., and Perper, R. J., 1973b, *J. Exp. Med.* **138**:461–472.
Pabst, H. F., and Crawford, J. A., 1974, *Pediatr. Res.* **8**:416.
Pachman, L. M., Esterly, N. B., and Peterson, R. D. A., 1971, *J. Clin. Invest.* **50**:226–230.
Page, A. R., Condie, R. M., and Good, R. A., 1962, *Am. J. Pathol.* **40**:519–530.
Page, R. C., Davies, P., and Allison, A. C., 1974, *Lab. Invest.* **30**:568–581.
Pantalone, R. M., and Page, R. C., 1975, *Proc. Natl. Acad. Sci. U.S.A.* **72**:2091–2094.
Perper, R. J., and Oronsky, A. L., 1974, *Arthritis Rheum.* **17**:47–55.

Perper, R. J., Alvarez, B., Colombo, C., and Schroeder, H., 1971, *Proc. Soc. Exp. Biol. Med.* **137**:506–512.
Perper, R. J., Sanda, M., Chinea, G., and Oronsky, A., 1974, *J. Lab. Clin. Med.* **84**:394–406.
Perper, R. J., Sanda, M., Stecher, V. J., and Oronsky, A. L., 1975, *Ann. N.Y. Acad. Sci.* **256**:190.
Peter, J. B., 1971, *Cell. Immunol.* **2**:199–202.
Phillips, S. M., and Zweiman, B., 1973, *J. Exp. Med.* **137**:1494–1510.
Raff, M. C., and Owen, J. J. T., 1971, *Eur. J. Immunol.* **1**:27–30.
Reich, E., 1975, in: *Proteases and Biological Control* (E. Reich, D. B. Rifkin, and E. Shaw, eds.), pp. 333–341. Cold Spring Harbor Laboratory, Cold Spring Harbor, New York.
Renoux, G., and Renoux, M., 1973, *Infect. Immun.* **8**:544–548.
Rinehart, J. J., Balcerzak, S. P., Sagone, A. L., and Lobuglio, A. F., 1974, *J. Clin. Invest.* **54**:1337–1343.
Ringrose, P. S., Parr, M. A., and McLaren, M., 1975, *Biochem. Pharmacol.* **24**:607–614.
Rosenthale, M. E., and Nagra, C. L., 1967, *Proc. Soc. Exp. Biol. Med.* **125**:149–153.
Sampson, D., and Lui, A., 1976, *Cancer Res.* **36**:952–955.
Sandberg, A. A., and Slaunwhite, W. R., Jr., 1963, *J. Clin. Invest.* **42**:51–54.
Schreiber, A. D., Parsons, J., McDermott, P., and Cooper, R. A., 1975, *J. Clin. Invest.* **56**:1189–1197.
Schuermans, Y., 1975, *Lancet* **1**:111.
Schumacher, K., Maerker-Alzer, G., and Preuss, R., 1975, *Arzneim.-Forsch.* **25**:603–606.
Schwab, J. H., Cromartie, W. J., and Robertson, B. S., 1959, *J. Exp. Med.* **109**:43–54.
Seeger, R. C., and Oppenheim, J. J., 1970, *J. Exp. Med.* **132**:44–65.
Segal, S., Cohen, I. R., and Fildman, M., 1972, *Science* **175**:1126–1128.
Smith, M. J., Hoth, M., and Davis, K., 1975, *Ann. Intern. Med.* **83**:509–511.
Stecher, V. J., Morse, J. H., and Thorbecke, J. H., 1967, *Proc. Soc. Exp. Biol. Med.* **124**:433.
Thompson, E. B., and Lippman, M. E., 1974, *Metabolism* **23**:159–202.
Thompson, J., and Van Furth, R., 1970, *J. Exp. Med.* **131**:429–442.
Thompson, J., and Van Furth, R., 1973, *J. Exp. Med.* **137**:10–21.
Tripodi, D., Parks, L. C., and Brugmans, J., 1973, *N. Engl. J. Med.* **289**:354–357.
Tuchinda, M., Newcomb, R. W., and DeVald, B. L., 1972, *Int. Arch. Allergy Appl. Immunol.* **42**:533–544.
Unanue, E. R., 1972, *Adv. Immunol.* **15**:95–165.
Unkeless, J. C., Gordon, S., and Reich, E., 1974, *J. Exp. Med.* **139**:834–850.
Van Furth, R., 1970, in: *Mononuclear Phagocytes* (R. Van Furth, ed.), p. 151, Blackwell, Oxford.
Van Furth, R., and Cohn, Z. A., 1968, *J. Exp. Med.* **128**:415–435.
Van Furth, R., and Jones, T. C., 1975, *Infect. Immun.* **12**:888–890.
Van Furth, R., Cohn, Z. A., Hirsch, J. G., Humphrey, J. H., Spector, W. G., and Langevoort, H. L., 1972, *Bull. WHO* **46**:845–852.
Van Furth, R., Gassmann, A. E., and Diesselhoff-Den Dulk, M. M. C., 1975, *J. Exp. Med.* **141**:531–546.
Vann, D. C., 1974, *Cell. Immunol.* **11**:11–18.
Van Zwet, T. L., Thompson, J., and Van Furth, R., 1975, *Infect. Immun.* **12**:699–705.
Virolainen, M., 1968, *J. Exp. Med.* **127**:943–953.
Volkman, A., and Gowans, J. L., 1965, *Br. J. Exp. Pathol.* **46**:62–70.
Wahl, L. M., Wahl, S. M., Mergenhagen, S. E., and Martin, G. R., 1974, *Proc. Natl. Acad. Sci. U.S.A.* **71**:3598–3061.
Wahl, L. M., Wahl, S. M., Mergenhagen, S. E., and Martin, G. R., 1975, Science **187**:261–263.
Waksman, B. H., and Namba, Y., 1976, *Cell. Immunol.* **21**:161–176.
Walz, D. T., DiMartino, M. J., and Misher, A., 1971, *J. Pharmacol. Exp. Ther.* **178**:223–231.
Wang, P., Franson, R. C., DeChatelet, L. R., Waite, M., and McCall, C. E., 1972, *Infect. Immun.* **6**:982–987.
Ward, P. A., Offen, C. D., and Montgomery, J. R., 1971, *Fed. Proc. Fed. Am. Soc. Exp. Biol.* **30**:1721–1724.
Weissmann, G., Goldstein, I., Hoffstein, S., Chauvet, G., and Robineaux, R., 1975, *Ann. N.Y. Acad. Sci.* **256**:222–231.
Werb, Z., and Gordon, S., 1975a, *J. Exp. Med.* **142**:346–360.
Werb, Z., and Gordon, S., 1975b, *J. Exp. Med.* **142**:361–377.
Weston, W. L., Mandel, M. J., Krueger, G. G., and Claman, H. M., 1972, *J. Invest. Dermatol.* **59**:345–348.
Weston, W. L., Claman, H. M., and Krueger, G. G., 1973, *J. Immunol.* **110**:880–883.

White, A., 1948, *Harvey Lect.* **43**:43–70.
Wibo, M., and Poole, B., 1974, *J. Cell. Biol.* **63**:430–440.
Wiener, E., and Marmary, Y., 1969, *Lab. Invest.* **21**:505–511.
Wiener, E., Marmary, Y., and Curelaru, Z., 1972, *Lab. Invest.* **26**:220–226.
Wills, E. D., Davies, P., Allison, A. C., and Haswell, A. D., 1972, *Nature (London) New Biol.* **240**:58–60.
Winchester, R. J., 1975, *Ann. N.Y. Acad. Sci.* **256**:73–81.
Winder, C. V., Lembke, L. A., and Stephens, M., 1969, *Arthritis Rheum.* **12**:472–482.
Wood, D. D., Cameron, P. M., Poe, M. T., and Morris, C. A., 1976, *Cell. Immunol.* **21**:88–96.
Zucker, J., Ramsey, R. H., Dorner, R. W., and Gantner, G. E., Jr., 1970, *Arthritis Rheum.* **13**:131–138.

13

Immunosuppressive Agents

FEDERICO SPREAFICO and ALESSANDRO ANACLERIO

1. Introduction and General Remarks

A reduction in immune reactivity can result from the exposure of the organism to a relatively large number of physical, chemical, or biological agents, or from the application of different types of immunologic or nonimmunologic maneuvers. Even restricting our interest to immunodepressive chemicals, i.e., to the type of agents most frequently employed clinically to obtain immunodepression, the literature is now so large that it would be impossible to analyze every facet of the field in depth in this chapter. Since a number of recent reviews of the subject are available (Berenbaum, 1965; Gabrielsen and Good, 1967; Schwartz, 1968; Makinodan *et al.*, 1970; Chalmers *et al.*, 1972; Hersh, 1974; J. F. Bach, 1975), we will consider in this survey only selected aspects of nonspecific immunodepressive intervention, and will concentrate on recent developments of those agents that are at present in experimental and clinical use.* In the attempt to reflect the historical evolution of immune manipulation toward the less "destructive" and the more selective and "physiologic," we will also briefly present newer substances or approaches that now appear to have great potential for practical exploitation. Further, we will not discuss such approaches to immunodepression as whole-body, local, or extracorporeal irradiation, thoracic duct drainage, or organ excision, since they are only of historical interest or have limited current value. Last, no discussion of the current status of clinical immunodepression will be attempted. As repeatedly emphasized by various investigators, the large number of uncontrolled clinical trials in disorders in which the immunologic basis is often undefined, the frequent absence of objective criteria for evaluating drug efficacy, and the large variability in the treatments employed preclude, in most cases, sound conclusions.

*Among the therapeutic agents, we have deliberately excluded antilymphocyte serum (ALS), since it is the subject of recent reviews (Lance *et al.*, 1970; Spreafico, 1972; J. F. Bach, 1975).

FEDERICO SPREAFICO and ALESSANDRO ANACLERIO • Laboratory of Tumor Chemotherapy and Immunology, Istituto di Ricerche Farmacologiche "Mario Negri", Milan, Italy 20157.

The existence of a large number of substances capable of interfering with immune reactivity at different levels raises the problem of defining exactly what an immunodepressive agent is. This difficulty reflects, on one hand, our ignorance of the mechanism of action of even the widely used immunodepressants and, on the other, the complexity of the immune reaction in its specific and nonspecific aspects. Both antigen and antibody can, in selected conditions, be employed for immunodepression. At the other extreme, agents that inhibit platelet aggregation, which plays an important role in organ graft rejection, can result in an "immunodepressive" effect. In addition, the manifestations of immune reactivity in both animals and man are often the result of an inflammatory reaction; thus, antiinflammatory agents may exert an immunodepressive effect although the specific activity of the immune cells is not modified. Conversely, bona fide immunodepressants frequently possess antiinflammatory capacity the relevance of which is often difficult to define, a point that has a number of important practical implications in the testing, evaluation, and rational use of such agents. Although we would favor the pragmatic approach of considering as immunodepressants those chemical or biological substances capable of reducing, with an acceptable therapeutic index, the development or expression of at least one type of immune reactivity and through mechanisms not involving exclusively the nonspecific consequences of this reactivity, it is clear that this restriction is only operational. Implicit is the concept that the mechanisms at work may be multiple, that the specificity of many immunodepressive products is only relative, and that the different types of immune responses may exhibit different sensitivity to interference.

The difficulty of definition is reflected in the unsatisfactory classification of immunodepressants. Considering only nonspecific immunodepressants, an ideal classification should take into account a complex series of points such as the nature and origin (physical, chemical, or biological) of the substance, the type of immune cell(s) involved and the level at which interference is exerted (e.g., antigen processing or recognition, lymphocyte activation or proliferation, intercellular cooperation or regulation, production or release of antibody or other mediators, and the effects of the latter on target cells or on amplifying cellular and humoral systems), and the biochemical mechanisms through which the activity is expressed. In view of our substantial ignorance on many of these aspects, no such classification is yet possible. In the past, these agents have been grouped either according to their presumed major biochemical mechanism of action at the cell level (e.g., alkylators, antimetabolites), an approach that obscures the fact that agents with the same mechanism may have different characteristics, and that does not encompass most of the newer biological agents or account for the phase of the immune process presumed as preferentially affected (Hersh, 1974). Makinodan *et al.* (1970) categorized immunodepressants according to their preferential activity with respect to the timing of antigen stimulation. Although this approach has practical appeal and permits at least a degree of definition as to the stage of the immune response inhibited, it cannot be forgotten that for many immunodepressants this preferential activity is heavily influenced by the test system and treatment conditions employed.

The levels at which an immune response can be inhibited are multiple; it can thus be easily perceived that in the screening and characterization of new putative immunodepressants, a variety of immunologic systems, including both cell-mediated and humoral reactivities, should be investigated employing a number of

TABLE 1. Factors That Influence the Effects of Immunodepressive Agents on Antibody Production

Type of antigen (thymus-dependent or independent)
Dose and route of antigen administration
Strength of antigen
Primary or secondary response
Use of adjuvant
Dose and route of agent administration
Schedule of treatment
Timing in relation to antigen
Assay of antibody production: serologic (e.g., precipitation, agglutination, cytolysis, complement fixation), cellular [plaque-forming cells (PFC), rosette-forming cells (RFC)], *in vivo* (clearance of antigen)
Day of assay
Type of Ig investigated
Association with other immunodepressive procedures (e.g., thymectomy, other drugs)
Association with physiologic or pathologic conditions, or both (e.g., host age and nutritional status, presence of neoplasms, postsurgical stress)

testing conditions regarding doses, schedules, and timing of injection relative to antigen stimulation. By way of example, a list of factors that influence the effects of immunodepressive compounds on antibody production is given in Table 1. Since the main experimental approaches to the screening and evaluation of immunodepressants have recently been extensively discussed (M. S. Mitchell, 1974; J. F. Bach, 1975), no detailed analysis of these aspects will be attempted here. Tables 2–4 present the systems that can be employed and parameters to be considered for a characterization of these types of compounds.

Taking into account the varied nature of immunodepressants and the multiplicity of levels at which they may act, no set of rules can be recommended, and a flexible combination of *in vitro* and *in vivo* investigations is often necessary. Although *in vitro* systems can frequently offer essential elements for the elucidation of the mechanisms of action of immunodepressants, even the more complex systems now available do not comprise all levels at which inhibition can be exerted. In addition, opposite activities can be seen between *in vitro* and *in vivo* conditions, as first observed with the mitogen phytohemagglutinin (PHA) (Spreafico and Ler-

TABLE 2. *In Vivo* Methods for Characterization of Immunodepressive Agents in Animals

Primary and secondary humoral immune response to thymus-dependent antigens (SRBC, serum proteins)
Primary response to thymus-independent antigens (*Escherichia coli* lipopolysaccharide, pneumococcal polysaccharide, polyvinylpyrrolidone)
Delayed type hypersensitivity (SRBC, oxazolone, methylated serum albumin)
Allograft rejection (*H-2* and non-*H-2* incompatible tissues or tumors)
Graft-vs.-host reaction
Autoimmune diseases [allergic encephalomyelitis, autoimmune thyroiditis, New Zealand Black (NZB) mouse diseases]
RES function (clearance of colloidal carbon, labeled albumin or erythrocytes)
Nonspecific inflammation (turpentine, cotton pellets, injection of Freund's adjuvant)
Myelotoxicity (^{59}Fe incorporation in bone marrow stem cells)

TABLE 3. *In Vitro* Methods for Evaluation of Immunocyte Subpopulations

Sensitivity to anti-*Thy 1,2* serum (T cells) and to anti-Ig serum or to anti-MBLA (B cells)
Rosette-forming cells
Response to mitogens: Con A, PHA (T cells), lipopolysaccharide (B cells), pokeweed mitogen (T and B cells)
Suppressor cells on humoral and cell-mediated responses (T cells)
Mixed lymphocyte reactivity (T cells)
Antibody response (T and B cells and macrophages)
Antigen-induced inhibition of leucocyte or macrophage migration (T cells)
Lymphotoxin production (T cells)
Antigen-induced DNA synthesis (T or B cells)
Cytotoxicity: against specific target cells (T cells), against antibody-coated target cells ("K" cells), by PHA- or Con-A-activated, nonsensitized lymphocytes (T cells)
Natural cytotoxicity: against C-positive tumor cells ("null" cells)
Phagocytosis: of colloidal carbon, latex particles, antigen–antibody complexes (macrophages, polymorphs)

ner, 1967). It is obviously only through *in vivo* studies that information can be obtained on classic pharmacological parameters, such as drug distribution and disposition, information that is crucial not only for a sound evaluation of the compound's therapeutic potential, but also for a clear understanding of its mode of action and the basis for a rational exploitation of these compounds. It cannot be overemphasized that, as is true for many pharmacological agents, the definition of the therapeutic index of the substance under study should be an essential element in the characterization of immunodepressive compounds, especially since many of these agents have significant activity only at doses close to toxicity. Unfortunately,

TABLE 4. Tests for Evaluation of Immunodepression in Humans

In vivo tests
Primary antibody responses: hemocyanin, T4 phage, influenza vaccine, xenogeneic erythrocytes
Secondary antibody responses: tetanus or diphtheria toxoids, polio, influenza or vaccine viruses, *Salmonella typhi* 4 antigen
Primary cellular immunity: skin reaction to DNCB, hemocyanin
Secondary cellular immunity: skin reaction to tuberculin, mumps, candidin, trichophyton, streptokinase-streptodornase
Nonimmunologic inflammatory response: Rebuck–Crowley "skin window"
In vitro tests
Mixed lymphocyte reaction
Blastogenesis after exposure to specific antigen
Responsiveness to mitogens such as PHA, Con-A, pokeweed mitogen
Natural cytotoxicity against various tumor lines
Leukocyte cytotoxicity against antibody-coated target cells
Mitogen-induced leucocyte cytotoxicity against nonspecific target cells
Cytotoxicity after *in vitro* sensitization to allo- or xenogeneic target cells
Number of T and B cells: rosette formation with SRBC (E-RFC), antibody-coated SRBC (EA-RFC), complement-coated SRBC (EAC-RFC); membrane Ig-bearing cells; use of specific cytotoxic xenoantisera
MIF production
Macrophage phagocytic capacity

these concepts, and thus the possibility of distinguishing between true and potential immunodepressants, are not frequently considered. Too often, for instance, *in vitro* studies employ nonphysiologic drug concentrations, or do not express the therapeutic dose as a fraction of the LD_{50} or of other more specific parameters of toxicity (e.g., myeloid inhibition), thus making comparisons between compounds difficult.

That immune mechanisms play a crucial and complex role in the control of neoplastic progression has now been clearly established; accordingly, a complete characterization of both the qualitative and quantitative aspects of the interaction of the tumor with the immune system should be a basic point for the investigation of these agents. Potency attained at the price of an excessive and/or a nonselective inhibition of host reactivities may not represent the most fruitful approach in this field. For example, the immunodepressive capacity of daunomycin may be the important determinant of the lower therapeutic activity of this agent in comparison with its structural analogue adriamycin (Mantovani *et al.*, 1976). Complete characterization of antineoplastic agents in this regard is in its infancy despite the direct relevance of such studies to more rational chemoimmunotherapeutic approaches.

If the ideal immunodepressant should induce the rapid, effective, and, if necessary, reversible abrogation of the response to a given antigen while otherwise sparing host capacity to react immunologically and with minimum host toxicity, it has to be concluded that present methods of immunodepression are still imperfect in many respects, since they are mostly based on "indiscriminate and destructive" approaches to immune interference, with the inescapable consequences of limited selectivity and low therapeutic indexes.

In recent years, a number of alternative biological substances and methods for inducing immunodepression that appear to offer greater selectivity and safety of application have been described. While waiting for practical methods for reliable induction of immune tolerance, it seems reasonable to predict that for a number of years, the more traditional use of cytotoxic chemicals will prevail.

This background suggests that a number of points should be given high investigative priority to increase the effectiveness of these treatments. Among these points, one could cite the problems of drug scheduling and of drug combinations. It has been shown repeatedly in both experimental and clinical oncology that the design of the dose regimen can considerably influence therapeutic efficacy, yet the elegant theoretical studies of Berenbaum (1967) on the possibility of designing treatment schedules that selectively inhibit immunocompetent cells more than other tissues (e.g., bone marrow) have not been followed up experimentally. Similarly, despite the undeniable success obtained in cancer treatment through the use of cytotoxic drug combinations, this aspect has received only superficial attention in immunologic manipulation.

2. Steroids

Despite more than two decades of wide empirical use of these agents, the precise mechanisms through which glucocorticoids depress immune reactivity are still uncertain (Claman, 1972). One obstacle is the marked species differences in the *in vitro* and *in vivo* sensitivity to these agents, the mouse, rat, and rabbit exhibiting a high degree of steroid sensitivity, while man, primates, and the guinea pig are highly steroid-resistant. Since most of the data on steroid effects on lymphoid cells and immunity have been obtained in sensitive species, extrapolation of specific conclusions to man has been difficult. Second, functionally distinct subpopulations and subsets of lymphocytes within a species appear to have varying degrees of steroid sensitivity, and conclusions on the effects exerted at each given level are additionally complicated by the variations in drug treatments and experimental systems employed. A third obstacle lies in the known nonspecific antiinflammatory effect of these steroids, which is the result of a multiplicity of activities including depression of granulocyte function (Mandell *et al.,* 1970) and a reduction in complement levels (Atkinson and Frank, 1973).

At the biochemical level, steroids have been shown to induce in lymphoid cells various modifications, the importance of which in mediating the *in vivo* effects of these agents is still incompletely understood. Such is the case for the reported increase in acid ribonuclease and hydrolases (Sachs *et al.,* 1962; McLeod *et al.,* 1963) and the reduction in aminoisobutyric acid transport (Frengley *et al.,* 1973) and RNA polymerase activity (K. E. Fox and Gabourel, 1967). Of greater importance may be the inhibition of DNA, RNA, and protein synthesis seen *in vitro* and *in vivo* in sensitive species (Kidson, 1967; Kirkpatrick *et al.,* 1971), dividing cells being arrested in the G_1 phase, possibly also as a result of interference with a chalone mechanism (Thompson and Van Furth, 1973). While these modifications may be the consequence of the binding of the hormone to the specific cytosol receptors and subsequent interaction of the complex with DNA, it seems that two other biochemical changes that could play important roles in the effects of these hormones on lymphoid cells are not dependent on an ultimate interaction with DNA. We refer to the inhibition of glucose uptake observed after steroid exposure in lymphocytes of many species including man (Baxter and Forsham, 1972), possibly mediated by the synthesis of a specific inhibitory protein (Munck *et al.,* 1972). This activity could explain in part the catabolic and cytolytic effects of these drugs. The apparently permissive activity of steroids on the cyclic 3′,5′-adenosine monophosphate (cAMP) system (Mendelsohn *et al.,* 1973) could be a mechanism of importance considering the relationships between the intracellular equilibrium of cyclic nucleotides and lymphocyte function as examined elsewhere in this volume.

This multiplicity of biochemical changes might explain the complexity of steroid effects at the cell level, where cell lysis is only one of the possible mechanisms. Alterations, possibly even reversible, of cellular metabolism could in fact play an important role in steroid immunodepressive activity. The importance of a redistribution of lymphocytes from the circulation into other body compartments, although very suggestive, remains to be more clearly assessed.

The *in vivo* effects of steroids on immunity are multiple and complex, and to define the target cell of these activities is very difficult and sometimes impossible, in view of the frequently contrasting results reported by various investigators.

An effect on T cells is clear, as indicated many years ago by the exquisite sensitivity of the thymus to these agents; the thymolytic effect of glucocorticoids is not indiscriminate, however, since it is exerted on the cortical elements, i.e., on cells that possess potential but not actual immunocompetence, and spares the immunocompetent medullary elements. Indeed, because of the destruction of inactive cells, the thymus of steroid-treated animals shows an apparent, relative increase in T-cell functions such as PHA and mixed leukocyte reaction (MLR) reactivities, helper cell activity, and the capacity to mount a graft-vs.-host reaction (GVH) (Blomgren and Svedmyr, 1971; J. J. Cohen and Claman, 1971a; Janossy and Greaves, 1972; Rühl *et al.*, 1973). A further indication of the relatively immature stage of steroid-sensitive thymocytes is the recent demonstration by Trainin *et al.* (1974) that incubation with thymus humoral factor transforms the sensitive elements into hormone-resistant cells. Mature T suppressor cells in the thymus appear to belong preferentially to the steroid-resistant population (Nachtigal *et al.*, 1975), although they appear to be the progency of steroid-sensitive thymocytes, a fact that can explain the finding that steroids, at variance with other immunosuppressants such as cytoxan (cyclophosphamide, Cy) or radiation, can actually antagonize the induction of tolerance in systems in which T suppressors operate (Dukor and Dietrich, 1970; Zan-bar *et al.*, 1975). In parallel, helper and GVH-producing splenocytes are steroid-resistant, as would be expected of long-lived elements that survive in environments that can contain high concentrations of these hormones. It should be noted, however, that GVH-initiator cells are also insensitive to steroids during the education phase (J. J. Cohen and Claman, 1971b), but the GVH itself is steroid-sensitive. The level at which steroids act in this circumstance is still unclear; the educated effector cells are just one of multiple possible targets.

Somewhat confusing data exist on the effects of steroids on the lymphocyte activation process by antigen or by mitogens. In fact, these agents did not reduce the *in vitro* sensitization of rat lymphoid cells to foreign fibroblast monolayers (Stavy *et al.*, 1973) or the *in vivo* sensitization of mouse T cells to sheep erythrocytes (SRBC) (Claman, 1972), whereas both the MLR and the *in vitro* stimulation by antigen or mitogens are steroid-sensitive both in animals and in man (Heilman and Leichner, 1972; Fauci and Dale, 1974). The hormone concentrations inhibitory of the PHA response are in the 1–100 μg/ml range, i.e., levels that do not affect cell viability, and the effect is seen only when steroids are added before or simultaneously with the stimulant. Even with optimum drug concentrations in the culture, blast transformation is not totally suppressed, a finding that is suggestive of the existence of antigen- or pokeweed-sensitive cells that are steroid-resistant (Heilman, 1972). After *in vivo* steroid treatment of mice, the PHA response is decreased in spleen but increased in bone marrow, possibly because of a migration of a PHA-responsive population (J. W. Moorhead and Claman, 1972). These authors thus postulated the existence of three subsets of peripheral T cells. One, present in the spleen, is theta-positive and PHA-responsive, steroid-sensitive, and not implicated in GVH or helper functions. A second, also present in the spleen, is theta-positive, steroid-resistant, PHA-responsive, and capable of initiating a GVH, expressing helper function, and migrating to the bone marrow. A third subpopulation is lodged in the bone marrow, theta-negative, PHA-responsive, and steroid-resistant.

As regards the effector mechanisms of T cells, it has been observed in various systems (I. R. Cohen *et al.*, 1970; Stavy *et al.*, 1973) that *in vitro* cytotoxicity can be reversibly inhibited by steroid doses that do not modify nucleic acid or protein synthesis. Since the binding to the target is not affected and the inhibition is seen when the drug is added at the beginning of incubation, indicating absence of effects on cytolysis itself, it has to be concluded that the steroid-sensitive step is the activation of the cytotoxic reaction. Among the effects on lymphocyte mediators, an effect on lymphotoxin production is controversial (Williams and Granger, 1969; Peter, 1971). Release of migration-inhibitory factor (MIF) is essentially unchanged

(Balow and Rosenthal, 1973; Weston *et al.*, 1973); however, the macrophage response to MIF is apparently inhibited. This capacity of steroids to prevent the recruitment and activation of macrophages is probably an important mechanism through which these agents suppress delayed hypersensitivity (DH) reactions, a well-known biological activity of these hormones *in vivo*. It should be recalled, however, that prolonged courses with relatively high doses are required to produce this effect in humans (Claman, 1972). Although local injection of steroids can inhibit cutaneous DH reactions, the antiinflammatory capacity of these agents is not the only mechanism operative in these conditions. In addition to the fact that steroids are also active when given at the sensitization stage (Fachet and Parrott, 1972), it has been shown that DH-depressive doses are ineffective in interfering with nonimmune inflammation (Brandriss *et al.*, 1965).

Skin allograft rejection can be delayed with appropriate treatment with these agents in steroid-sensitive species, although it should be noted that a local effect on the graft cannot be excluded, since the incubation of allogeneic skin with steroids can delay its rejection (Klane *et al.*, 1971). This effect on the graft itself is not limited to steroids, but has also been described with other agents such as irradiation, antilymphocyte serum (ALS), and Cy (Guttmann and Lindquist, 1969), and has been attributed to a destruction of "passenger" leukocytes that, carried over in the skin or organ allograft, could represent an important part of the immunogenicity of the graft. The mechanism at the basis of such an activity is not clear, however, and it should be noted that the perfusion of donor organs with immunosuppressants is not always effective in prolonging their acceptance by the host (Tremann *et al.*, 1975). The data on steroid effectiveness in organ transplantation in animals are contrasting: in dogs, an increase in kidney allograft survival was seen by Zukoski *et al.* (1963a), whereas Marchioro *et al.* (1964) could see effects only on the histology of acute rejection. Similarly, the positive effects found by Tinbergen (1968) in rats are to be contrasted with the negative ones found by Shehadeh *et al.* (1970). Among other experimental factors, the dependence of steroid immunodepression on antigenic strength could possibly explain such discrepancies in conditions in which histoincompatibility was not carefully controlled. While steroids are doubtfully active on organ grafts in animals, they synergize well in these conditions with other chemical or biological immunodepressants such as ALS (Lance *et al.*, 1970). In man, steroids have a documented beneficial activity on the rejection crises of kidney transplants (Hamburger *et al.*, 1972), an activity that is observable soon after treatment with high doses, so that it seems likely that the effects are exerted on the immune effector phase or on the nonspecific inflammatory components of rejection, or on both. It is relevant to note here that the injection of 100–400 mg hydrocortisone into humans was found to produce a profound decrease in circulating lymphocytes and monocytes, with a return to normal values within 24 hr (Fauci and Dale, 1974).

In sensitive species, steroids are good suppressors of humoral antibody production, the degree of inhibition being dependent on the strength of antigenic stimulation, and more so than, for instance, with Cy. The timing of treatment in relation to challenge is also crucial; the highest reduction in anti-SRBC primary antibody production by mice is observed with cortisone injections 48 or 24 hr before antigen, whereas drug pretreatment is only effective in suppressing late antibody production. In fact, both IgM and IgG responses can be suppressed by cortisone, and late IgG antibody levels can be reduced when drug treatment is delayed until 15 days after SRBC, thus showing a much greater sensitivity of this antibody response than for IgM antibodies to these drugs. Recovery from steroid immunosuppression is relatively rapid, especially when antigenic stimulation is strong. The secondary response is significantly more difficult to inhibit. In man, most authors have found no reduction in primary responses to standard stimuli such as pertussis, typhoid, or tetanus vaccines (David *et al.,* 1970). However, decreases in antinuclear antibody titers have been described in patients with lupus erythematosus under steroid treatment (Cruchaud, 1971). Again, differences in the steroid type and treatment employed make it impossible to compare the various studies. The reduction in circulating antibody observed in animals is not the result of an effect on mature antibody-forming cells (AFC), which are corticoresistant both *in vitro* and *in vivo* (Elliott and Sinclair, 1968), and the same seems to apply for AFC-progenitors in the spleen and bone marrow, although this point is still controversial. In fact, Segal *et al.* (1972) reported that hydrocortisone treatment did not depress the *in vitro* response of spleen cells to a T-independent antigen, a finding that would support a substantial insensitivity of B lymphocytes to steroids.

J. J. Cohen and Claman (1971a) observed that the depressed capacity of splenocytes from steroid-treated mice to transfer adoptive immunity to SRBC could be restored by bone marrow cells, but not by thymocytes.

While effects of steroids on B cells and T cells are not clear, a somewhat less clouded picture appears to hold for the monocyte–macrophage system. At the subcellular level, in addition to inhibition of amino acid incorporation and modification in intracellular enzyme distribution (Gray and Koeppe, 1966; Epstein *et al.,* 1967), the change that has received most attention is lysosomal stabilization (Weissmann and Thomas, 1963) because of the possible role of these organelles in inflammation. A depression in phagocytosis was described by some groups (Benveniste *et al.,* 1970; Wiener *et al.,* 1972; Atkinson *et al.,* 1973), both *in vivo* and *in vitro.* Craddock *et al.* (1967) reported that normal macrophages reconstituted immunocompetence of steroid-treated rats. Others, however, found an absence of significant effects on phagocytosis and antigen processing (J. G. Hirsch and Church, 1961; Allison and Addock, 1965; Gemsa *et al.,* 1973), and J. J. Cohen and Claman (1971a) could not confirm Craddock's findings in mice. Steroids have clear effects on monocyte–macrophage kinetics and accumulation in peripheral sites, as described by Van Furth and his colleagues (Thompson and Van Furth, 1973; Van Furth *et al.,* 1973). Both in normal conditions and after inflammation, steroids depress monocyte influx at the inflammatory site as a consequence of a marked reduction of circulating monocytes, which is in turn attributable to the sequestration of these elements in unknown sites, rather than to a decrease in monocyte production (Van Furth *et al.,* 1973). Essentially similar findings (suppression of macrophage infiltrates in the lesions possibly secondary to the inhibition of lymphocyte proliferation) were obtained by North (1972) in studying cortisone suppression of the cell-mediated immunity to *Lysteria monocytogenes* in mice, an infection that, like many others by bacteria, viruses, fungi, or parasites, can be increased in severity or incidence or both by steroid treatment (David *et al.,* 1970).

Considering that macrophages are necessary for the development and expression of cellular immunity (Unanue, 1972), the capacity of steroids to compromise host ability to mobilize these cells into inflammatory sites and to recruit and activate those already present in the tissues (Balow and Rosenthal, 1973) plays an important role in the depression of delayed reactivities by these agents.

3. Azathioprine and 6-Mercaptopurine

Although a number of other compounds considered to act mainly if not exclusively as antimetabolites have been shown to possess immunodepressive activity (Makinodan *et al.*, 1970), this discussion will consider mainly 6-mercaptopurine (6-MP) and its nitroimidazole derivative, azathioprine (AZA), which are practically the only members of this class of agents to have had extensive clinical use as immunodepressants. This clinical preference for AZA over other thiopurines, or other drugs with different biochemical modes of action, is to a certain degree surprising. Other compounds with greater immunodepressive activity are available, and at least in the mouse, the inhibitory activity of these thiopurines on the lymphoid system, in comparison with their activity on the erythropoietic system (Floersheim, 1970), is certainly less selective than that of other agents such as Cy or methotrexate (MTX). Since, as proved in the study of antineoplastic agents, animal toxicity, if adequately performed, is representative of the clinical response (Mellett, 1974), the failure to extend clinical trial of agents other than thiopurines is just another indication of the lack of a rational immunodepressive therapy based on sound pharmacological considerations. The preferential clinical use of thiopurines can thus be related to the historical observations by Schwartz *et al.* (1958), which started the modern era of chemical immunosuppression, particularly in organ transplantation.

In vitro, AZA was reported to be more active than 6-MP in inhibiting protein and antibody synthesis (Forbes and Smith, 1967; Leung and Vas, 1968); the *in vivo* results, however, are much less clear. The earlier indications of greater immunodepression with AZA were not confirmed (Berenbaum, 1971; Spreafico *et al.*, 1973), since equimolar doses of 6-MP were significantly more potent than AZA after parenteral treatment of rodents. Since the imidazole group was inserted with the intent of protecting the sulfydryl group of 6-MP from rapid methylation, AZA was thought to be a slow-release form of 6-MP. Elion (1967) proved this idea untenable, since 70% of the drug is nonenzymatically transformed into 6-MP within 5 min of injection into mice. The nitroimidazole moiety was additionally capable of reducing the immunodepression induced by a concomitant injection of 6-MP. In addition to an alleged lower toxicity (Elion and Hitchings, 1975), the only clearly demonstrated advantage of AZA is thus its better gastrointestinal absorption in animals and in man (Elion, 1969). The debate is still open on whether AZA activity is mediated entirely by the formation of 6-MP. In studies employing radioactive drugs, no differences in the kinetics of ^{35}S turnover were seen between AZA and 6-MP in man, a species in which it seems probable that a rapid splitting of AZA also occurs (Elion, 1972). Because of their advocated clinical significance, it may be worth noting that two types of bioassays have been described for an evaluation of AZA pharmacokinetics in man: the capacity of the serum of treated individuals to inhibit rosette formation by mouse splenocytes or to inhibit MLR (J. F. Bach, 1975). Although the second technique has been claimed to be more sensitive, the former technique has been employed more extensively because of its greater technical simplicity. Its proponents have shown that the rate of disappearance of AZA (or its metabolites, or both) from plasma as determined by rosette inhibition was essentially similar to that found with the labeled drug. Although this bioassay is not without criticisms, based essentially on the fact that it exploits a biological activity apparently unique to AZA and not shared by 6-MP and the significance of which in AZA immunodepression is still undetermined (see below), it would nevertheless appear to have a degree of clinical potential. For instance, it was shown by J. F. Bach and Dardenne (1971) that renal failure markedly modifies the persistence of the drug in the circulation, a finding in keeping with clinical reports by some groups (but not all) of significantly higher toxicity of AZA in patients with impaired kidney function (J. F. Bach, 1975). On the other hand, abnormalities in the apparent AZA metabolism evaluated by this bioassay were reported in liver disease (J. F. Bach, 1975), a fact that should caution against the use of this compound in autoimmune hepatic conditions (Soloway *et al.*, 1971).

As seen also in various *in vitro* conditions (Berenbaum, 1961; Frisch and Davies, 1962; Sahiar and Schwartz, 1966), 6-MP and AZA can inhibit antibody production *in vivo,* primary responses appearing much more sensitive than secondary. The dose–response curve is clearly hyperbolic (Figure 1) (Spreafico *et al.*, 1973), as expected for an antimetabolite. IgG production is more easily suppressed than IgM production, and it is also possible in selected experimental conditions (e.g., low antigen and drug doses) to totally suppress the former type of antibodies while sparing the latter. The timing of drug treatment relative to antigenic challenge is critical in all animal species and with all defined antigens investigated. The optimum time for observing significant immunodepression is within 48 hr of antigen injection. Pretreatment, even prolonged, is generally much less effective, and indeed can lead to a stimulation of antibody production (Schwartz, 1966). In man, antibody production is relatively resistant, since a depression in titers to primary or recall antigens is observable only when these agents are administered in high doses (Santos *et al.*, 1964; Hersh *et al.*, 1966). Following drug cessation, recovery appears to be rapid. With the lower doses generally employed in chronic treatments, the effects are modest or negative (Denman *et al.*, 1970; Lee *et al.*, 1971), and also in patients with kidney grafts under treatment with AZA, there is usually little or no depression of humoral immunity (Waller *et al.*, 1972).

Various studies showed that thiopurines can depress cell-mediated reactivities in animals ranging from DH to the more common antigens (Borel and Schwartz, 1964; Dietrich and Hess, 1970; Phillips and Zweiman, 1973), to GVH (Barnes *et al.*, 1966), and various experimental autoimmune diseases (Spiegelberg and Miescher, 1963; Vogel and Calabresi, 1969). It should be noted that for most of these reactivities negative results were also observed. Comparisons among the various

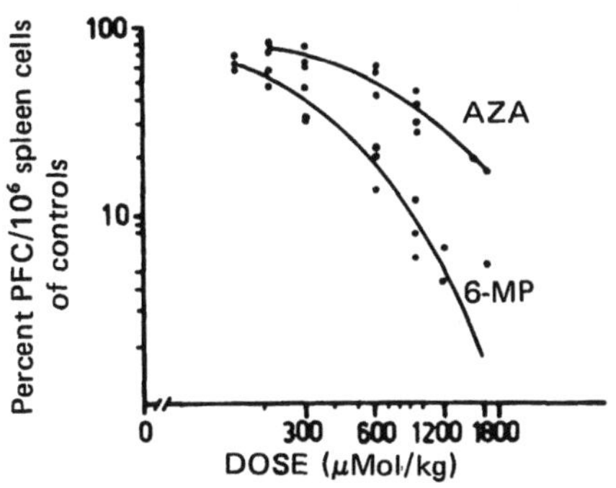

Figure 1. Comparative depression of peak anti-SRBC splenic PFC response after intravenous treatment with AZA or 6-MP in mice.

studies are frequently very difficult in view of the differences in the sensitization procedures and in the drug treatments employed. The action of 6-MP in depressing DH is complex, with effects on both specific and nonspecific mechanisms. With treatments initiated at the time of antigenic stimulation, blocking of sensitization can be obtained (Borel and Schwartz, 1964), with reduction of the *in vitro* lymphocyte proliferative response to antigen (Winkelstein *et al.*, 1973), but with no effects on MIF release (Brown *et al.*, 1976). Effects on the efferent phase are also recognizable, although it is still unclear whether these effects involve only nonspecific mechanisms. In a careful study, Phillips and Zweiman (1973) obtained evidence favoring the latter view, identifying bone-marrow-derived nonsensitized cells (most probably monocytes) recruited in the periphery by the lymphocyte–antigen interaction as the primary target of 6-MP-induced depression of DH in the guinea pig. Although the effect on mononuclear phagocytes still needs further development, the depression in promonocyte production and marked monocytopenia (Van Furth *et al.*, 1973) following AZA is probably one of the major mechanisms underlying the antiinflammatory activity of these agents. As regards *in vitro* cellular responses, AZA can inhibit MLR (M. A. Bach and Bach, 1972) when the drug is added at the beginning of the cultures. Delayed introduction of the chemical when DNA synthesis is at its peak is ineffective, a finding that was interpreted by these authors as implying a blockade of cell recognition. The generation under these conditions of killer cells, a process that requires cell proliferation, is also prevented by early AZA treatments. However, no effects of AZA are seen in cell-mediated cytotoxicity tests when presensitized cells are used (Brown *et al.*, 1976), findings that would support an antiproliferative effect by this agent. The PHA response *in vitro* of human and animal cells can also be blocked by similar early AZA treatment, although the doses required are relatively high. The requirement of significantly higher drug concentrations to inhibit the response to pokeweed mitogen (a T and B lymphocyte stimulant) may indicate a lower sensitivity of B cells to the drug. The PHA or antigen responsiveness of lymphocytes from patients or animals under AZA treatment is very controversial, since both show significant depressions and no decreases have been reported.

Since the first studies of Calne *et al.* (1962) showing the possibility of prolonging kidney allograft survival in dogs with 6-MP or AZA, various other groups have confirmed the effects of these agents on skin and organ grafts. Again, positive results have not been obtained in every case (see J. F. Bach, 1975), large doses being necessary especially when strong histocompatibility differences are involved. A great deal of effort has been made to correlate various *in vitro* tests with the immune status of the kidney allograft recipient. So far, none of the tests employed has revealed a satisfactory method for predicting the outcome of the transplant, while at the same time, the tests have shown that the immunodepression given by AZA in these patients is at best partial. That AZA treatment in this condition is undoubtedly effective indicates that the mechanisms responsible for the prolonged survival of kidneys obtained with this agent are still imperfectly understood, a conclusion that is true not only for man but also for animals (Simonian and Murray, 1971).

As regards the effects of these thiopurines on lymphocyte subpopulations, there now exists a reasonably large body of evidence favoring an activity of AZA and 6-MP on T cells. As extensively reviewed by J. F. Bach (1975), this conclusion rests essentially on the findings that these agents appear to be more active both in man and in rodents on T-cell-mediated responses (MLR, blast transformation by antigens or nonspecific stimulants, cell-mediated lymphotoxicity, DH, and organ graft rejection) than on humoral antibody production. There is also an effect on cell-mediated autoimmune diseases in animals, whereas no clear effects were seen in the autoimmune disease of NZB mice (Gelfand and Steinberg, 1972), which is associated with B-cell hyperactivity. In parallel, AZA treatments are accompanied by a greater increase in T-cell-dependent viral infections than in B-cell-dependent bacterial infections (Fournier *et al.*, 1973). More directly, one could also cite the preferential inhibition of IgG antibody production, known to be more T-dependent than IgM synthesis, and the inability of AZA to suppress *in vitro* responses to T-independent antigens even at doses much higher than those capable of suppressing the response to T-dependent stimuli (Rollinghoff *et al.*, 1973). Last, AZA has a selective inhibitory capacity on T-rosette-forming cells, a sensitivity that is lost after thymectomy, is absent in nude mice, and reappears after treatment with thymic hormone (J. F. Bach, 1975). It is still possible, however, that this selectivity is relative rather than absolute, and that other immunocyte subpopulations may also be affected, e.g., killer (K) cells, which, although resistant *in vitro* (Brown *et al.*, 1976), are inhibited by AZA treatments *in vivo* (Purves and Berenbaum, 1975).

If the cellular basis for immunodepression by AZA and 6-MP has not been entirely clarified, the same conclusion also applies for the mechanisms of these agents at the subcellular level. In fact, while inhibition of DNA, RNA, and protein synthesis obtained by blocking *de novo* purine synthesis and interconversion (Elion and Hitchings, 1975) may account for many aspects of immunodepression by these drugs, other biological activities are difficult to reconcile with an inhibition of DNA synthesis. We are referring, for instance, to the very rapid and reversible inhibition of rosette-forming T cells and of MLR *in vitro* (M. A. Bach and Bach, 1972; Debray-Sachs *et al.*, 1973; Rollinghoff *et al.*, 1973), findings that have been taken as indications of an interference with antigen recognition and the biochemical basis of which is still unknown. Thus, whether the antiproliferative activity is the sole basis for the immunodepression by these thiopurines is still an open question.

4. Cyclophosphamide

Alkylating agents were among the first chemicals to be investigated for their immunodepressive capacity, since in 1921 Hektoen and Corper (1921) showed a reduction in hemolysin and agglutinin formation in rabbits stimulated with SRBC after the injection of toxic doses of nitrogen mustard. Despite this finding, comparatively less attention has been devoted to the immunodepressive activity of alkylating agents than to other classes of compounds. This lack of attention is difficult to understand considering that although a number of alkylating drugs are weak immunodepressants or possess low therapeutic indexes (e.g., uracil mustard, triethylene melanine, chlorambucil), others such as Cy, imidazole-4-carboxamide-5-(3,3-dimethyl-1-triazeno) (DTIC), and melphalan have remarkable characteristics in this sense. Among the latter drugs, Cy is by far the most extensively investigated because of its potency. It is probably the most potent chemical immunodepressant so far available. With appropriate treatment as regards dose and schedule, it has broad and marked effects on immunologic responsiveness that are obtained with

TABLE 5. Effect of Antitumor Drugs on Spleen Cellularity, Antibody-Forming Cells, and ^{59}Fe Uptake of Erythroid Cells

Drug	Δ log number of spleen cells	Δ log CPM	Δ log PFC/spleen	δ = Δ log PFC − Δ log CPM
300 R	0.662	0.721	0.945	0.224
600 R	1.195	0.998	1.427	0.429
Cyclophosphamide	0.538	0.750	2.355	1.605
Demecolcine	0.156	0.224	1.114	0.890
Methotrexate	0.115	1.887	2.329	0.442
BCNU	0.196	0.567	0.996	0.429
Busulphan	0.437	0.162	0.551	0.388
Cytosine arabinoside	0.776	1.135	0.178	0.357
Orthomerphalan	0.539	1.263	1.429	0.166
6-Mercaptopurine	0.133	0.374	0.480	0.106
Procarbazine	0.375	1.093	0.749	−0.344
Aminochlorambucil	0.449	0.779	0.334	−0.445
Prednisolone	0.346	0.615	0.155	−0.460
Actinomycin D	0.110	0.483	−0.025	−0.508
Mitomycin C	0.236	1.393	−0.611	−0.782
Vinblastine	0.277	1.279	0.269	−1.010
Vincristine	0.018	1.357	0.032	−1.325

relatively lower general toxicity. In an elegant series of studies in which the bone marrow proliferative capacity, assessed by the appearance of ^{59}Fe-incorporating cells in the circulation, was evaluated simultaneously with the effects on spleen PFC, Floersheim (1970) determined that Cy possesses the more favorable index in comparison with radiation, MTX, 6-MP, procarbazine, cytosine arabinoside (ara-C), prednisolone, and the vinca alkaloids (Table 5).

Single Cy injections in relatively low doses will induce a marked and rapid decrease in cellularity in lymphoid organs with a profound lymphopenia characterized predominantly by a decrease in small- and medium-sized lymphocytes (Turk and Poulter, 1972). In constrast, equitoxic doses of 6-MP do not cause marked changes in the circulating levels of the same cells in the mouse; the reductions are essentially in the number of polymorphs, monocytes, and large lymphocytes (Lemmel *et al.,* 1971). In addition, 6-MP causes a reduction in the hematocrit not seen with Cy, a further indication of the relatively greater selectivity of the latter for the lymphoid tissue. The selective efficacy ratio—i.e., the ratio between the doses that reduce hematopoietic stem cells and those that reduce by 50% primary PFC precursors is in fact 8.9 for Cy in the mouse (Vecchi *et al.,* 1976b).

Another important and distinguishing property of Cy is that immunodepression is obtainable with drug injections administered either before or after antigen stimulation, as would be expected from a cell-cycle-nonspecific agent. Considering, however, that Cy is clearly proliferation-dependent (Bruce *et al.,* 1966) and that in nonproliferating elements the damaged DNA, the main biochemical target of alkylators, stands a better chance of being repaired, it is not surprising that the greatest immunodepression is seen with Cy treatments given after antigen, the most sensitive period being between 48 hr before and 2 days after challenge. Figure 2 (Vecchi *et al.,* 1976b) shows the high potency of Cy in depressing a primary antibody response and the steep exponential dose–response curve present in these conditions and compares these effects with the inhibitory ones induced by DTIC. Cy does not suppress only primary IgM and IgG antibody production. It suppresses secondary responses to a lesser degree than the primary response, with a ratio of approximately 1.3 between the doses that cause 50% reduction of total primary and those that determine 50% reduction of secondary anti-SRBC AFC in the mouse. According to our experience, this differential is more favorable for Cy than for other chemicals such as AZA, MTX, or steroids. This inhibition of antibody response, which is also observable in man when appropriate doses are used, is not mediated by an effect on mature AFC, which, as intermitotic cells, are relatively resistant to Cy, but is rather attributable to the antiproliferative activity of the agent. In addition, Cy can decrease DH in several species (Winkelstein *et al.*, 1972), including man (Santos *et al.*, 1971), in whom treatment with this agent can be associated with a reduction in PHA (Alepa *et al.*, 1970), antigen-induced lymphocyte transformation (Stockman *et al.*, 1973), and possibly MIF production (Winkelstein *et al.*, 1973). Under selected conditions, Cy can also increase DH reactions, possibly as the consequence of the interruption of a feedback control exerted by B (Turk *et al.*, 1972) or suppressor T cells (Mitsuoka *et al.*, 1976) on effector T cells. Since the main consequence of Cy effects on cells is to restrict their ability to complete mitosis, damaged lymphocytes may retain the capacity to function normally in the nondividing state. This may explain the observations of a dichotomy between a depressed *in vitro* antigen-induced lymphocyte replication and the preserved activity of sensitized cells to function in cell-mediated reactions or antibody production (Winkelstein *et al.*, 1974). In this depression of DH, the antiinflammatory activity that Cy possesses, which is less than that of other chemical immunodepressants (Perper *et al.*, 1971), does not appear to play a major role. The same conclusion would also seem to apply for the favorable activity obtained with this agent in various experimental autoimmune conditions with an effect not only in the prevention of disease induction, but also on established disease (Paterson *et al.*, 1971), the signs and symptoms of which can be significantly ameliorated for long periods even with relatively short courses of treatments. Of relevance for its practical implications is the fact that Cy is capable of influencing the autoimmune disease of NZB and B/W mice. Appearance of disease can be

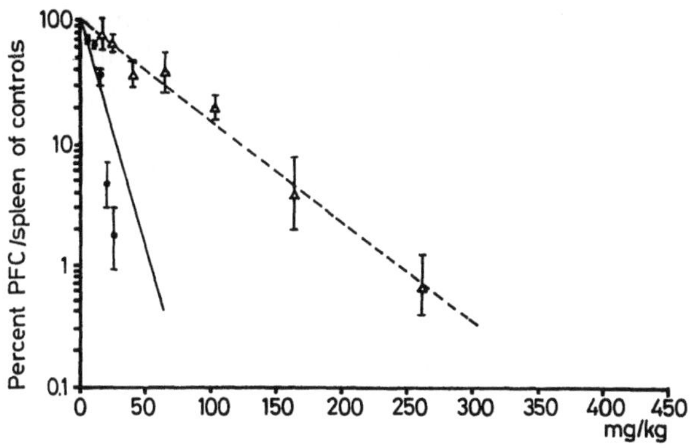

Figure 2. Depression of peak anti-SRBC splenic PFC response after intraperitoneal treatment with Cy or DTIC in mice. (•———•) Cy; (∇———∇) DTIC. The vertical brackets denote S.E.M.

blocked with treatments initiated early in life (Morton *et al.*, 1972), and active disease can be significantly ameliorated when later treatments are used (Russel and Hicks, 1968). In comparison with other drugs, Cy was found to be superior to AZA or methylprednisolone in the treatment of this autoimmune disease, but a combination of Cy and steroids is more effective, and the combination of the three agents is the most effective (Gelfand and Steinberg, 1972). It should also be noted that in this condition, which bears a number of resemblances to human lupus erythematosus, injections of Poly I:Poly C followed by Cy can lead to very marked reductions in the titers of antinuclear antibodies (Steinberg and Talal, 1970). A similar observation was made in animals with established autoimmune thyroiditis in which repeated courses of thyroid antigens followed by Cy led to a suppression of antithyroid autoantibodies (Nakamura and Weigle, 1970), a finding that was interpreted as the progressive extinction by the drug of the memory clones stimulated by the repeated antigen injection. Although controlled studies are still limited in number, Cy showed significant activity in various autoimmune diseases, including systemic lupus erythematosus (Feng *et al.*, 1973), the nephrotic syndrome (Drummond *et al.*, 1968), and rheumatoid arthritis (Fosdick, 1971). On theoretical grounds, this agent, the half-life of which in man is of the order of 4–6 hr, should be employed with caution in autoimmune liver disease, considering that it is in this organ that the biotransformation of Cy, which is inactive *per se*, occurs.

Although a few negative reports have appeared (Zukoski *et al.*, 1963b), a general consensus exists that Cy can significantly prolong the survival of organ or skin allografts in various species (Berenbaum and Brown, 1963; Santos, 1967; Silvers *et al.*, 1967). This effect is not mediated by tolerance induction or by enhancing antibodies, but would rather seem to be due to a depression of cell-mediated cytotoxicity, as directly demonstrated by Husberg (1972). The possible role played by a reduction by Cy of graft "immunogenicity" (Guttmann and Lindquist, 1969) remains to be evaluated. These positive results in animals were confirmed by Starzl *et al.* (1973) in liver and kidney transplant patients in whom combined treatments of Cy with antilymphocyte globulin (ALG) and prednisone appeared superior to previous experience with the standard treatment (AZA, ALS, and steroids). Another cell-mediated reactivity that can be suppressed by Cy even with late treatment is GVH (Santos and Owens, 1966). This effect is seen not only in rodents and chickens, but also in monkeys. More important for its therapeutic potential is the capacity of Cy to facilitate the induction of tolerance not only to soluble antigens, a result that can also be obtained with other chemicals (although with less ease and for shorter periods than with Cy), but also to particulate antigens (Frisch and Davies, 1966; Many and Schwartz, 1970a,b; Aisenberg and Murray, 1973). This state of specific unresponsiveness, the cellular basis of which in terms of the lymphocyte population(s) involved is still unclear (Aisenberg and Murray, 1973), occurs normally with the administration of relatively high Cy doses very near to antigen injection, and presumably results in the elimination by the drug of the relevant stimulated, proliferating clones. Unresponsiveness can be very long-lasting, its duration being dependent on the use of high doses of weak antigens, a repetition of antigen administration, and thymectomy. This capacity of Cy was employed by Santos and his group (Santos, 1972) in the first reasonably effective protocol for bone marrow transplantation in man. The recipient is primed with blood from the donor, followed 24 hr later by the first of 4 Cy injections at 40 mg/kg, to inactivate the stimulated lymphocytes and to create the "space" for the actual bone marrow transplant performed on day 6. Although good results were reported for the majority of patients in terms of graft take, the necessity for very high and toxic drug doses in cases of a GVH resulting from the inability of serologically defined histocompatibility antigens to assure the appropriate matching between donor and recipient (F. H. Bach *et al.*, 1976) is still a major problem to be overcome in this field. A similar approach with Cy was used to induce tolerance to solubilized histocompatibility antigens prior to mouse skin grafts (Halle-Pannenko *et al.*, 1970) or to equine γ-globulin prior to initiation of therapy with ALS (Stockman *et al.*, 1972).

The last point to be considered in this brief review of Cy immunodepression concerns its effects on lymphocyte subpopulations. Although a possible effect of Cy on macrophages is indicated by a reduction in antigen-trapping in lymph nodes (Nettesheim and Hammons, 1970), this drug is classically considered to be selectively toxic for B cells. The initial evidence in favor of this conclusion derives from the work of Turk and his colleagues (Turk *et al.*, 1972; Turk and Poulter, 1972) showing the occurrence after single high doses of a specific depletion of non-thymus-dependent areas of the lymphoid tissue, with a marked enrichment in the percentage of T cells. As might have been expected, remembering the preferential effect of Cy on proliferating cells, treatment with this drug is followed by a marked destruction of short-lived lymphocytes, a population mainly composed of non-T cells. In addition, one may cite the synergism of Cy with thymectomy or ALS in inducing peripheral lymphoid depletion and the possibility of obtaining with this drug a true chemical bursectomy in neonatal chickens (Lenna *et al.*, 1972). Functionally, this selectivity would explain various *in vivo* activities of this agent already mentioned, such as its effects on the autoimmune disease of NZB mice, which is associated with B-cell hyperactivity and T-cell deficiency, or the possibility of curing Cy-promoted viral infections with passive antibody. It should be emphasized, however, that this selectivity for B cells is far from absolute; T lymphocytes are also sensitive to Cy even when the drug is administered in a single high dose, as indicated, for instance, by the necessity for both T and B cells to reconstitute the immune capacity of Cy-treated mice (J. F. Bach and Dardenne, 1972). An effect on T cells is also shown by the inhibitory activity of Cy on clearly T-dependent reactivities such as experimental allergic encephalomyelitis and autoimmune thyroiditis, PHA- and antigen-induced blast transformation, and allograft survival. Recent information suggests that a subpopulation of T lymphocytes is rapidly dividing (J. W. Moorhead and Claman, 1974), and thus probably sensitive to Cy. Treatment conditions will thus influence very much the selectivity of its action on one or the other of the lymphocyte populations. The final result will be the sum of the interplay of a series of complex factors, such as the relative turnover rates and proliferative status of the relevant populations, drug dose, course, and timing in respect to antigen, and the relative roles played by cellular and humoral mechanisms in any given reactivity.

Among the other immunodepressive alkylating agents, two deserve brief mention mainly to reemphasize the interesting properties of this class of compounds. The first is melphalan, which, although it was reported to have a high therapeutic index in mice and to be immunodepressive in man (Makinodan *et al.*, 1970), has not been investigated extensively. The second is DTIC, a compound widely employed in the treatment of human melanoma, which has shown a remarkably long-lasting immunodepressive activity on both humoral and cell-mediated responsiveness, especially when it is injected before antigen. Single nontoxic injections depress allograft reactivity across the *H-2* barrier in mice for 2 months, through a mechanism that does not involve extensive cellular destruction (Vecchi *et al.*, 1976b). In view of its immunodepressive activity on both cellular and humoral responses exerted when given before or after antigen stimulation, the antitumor agent procarbazine has a number of similarities to Cy and other alkylators. This agent has not, however, been submitted to a more detailed analysis, even though it is employed on a relatively large scale for the treatment of lymphoid malignancies, possibly because it is a relatively potent carcinogen in animals.

The crucial steps in the metabolism of Cy occur at the level of the liver microsomal enzymes (Figure 3) (Hohorst *et al.*, 1976), i.e., the enzymatic system, which is generally considered to play the major role in the biotransformation of a large variety of both exogenous and endogenous substances, rendering this drug a very suitable one for investigation of drug interactions in cytotoxic treatment, considering that a number of agents can modify the activity of the liver microsomes. The problem of drug interactions has not received systematic analysis in the pharmacology of immunodepression, although it should have considerable clinical interest, since the patient under immunodepressive therapy is most often given multiple medications directed against his major immunologic disturbance, for the treatment of other concomitant diseases, and/or in the frame of a general supportive therapy. In considering this problem, one can expect both interactions between immunodepressants and interactions between immunodepressants and other, non-immunodepressive, agents. This second consideration in turn has two aspects, namely, the effects of other drugs on the activity of the immunodepressant and the consequences of a concomitant or previous administration of cytotoxic agents on the activity of other drugs. It is known from experimental cancer chemotherapy that a combination of two effective cytotoxics will not always result in greater cell-killing than seen with either drug alone; schedule-dependent antagonisms have been described between MTX and 5-fluorouracil (5-FU), MTX and ara-C, and MTX and L-asparaginase (Goldin *et al.*, 1974). This type of interaction is also seen with the immunodepressive effect of these agents, which is illustrated in Table 6 for the MTX–L-asparaginase combination as well as the combinations between steroids and MTX (Garattini *et al.*, 1975). The mechanisms of these interactions are varied and not entirely elucidated. They range from reciprocal interferences with the biochemical modes of cell-killing or with drug uptake by the cells or with both, as for the MTX–L-asparaginase and steroid–MTX antagonisms, to modifications in the rate of drug biotransformation, as for the Cy–steroid interaction. Qualitative or quantitative changes in drug metabolism, or both, are the explanations of the interaction observed when phenobarbital, a typical microsomal "inducer," is given with various chemical immunodepressants (Spreafico *et al.*, 1974). It may be of interest that a number of agents possess a "latent" immunodepressive activity, so that they should be used with some caution in patients already undergoing "overt" immunodepressive treatment or in those conditions in which immune defenses are physiologically or pathologically lowered. Drugs of the phenothiazine class are perhaps the best known in this category (Garry and Ukeyi, 1972), but the list has been growing in recent years to include agents of different pharmacological classes

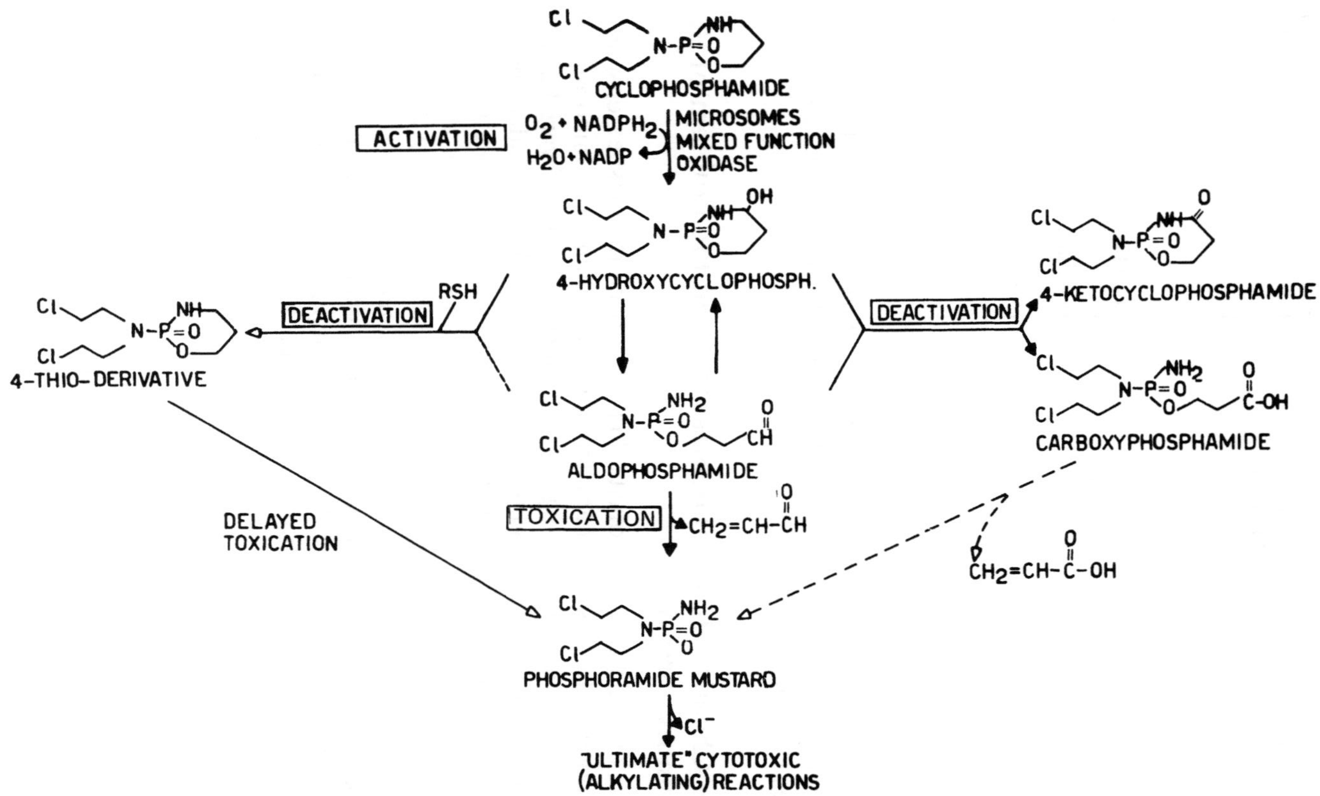

Figure 3. Routes of metabolic activation and deactivation of Cy in the light of reactions that have been postulated or identified either *in vivo* or *in vitro*.

TABLE 6. Drug Antagonism in Immunodepressive Treatments[a]

Experimental group	Drug dose	Day of treatment	PFC/spleen ($\times 10^{-3}$)
Controls	—	—	420
L-Asparaginase	50 IU	1	60
Methotrexate	20 mg/kg	1	6
L-Asparaginase + Methotrexate	50 IU / 20 mg/kg	1 / 1	56
Controls	—	—	58
Prednisone	30 mg/kg	1 (−4 hr)	64
Methotrexate	10 mg/kg	1	9
Prednisone + Methotrexate	30 mg/kg / 10 mg/kg	1 (−4 hr) / 1	43

[a] 4×10^8 SRBC given on day 0.

such as griseofulvin (F. Mitchell *et al.*, 1973), rifampicin (Spreafico *et al.*, unpublished observations), steroid contraceptive agents (Vecchi *et al,*, 1976a), and anesthetic gases (Viljanen *et al.*, 1973).

5. Other Chemical Immunodepressants and the Problem of Selective Immunosuppression

Among the folic acid antagonists, MTX has been the most extensively investigated compound, although its characterization in a number of important aspects is more incomplete than for other agents. Although a degree of variability has been described in different species and test systems, it may be concluded that MTX is a potent immunodepressant with a relatively favorable therapeutic ratio in both animals and man (Hersh, 1974), suggesting that in treatment of autoimmunity the therapeutic value of MTX may in effect be better than of AZA or Cy. This immunodepressive activity is characterized by a marked capacity to interfere with antibody production, especially when the drug, which is known to be cell-cycle-specific, is given at the height of the proliferation phase of the response. Treatment prior to the antigen is ineffective or may even lead to an increase in antibody production (Uyeki, 1967). The latter paradoxical phenomenon is known to occur in animals and in man after treatment with other immunodepressants, and is possibly to be linked with the "overshoot" in immune reactivity described after interruption of therapy in patients. Although a hypothetical mechanism was discussed by Makinodan *et al.* (1970), the basis for these effects remains essentially unknown. Although comparisons with other agents are often difficult, MTX is generally considered to be one of the most potent inhibitors of the establishment of DH, although its antiinflammatory activity probably plays a role in this capacity. The drug is effective in GVH and autoimmune conditions, although it is perhaps not a good suppressor of the allograft rejection, a finding that has led to the contention by some groups that cellular reactivities may be more resistant than humoral responses to this agent.

An important feature of pharmacological activity of MTX is the availability of a specific antidote, folinic acid. By analogy with what is known of its antitumor effect, by an appropriate scheduling of the two agents, inhibition of the toxic effects with a maintenance of MTX immunodepression can be obtained, as first described in mice by Berenbaum and Brown (1965). Although the applicability of this principle to man was confirmed by M. S. Mitchell *et al.* (1969), this approach seems, somewhat surprisingly, not to have been explored for human therapy. It is possible that the favorable effects recently obtained with folinic acid rescue after high-dose MTX treatment in certain human neoplastic conditions may induce a reevaluation of the use of this agent in immunosuppressive therapy. The renal route of drug excretion may represent an important limitation in kidney transplants.

The vinca alkaloids deserve only brief mention in this context in view of their low therapeutic ratio as immunodepressants in animals; generally, high doses are required to observe an effect, and the myelodepressive activity is much higher than the immunodepressive one. Even though one study (Santos *et al.*, 1964) found no immunodepression in man, considering its relatively widespread use in clinical oncology, a reconsideration of immunodepressive activity, especially in combination therapy, would not seem unwarranted. A low therapeutic ratio is also the main limiting characteristic of agents such as puromycin, mitomycin C, azaserine, and actinomycin D, the last being the only one among these antibiotics to have been employed clinically on a relatively large scale for the treatment of acute rejection crises. Its activity has never really been proved, however, and its therapeutic use has been practically abandoned. Actinomycin D is thus exploited only as a tool to analyze selected aspects of the biochemistry and molecular biology of immunocyte activity, taking advantage of the selective action of this compound on DNA-dependent RNA synthesis.

Although the nucleoside analogue and specific inhibitor of DNA synthesis ara-C is immunodepressive, its short half-life is a limit to practical exploitation. This agent can inhibit humoral antibody responses in both animals and man; however, ara-C does not appear to prolong allograft survival in rodents or dogs, and its suppression of GVH development is moderate (Hersh, 1974). Thus, this compound has a comparatively low therapeutic index as an immunodepressant. In this regard, the recent ester derivatives that act by slowly releasing ara-C in the circulation appear more interesting, and the palmitate derivative was reported to possess a remarkable potency in animals (Gray *et al.*, 1972) and deserves more careful investigation for a possible human use, considering the availability of a specific antidote, deoxycytidine, for this class of compounds. A potentially important property of the adamantoyl derivative of ara-C is its preferential activity on cellular vs. humoral responses (Gray *et al.*, 1972), a type of differential activity similar to that displayed by ALS (Spreafico, 1972) and, among the newer chemical immunodepressants, by niridazole and oxisuran. Treatments with both agents have in fact been shown to prolong allograft survival while being less inhibitory for humoral responses (Pelley *et al.*, 1975; A. E. Fox *et al.*, 1973). Although comparatively little information is available, chemicals that exhibit a preferential suppressive activity on humoral vs. cellular responsiveness are also known. As already noted, Cy, in selected conditions of drug dose, schedule, and timing with respect to antigen, can be a selective B-cell depressant (Dennert *et al.*, 1975). The bisdioxopiperazines ICRF 154 and 159 may be very similar, as suggested by their effectiveness in depressing antibody formation while not prolonging allograft survival (Duke *et al.*, 1973). The interest in this type of finding derives from the more immediate goals of a more rational immunodepression with greater selectivity in immunologic manipulation, so as to eliminate those components of the immune reactivity that play a pathogenetic role while sparing others that could be of therapeutic value.

So far, the only attempts to exploit selective immunodepression therapeutically in conditions in which humoral and cell-mediated reactivities have contrasting effects appear to be those of Calabresi, Heppner, and associates employing a solid tumor in which serum factors block the expression of cell-mediated immunity (CMI) (Heppner *et al.*, 1974). By a careful choice of ara-C dose and schedule, they could obtain a significant delay in mammary carcinoma progression due to an inhibition in the development of blocking serum factors and a sparing of CMI. Conditions of treatment with ara-C are very stringent, however, and in the more recent studies of this group, 5-FU was found to have a somewhat greater flexibility. The best results to date were obtained with the complex MTX–folinic acid–5-FU combination. Although these data are obviously partial and need to be extended to other conditions in which even limited degrees of selectivity would be of therapeutic interest (e.g., the sparing of enhancing serum activity in kidney transplantation), it should be concluded that a more on-target immune manipulation is possible employing the relatively "crude" agents now available.

Selectivity in immunodepression of antineoplastic agents alone and in combination with nonspecific immunotherapy has clear implications for more effective cancer therapy. The differential capacity of antitumor agents to affect the various lymphocyte subpopulations and, consequently, the various immune effector mechanisms should be considered in light of the fact that immunostimulants also vary in their effects on the different specific and nonspecific effector mechanisms (see Chapter 14). The goal would thus be not only to employ less immunodepressive chemotherapy agents or more selective treatments, but also to pair these drugs rationally with immunostimulants that act on mechanisms not affected by the previous or concomitant chemotherapy. Such "complementary" types of chemoimmunotherapy are probably the explanation for the marked synergism observed between adriamycin and the immunomodulator *Corynebacterium parvum* (Tagliabue *et al.*, 1977). Not even additive effects are seen when equiactive doses of daunomycin are used. As mentioned, adriamycin spares macrophages and antibody-dependent cellular cytotoxicity, which are both important targets in the immunostimulatory mode of action of this adjuvant (Mantovani, 1977).

The mechanisms by which chemical immunodepressants exert such preferential activity on different lymphocyte subpopulations remain essentially unknown. Since both phase-specific and -nonspecific agents with biochemical modes of action have been found to have this activity, this property does not seem to be specific for any single class of compounds. Most of the selective chemical agents appear to preferentially affect proliferating rather than resting cells, a fact that may explain a preferential sensitivity of B cells and of the rapidly proliferating proportion of T cells; however, purely cytokinetic mechanisms do not account for all known aspects of this phenomenon. The distribution in the various lymphoid organs of the different agents as well as of those enzymes involved in their activation or inactivation is largely unknown. It may be relevant in this connection to mention that the thymus has a high activity of deoxycytidine kinase, the enzyme that activates ara-C, which perhaps accounts for the preferential activity of adamantoyl-ara-C on CMI (Gray *et al.*, 1972). It is possible that various lymphocyte subpopulations at rest or after immune activation differ in certain metabolic aspects, and that mechanisms other than cell-killing are operative to account for the very high sensitivity of macrophages to daunomycin. The activity of these drugs on the production or activity or both of the various factors recently proposed as physiologic regulators of the immune response has not yet been explored. Thus, until more basic information on the normal regulation of immunity and on what agents are selective in which conditions is obtained, the basis for this preferential activity will remain speculative.

6. Nonspecific Biological Immunodepressants

The prototype of this class of immunodepressants is ALS, which has been extensively investigated in both animals and man and the use of which has become a "staple" in a number of clinical immunodepressive treatments. More recently, a series of other factors of biological origin have also been described as having immunodepressive or immunoregulatory activity. They represent a group of agents the characteristics and properties of which require more extensive investigation. Accordingly, their true physiologic relevance and therapeutic potential are still undetermined. Although some of these materials will find their major usefulness as probes in the unraveling of the basic regulatory mechanisms of the immune response, others may find future practical exploitation, since, at least in principle, they are closer to the ideal "physiologic" immunodepressant. Without exhaustive review, we will touch on those factors for which sufficient basis for preliminary conclusions appears to exist.

6.1. Interferon

For many years, interferons, a group of proteins ranging from 20,000 to 100,000 in molecular weight, have been investigated for their antiviral activity. More recently, however, evidence has been produced suggesting complex immunoregulatory activity of these substances. It is now established that in addition to being produced by nonlymphoid cells, interferon is released by lymphoid cells in response to various types of inducers, including not only DNA and RNA viruses, but also both T- and B-cell mitogens and specific antigens (Rasmussen *et al.*, 1974). In addition, interferon or substances present in the preparation can increase the cytotoxicity of sensitized splenocytes and enhance phagocytosis; conversely, different nonspecific immunomodulators (e.g., endotoxin, polynucleotides) are all good interferon inducers (Huang *et al.*, 1971; Lindhal-Magnusson *et al.*, 1972). More recently, interferon was shown to depress immune reactivity, including GVH, allograft rejection, lymphocyte recognition *in vitro* and *in vivo* of alloantigens, and the primary or secondary anti-SRBC response (Chester *et al.*, 1973; Brodeur and Merigan, 1974; M. S. Hirsch *et al.*, 1974). Low concentrations (10 U/ml) of partially purified human type I interferon will suppress the *in vitro* lymphocyte response to PHA and Con A and allogeneic stimulation, whereas 1000 U/ml is required to suppress the stimulation by pokeweed mitogen (Blomgren *et al.*, 1974). Suppression of both *in vitro* and *in vivo* antibody production is observed with treatments during the inductive period, whereas the phase of antibody synthesis appears to be insensitive; indeed, in *in vitro* systems, late treatments can lead to an increase in the detectable AFC number, followed later by an apparent exhaustion of the response (Gisler *et al.*, 1974).

The precise mechanism of interferon-induced immunosuppression of both T and B cells is not known. The effects on the inductive phase of the immune response, the multiplication of mouse cells in culture (Lindhal-Magnusson *et al.*, 1971), and the replication of lymphocytes transferred to lethally irradiated recipients (Cerottini *et al.*, 1973) would indicate an antiproliferative action. However, that interferon can also be immunostimulatory suggests that a multiplicity of mechanisms are operative. This biological activity of interferon may provide an explanatory basis for the immunodepression observed during certain viral infections or found after treatment with nonspecific mitogens. However, since interferon is both produced by and has complex effects on lymphoid cells, we are tempted to suggest that it has a locally important immunoregulatory role in the response to viral and nonviral antigens.

6.2. Chalones

Other factors that presumably play a role in the complex control of the immune response are the lymphocytic chalones. By definition, a chalone is a non-species-specific, tissue-specific endogenous mitotic inhibitor; i.e., it is present in and synthesized by the tissue on which it exerts an antiproliferative activity through a noncytotoxic mechanism (Bullough, 1975). On this basis, it is understandable that lymphocyte chalones have attracted interest in the hope of obtaining a physiologic immunosuppressant. After the initial observations of J. F. Moorhead *et al.* (1969), various other *in vivo* and *in vitro* immune reactivities were shown to be inhibited by such materials, which, chemically, are glycoproteins of molecular weight 30,000–50,000. These activities include a decrease in PHA reactivity with a block in MIF release obtained *in vitro* with concentrations of 50 μg/ml, and depressions of anti-SRBC responsiveness, allograft rejection, and GVH. The latter reactivity is inhibited either by *in vitro* pretreatment of the cells to be infused or by early treatments of the recipient (Houck *et al.*, 1973; Kiger *et al.*, 1972; Florentin *et al.*, 1973). Using an alcohol extract from lamb thymus, Florentin and associates showed an inhibition of the response to T-dependent antigens with sparing of antibody production to T-independent stimuli, thus suggesting a T-lymphocyte specificity for thymus product. However, similar chalones extracted from the spleen can apparently act on both T and B cells, as might have been expected considering the mixed composition of this organ. It would thus appear that the duality of the lymphoid system is also expressed in the chalone regulatory mechanism, with specific factors for each of the main cell lineages.

The mechanism of action of chalones is still undetermined. The capacity to block, through a noncytotoxic mechanism, spontaneous DNA synthesis of lymphocytes in short-term culture (Houck *et al.*, 1973) may be taken as indicative of an activity on cell proliferation rather than on antigen recognition, by analogy with what is known for other chalones (Bullough, 1975). Considering the role of cyclic nucleotides in lymphocyte function, it is not surprising that an interaction of the epidermal chalone with the cyclic nucleotide system was recently observed (Elgjö,

1975). However, the biochemical basis of chalone activity remains to be clarified. Also, it is not known whether there exists a single compound or a family of chalones, possibly blocking the cells in different phases of the cell cycle. Ignorance also surrounds the relationships between chalones and mitosis-promoting mesenchymal factors, which seem to constitute the other component that intervenes in the regulation of tissue mass.

6.3. Low-Molecular-Weight Lymphoid Inhibitor

Since chalones are heat-labile, protease-sensitive, high-molecular-weight factors, they should be distinguished from the heat-stable, protease-resistant, low-molecular-weight inhibitor of lymphoid proliferation, which was recently discussed by Ranney (1975) and which is probably identical to the cell-proliferation-inhibitory factor of macrophagic origin described by Waldman and Gottlieb (1973). This chemically unidentified inhibitor(s), which appears to be synthetized and spontaneously released in the supernatant by cultures of unstimulated cells (probably macrophages) of peripheral lymphoid organs of various animal species, is capable of producing a progressive decrease in DNA synthesis and of blocking the division of stimulated or resting B and T lymphocytes. This inhibitor is maximally released in crowded cultures, and appears to act specifically on lymphocytes through a noncytotoxic mechanism that spares protein synthesis, the latter process being, on the other hand, necessary for its production or release or both. Since the release of this non-species-specific inhibitor is blocked by antigenic or mitogenic stimulation, it has been suggested to be a potential feedback regulator of lymphocyte proliferation, acting as a modulator of DNA synthesis and cell division, rather than of the antigen-recognition or lymphocyte-activation phases.

Considering its properties and that the cells that release this inhibitor are widespread in lymphoid organs in proximity to both T and B cells, it was also suggested (Ranney, 1975) that the peripheral lymphoid system may normally be under a nonspecific negative influence lifted by antigen introduction, which is in turn followed by the production by the stimulated cells of additional specific (e.g., antibody, antigen–antibody complexes) and nonspecific antiactivating factors that prevent excessive responses by residual lymphocytes.

In addition to the growth-inhibitory factor described, macrophages also appear to produce a cytotoxic activity. Kramer and Granger (1972) described a "toxin" in cultures of immune macrophages and active against a number of cells. In the past, many investigators have found inhibition of lymphocyte function by the addition of macrophages to the cultures (Unanue, 1972; Keller, 1973). To compound the complexity, it should be recalled that these same cells also appear to release substances that stimulate lymphocyte proliferative capacity in response to lectins (Gery and Waksman, 1972).

6.4. Immunoregulatory α-Globulin

Beginning with the work of Kamrin (1959) showing that circulating rodent α-globulins could prolong the survival of histoincompatible skin grafts, various groups have described the presence in normal mammalian serum of factors migrating in the same region and capable of suppressing immunity. On the basis of available evidence, the responsible substance would appear to be an α-globulin that is not cytotoxic, does not contain cortisol, is heat-stable, lacks protease and ribonuclease activity, and is not species-specific. Immunoregulatory α-globulin (IRA) is a suppressor of T-dependent reactivities, including the *in vitro* response of lymphocytes to mitogens, specific antigens, or tumor cells, spontaneous T-rosette formation, and the release of MIF by sensitized lymphocytes (Cooperband *et al.*, 1972; Glaser and Herberman, 1974). Parallel data have been obtained for its *in vivo* immunodepressive activity as indicated by its capacity to prolong allograft survival and to suppress primary and secondary response to T-dependent but not to T-independent antigens (Menzoian *et al.*, 1974). In inhibiting the mouse anti-SRBC response, only pretreatment with IRA is required. Single doses of 20 mg IRA-protein reduce the peak response by 80–90%. This fact, together with the finding of an inhibition by IRA of specific antigen but not of mitogen binding to lymphocytes at 4°C (Glasgow *et al.*, 1972) and the finding that its addition to cultures after the activation phase does not modify lymphocyte proliferation (Cooperband *et al.*, 1972), suggests that IRA may act as a reversible inhibitor of lymphocyte recognition and activation, rather than of cell division. The ease with which its *in vitro* activity can be reversed by washing suggests a loose binding of IRA to the lymphocyte surface.

It appears that the immunodepressive activity of IRA is contained in a polypeptide of low molecular weight (2000–5000) noncovalently bound to carrier α-globulins (Occhino *et al.*, 1973). This very incomplete characterization of IRA prevents definite conclusions as to its relationships with other serum immunosuppressive factors such as those described by Milton (1971) and Carpenter *et al.* (1971). On the other hand, IRA appears to be very similar, if not identical, to the serum factor of Veit and Michael (1973). That the "antibody-inhibitory factor" described by Ambrose (1973) in serum-free medium of antigen-stimulated rabbit lymphnode cultures is sensitive to ribonuclease indicates that it is different from IRA. The absence of RNAse activity in IRA would also distinguish it from the serum factor of Mawbray (1967). The relationship of IRA to the T-cell chalone is unknown, since its cellular site of origin is undetermined. The finding of an increase in IRA-like activity in both mouse and human serum after antigenic stimulation (Riggio *et al.*, 1969; Veit and Michael, 1973) led to the hypothesis that IRA, or similar factors, may participate in the normal feedback control of T-cell responses. Its capacity to permit the proliferation of a stimulated clone while inhibiting the activation of unstimulated cells could in principle also fit the requirements of the humoral factor postulated by Möller and Sjöberg (1971) as playing a role in antigenic competition among T-cell-dependent antigens.

Since IRA is found in trace amounts in normal human blood, a potentially interesting source for its isolation could be the serum of cancer patients in whom an immunodepressive, non-species-specific peptide that physicochemically resembles IRA can be found in high quantities (Nimberg *et al.*, 1975), possibly as a response to an antigenic load. This factor could presumably play a role in the failure of cancer patients to respond immunologically.

6.5. α-Fetoprotein

Another factor for which a nonspecific immunoregulatory function has been advanced is α-fetoprotein (AFP). This glycoprotein, which represents the dominant serum protein in early embryonic life, was recently shown to be synthesized not only by the liver, but also by immunologically activated spleen and lymph node mononuclear cells (Keller and Tomasi, 1976). AFP has been shown to suppress, through a noncytotoxic mechanism, a variety of experimental immune responses such as primary and secondary anti-SRBC responses and MLR and blastogenesis induced by T-cell mitogens such as Con A (Murgita and Tomasi, 1975). The inhibition seems to be exerted at the recognition or activation phase, since the *in vitro* sensitization of T cells to alloantigens is blocked, whereas the cytotoxicity of activated T cells is unimpaired (Dattwyler and Tomasi, 1975). AFP is not only synthesized by but also binds to lymphocytes, specifically to T cells, as shown indirectly by an analysis of its functional activities and directly by immunofluorescence. Some 20% of purified mouse peripheral T cells bind AFP, but bone marrow cells or lymphocytes from nude mice do not.

The mechanism(s) through which AFP exerts its inhibition of lymphocytes is unknown. It appears to act as a negative-feedback signal for the lymphocyte, since an inverse relationship exists between the quantity of membrane-bound AFP and protein synthesis. Similarly, its physiologic role is still speculative.

Since the inhibitory effect of AFP on lymphocytes is proportional to the intensity of stimulation, this protein may serve as a natural mechanism that helps in the establishment of tolerance to autologous antigens, or in protecting the fetus from the effects of maternal immune mechanisms, or in both. Its disappearance at birth may in addition contribute to the gradual maturation of immunity occurring in the first weeks of life (Murgita and Tomasi, 1975). Serum factors capable of suppressing lymphocyte reactivity to mitogens or antigens were reported to be present in hepatitis, alcoholic and primary biliary cirrhosis, gastrointestinal cancer, and ataxia telangectasia (Yachnin, 1975), all conditions in which increased levels of AFP are found in the circulation. However, considering the minute amounts of AFP that are sufficient to inhibit *in vitro* antibody formation (1 μg/ml, i.e., concentrations that are 1000 times lower than those found in mouse serum at birth), it is possible that local increases in AFP not systemically detectable may play a role in a number of conditions associated with a deficient immune reactivity. In addition to cancer, in which AFP could be produced by the tumor as well as by the stimulated lymphocytes, another condition in which AFP could be a partial explanation is the immunodepression associated with GVH, which is known to be more profound and long-lasting for T-mediated reactivities. Although viruses, T suppressor cells, and macrophages have all been implicated, an immunodepressive factor produced by, and preferentially acting on, T cells was recently described by Phillips *et al.* (1975). Last, it is possible that the immunodepressive activity exerted by certain liver fractions (Mandel *et al.*, 1965; Schumacher *et al.*, 1974), which has been implicated in the longer survival of liver allografts in comparison with those of other organs, may in reality be represented by AFP.

6.6. Phytomitogens

Since the initial demonstration that PHA could exert an immunodepressive activity *in vivo* (Spreafico and Lerner, 1967), a number of other reports have confirmed this activity in various systems. As reviewed by Makinodan *et al.* (1970), this lectin can reduce both skin and organ allograft rejection and the humoral response to various antigens when administered during the sensitization phase. Similar activity is also possessed by other mitogens such as Con A. This substance has been shown to delay allograft rejection in rodents and primates, to inhibit DH reactions and humoral antibody responses, and to decrease the requirement of other immunodepressants in canine renal transplants (Markowitz *et al.*, 1969; Weil *et al.*, 1974; Narayan *et al.*, 1976).

The mechanism of action of these agents is undetermined. Mention has been made of the production of various immunodepressive factors by mitogen-stimulated lymphocytes; however, lymphopenia has also been described by some authors as following Con A treatments (Nirmul *et al.*, 1972). The possibility of an activation of T suppressor cells is suggested. Another potentially interesting use of Con A was recently proposed by Tyan (1974), who observed that because myeloid and erythroid precursors are more resistant to the "toxic" effect of *in vitro* incubation with Con A than mature immunocompetent cells in the bone marrow, Con A reduces the GVH potential of the treated allogeneic marrow preparations. In comparison with physical or immunologic methods of eliminating mature T cells from the bone marrow (e.g., separation by density-gradient centrifugation, alloantisera against T-cell-specific antigens, specific adsorption of lymphocytes by monolayer of host fibroblasts), this approach would seem to offer a number of practical advantages. The use of those physiologic factors that mimic the T-cell-inhibitory effects of Con A without manifesting its toxic properties would be even more ideal.

7. Perspective for Immunologic Control

As repeatedly mentioned in the preceding sections, although beneficial effects have frequently been obtained both in the treatment of autoimmune disease and in the prevention of graft rejection by the use of available chemical and biological immunodepressants, the main limiting feature of such therapeutic intervention is its nonspecific diminution in immune resistance, marked damage to nonlymphoid organs, and an apparent increase in the incidence of neoplasms. Although there is much room for improving existing modalities and developing newer, less toxic, nonspecific immunodepressants for more effective and safe application of immunodepression, it seems clear that the ultimate objective of intervention in this field is to obtain specific suppression of unwanted immune responses. Since the first demonstration of immune tolerance (Owen, 1945), it has become increasingly clear that one can inactivate the cells capable of responding to a particular antigen, or determinant, without interfering with the responses to other antigenic stimuli. A number of possible approaches have now been proposed to produce such selective immune depression.

One of the classic models for tolerance induction in the mature animal involves the injection of high antigen doses in the appropriate physical form. Before this approach can be therapeutically applied, both the histocompatibility and tissue autoantigens to be employed need to be more fully characterized and made available in great quantities. Of potential interest as alternatives would be the use of nonmetabolizable antigens that could maintain the cells in the state of "chronic paralysis" of antigen excess or the use of toxic antigens. The possibility of specifically blocking for extended periods an ongoing response to hapten–protein complex by the injection of hapten-substituted copolymers of D-amino acids was described by Katz *et al.* (1972). Poly-D-amino acids are known to be poorly immunogenic because of their slow metabolism. The use of toxic antigens is, in principle, another attractive approach. As recently reviewed by Lyle and Parker (1974), a number of possibilities already exist for rendering an antigen capable of destroying rather than stimulating antigen-reactive cells, such as the incorporation in the antigen of a radiolabel of high specific activity, or the coupling of antigen to a toxin or to a nontoxic enzyme capable of locally activating a toxic compound from a nontoxic substrate. Although some of these systems have been shown to be effective in well-controlled *in vitro* conditions, formidable problems will have to be solved before the potential of this form of affinity cytotoxicity can be assessed *in vivo* in man.

Extensive work has been published on the manner by which antibody may influence antibody production (Uhr and Möller, 1968; Schwartz, 1971). A growing number of experimental demonstrations indicate that antibody may modulate T-cell function; antibody will thus probably be a very powerful tool for a selective immune manipulation, as exemplified by the effectiveness of specific antibody in the prevention of clinical Rh isoimmunization. While the mechanisms by which enhancing antibodies prolong allograft survival are still unclear and their relationship to serum blocking factors a matter of dispute (Carpenter *et al.*, 1976), it is now established that antidonor antibody can prolong the survival of organ grafts. Recently, much interest has centered on the possible use of antiidiotypic antibodies as a means of obtaining selective immunodepression (McKearn, 1974; Binz and Wigzell, 1976). These antibodies combine with the antigenic determinants expressed by the receptor sites of other antibodies, which are possibly identical with the receptor sites carried by lymphocytes. Although antiidiotypic responses have been shown to prolong allograft survival, the complexity of the manipulations involved in preparing these antibodies is considerable, and, more important for clinical application, their production depends on the specific pretreatment of the recipient. This requisite would be a severe obstacle in the case of cadaver kidney grafts. A more likely application in man may be in the control of autoimmune diseases. The exquisite specificity of antibody provides two other potential ways for a selective immunologic control: the use of antibodies as carriers of toxic compounds or as immunoadsorbents for the removal of unwanted molecules in a kind of immune dialysis. This approach could also be applied with immunoadsorbent-antigen-containing columns for the specific removal of antigen-reactive cells. This type of approach could additionally be of great potential in other, nonimmune pathologic conditions, e.g., in the treatment of endotoxin shock with antianaphylatoxin antibody or for the removal of poisons, mediators of inflammation, or hormones. Antibody may also be used to modulate hyperfunctioning organs following the concept already employed to induce immune sympathectomy employing antisera to nerve growth factor. Once the purification of specific lymphocyte chalones and of lymphocyte products is achieved, the immune response may be controlled either through the activation of specific lymphocyte populations or through the injection of antibodies specifically raised against lymphocytes involved in the immune reaction or against their products. Examples of the latter would be the inhibition of the T-cell substituting factor(s) that mediates the T–B cell interactions, of soluble lymphocyte products capable of destroying specific target cells (lymphotoxins), or of MIF. The use of such antibodies represents a further attempt to selectively depress unwanted humoral or cell-mediated immune responses.

In conclusion, it appears that approaches to specific immunodepression, although still in their infancy, are no longer the object of pure speculation, and that a sounder knowledge of the immune system and of its mechanisms of regulation will be needed before these approaches can be applied to man.

References

Aisenberg, A. C., and Murray, C., 1973, *Cell. Immunol.* **7**:143–151.

Alepa, F. P., Zvaifler, N. J., and Sliwinski, A. J., 1970, *Arthritis Rheum.* **13**:754–760.

Allison, F., Jr., and Adcock, M. H., 1965, *J. Bacteriol.* **89**:1256–1261.

Ambrose, C. T., 1973, *J. Exp. Med.* **137**:1369–1392.

Atkinson, J. P., and Frank, M. M., 1973, *J. Immunol.* **111**:1061–1066.

Atkinson, J. P., Schreiber, A. D., and Frank, M. M., 1973, *J. Clin. Invest.* **52**:1509–1515.

Bach, F. H., Bach, M. L., and Sondel, P. M., 1976, *Nature (London)* **259**:273–281.

Bach, J. F., 1975, *The Mode of Action of Immunosuppressive Agents*, North-Holland Publishing Co., Amsterdam.

Bach, J. F., and Dardenne, M., 1971, *Transplantation* **12**:253–259.

Bach, J. F., and Dardenne, M., 1972, *Cell. Immunol.* **3**:1–10.

Bach, M. A., and Bach, J. F., 1972, *Clin. Exp. Immunol.* **11**:89–98.

Balow, J. E., and Rosenthal, A. S., 1973, *J. Exp. Med.* **137**:1031–1041.

Barnes, B. A., Schad, P. B., and Pinn, V. W., 1966, *Transplantation* **4**:154–208.

Baxter, J. D., and Forsham, P. H., 1972, *Am. J. Med.* **53**:573–589.

Benveniste, J., Higounet, F., and Solomon, J. C., 1970, *J. Reticuloendothel. Soc.* **8**:499–507.

Berenbaum, M. C., 1961, *Pathol. Biol.* **9**:963–966.

Berenbaum, M. C., 1965, *Br. Med. Bull.* **21**:140–160.

Berenbaum, M. C., 1967, *J. Clin. Pathol. Suppl.* **20**:471–492.

Berenbaum, M. C., 1971, *Clin. Exp. Immunol.* **8**:1–8.

Berenbaum, M. C., and Brown, I. N., 1963, *Nature (London)* **200**:84.

Berenbaum, M. C., and Brown, I. N., 1965, *Immunology* **8**:251–259.

Binz, H., and Wigzell, H., 1976, *Nature (London)* **262**:294, 295.

Blomgren, H., and Svedmyr, E., 1971, *Cell. Immunol.* **2**:285–299.

Blomgren, H., Strander, H., and Cantell, K., 1974, *Scand. J. Immunol.* **3**:697–705.

Borel, Y., and Schwartz, R., 1964, *J. Immunol.* **92**:754–761.

Brandriss, M. W., Smith, J. W., and Friedman, R. M., 1965, *Ann. N. Y. Acad. Sci.* **122**:356–368.

Brodeur, B. R., and Merigan, T. C., 1974, *J. Immunol.* **113**:1319–1325.

Brown, T. E., Ahmed, A., Filo, R. S., Knudsen, R. C., and Sell, K. W., 1976, *Transplantation* **21**:27–35.

Bruce, W. R., Meeker, B. E., and Valeriote, F. A., 1966, *J. Natl. Cancer Inst.* **37**:233–245.

Bullough, W. S., 1975, *Life Sci.* **16**:323–330.

Calne, R. Y., Alexandre, G. P., and Murray, J. E., 1962, *Ann. N. Y. Acad. Sci.* **99**:743–761.

Carpenter, C. B., Boylston, A. W., II, and Merrill, J. P., 1971, *Cell. Immunol.* **2**:425–434.

Carpenter, C. B., D'Apice, A. J. F., and Abbas, A. K., 1976, *Adv. Immunol.* **22**:1–65.

Cerottini, J.-C., Brunner, K. T., Lindahl, P., and Gresser, I., 1973, *Nature (London)* **242**:152, 153.

Chalmers, A. H., Burgoyne, L. A., and Murray, A. W., 1972, *Drugs* **3**:227–253.

Chester, T. J., Pancker, K., and Merigan, T. C., 1973, *Nature (London)* **246**:92–94.

Claman, H. N., 1972, *N. Engl. J. Med.* **287**:388–397.

Cohen, J. J., and Claman, H. N., 1971a, *J. Exp. Med.* **133**:1026–1034.

Cohen, J. J., and Claman, H. N., 1971b, *Nature (London)* **229**:274–275.

Cohen, I. R., Stavy, L., and Feldman, M., 1970, *J. Exp. Med.* **132**:1055–1070.

Cooperband, S. R., Badger, A. M., Davis, R. C., Schmid, K., and Mannick, J. A., 1972, *J. Immunol.* **109**:154–163.

Craddock, C. G., Winkelstein, A., Matsuyuki, Y., and Lawrence, J. S., 1967, *J. Exp. Med.* **125**:1149–1272.

Cruchaud, A., 1971, in: *New Concepts in Allergy and Clinical Immunology* (U. Serafini, A. W. Frankland, C. Mazala, and J. M. Jamar, eds.), pp. 417–450, Excerpta Medica, Amsterdam.

Dattwyler, R. J., and Tomasi, T. B., 1975, *Int. J. Cancer* **16**:942–945.

David, D. S., Grieco, H., and Cushman, P., Jr., 1970, *J. Chronic Dis.* **22**:637–711.

Debray-Sachs, M., Dimitriu, A., Bach, M. A., and Hamburger, J., 1973, *Cell. Immunol.* **7**:181–183.
Denman, E. J., Denman, A. M., Greenwood, B. M., Gall, D., and Heath, R. B., 1970, *Ann. Rheum. Dis.* **29**:220–231.
Dennert, G., Hatlen, L. E., and Tucker, D. F., 1975, *J. Natl. Cancer Inst.* **54**:621–629.
Dietrich, F. M., and Hess, R., 1970, *Int. Arch. Allergy* **38**:246–251.
Drummond, K. N., Hillman, D. A., and Marchessault, J. H., 1968, *Can. Med. Assoc. J.* **98**:524–531.
Duke, D. I., Field, E. O., Finch, M., Hellman, K., Tucker, A. S. B., and Tucker, D. F., 1973, *Biomedicine* **18**:199–205.
Dukor, P., and Dietrich, F. M., 1970, *J. Immunol.* **105**:118–125.
Elgjö, K., 1975, *J. Invest. Dermatol.* **64**:14–18.
Elion, G. B., 1967, *Fed. Proc. Fed. Am. Soc. Exp. Biol.* **26**:898–904.
Elion, G. B., 1969, *Proc. Am. Assoc. Cancer Res.* **10**:21.
Elion, G. B., 1972, *Proc. R. Soc. Med.* **65**:257–260.
Elion, G. B., and Hitchings, G. H., 1975, in: *Antineoplastic and Immunosuppressive Agents, Part II* (A. C. Sartorelli and D. G. Johns, eds.), pp. 404–425, Springer-Verlag, Berlin.
Elliott, E. V., and Sinclair, N. R., 1968, *Immunology* **15**:643–652.
Epstein, S. M., Verney, E., Miale, T. D., and Sidransky, H., 1967, *Am. J. Pathol.* **51**:769–788.
Fachet, J., and Parrott, D. M., 1972, *Clin. Exp. Immunol.* **10**:661–672.
Fauci, A. S., and Dale, D. C., 1974, *J. Clin. Invest.* **53**:240–246.
Feng, P. H., Jayaratnam, F. J., Tock, E. P. C., and Seah, C. S., 1973, *Br. Med. J.* **2**:450–452.
Floersheim, G. L., 1970, *Clin. Exp. Immunol.* **6**:861–870.
Florentin, I., Kiger, N., and Mathé, G., 1973, *Eur. J. Immunol.* **3**:624–627.
Forbes, I. J., and Smith, J. L., 1967, *Lancet* **2**:334–337.
Fosdick, W. H., 1971, *Arthritis Rheum.* **14**:363–364.
Fournier, C., Bach, M. A., Dardenne, M., and Bach, J. F., 1973, *Transplant. Proc.* **5**:523–526.
Fox, A. E., Gawlak, D. L., Ballantyne, D. L., Jr., and Freedman, H. H., 1973, *Transplantation* **15**:389–394.
Fox, K. E., and Gabourel, J. D., 1967, *Mol. Pharmacol.* **3**:479–486.
Frengley, P. A., Lichtman, M. A., and Peck, W. A., 1973, *J. Clin. Invest.* **52**:1518–1525.
Frisch, A. W., and Davies, G. H., 1962, *J. Immunol.* **88**:269–273.
Frisch, A. W., and Davies, G. H., 1966, *J. Lab. Clin. Med.* **68**:103–112.
Gabrielsen, A. E., and Good, R. A., 1967, *Adv. Immunol.* **6**:91–229.
Garattini, S., Bartosek, I., Donelli, M. G., and Spreafico, F., 1975, in: *Pharmacological Basis of Cancer Chemotherapy,* pp. 565–593, Williams & Wilkins, Baltimore.
Garry, V. F., and Uyeki, E. M., 1972, *Biochem. Pharmacol.* **21**:2801–2804.
Gelfand, M. C., and Steinberg, A. D., 1972, *Arthritis Rheum.* **15**:247–252.
Gemsa, D., Woo, C. H., Fudenberg, H. H., and Schmid, R., 1973, *J. Clin. Invest.* **52**:812–822.
Gery, I., and Waksman, B. H., 1972, *J. Exp. Med.* **136**:143–155.
Gisler, R. H., Lindhal, P. and Gresser, I., 1974, *J. Immunol.* **113**:438–444.
Glaser, M., and Herberman, R. B., 1974, *J. Natl. Cancer Inst.* **53**:1767–1769.
Glasgow, A. H., Cooperband, S. R., Schmid, K., and Mannick, J. A., 1972, *J. Clin. Invest.* **51**:36a, 37a.
Goldin, A., Venditti, J. M., and Mantel, N., 1974, in*Antineoplastic and Immunosuppressive Agents, Part I,* (A. C. Sartorelli and D. J. Johns, eds.), pp. 411–448, Springer-Verlag, Berlin.
Gray, G. D., and Koeppe, O. J., 1966, *Proc. Soc. Exp. Biol. Med.* **122**:950–952.
Gray, G. D., Nichol, F. R., Mickelson, M. M., Camieuer, G. W., Gish, D. T., Kelly, R. C., Wechter, W. J., Moxley, T. E., and Neil, G. L., 1972, *Biochem. Pharmacol.* **21**:465–475.
Guttmann, R. D., and Lindquist, R. R., 1969, *Transplantation* **8**:490–495.
Halle-Pennenko, O., Martyré, M.-C., and Chanvanet, M., 1970, *Rev. Eur. Etud. Clin. Biol.* **15**:1090–1093.
Hamburger, J., Crosnier, J., Dormont, J., and Bach, J. F., 1972, *Renal Transplantation Theory and Practice,* Williams & Wilkins, Baltimore.
Heilman, D. H., 1972, *Clin. Exp. Immunol.* **11**:393–403.
Heilman, D. H., and Leichner, J. P., 1972, in: *Proceedings of the Sixth Leukocyte Culture Conference* (M. R. Schwarz, ed.), p. 581, Academic Press, New York.
Hektoen, L., and Corper, H. J., 1921, *J. Infect. Dis.* **28**:279–283.
Heppner, G. H., Griswold, D. E., Di Lorenzo, J., Poplin, E. A., and Calabresi, P., 1974, *Fed. Proc. Fed. Am. Soc. Exp. Biol.* **33**:1882–1885.

Hersh, E. M., 1974, in: *Antineoplastic and Immunosuppression Agents, Part I* (A. C. Sartorelli and D. G. Johns, eds.), pp. 577–617, Springer-Verlag, Berlin.
Hersh, E. M., Carbone, P. P., and Freireich, E. J., 1966, *J. Lab. Clin. Med.* **67**:566–572.
Hirsch, J. G., and Church, A. B., 1961, *J. Clin. Invest.* **40**:794–798.
Hirsch, M. S., Ellis, D. A., Black, P. H., Monaco, A. P., and Wood, M. L., 1974, *Transplantation* **17**:234–236.
Hohorst, H. J., Dreager, U., Peter, G., and Voelcker, G., 1976, *Cancer Treat. Rep.* **60**:309–315.
Houck, J. C., Attallah, A. M., and Lilly, J. R., 1973, *Nature (London)* **245**:148–150.
Huang, K.-J., Donahoe, R. M., Gordon, F. B., and Dressler, H. R., 1971, *Infect. Immun.* **4**:581–588.
Husberg, B. S., 1972, *Clin. Exp. Immunol.* **10**:697–711.
Janossy, G., and Greaves, M. F., 1972, *Clin. Exp. Immunol.* **10**:525–536.
Kamrin, B. B., 1959, *Proc. Soc. Exp. Biol. Med.* **100**:58–61.
Katz, D. H., Hamaoka, T., and Benacerraf, B., 1972, *J. Exp. Med.* **136**:1404–1429.
Keller, R., 1973, *J. Exp. Med.* **138**:625–644.
Keller, R. H., and Tomasi, T. B., 1976, *J. Exp. Med.* **143**:1140–1153.
Kidson, C., 1967, *Nature (London)* **213**:779–782.
Kiger, N., Florentin, I., and Mathé, G., 1972, *Transplantation* **14**:448–454.
Kirkpatrick, A. F., Milholland, R. J., and Rosen, F., 1971, *Nature (London)* **232**:216–218.
Klane, P., Jolley, W. B., and Hinshaw, D. B., 1971, *Transplant. Proc.* **3**:323–326.
Kramer, J. J., and Granger, G. A., 1972, *Cell. Immunol.* **3**:88–100.
Lance, E. M., Medawar, P. B., Nehlsen, S. L., Cooper, S., and Gunn, A., 1970, in: *International Symposium on Antilymphocyte Serum* (J. F. Bach, J. Dormont, A. Eyquem, M. Roynaud, and R. H. Regamey, eds.), pp. 231–250, S. Karger, Basel.
Lee, A. K., Mackay, I. R., Rowley, M. J., and Yap, C. Y., 1971, *Clin. Exp. Immunol.* **9**:507–518.
Lemmel, E., Hurd, E. R., and Ziff, M., 1971, *Clin. Exp. Immunol.* **8**:355–362.
Lenna, T. J., Frommel, D., and Good, R. A., 1972, *Int. Arch. Allergy* **42**:20–39.
Leung, F. C., and Vas, S. I., 1968, *Can. J. Microbiol.* **14**:7–11.
Lindhal-Magnusson, P., Leary, P., and Gresser, I., 1971, *Proc. Soc. Exp. Biol. Med.* **138**:1044–1050.
Lindhal-Magnusson, P., Leary, P., and Gresser, I., 1972, *Nature (London) New Biol.* **237**:120–121.
Lyle, L. R., and Parker, C. W., 1974, *Fed. Proc. Fed. Am. Soc. Exp. Biol.* **33**:1889–1893.
Makinodan, T., Santos, G. W., and Quinn, R. P., 1970, *Pharmacol. Rev.* **22**:189–247.
Mandel, M. A., Monaco, A. P., and Russell, P. S., 1965, *J. Immunol.* **95**:673–682.
Mandell, G. L., Rubin, W., and Hook, E. W., 1970, *J. Clin. Invest.* **49**:1381–1388.
Mantovani, A., 1977, *Cancer Res.*, in press.
Mantovani, A., Vecchi, A., Tagliabue, A., and Spreafico, F., 1976, *Europ. J. Cancer* **12**:371–379.
Many, A., and Schwartz, R. S., 1970a, *Proc. Soc. Exp. Biol. Med.* **133**:754–757.
Many, A., and Schwartz, R. S., 1970b, *Clin. Exp. Immunol.* **6**:87–99.
Marchioro, T. L., Axtell, H. K., La Vie, M. F., Waddell, W. R., and Starzl, T. E., 1964, *Surgery* **55**:412–417.
Markowitz, H., Person, D. A., Gitnick, G. L., and Ritts, R. E., Jr., 1969, *Science* **163**:476.
Mawbray, J. F., 1967, *J. Clin. Pathol.* **20**:499.
McKearn, T. J., 1974, *Science* **183**:94–96.
McLeod, R. M., King, C. E., and Hollander, V. P., 1963, *Cancer Res.* **23**:1045–1050.
Mellet, L. B., 1974, *Clin. Pharmacol. Ther.* **16**:230–242.
Mendelsohn, J., Multer, M. M., and Boone, R. F., 1973, *J. Clin. Invest.* **52**:2129–2137.
Menzoian, J. O., Glasgow, A. H., Nimberg, R. D., Cooperband, S. R., Schmid, K., Saporoschetz, I., and Mannick, J. A., 1974, *J. Immunol.* **113**:266–273.
Milton, J. D., 1971, *Immunology* **20**:205–212.
Mitchell, F., Yamamoto, R. S., and Weisburger, J. H., 1973, *Proc. Soc. Exp. Biol. Med.* **143**:165–167.
Mitchell, M. S., 1974, in: *Antineoplastic and Immunosuppressive Agents, Part I* (A. C. Sartorelli and D. G. Johns, eds.), pp. 555–576, Springer-Verlag, Berlin.
Mitchell, M. S., Wade, M. E., and De Conti, R. C., 1969, *Ann. Intern. Med.* **70**:535–547.
Mitsuoka, A., Baba, M., and Marikawa, S., 1976, *Nature (London)* **262**:77, 78.
Möller, G., and Sjöberg, O., 1970, *Immunology* **1**:110.
Moorhead, J. F., Paraskova-Tchernozenska, E., Pirrie, A. J., and Hayes, C., 1969, *Nature (London)* **224**:1207–1208.
Moorhead, J. W., and Claman, H. N., 1972, *Cell. Immunol.* **5**:74–86.

Moorhead, J. W., and Claman, H. N., 1974, *J. Exp. Med.* **112**:333–338.
Morton, J. I., Brown, M., and Siegel, B. V., 1972, *Proc. Soc. Exp. Biol. Med.* **139**:1417–1420.
Munck, A., Wira, C., Young, D. A., Mosher, K. M., Hallahan, C., and Bell, P. A., 1972, *J. Steroid Biochem.* **3**:567–578.
Murgita, R. A., and Tomasi, T. B., 1975, *J. Exp. Med.* **141**:440–452.
Nachtigal, D., Zan-Bar, I., and Feldman, M., 1975, *Transplant. Rev.* **26**:87–105.
Nakamura, R. M., and Weigle, W., 1970, *Clin. Exp. Immunol.* **7**:541–550.
Narayan, R. K., Job, C. K., Mani, M. M., and Bachhawat, B. K., 1976, *Transplantation* **21**:370–374.
Nettesheim, P., and Hammons, A. S., 1970, *Proc. Soc. Exp. Biol. Med.* **133**:696–701.
Nimberg, R. B., Glasgow, A. H., Menzoian, J. O., Constantian, M. B., Cooperband, S. R., Mannick, J. A., and Schmid, K., 1975, *Cancer Res.* **35**:1489–1494.
Nirmul, G., Severin, G., and Taub, R. N., 1972, *Transplantation* **14**:91–95.
North, R. J., 1972, *Cell. Immunol.* **3**:501–515.
Occhino, J. C., Glasgow, A. M., Cooperband, S. R., Mannick, J. A., and Schmid, K., 1973, *J. Immunol.* **110**:685–694.
Owen, R. D., 1945, *Science* **102**:400–401.
Paterson, P. Y., Drobish, D. G., and Biddick, A. S., 1971, *J. Immunol.* **106**:570–572.
Pelley, R. P., Pelley, R. J., Stavitsky, A. B., Mahmoud, A. A. F., and Warren, K. S., 1975, *J. Immunol.* **115**:1477–1482.
Perper, R. J., Alvarez, B., Colombo, C., and Schroder, H., 1971, *Proc. Soc. Exp. Biol. Med.* **137**:506–512.
Peter, J. B., 1971, *Cell. Immunol.* **2**:199–202.
Phillips, S. M., and Zweiman, B., 1973, *J. Exp. Med.* **137**:1494–1510.
Phillips, S. M., Gleichmann, H., Hirsch, M. S., Black, P., Merrill, J. P., Schwartz, R. S., and Carpenter, C. B., 1975, *Cell. Immunol.* **15**:152–168.
Purves, E. C., and Berenbaum, M. C., 1975, *Transplantation* **19**:274–276.
Ranney, D. F., 1975, *Adv. Pharmacol. Chemother.* **13**:359–408.
Rasmussen, L. E., Jordan, G. W., Stevens, D. A., and Merigan, T. C., 1974, *J. Immunol.* **112**:728–736.
Riggio, R. R., Schwartz, G. H., Bull, F. G., Stenzel, K. H., and Rubin, A. L., 1969, *Transplantation* **8**:689–694.
Rollinghoff, M., Schroder, J., and Wagner, H., 1973, *Clin. Exp. Immunol.* **15**:261–269.
Rühl, H., Vogt, W., Rühl, U., Bochert, G., and Schmidt, S., 1973, *Immunology* **25**:753–760.
Russel, P. J., and Hicks, J. D., 1968, *Lancet* **1**:440–446.
Sachs, G., Deduve, C., Dvorkin, B. S., and White, A., 1962, *Exp. Cell Res.* **28**:597–600.
Sahiar, K., and Schwartz, R. S., 1966, *Int. Arch. Allergy* **29**:52–68.
Santos, G. W., 1967, *Fed. Proc. Fed. Am. Soc. Exp. Biol.* **26**:907–913.
Santos, G. W., 1972, in: *Current Problems in Immunobiology* (M. G. Hanna, Jr., ed.), p. 143, Plenum Press, New York.
Santos, G. W., and Owens, A. H., Jr., 1966, *Nature (London)* **210**:139–140.
Santos, G. W., Owens, A. H., Jr., and Sensenbrenner, L. L., 1964, *Ann. N. Y. Acad. Sci.* **114**:404–423.
Santos, G. W., Sensenbrenner, L. L., Burke, P. J., Colvin, M., Owens, A. H., Jr., Bias, N. B., and Slavin, R. E., 1971, *Transplant. Proc.* **3**:400–404.
Schumacher, K., Maerker-Alzer, G., and Wehmer, U., 1974, *Nature (London)* **251**:655–656.
Schwartz, R. S., 1966, *Fed. Proc. Fed. Am. Soc. Exp. Biol.* **25**:165–168.
Schwartz, R. S., 1968, in: *Human Transplantation* (F. T. Rapaport and J. Dausset, eds.), pp. 440–449, Grune & Stratton, New York.
Schwartz, R. S., 1971, *Prog. Immunol.* **1**:1081–1092.
Schwartz, R. S., Stack, J., and Dameshek, W., 1958, *Proc. Soc. Exp. Biol. Med.* **99**:164–170.
Segal, S., Cohen, I. R., and Feldman, M., 1972, *Science* **175**:1126–1128.
Shehadeh, I. H., Guttmann, R. D., and Lindquist, R. R., 1970, *Transplantation* **10**:66–74.
Silvers, W. K., Wilson, D. B., and Palm, J., 1967, *Science* **155**:703–704.
Simonian, S. J., and Murray, J. E., 1971, *Transplant. Proc.* **3**:470–472.
Soloway, R. D., Baggenstoss, A. H., Elveback, L. R., Schoenfield, L. J., Stubbs, B. L., and Summerskill, W. H. J., 1971, *Gastroenterology* **60**:167–172.
Spiegelberg, H. L., and Miescher, P. A., 1963, *J. Exp. Med.* **118**:869–890.
Spreafico, F., 1972, *Adv. Pharmacol.* **10**:257–338.
Spreafico, F., and Lerner, E. M., 2nd., 1967, *J. Immunol.* **98**:407–416.

Spreafico, F., Donelli, M. G., Bossi, A., Vecchi, A., Standen, S., and Garattini, S., 1973, *Transplantation* **16**:269–278.

Spreafico, F., Donelli, M. G., Vecchi, A., Bossi, A., and Garattini, S., 1974, in: *Recent Results in Cancer Research,* Vol. 49, (G. Mathé, and R. K. Oldham, eds.), p. 88, Springer-Verlag, Berlin.

Starzl, T. E., Groth, C. G., and Putnam, C. W., 1973, *Transplant. Proc.* **5**:511–516.

Stavy, L., Cohen, I. R., and Feldman, M., 1973, *Cell. Immunol.* **7**:302–312.

Steinberg, A. D., and Talal, N., 1970, *Clin. Exp. Immunol.* **7**:687–691.

Stockman, G. D., Judd, K. P., and Trentin, J. J., 1972, *Transplantation* **13**:66–71.

Stockman, G. D., Heim, L. R., South, M. A., and Trentin, J. J., 1973, *J. Immunol.* **110**:277–282.

Tagliabue, A., Polentarutti, N., Vecchi A., Mantovani, A., and Spreafico, F., 1976, *Europ. J. Cancer,* in press.

Thompson, J., and Van Furth, R., 1973, *J. Exp. Med.* **137**:10–21.

Tinbergen, W. J., 1968, *Transplantation* **6**:203–207.

Trainin, N., Levo, Y., and Rotter, V., 1974, *Eur. J. Immunol.* **4**:634–637.

Tremann, J. A., Haines, J. G., Bleifuss, J. H., Agodoa, L. C. Y., and Marchioro, T. L., 1975, *Transplantation* **19**:520–522.

Turk, J. L., and Poulter, L. W., 1972, *Clin. Exp. Immunol.* **10**:285–296.

Turk, J. L., Parker, D., and Poulter, L. W., 1972, *Immunology* **23**:493–501.

Tyan, M. L., 1974, *Transplantation* **18**:305–312.

Uhr, J. W., and Möller, G., 1968, *Adv. Immunol.* **8**:81–127.

Unanue, E. R., 1972, *Adv. Immunol.* **15**:95–165.

Uyeki, E. M., 1967, *Biochem. Pharmacol.* **16**:53–58.

Van Furth, R., Thompson, J., and Gassmann, A. E., 1973, in: *Non-Specific Factors Influencing Host Resistance* (W. Braun and J. Unger, eds.), p. 79, Karger, Basel.

Vecchi, A., Tagliabue, A., Mantovani, A., Anaclerio, A., Barale, C., and Spreafico, F., 1976a, *Biomedicine* **24**:231–237.

Vecchi, A., Fioretti, M. C., Mantovani, A., Barzi, A., and Spreafico, F., 1976b, *Transplantation* **22**:49–54.

Veit, B., and Michael, J. G., 1973, *J. Immunol.* **111**:341–351.

Viljanen, M. K., Kanto, J., Vapaavuori, M., and Toivanen, P., 1973, *Br. Med. J.* **3**:499–500.

Vogel, C. L., and Calabresi, P., 1969, *Proc. Soc. Exp. Biol. Med.* **131**:251–256.

Waldman, S. R., and Gottlieb, A. A., 1973, *Cell. Immunol.* **9**:142–156.

Waller, M., Pierce, J. C., Moncure, C. W., and Hume, D. M., 1972, *Clin. Exp. Immunol.* **11**:173–186.

Weil, R., III, Nozawa, M., Chernack, W., Weber, C., Reemtsma, K., and McIntosh, R., 1974, *Transplantation* **17**:600–604.

Weissmann, G., and Thomas, L., 1963, *J. Clin. Invest.* **42**:661–669.

Weston, W. L., Claman, H. N., and Krueger, G. G., 1973, *J. Immunol.* **110**:880–883.

Wiener, E., Marmary, Y., and Curelaru, Z., 1972, *Lab. Invest.* **26**:220–226.

Williams, T. W., and Granger, G. A., 1969, *J. Immunol.* **103**:170–178.

Winkelstein, A., Mikulla, J. M., Nankin, H. R., Pollock, B. H., and Stolzer, B. L., 1972, *J. Lab. Clin. Med.* **80**:506–513.

Winkelstein, A., Nankin, H. R., and Mikulla, J. M., 1973, in: *Proceedings of the Seventh Leukocyte Culture Conference* (F. Daguillard, ed.), p. 429, Academic Press, New York.

Winkelstein, A., Ruben, R. L., Tolchin, S. F., and Pollock, B. H., 1974, *J. Lab. Clin. Med.* **83**:504–510.

Yachnin, S., 1975, *J. Exp. Med.* **141**:242–256.

Zan-Bar, I., Nachtigal, D., and Feldman, M., 1975, *Cell. Immunol.* **17**:215–230.

Zukoski, C. F., Callaway, J. M., and Rhea, W. G., Jr., 1963a, *Surg. Forum* **14**:208–210.

Zukoski, C. F., Callaway, J. M., and Rhea, W. G., Jr., 1963b, *Transplantation* **1**:293–297.

14

Mechanisms of Immunopotentiation

JOHN W. HADDEN, LILIAN DELMONTE, and
HERBERT F. OETTGEN

1. Introduction

Immunopharmacology, as defined by the contents of this volume, represents a broad endeavor to elucidate the basic molecular aspects, both intercellular and intracellular, of the regulation of immune response. While this scientific enterprise is in its infancy, perhaps the most critical evaluation of its progress to date lies in the appreciation of the extent to which principles have emerged that will be therapeutically useful. The application of therapeutic agents that suppress the immune response and its associated inflammation has developed empirically, as a result of the need for symptomatic relief, effective organ transplantation, and amelioration of immunopathologic processes such as allergy and autoimmunity. In contrast, the development of agents that augment immune responses has been more recent, as a result of the need to combat cancer, to reverse iatrogenic immunosuppression, and to treat immunodeficiency and chronic infection. As is always the case with therapeutic endeavors, it turns out to be far easier to generate agents that inhibit than agents that augment physiologic functions. This chapter will attempt to summarize the progress that has been made in the development of approaches to the potentiation of immune responses, with the ultimate goal of effective therapy.

We use the term "immunopotentiator" to define a large category of therapeutic agents, recognizing that it does not describe their actions adequately. Clearly, many of these agents are immunomodulatory in that they augment one immunologic function at the expense of another, or stimulate or inhibit immune responses depending on the time of administration with respect to antigen. Others might be better described as "immunoadjuvants," in the sense that they have relatively little effect in the absence of antigen and act principally to expand the immune response

JOHN W. HADDEN, LILIAN DELMONTE, and HERBERT F. OETTGEN • Memorial Sloan-Kettering Cancer Center, New York, New York 10021.

to antigenic stimulation. Still other agents might be termed "immunonormalizing," in that they seem to augment a depressed response, but have little effect on the optimal or normal response. Still others qualify as "immunosubstituting," in that they appear to substitute for biological factors. For lack of a better term to encompass these different types of action, we will continue to use the term "immunopotentiator."

The agents to be discussed include bacteria, bacterial products, plant products, synthetic agents, and products of the immune system itself. They are evaluated in terms of their actions *in vivo* and *in vitro*. We have attempted, as much as possible, to address ourselves to the molecular aspects of their actions, and to integrate them with the observations detailed in other chapters of this volume. Finally, we have outlined current therapeutic applications of these agents, and have offered speculation on their analysis and future applications.

2. Biological Substances

2.1. Bacillus Calmette-Guérin and Mycobacterial Fractions

The history of awareness of a role for mycobacteria in cell-mediated immunity (CMI) dates back to Koch, who, in 1880, during early attempts to develop a vaccine against tuberculosis, observed the phenomenon now known as delayed-type hypersensitivity (DTH). Forty-one years elapsed before Calmette and Guérin succeeded in developing a vaccine against tuberculosis, now known as bacillus Calmette-Guérin (BCG). Soon thereafter, Lewis and Loomis (1924) found that Mituberculosis could act as an adjuvant. In 1942, Freund and McDermott (1942) found that immune responses to many antigens were enhanced by mixing the antigen with water, suspending mycobacteria in oil, and combining the two in an oil-in-water emulsion (complete Freund's adjuvant, CFA). Halpern *et al.* (1959) and Old *et al.* (1959, 1961) demonstrated the stimulatory effects of BCG on the reticuloendothelial system (RES), and related this phenomenon to increased "nonspecific" resistance to antigenically unrelated microorganisms and tumor cells. BCG has come to be known as the prototype of immunopotentiators, because it stimulates humoral and cellular immune responses to unrelated antigens in addition to its own antigenic determinants. More recently, several other mycobacterial strains, both pathogenic and nonpathogenic, have also been shown to possess immunomodulating activity and to inhibit growth of tumors.

In view of the disadvantages of a live vaccine, interest has been directed more recently toward mycobacterial cell wall fractions with similar but more reproducible biological activities. Table 1 lists preparations that have been evaluated as immunopotentiators for possible clinical use.

The immunomodulatory characteristics of BCG and various mycobacterial cell wall fractions include potentiation of cellular immune responses, augmentation of humoral immune responses (primarily to T-cell-dependent antigens), and stimulation of the RES. As an adjuvant that acts primarily on T-cell-mediated functions, BCG: (1) stimulates T-cell proliferation (Mackaness *et al.*, 1973); (2) amplifies T-cell-dependent humoral responses (Stjernswärd, 1966; Miller *et al.*, 1973); (3) augments cellular immune responses such as DTH (Miller *et al.*, 1973), skin allograft rejection (Vitale and Allegretti, 1963; Peters *et al.*, 1974), and male-to-

TABLE 1. **Biologically Active Mycobacterial Fractions**

Mycobacterial fraction	Chemical nature	References
Cell wall skeleton (CWS)	Insoluble peptidoglycolipid	Ribi *et al.* (1973)
Cord factor (CF, P_3)	6,6-Dimycolate of trehalose	Bekierkunst *et al.* (1969), Ribi *et al.* (1973)
Methanol extraction residue (MER)	Methanol-insoluble fraction of phenolated organisms	Weiss and Wells (1960)
Interphase material (IPM)	Muramic acid, glucosamine, α,α'-diaminopimelic acid, neutral carbohydrates, lipids	Lamensans *et al.* (1975)
Water-soluble adjuvant (WSA)	Muramic acid-containing polymer linked to arabinogalactan	Chedid *et al.* (1972)
WSA analogue (WSA_1)	Muramic dipeptide (*n*-acetyl-muramyl-L-analyl-D-isoglutamine)	Juy and Chedid (1975)

female skin isograft rejection (Balner *et al.*, 1962); and (4) breaks induced tolerance to skin allografts (Clark and Monaco, 1974).

BCG was found to render poorly immunogenic antigens immunogenic (Green *et al.*, 1969), and to potentiate the cell-mediated immune response to poorly immunogenic tumor antigens (Hawrylko, 1975). In hyperimmunized animals, the T-cell responses of which are blocked by circulating antigen–antibody complexes, BCG restores CMI, probably by accelerating the clearance of circulating immune complexes by the RES (Mackaness *et al.*, 1974). In this sytem, the effectiveness of BCG is increased by concomitant administration of cyclophosphamide. This suggests that combination treatment with BCG and cyclophosphamide might be useful in the clinic.

Route and time of administration are important. In general, direct contact between BCG and antigen or injection into sites drained by the same lymph nodes is favorable. It has been noted that cellular proliferation within the draining lymph nodes correlates well with cellular immune reactions, but not, apparently, with the antibody responses (Miller *et al.*, 1973).

While repeated scarification with BCG enhances skin hypersensitivity to sheep erythrocytes (SRBC) and depresses the humoral immune response (Peters *et al.*, 1974), a single dose of BCG given intravenously before immunization has the opposite effect (Toujas *et al.*, 1973).

BCG activates macrophages, as evidenced by (1) increased phagocytic activity (Old *et al.*, 1961), (2) increased activity of lysosomal enzymes (Thorbecke *et al.*, 1961), (3) activation of phospholipase A (Munder and Modollel, 1974), (4) production of lymphocyte-activating factor (LAF) that enhances T-cell helper function and T-cell cytotoxicity (Mitchell *et al.*, 1973), (5) increased chemotaxis (Meltzer *et al.*, 1975), and (6) selective toxicity for tumor cells (Hibbs *et al.*, 1972; Cleveland *et al.*, 1974).

2.1.1. Mycobacterial Fractions

Concentrated efforts to isolate the component(s) responsible for the immunopotentiative and antitumor activities of mycobacteria have yielded a variety of fractions (Table 1). With the exception of MER and WSA, the biological activities of these agents have not yet been characterized sufficiently for us to attempt to predict their clinical potential.

CWS and *CF* are two mycobacterial fractions with actions similar to those of living BCG. When administrered in an oil-in-water emulsion both induce a granulomatous and proliferative reaction in regional lymph nodes (Mackaness *et al.*, 1973; Bekierkunst, 1974; Champlin and Hunter, 1975) and enhance cell-mediated immune responses in a way comparable to CFA (Bekierkunst, 1974; Taniyama *et al.*, 1975; Y. Yamamura *et al.*, 1975).

IPM, a complex mycobacterial cell wall component, has been shown to be nonantigenic, to increase nonspecific resistance to viral infections, to activate macrophages, and to stimulate antibody production and DTH to ovalbumin to the same degree as CFA (Lamensans *et al.*, 1975; Juy and Chedid, 1975; Chedid, personal communication).

MER is the most extensively studied mycobacterial fraction. Its immunomodulatory and antitumor activities, which are similar to those of BCG, are the subject of a recent review by Weiss (1976).

MER stimulates both B and T lymphocytes. In mice, it has a direct mitogenic effect on B cells, as demonstrated in cultures of macrophage-depleted spleen cells of nude mice (Ben-Efraim and Diamantstein, 1977). In addition, lymphocytes from mice treated with MER show an increased blastogenic response to lipopolysaccharide (LPS) *in vitro* (Gery *et al.*, 1974). MER promotes mitosis of T cells indirectly, by inducing macrophages to produce a T-cell-activating factor (LAF) (Gery *et al.*, 1974). MER promotes nonspecific resistance to a variety of pathogenic microorganisms (Weiss *et al.*, 1964), enhances phagocytic activity of macrophages *in vivo* (Steinkuller *et al.*, 1969) and *in vitro* (Gallily and Ben-Ishay, 1976), and induces an increase of lysosomal enzyme activity in macrophages (Yagel *et al.*, 1975).

In rodents, MER given before or after administration of a variety of antigens stimulates humoral and cellular immune responses. Specifically, MER: (1) accelerates and augments the primary and secondary antibody response; (2) renders subimmunogenic doses of antigens immunogenic; (3) breaks tolerance induced in neonates; (4) prevents induction of tolerance in adults; (5) stimulates cell-mediated immune reactions; (6) accelerates allograft rejection; (7) accelerates rejection of male skin isografts by females; (8) reverses the immunosuppressive effects of X-ray irradiation, cortisone, and antithymus serum (Weiss and Yashpe, 1973; see Weiss, 1976); and (9) partially reverses the depression of antibody formation and DTH by immunosuppressive chemotherapeutic agents such as cyclophosphamide and methotrexate (see Weiss, 1976).

WSA, a water-soluble polymer that contains muramic acid, has the immunoadjuvant properties of CFA, but does not induce granulomas when administered in either oil or water (Chedid *et al.*, 1972; Parant and Chedid, 1974). WSA does not increase the phagocytic activity of the RES, cause hepatosplenomegaly, or induce hypersensitivity to endotoxin (Chedid *et al.*, 1972; Parant and Chedid, 1974), but does activate macrophages *in vivo* and *in vitro* with respect to rendering them nonspecifically cytotoxic for tumor cells (Juy and Chedid, 1975). WSA augments the primary humoral immune response to both T-cell-dependent and T-cell-independent antigens *in vivo* and *in vitro* (Parant and Chedid, 1974). Administration of WSA *in vivo* augments mixed lymphocyte culture (MLC) reactions *in vitro* (Bona *et al.*, 1974).

Chedid and his associates (Juy and Chedid, 1975; Chedid, personal communication) synthesized several low-molecular-weight muramic acid analogues, one of which, *WSA*$_1$, has essentially the same immunopotentiating activity as native WSA; it is highly effective when given orally without direct contact with antigen. WSA$_1$ activates macrophages *in vivo,* but only when administered at low doses. In addition, it augments the mitogenic effect of concanavalin A (Con A) on lymphocytes (Muscoplat and Chedid, personal communication).

WSA is of potential clinical interest, since (1) it has an immunopotentiative and antitumor spectrum similar to that of BCG; (2) it is active in aqueous solution and hence does not induce hepatic or pulmonary granulomas (unlike mycobacterial preparations suspended in oil); and (3) its synthetic analogue, WSA$_1$, which is nonimmunogenic and nontoxic, has the same immunopotentiative and antitumor spectrum as native WSA and, unlike other mycobacterial preparations, is effective orally (Chedid *et al.,* 1972; Parant and Chedid, 1974; Juy and Chedid, 1975).

2.1.2. Mechanism of Action

Although antigenicity has been correlated with immunoadjuvancy of mycobacteria (Mackaness *et al.,* 1973), that fractions such as WSA and its analogue WSA$_1$ possess adjuvant activity in the absence of antigenicity indicates that these attributes are separable. The mechanism by which immunogenic mycobacterial preparations augment immune responses to unrelated antigens are reviewed by Hadden and Englard in Chapter 5. Briefly, the principal effects of BCG and related mycobacteria and of other microorganisms such as *Listeria, Brucella,* and *Salmonella* appear to be an initial stimulation of T-lymphocyte proliferation (which is antigen-specific), followed by macrophage proliferation and activation (which is nonspecific). The stimulation of T cells results in the elaboration of a variety of soluble mediators that act on macrophages. They include macrophage chemotactic factor, aggregating factor, migration-inhibitory factor (MIF), mitogenic factor, activating factor, and colony-stimulating factor (CSF). Stimulated macrophages, in turn, elaborate CSF, initiating an autofeedback regulation of their own proliferation and activation, and LAF, initiating a feedback loop to T lymphocytes that further promotes their proliferation. The principal effector of the enhanced nonspecific immune response is the "activated" macrophage, which is characterized by being more aggressively phagocytic and bactericidal for resistant pathogens (presumably as a result of intracellular accumulation of lysosomal enzymes), and being nonspecifically cytotoxic for tumor cells, but not for normal cells.

Both the specific effects of BCG on T cells and its nonspecific effects on macrophages may be mediated by cyclic GMP (cGMP) (see Chapters 1 and 5).

2.1.3. Therapeutic Uses of Bacillus Calmette-Guérin

(a) Effects on Immune Response. Clinical investigations of the effects of mycobacteria on the immune system have so far been limited to trials with BCG and MER in cancer patients. Observed effects include the conversion of initially negative DTH to dinitrochlorobenzene (DNCB) (Eilber *et al.,* 1975), and apparently dose-dependent increases of the lymphocyte response to lectin mitogens and purified protein derivative (PPD) in melanoma patients given intralesional injections (Gutterman *et al.,* 1973; Seigler *et al.,* 1975). Bluming *et al.* (1972) reported that

BCG (Pasteur) given by scarification potentiated DTH responses to common antigens, whereas BCG (Glaxo) given intradermally did not. In preliminary studies with patients with malignant melanoma stage 2 treated surgically, we (Pinsky *et al.*, 1976) have not observed any consistent immunologic effect of intradermal BCG (Tice) other than induction of DTH to PPD after prolonged percutaneous vaccination. Issues concerning variability in the immunostimulatory potency of different strains of BCG, as well as issues of optimal route, site, and dose of administration of BCG and the patient's initial immune status, must be resolved before meaningful interpretation can be made of the clinical effects of BCG on immune responses.

MER appears to increase DTH to new and recall antigens in immunodepressed cancer patients (Moertel *et al.*, 1975; Richman, 1975; Robinson *et al.*, 1975; Stupp *et al.*, 1975, 1977). While Moertel *et al.* (1975) observed increases in serum Ig levels and circulating T cells as well as increases in *in vitro* lymphocyte blastogenesis in response to lectin mitogens, Richman (1975) and Stupp *et al.* (1975;1977) found both increases and decreases in mitogen responsiveness of lymphocytes. This discrepancy may be due to the fact that the patients in the two latter studies received chemotherapy concurrently with MER.

(b) Effects on Cancer. Historically, the first attempts to treat cancer patients with BCG (Holmgren, 1935) antedate the discovery of its antitumor effects in animals (Halpern *et al.*, 1959; Old *et al.*, 1959) by a quarter of a century. Holmgren (1935) reported "a certain retardation of disease" and induction of tuberculin sensitivity in tuberculin-negative patients. This report went largely unnoticed until the discovery that BCG inhibits tumors in experimental animals (Halpern *et al.*, 1959; Old *et al.*, 1959) led to a resurgence of investigation in laboratory animals (see Bast *et al.*, 1976) and in man (see Mastrangelo *et al.*, 1976).

In experimental animals, BCG has been shown to inhibit the development and progression of spontaneous, induced, and transplanted solid tumors and leukemias (see Bast *et al.*, 1976). CWS, CF, MER, and WSA have shown similar antitumor effects in laboratory animals (Bekierkunst *et al.*, 1969; Zbar *et al.*, 1972a; Chedid *et al.*, 1973; Ribi *et al.*, 1973; Chedid and Lamensans, 1974; Bekierkunst *et al.*, 1974; Weiss, 1976). In animals with established tumors, best results were obtained by intralesional injection of BCG or its fractions; in general, systemic administration of BCG had little effect on established tumor grafts (Zbar *et al.*, 1972b; T. Yamamura *et al.*, 1974; Proctor *et al.*, 1976).

Modern efforts to determine the value of BCG in the treatment of human cancer began less than 10 years ago. In 1969, Mathé *et. al.* (1969) first reported that percutaneous vaccination with BCG prolonged chemotherapy-induced remissions in children with acute lymphoblastic leukemia (ALL). Later reports by others indicate that BCG has little if any effect in the treatment of ALL (Medical Research Council, 1971; Heyn *et al.*, 1973; Gutterman *et al.*, 1974) but, given alone or combined with irradiated leukemia cells, potentiates the effects of chemotherapy in patients with acute myeloblastic leukemia (Powles *et al.*, 1973; Gutterman *et al.*, 1974) and, possibly, chronic myelogenous leukemia (Sokal *et al.*, 1973; Vogler and Chan, 1974). Administration of BCG by percutaneous vaccination was variously reported to delay (Gutterman *et al.*, 1973; Morton *et al.*, 1974) or not to affect (Pinsky *et al.*, 1976) recurrence after surgery in patients with malignant melanoma stage 2-3, as well as to delay postsurgical recurrence in patients with colon cancer (Maviglit *et al.*, 1976). In combination with chemotherapy, BCG was shown to prolong drug-induced responses in patients with metastatic melanoma (Reed *et al.*, 1975) and metastatic breast cancer (Cardenas *et al.*, 1976).

Another application of BCG has been direct injection into skin metastases. In 1970, Morton *et al.*, (1970) first observed regression of cutaneous melanoma metastases after intratumoral injection of BCG. Skin metastases from other types of cancer, including breast cancer and sarcomas, were also found to regress after intralesional injection of BCG (E. Klein and Holtermann, 1972; Smith *et al.*, 1973). The overall experience with intratumoral injection of BCG has been that (1) approximately 50% of all injected skin lesions regress; (2) intradermal metastases regress more often than subcutaneous lesions; (3) regression of skin lesions occurs less frequently in patients who also have visceral metastases; and (4) noninjected skin lesions regress occasionally in patients whose injected skin lesions regress, but visceral metastases do not (Nathanson, 1974; Mastrangelo *et al.*, 1976).

Of the mycobacterial fractions, only MER is currently being investigated in large-scale clinical trials. These trials are still in an early stage, but some of the preliminary results appear "promising" (see Weiss, 1976). In a pilot study of adults with acute myelocytic leukemia, Cuttner *et al.* (1975) observed longer persistence of drug-induced remission in patients maintained with combination chemotherapy and MER than in those maintained with chemotherapy alone.

The mechanisms of the antitumor effects of BCG are thought to be related, on one hand, to the nonspecific tumoricidal effects of activated macrophages and soluble mediators (see Chapter 5) and, on the other, to an amplification of humoral and cellular immune responses to tumor-specific antigens (Balner *et al.*, 1962; Amiel and Bérardet, 1972; Zbar *et al.*, 1972b; Harmel *et al.*, 1975). Although, in special instances, a fortuitous cross-reactivity between BCG and tumor-specific antigens was observed in animals (Borsos and Rapp, 1973; Bucana and Hanna, 1974; Minden *et al.*, 1974), the majority of studies in both laboratory animals and man failed to show such cross-reactivity.

2.2. Corynebacteria

During a systematic search for other microorganisms that, like BCG, stimulate the immune system nonspecifically, killed *Corynebacterium parvum* was found to be a potent stimulator of the RES (Prévot *et al.*, 1958; Halpern *et al.*, 1964) and to have immunoadjuvant activity (Neveu *et al.*, 1964). Subsequent investigation revealed that *C. parvum* inhibits the growth of tumors in experimental animals (Halpern *et al.*, 1966; Woodruff and Boak, 1966). It has since been found that several other species of anaerobic corynebacteria also have immunomodulatory properties (Prévot and Tran Van Phi, 1964; Raynaud *et al.*, 1972; Adlam and Scott, 1973; O'Neill *et al.*, 1973), and that at least one other species, *C. granulosum,* also has marked antitumor activity in laboratory animals (Halpern *et al.*, 1973; Mathé *et al.*, 1973). *C. parvum* and *C. granulosum* were shown to affect immune parameters and to potentiate the effects of chemotherapy in cancer patients (Halpern and Israël, 1971; Israël, 1974, 1975; Reed *et al.*, 1975). (*C. parvum* and *C. granulosum* will hereafter be referred to collectively as CP.)

The observations cited above and the fact that corynebacteria, unlike BCG, are effective in the form of a killed vaccine account for the current interest in therapeutic trials of CP in patients with cancer and immunodeficiency diseases. Since CP has side effects common to crude bacterial preparations (Oettgen *et al.*, 1976), efforts are in progress to purify and characterize fractions of corynebacterial cell walls that show immunomodulatory activity but are less toxic than the intact microorganism (Kouznetzova *et al.*, 1974; Nguyen-Dang *et al.*, 1973; Adlam *et al.*, 1975).

2.2.1. Effects on the Immune System of Animals

In animals, CP was shown to increase the production of antibody to both T-cell-dependent and T-cell-independent antigens (Pinckard *et al.*, 1967; Pinckard and Halonen, 1971; Del Guercio, 1972; Raynaud *et al.*, 1972; Howard *et al.*, 1973; Warr and Sljivic, 1974). CP renders tolerogenic doses of antigens immunogenic (Pinckard *et al.*, 1967; Wiener and Bandieri, 1975), but fails to break established tolerance. Transfer experiments suggest that activated macrophages may mediate the T-cell-independent effects of CP on antibody production (Howard *et al.*, 1973; Wiener, 1975). Another mechanism whereby CP may augment the effects of the humoral immune response may be its capacity to activate the classical and alternate pathways of complement (McBride *et al.*, 1975).

CP treatment of the recipient depresses allograft rejection (Castro, 1974) and graft-vs.-host (GVH) reactions (Howard *et al.*, 1967; Cudkowicz, 1968; Scott, 1972). The cell-mediated immune response of sensitized mice is depressed by CP injected intravenously but not subcutaneously (Asherson and Alwood, 1971; Scott, 1974). The depression of the cellular immune response occurs simultaneously with stimulation of the humoral response, indicating that CP does not depress T-cell helper function (Howard *et al.*, 1973; Toujas *et al.*, 1973). Silica-induced destruction of macrophages reverses CP-induced inhibition of GVH disease (Lotzova and Cudkowicz, 1974), and splenectomy prior to intravenous injection of CP abrogates its inhibitory effect on CMI (Scott, 1974), suggesting that "suppressor" macrophages mediate CP-induced inhibition of cellular immunity.

Splenic and bone marrow lymphocytes from CP-treated mice show impaired MLC reactivity and respond poorly to phytohemagglutinin (PHA), a T-cell mitogen), but normally to pokeweed mitogen (PWM), a mixed T- and B-cell mitogen, and LPS (a B-cell mitogen) (Scott, 1972; Howard *et al.*, 1973). Impairment of the response of splenic T cells to PHA is reversed by removal of macrophages from the cell suspension; addition of macrophages from CP-treated mice inhibits the PHA reactivity of splenic lymphocytes from normal mice. Conversely, lymph node lymphocytes from CP-treated mice respond well to PHA (Scott, 1972) and show increased cytotoxicity for syngeneic tumor cells (Halpern *et al.*, 1973; Fisher *et al.*, 1974).

Stimulation of the RES by CP is manifested by hepatosplenomegaly and accelerated clearance of particles from the circulation (Halpern *et al.*, 1964), as well as by increased resistance to unrelated bacterial (Adlam *et al.*, 1972) and viral infections (Halpern *et al.*, 1973). CP induces macrophages to proliferate, as evidenced by their increased cloning efficiency *in vitro* (Wolmark *et al.*, 1974; Dimitrov *et al.*, 1975), and to become activated. The characteristics of macrophages activated by CP include increased phagocytic and bacteriostatic activity (Fauve and Hévin, 1971), augmented antigen-processing efficiency (Wiener and Bandieri, 1975), accumulation of lysosomal enzymes (Wilkinson *et al.*, 1973; Olivotto and Bomford, 1974), activation of phospholipase A (Munder and Modolell, 1974), and nonspecific cytostatic activity directed against tumor cells (Ghaffar *et al.*, 1975; Olivotto and Bomford, 1974; Scott, 1974). Increased nonspecific resistance to infections may be correlated with the enhanced bacteriostatic and lysosomal enzyme activity of macrophages. In addition to T-cell-mediated activation, macrophage activation may also be mediated by a corynebacteria-elaborated macrophage-specific chemotactic factor. Its production correlates with increased phagocytosis and macrophage-initiated release of lysosomal enzymes from neutrophils, but not with the immunoadjuvant effect (Wilkinson *et al.*, 1973). Thus, both direct and T-cell-mediated mechanisms appear to be involved in the activation of macrophages by CP (Bomford and Christie, 1975; Christie and Bomford, 1975; Ghaffar *et al.*, 1975) (See Chapter 5 for further discussion of the mechanisms involved in macrophage proliferation and activation.)

2.2.2. Effects on Immune Parameters in Man

Information concerning the action of CP on immune parameters in man comes from studies of its therapeutic and toxic effects in cancer patients. Reed *et al.* (1975) reported that DTH reactions to common antigens are increased after intravenous but not after subcutaneous administration of CP. Israël (1974) and our own group at Memorial Hospital were unable to demonstrate a consistent effect of parenterally administered CP on dermal DTH reactions in man. Israël observed that skin test reactivity tended to remain stable or improve in patients treated with CP alone or in conjunction with chemotherapy, but to remain unchanged or become depressed in those treated with chemotherapy alone. Our own experience at Memorial Hospital is still at a preliminary stage; so far, we have not been able to define a clear-cut pattern of CP-induced changes.

2.2.3. Effects on Cancer

The antitumor effects of CP were reviewed by Scott (1974) and Oettgen *et al.* (1976). Briefly, CP injected intravenously or intraperitoneally inhibits tumor growth in mice, if given prior to tumor transplantation, but not after the tumor has already become established. Intralesional injection of CP, which affords close contact between immunopotentiator and tumor antigens, has been shown to induce rejection not only of the injected tumor, but also, in some instances, of distant metastases. Systemic administration of CP has proved most effective when combined with cytotoxic chemotherapy or radiotherapy. In man, initial trials reported by Israël (1975), who treated over 400 patients with various types of malignancies, indicated promising results that have yet to be fully confirmed. In a small group of patients, Band *et al.* (1975) observed partial tumor regression in 3 of 18 patients with chemotherapy-resistant metastatic disease after intravenous infusion of CP. At this center, we have observed complete or partial regression of injected cutaneous metastases (mostly malignant melanoma) in 6 of 14 patients; uninjected lesions failed to regress. Thus, the available data appear to suggest that CP may be useful in potentiating the antitumor effects of conventional therapy, and that intralesional treatment may be beneficial for local but not for distant metastases.

2.3. Lipopolysaccharides

Lipopolysaccharides (LPS) are responsible for the characterisic biological activities of endotoxins of gram-negative bacteria. The marked similarity of the biological activities of various LPS is attributable to their common Lipid A structure, and contrasts with the antigenic diversity of their polysaccharide moieties.

LPS has long been known to be a potent modulator of immune reactions, and to induce regression of spontaneous, induced, and transplanted tumors in laboratory animals. Its toxicity has limited exploration of its therapeutic potential in man. For this reason, the mechanism of action of LPS on the immune system and on tumors has been the subject of intensive investigation aimed at circumventing unacceptable toxicity by modifying the LPS molecule or by identifying LPS-induced mediators of desirable biological activities.

In addition to its effects on the immune system and on tumors, LPS induces (1) release of pyrogens and lysosomal enzymes from phagocytic cells; (2) production of interferon; (3) endocrine changes; (4) granulocytosis and proliferation of hemopoietic stem cells; (5) release of vasomotor agents, resulting in progressive hypotension and shock; and (6) changes in the clotting system, associated with disseminated intravascular coagulation.

LPS is not only a potent immunogen and tolerogen in itself (Britton and Möller, 1968; Möller *et al.*, 1973), but also affects the immune response to unrelated antigens. Depending on the experimental conditions, LPS may enhance or depress immune reactions *in vivo* (Franzl and McMaster, 1968; Allison and Davies, 1971; Jones and Kind, 1972; Schmidtke and Dixon, 1972; Hamaoka and Katz, 1973; Dresser and Phillips, 1973) and *in vitro* (Ortiz-Ortiz and Jaroslow, 1970; Sjöberg *et al.*, 1972; Bullock and Andersson, 1973; Hoffmann *et al.*, 1973; Watson *et al.*, 1973). Under appropriate conditions, LPS enhances both T-cell-dependent and T-cell-independent antibody production (Ortiz-Ortiz and Jaroslow, 1970). It restores the humoral immune response in aged mice (Strausser *et al.*, 1971), enhances the response to weak antigens (Chiller *et al.*, 1973), renders tolerogenic doses of antigen immunogenic (Chiller *et al.*, 1973), and prevents induction of B-cell but not of T-cell tolerance (Louis *et al.*, 1973).

Treatment of mice with LPS enhances the cellular immune response to SRBC if LPS is administered after antigen (efferent arc), but suppresses the response if LPS is administered before antigen (afferent arc) (Lagrange *et al.*, 1975; Lagrange and Mackaness, 1975). GVH, allograft rejection, and antibody-dependent cell-mediated cytotoxicity were reported to be enhanced by LPS (Al-Askari *et al.*, 1964; Pudifin *et al.*, 1971; Skopinska, 1972).

A major target of LPS appears to be the B lymphocyte. LPS is a mitogen for B cells from murine and human spleen and avian peripheral blood (Peavy *et al.*, 1970, 1973; W. T. Weber, 1973; Greaves *et al.*, 1974), but is not mitogenic for B cells from the avian bursa or human peripheral blood, or for T cells from murine thymus (Peavy *et al.*, 1971; Gery *et al.*, 1972; W. T. Weber, 1973). LPS may modify T-cell responses to mitogens, either directly or indirectly through effects on macrophages (Schmidtke and Najarian, 1975). *In vitro,* LPS induces differentiation of B-cell precursors from spleen and fetal liver (Hämmerling *et al.*, 1975; Kearney and Lawton, 1975), as well as differentiation of splenic T-cell precursors (Scheid *et al.*, 1973), as shown by the appearance of characteristic markers on the surfaces of these cells. For the B cell, this includes both surface Ig and a C3 receptor. With the acquisition of a C3 receptor, the B lymphocyte becomes responsive to the mitogenic effect of LPS.

In the presence of antigen, LPS stimulates clonal expansion of antigen-reactive

B cells and accelerates their differentiation into antibody-secreting cells (Möller *et al.*, 1973; Quintans and Lefkovits, 1974). *In vitro* studies with splenic B lymphocytes showed that LPS initiates both proliferation and postmitotic synthesis of Ig (Melchers and Andersson, 1974).

LPS permits T-cell-dependent antigens to initiate antibody synthesis in mice depleted of helper T cells, provided they either possess a residual pool of T-cell precursors or are capable of responding to the T-cell-inducing effect of LPS. An immune response to LPS itself is not involved in this phenomenon.

The effect of LPS on antibody formation *in vitro* appears to depend on the functional state of the responding cell population. LPS suppresses antibody formation when added to spleen cell cultures before or together with antigen, but stimulates antibody production when added after antigen (Ortiz-Ortiz and Jaroslow, 1970; Hoffmann *et al.*, 1975). Addition of antigen-primed T cells fails to reverse the LPS-induced inhibition of antibody production (Hoffmann *et al.*, 1975). This finding suggests that LPS may interfere with antigen recognition by antigen-reactive helper cells or prevent these cells from achieving appropriate expression of the antigen signal (suppressor function?). Once T helper cells are antigen-activated, LPS acts to expand the B-cell compartment.

LPS promotes marked consumption of complement fractions C3–9, but little consumption of C1, C4, and C2, *in vitro* (Gewurz *et al.*, 1968). Mergenhagen *et al.* (1973) proposed that endotoxin may act either via the classical pathway, which involves the formation of C3 convertase ($C\overline{42}$) in the presence of a γ-2-globulin or via the alternate pathway, by activating a proenzyme of C3 activator that bypasses the requirement for C1, C4, and C2. Support for the latter concept is derived from the findings that LPS activates C3 in C4-deficient and cobra-venom-factor-treated guinea pig serum (Frank and May, 1973).

Recently, Dukor and Hartmann (1973) proposed that two signals, specific binding of antigen by Ig receptors and nonspecific interaction of activated C3 with its receptors, are required for specific triggering of B cells to proliferate and produce antibody. The observations of Dukor *et al.* (1973) and Bitter-Suermann *et al.* (1975) raise the possibility that nonspecific activation of B cells by LPS may also be controlled by dual signals: a direct effect due to attachment of LPS to putatively specific receptor sites and an indirect effect mediated by LPS activation of C3. While Janossy *et al.* (1973) and Waldmann and Lackmann (1975) contested this observation, this interpretation is consonant with the finding that LPS is mitogenic for mature B lymphocytes and macrophages, both of which have C3 receptors, but not for T lymphocytes, which lack C3 receptors.

In vivo studies suggest that macrophages play a role in mediating the adjuvant effect of LPS on T-cell-independent antibody responses (Spitznagel and Allison, 1970; Allison and Davies, 1971), but are not required to mediate the substitution of T-cell helper function by LPS (Sjöberg *et al.*, 1972). Injection of LPS is also associated with macrophage proliferation (Forbes, 1964) and activation in terms of tumoricidal capacity (Alexander and Evans, 1971). LPS *in vitro* induces a number of alterations of macrophages, including increased lysosomal enzyme content (Wiener and Levanon, 1968) and CSF production (Ruscetti and Chevernick, 1974), augmented glucosamine (Wilton *et al.*, 1975) and cytophilic antibody uptake (Tizard, 1971), secretion of a B-cell-activating factor (Wood and Cameron, 1976), and development of selective tumoricidal activity (Alexander and Evans, 1971).

2.3.1. Mechanism of Action on Cells of the Immune System

LPS is thought to act through receptors on the cell surface, although this idea has not been studied critically. Within this perspective, at least some of the effects of LPS can be compared with those of hormones and of other lectin mitogens the sites of action of which also lie at the cell surface. Bitensky *et al.* (1971) were the first to examine this possibility and to demonstrate that endotoxin treatment *in vivo* produces an enhanced sensitivity of the membrane enzyme adenylate cyclase to stimulation by epinephrine. This observation suggests that in liver and lymphoid cells, and possibly also in a number of other types of cells, LPS activity could be equated with an increase in cellular levels of cyclic AMP (cAMP). While De Rubertis *et al.* (1974) failed to find increases in adenylate cyclase activity or cAMP levels in unfractionated spleen cells, several other workers showed that in both B- and T-cell precursors from albumin-gradient-fractionated spleen cells, LPS-induced differentiation is closely paralleled by the effects of cAMP and a variety of agents known to increase cellular levels of cAMP (Scheid *et al.*, 1973; Hämmerling *et al.*, 1975). We observed that LPS, at concentrations that induce differentiation, does increase cAMP levels in precursor-cell-rich gradient fractions (Hadden, *et al.*, unpublished observations). Thus, it would appear that the differentiation-inducing capacity of LPS on lymphocyte precursors may be mediated by an increase in cellular levels of cAMP, presumably initiated by an action of LPS on adenylate cyclase.

Induction of proliferation of B lymphocytes, activation and possibly also proliferation of macrophages, and aggregation of platelets by LPS are consonant with events known or suspected to involve cGMP (see Chapters 1, 2, 4, and 5). Induction of proliferation of B cells by LPS is mimicked by cGMP (Weinstein *et al.*, 1974), and is associated with cellular increases in cGMP (Watson, 1975; Hadden and Coffey, unpublished observations) and decreases in levels of cAMP (Hadden *et al.*, unpublished observations). While LPS effects on levels of cGMP in macrophages and platelets have not been examined, agents with similar action on these cells increase levels of cGMP (Goldberg *et al.*, 1974; Hadden, unpublished observations). It should be noted that in cells in which LPS action is associated with a rise in cGMP, a complement receptor, thought to be related to LPS responsiveness, is invariably present on the cell surface. These correlative observations suggest that C3 activation may be involved in stimulating guanylate cyclase directly or indirectly through the influx of calcium.

While the action of LPS on cell-surface-related events appears to be probable, elucidation of the complexity of the effects of LPS on cellular levels of cyclic nucleotides and on the enzymes related to their generation, action, and catabolism is essential to clarify the pleomorphic action of this complex modulator on various components of the immune response.

2.3.2. Lipopolysaccharide in Cancer Therapy

The history of tumor regression associated with bacterial infection dates back more than 100 years (Busch, 1866). Between 1891 and 1935, Coley used first viable streptococci and later the mixed vaccines of *Streptococcus* and *Serratia marcescens* (Coley toxins) in over 400 cancer patients, obtaining striking results in some cases (Nauts *et al.*, 1953). The active antitumor principle (LPS) was isolated by Shear and his colleagues in 1943 (Shear *et al.*, 1943). Starting at the turn of the century and continuing well through the 1940s, numerous investigators confirmed the antitumor efficacy of a variety of bacteria and their products and, later, of LPS against a large spectrum of animal tumors. However, unacceptable toxicity of purified LPS and of its biologically active moiety, Lipid A, have precluded clinical use. Recently, it was reported that BCG-infected mice respond to injection of LPS by releasing into the serum a factor (tumor necrosis factor, TNF) that, like LPS, induces necrosis and occasional regression of murine tumor transplants, and unlike LPS, is cytotoxic for certain murine and human tumor cells *in vitro* (Carswell *et al.*, 1975; Helson *et al.*, 1976; Williamson *et al.*, personal communication). TNF has a variety of effects on immune responses *in vitro*, some similar to and others different from those of LPS (Hoffmann *et al.*, 1976), and is not toxic for animals. TNF appears to represent an endogenous mediator of the tumor-necrotizing activity of LPS, but to lack its prohibitive toxicity. The production, purification, and characterization of TNF and its application in cancer therapy represent one of the current challenges in LPS research.

2.4. Polysaccharides

In 1957, Benacerraf and Sebestyen (1957) demonstrated that zymosan, a cell wall preparation from the yeast *Saccharomyces cerevisiae*, has a marked stimulating effect on the RES. Almost simultaneously, Bradner *et al.* (1958) and Mankowski *et al.* (1957) discovered the antitumor activity of zymosan and a polysaccharide from another yeast (*Candida guilliermondi*) against two transplantable mouse tumors. Immunostimulatory and antitumor activities have since been demonstrated for a large variety of polysaccharides derived from natural sources (bacteria, fungi such as mushrooms and yeasts, lichens, and higher plants). Glucans possessing a linear β-1→3 glucose structure have, in general, been found to be particularly potent. Two examples are lentinan, a partially characterized, high-molecular-weight ($\pm 10^6$) preparation from the mushroom *Lentinus edodes* (Chihara *et al.*, 1970), and the glucan derived from zymosan (Riggi and Di Luzio, 1961; Di Luzio *et al.*, 1976).

Lentinan is an immunoadjuvant, but (unlike most other immunostimulatory agents such as BCG, LPS, *C. parvum*, and other polysaccharides) does not stimulate the RES or humoral immune responses (Maeda and Chihara, 1973; Dennert and Tucker, 1973). Lentinan normalizes depressed helper T-cell activity and potentiates antibody-dependent cell-mediated cytotoxicity, but has no effect on other T-cell functions such as allograft rejection, GVH reactions, and DTH (Dennert and Tucker, 1973; Maeda and Chihara, 1973; Haba *et al.*, 1976). Lentinan is not cytotoxic to tumor cells *in vitro*, indicating that its antitumor activity is exerted indirectly. T cells probably participate in mediating the agent's antitumor activity, since lentinan is ineffective against neoplasms in neonatally thymectomized mice, and only marginally effective in ALS-treated tumor-bearing mice (Maeda and Chihara, 1973).

The glucan derived from zymosan has been reported to have a different spectrum of activity. It augments the primary and secondary hemolysin response to T-cell-dependent antigens such as SRBC, and accelerates allograft rejection (Di

Luzio *et al.*, 1976). This glucan appears to exert at least part of its antitumor effect by means of nonspecific activation of macrophages, as indicated by (1) the absence of direct cytotoxicity against tumor cells *in vitro,* (2) tumor regression in mice and rats injected *in vivo* with glucan-activated macrophages, and (3) massive macrophage infiltration of rodent and human tumors that are regressing in response to intralesional injection of this agent (Mansell *et al.*, 1975; Di Luzio *et al.*, 1976).

Information on the polysaccharides is too preliminary and their actions too diverse to permit us to formulate a generalized concept of their mechanism of action. Possible mechansims of action of immunopotentiators on T cells and macrophages are discussed elsewhere in this chapter and in Chapter 5.

3. Chemical Immunopotentiators

The agents discussed up to this point represent bacteria or bacterial products that qualify both as immunopotentiators, in that they augment immune responses nonspecifically, and as immunoadjuvants, in that they augment specific immune responses when presented in conjunction with antigen. Although extensive animal studies have provided the rationale for employing these agents in immunotherapy in man, their toxicity has drastically limited their clinical application. Consequently, considerable efforts are being made to develop chemically defined immunopotentiators capable of achieving the same or greater effects on immune responses, with greater specificity for individual components of the immune system and less toxicity than cruder products discussed so far. Agents in this category include polynucleotides and levamisole. While these agents are currently being evaluated or considered in terms of their usefulness in the treatment of cancer, their eventual application may well include immunodeficiency diseases, chronic viral, bacterial, and fungal infections, and the so-called autoimmune disorders.

3.1. Polynucleotides

In 1963, Braun *et al.* (1963) observed that treatment with naturally occurring oligonucleotides delayed the onset of spontaneous mammary cancer in aging C3H mice. Subsequently, Braun and Nakano (1967) discovered that synthetic double-stranded complementary RNA homopolymers (dsRNA) such as poly I:C and poly A:U stimulated phagocytosis and augmented the antibody response to SRBC both *in vivo* and *in vitro*. Single-stranded homopolymers were found to be destroyed too rapidly *in vivo* to affect the immune system, although they were somewhat active *in vitro*. Independently, others discovered that dsRNA enhanced nonspecific resistance to viral (Lampson *et al.*, 1967) and bacterial infections (Fauve *et al.*, 1966), and that poly I:C was a potent inducer of interferon (Field *et al.*, 1967).

Animal and clinical studies have shown poly I:C to be toxic at doses required to induce interferon. On the other hand, poly A:U (which is a poor interferon inducer) is nontoxic, and has therefore had a more prominent role in recent investigations.

3.1.1. Effects of dsRNA on Immune Response

Treatment of mice with dsRNA affects the T-cell-dependent antibody response in various ways: (1) Both primary and secondary antibody response are enhanced (Braun *et al.*, 1971; Johnson *et al.*, 1971), and the induction period is shortened

(Johnson *et al.*, 1971). Contact between dsRNA and antigen is not essential for these effects, but timing is critical. For example, the time required for antibody induction is shortened if dsRNA is given within 0–2 hr after the antigen, but prolonged if dsRNA is given 12–24 hr before the antigen. There is no simple dose–response relationship; very high doses have no effect or even inhibit the response (Braun and Ishizuka, 1971). (2) The response to subimmunogenic doses of antigen and to weak immunogens is enhanced (Braun, 1969; Levy *et al.*, 1969; Braun *et al.*, 1971; Johnson *et al.*, 1971), induction of tolerance to T-cell-dependent antigens is inhibited (Kong and Capanna, 1974), and the induction period to subimmunogenic doses of antigen is shortened (Cone and Marchalonis, 1972). (3) A secondary response may be induced without antigen (Braun *et al.*, 1971; Johnson *et al.*, 1971). (4) The development of humoral immune competence in newborn mice is accelerated (Winchurch and Braun (1969) in a manner comparable to that induced by injection of adult peritoneal macrophages (Braun and Lasky, 1967; Argyris, 1968). (5) The impaired antibody responses of aged and genetically low responder mice are restored (Braun, 1970; Mozes *et al.*, 1970). Treatment with dsRNA is thought to expand the B-cell compartment and amplify antibody production without altering the number of antigen-reactive cells (Mozes *et al.*, 1973b).

Addition of poly A:U to tissue cultures was shown to modify the primary and secondary antibody response to SRBC *in vitro* (Cone and Marchalonis, 1972; Jaroslow and Ortiz-Ortiz, 1972). At optimum concentrations, the secondary response is augmented to a greater degree than the primary response. At higher concentrations, both responses are inhibited. The effect of poly A:U on antibody production *in vitro* has generally been attributed to increased helper function of T cells (Jaroslow and Ortiz-Ortiz, 1972). This view is confirmed by the finding that dsRNA markedly reduces the number of exogenous helper T cells required by T-cell-deficient mice to mount an antibody response to SRBC (Cone and Marchalonis, 1972). It was suggested that inhibition of antibody production by high concentrations of poly A:U is mediated by low levels of interferon (Johnson *et al.*, 1971).

dsRNA modulates cell-mediated immune responses. It augments GVH reactions and dermal DTH responses (Braun, 1970; Casavant and Youmans, 1975), but only if given 0–12 hr before antigen. *In vivo,* dsRNA restores immune competence to mice rendered T-cell-deficient by neonatal thymectomy or antithymus serum or both, by stimulating expansion of the residual T-cell compartment (Johnson *et al.*, 1971). *In vitro,* dsRNA induces T-cell differentiation from precursor cells in genetically athymic nude mice (Scheid *et al.*, 1973).

dsRNA exerts a number of effects on T lymphocytes *in vitro*. Cells from fractions of mouse spleens enriched in T-cell precursors can be induced with poly A:U to undergo differentiation, as evidenced by the expression of T-cell surface markers (Scheid *et al.*, 1973). Poly A:U enhances T-cell proliferative responses to recall antigens such as PPD and tetanus toxin (Chess *et al.*, 1972; Graziano *et al.*, 1974) and both proliferative and cytotoxic responses to allogeneic cells (Chess *et al.*, 1972; Wagner and Cone, 1974). Optimum concentrations of poly A:U stimulate, whereas supraoptimum concentrations inhibit, and responses to weak stimuli or suboptimum antigen concentrations are augmented, while those to optimum immunogenic concentrations of antigen are hardly affected. Responses of T cells to strong stimuli such as PHA are inhibited by poly A:U (Chess *et al.*, 1972). In general, the effects of poly A:U on T-cell functions *in vitro* occur at concentrations below those required to modify the humoral immune response *in vitro*.

Effects of dsRNA on the phagocytic system are indicated by increased nonspecific resistance to viral (Lampson *et al.*, 1967; Hamilton *et al.*, 1969) and bacterial infections (Mackaness, 1964; Fauve *et al.*, 1966), presumably due to accelerated clearance of infectious organisms (Braun and Nakano, 1967; Johnson *et al.*, 1971). The phagocytic effect is time-dependent, occurring only if the microorganisms are injected at least 60 min after dsRNA (Braun *et al.*, 1971). It does not require participation of T cells, since it can be elicited in nude mice (Cheers and Cone, 1974). Stimulation of macrophages involved in primary antigen processing is indicated by increased RNA synthesis (without increased antigen uptake or retention) in macrophage monolayers in the presence of dsRNA *in vitro*. Syngeneic mice injected with these macrophages show increased antibody production (Johnson *et al.*, 1971). Activation of macrophages by dsRNA is also manifested by the development of selective cytotoxicity for tumor cells (Alexander and Evans, 1971).

3.1.2. Mechanism of Action of dsRNA

On the suggestion of Kurt Hirschhorn, Werner Braun and his associates considered the possibility that the effects of poly A:U on the immune response might be mediated by cAMP. They (Ishizuka *et al.*, 1970, 1971; Braun and Ishizuka, 1971) observed that cAMP mimicked the effects of poly A:U on the antibody response to SRBC *in vivo* and *in vitro*, and that the phosphodiesterase inhibitor theophylline potentiated the effects of poly A:U. They further observed that adenylate cyclase activity was increased in spleen cells treated with poly A:U (Winchurch *et al.*, 1971). These observations were interpreted to indicate that poly A:U acts via cAMP. The effect of *in vivo* administration of poly A:U or cAMP *per se* on intracellular levels of cAMP has not been examined. It was shown, however, that administration of SRBC *in vivo* produces increases in cAMP levels in spleen cells during initiation of the immune response. These early increases in cAMP are thought to represent initiation of T-cell helper activity (Yamamoto and Webb, 1975). Mozes *et al.* (1973a) were unable to show that poly A:U increases cAMP levels in unfractionated spleen cells, thus casting doubt on this interpretation. More recently, however, Scheid *et al.* (1973) were able to show that poly A:U induces T-cell differentiation in mouse spleen cell fractions enriched in T-cell precursors, as do cAMP itself and a number of agents that increase cellular levels of cAMP. We observed a direct correlation between increased cAMP levels and *in vitro* induction of T-cell differentiation with poly A:U (Hadden *et al.*, unpublished observations). These observations suggest that poly A:U enhances the T-cell-dependent antibody response by increasing the number of T helper cells. The findings do not contribute to the understanding of the effects of poly A:U on the proliferation of T and B cells *in vitro* and on the function of macrophages. It seems reasonable to suggest that some actions of poly A:U, like those of LPS, may be linked to changes in cGMP levels in these cells. Other actions that might be considered include alterations of surface charge characteristics, antigen-binding, cell–cell interaction, and possibly cell-migration patterns.

3.1.3. Therapeutic Applications of dsRNA

Therapeutic trials of dsRNA have been limited to animals and patients with cancer. In rodents, dsRNA retards the development of primary spontaneous transplanted tumors (Youn *et al.*, 1968; Sarma *et al.*, 1969; Levy *et al.*, 1969; Braun, 1970; Vandeputte *et al.*, 1970; Mathé *et al.*, 1971; Lundy *et al.*, 1973; Drake *et al.*, 1974; Lacour *et al.*, 1975) and reduces the incidence of tumor recurrence after surgical excision of spontaneous and transplanted tumors (Braun, 1970; Lacour *et al.*, 1972). Preliminary trials in patients have been disappointing. Mathé *et al.* (1970) reported that induction of partial remission with chemotherapy, followed by treatment with poly A:U, resulted in complete remission in 5 of 15 patients with ALL. Others (De Vita *et al.*, 1970; Krakoff *et al.*, 1970) were unable to elicit antitumor responses in cancer patients with a large tumor load. Poly A:U, used at doses approximately 7 times lower than those reported effective against murine tumors, has not so far shown any antitumor effects in two other series of cancer patients (Wanebo *et al.*, 1975; J. Lacour, personal communication).

At first, it was thought that the antitumor effect of dsRNA was mediated by interferon. However, in view of the nature and timing of the antitumor effect and because poly A:U (a poor interferon inducer) has a spectrum of biological activity similar to that of poly I:C, an immunologic mechanism of action had to be considered. The clarification of the effects of poly A:U on the immune response has provided the rationale for considering its immunopotentiating action as the major mechanism for its antitumor action. Although its effects on the immune response are complex, its nontoxic adjuvant characteristics, coupled with its ability to abrogate tolerance and augment T-cell-dependent responses, make it an excellent candidate for use in combination with tumor cells or tumor-specific antigens for active immunotherapy.

In the realms of immunodeficiency and infectious disease, the therapeutic potential, in terms of induction of T cells from precursors and nonspecific augmentation of macrophage activity against viral and bacterial pathogens, warrants further investigation of this intriguing class of agents.

3.2. Levamisole

Levamisole is a phenylimidazothiazole that was developed as an antihelmintic agent. Its usefulness has been attributed to its capacity to inhibit the motility of parasites. It was fortuitously discovered by Renoux and Renoux (1971) that levamisole augments the protective effect of an anti-*Brucella* vaccine against challenge with virulent *Brucella*. In retrospect, it was realized that this discovery was preceded by related observations, including instances in which unrelated infectious diseases were ameliorated or cured in animals treated with levamisole for nematode infestation. The Renoux' observation stimulated many investigations aimed at defining the mechanism of action of levamisole and its immunotherapeutic effects.

The results of Renoux and Renoux (1971, 1972a,d,e, 1974a,b, 1977) and Renoux *et al.* (1976) indicate that levamisole treatment of mice augments the production of antibody to SRBC, enhances the GVH reaction, and increases nonspecific resistance to *Brucella* and *Rickettsia* infections. The latter findings have been extended by others. Fischer *et al.* (1975a,b) found that treatment of weanling rats with levamisole increased their resistance to inoculation with herpesvirus and staphylococci. Rojas (personal communication) observed that levamisole is effective in the treatment of hoof and mouth disease and, when combined with vaccination, also enhances resistance to primary infection. The Renoux' early studies revealed that a number of variables affect the response. For example, individuals with depressed immunocompetence seemed to respond better than those with normal or near-normal responsiveness; the response to suboptimum antigenic stimuli was often augmented, while the response to optimum stimuli remained relatively unaffected. These findings led to the concept that levamisole is an "immunonormalizing" rather than an immunopotentiating agent.

3.2.1. Effects on Immune Response

Levamisole has little effect on antibody production in immunocompetent animals and human subjects (cf. Symoens, 1977), but augments antibody production in mice that are immunodeficient because of genetic factors or old age (Renoux and Renoux, 1972b, 1974a,b, 1977; Spreafico *et al.*, 1975). At doses that augment antibody production, specific lymphocyte-mediated cytotoxicity for tumor cells is suppressed (Mantovani and Spreafico, 1975); at higher doses, however, it is augmented (Faanes *et al.*, 1977).

In man, levamisole was reported to restore and augment DTH responses to DNCB or PPD (Brugmans *et al.*, 1973; Renoux *et al.*, 1973; Tripodi *et al.*, 1973; Verhaegen *et al.*, 1973; Rojas *et al.*, 1976), and to increase the proliferative response of lymphocytes to mitogens or antigens *in vitro* (Sunshine *et al.*, 1977; Rojas, personal communication).

Added *in vitro*, levamisole augments DNA synthesis by mouse spleen cells and thymocytes in response to mitogens and alloantigens, as well as in the absence of these stimuli (Woods *et al.*, 1974, 1975; Hadden *et al.*, 1975; Merluzzi *et al.*, 1975). In most studies with human lymphocytes, levamisole was found to induce only small increases of the proliferative response to mitogens (Lichtenfeld *et al.*, 1974, 1977; Hadden *et al.*, 1975; Chan and Simons, 1975; Sampson and Lui, 1976; Goyanes-Villaescusa, 1976) and to alloantigens or allogeneic cells (Lichtenfeld, 1974; Pabst and Crawford, 1975). Levamisole was reported to augment mitogen-induced lymphokine production (Whitcomb *et al.*, 1976), E-rosette formation by T cells (Verhaegen *et al.*, 1975), and T-cell suppressor activity (Sampson and Lui, 1976). In these studies, supraoptimum concentrations of levamisole were found to be inhibitory. The relatively weak response to antigens was augmented more than the relatively strong response to mitogens, and the effects were demonstrable more easily with cells from immunosuppressed subjects than with cells from normal subjects. The accumulated evidence appears to indicate that the thymus-dependent lymphocyte is preferentially responsive to levamisole.

Treatment of mice with levamisole enhances RES activity, as is evident from beneficial effects on experimental infections with intracellular pathogens, increased carbon clearance (Hoebeke and Franchi, 1973), and enhanced phagocytic and bactericidal activity of peritoneal macrophages (Versijp *et al.*, 1975; Renoux *et al.*, 1976). Added *in vitro*, levamisole augments phagocytosis of opsonized SRBC by peritoneal macrophages of mice (Oliveira-Lima *et al.*, 1974) and phagocytosis and killing of *Listeria* by peritoneal macrophages of guinea pigs (see Chapters 4 and 5). Levamisole also augments the chemotactic response of neutrophils and monocytes from normal and immunodeficient patients (Wright *et al.*, 1977).

3.2.2. Mechanisms of Action

Levamisole is a derivative of imidazole, an agent known to act on cyclic nucleotide phosphodiesterases, that promotes increased breakdown of cAMP and decreased breakdown of cGMP. The effects of levamisole on the proliferative responses of mouse and human lymphocytes (Hadden *et al.*, 1975) and on phagocytosis by macrophages (Oliveira-Lima *et al.*, 1974) can also be induced with imidazole. As would be expected, theophylline, which decreases the breakdown of cAMP, reverses the levamisole-induced increase of antibody production to SRBC by mouse spleen cells (Renoux and Renoux, 1972c). The effects of levamisole on lymphocyte proliferation, lymphokine production, and cytotoxicity are also shared by imidazole and other agents that increase cGMP levels in lymphocytes (see Chapters 1–3). The increase in cGMP levels closely parallels effects of these agents on lymphocyte proliferation (Hadden *et al.*, 1975). Similarly, the levamisole-induced increase in cGMP levels in human mononuclear cells is paralleled by an augmentation of the chemotactic response of these cells (Wright *et al.*, 1977).

While some of the effects of levamisole may be mediated by its ability to increase cGMP in lymphocytes and macrophages, other effects may be more directly related to the sulfur-containing ring (see Section 3.3.1).

One action of levamisole, mobilization of polymorphonuclear leukocytes to sites of infection in weanling rats (Fischer *et al.*, 1975b), deserves special comment. The functional deficiency of leukocytes and monocytes from newborn animals is thought to represent a maturation-dependent impairment of nonspecific resistance. Aside from its direct effect on the chemotactic response of polymorphonuclear leukocytes and monocytes (Wright *et al.*, 1977), levamisole may also modify the generation of these two cell types. The growth and maturation of both cell lines is known to be under the regulation of CSF. We (Kurland *et al.*, 1977) observed that the action of CSF on the *in vitro* formation of colonies by these cells is augmented by imidazole and other agents that increase cellular levels of cGMP. The speculation that levamisole would have an imidazolelike action on granulopoiesis is relevant in terms of the possibility that it may enhance the recovery not only of immune responses, but also of bone marrow function following cytotoxic chemotherapy (Lods *et al.*, 1976).

3.2.3. Therapeutic Uses in Immunodeficiency, Infections, and Related Disorders

It appears that levamisole is not generally effective against primary bacterial or viral infections in immunocompetent adult animals, but may be of some benefit in the treatment of chronic or recurrent infections in immunodeficient patients or immature animals (Symoens and Brugmans, 1976). Since levamisole has no intrinsic antibacterial or antiviral properties, those effects must be mediated by its immunopotentiating activity. Immunodeficiency diseases that have been treated with some degree of success include Job's or hyperimmunoglobulin E syndrome, lazy leukocyte syndrome, Wiskott–Aldrich syndrome, ataxia telangectasia, chronic granulomatous disease, and cyclic neutropenia (Spitler *et al.*, 1977; Wright *et al.*, 1977). In recurrent herpes infections, levamisole reduced the frequency, duration, and severity of infectious episodes, and, in some studies, was associated with improvement of nonspecific and virus-specific immune parameters (Kint and Verlinden, 1974; O'Reilly *et al.*, 1977; Spitler *et al.*, 1977). In acne conglobata, recurrent furunculosis, and other chronic pyogenic skin infections, levamisole treatment improved or cleared the lesions (Ippen and Quadripur, 1975; Spitler *et al.*, 1977). In a controlled study, the majority of children with respiratory infections who had been treated with levamisole showed a reduction in the number, severity, and duration of infectious episodes (Van Eygen *et al.*, 1976). In a number of disorders suspected of representing infectious diseases commonly associated with selective immunologic defects, levamisole produced clinical improvement. These disorders include rheumatoid arthritis (C. M. Basch *et al.*, 1975; Schuermans, 1975; Trabert *et al.*, 1975; Huskisson *et al.*, 1976), Reiter's syndrome (Ippen and Quadripur, 1975; Trabert *et al.*, 1975), systemic lupus erythematosus (Gorden and Keenan, 1975), aphthous stomatitis (Symoens and Brugmans, 1976; Spitler *et al.*, 1977), and Crohn's disease (Bertrand *et al.*, 1974). Clinical testing of levamisole is still in an early stage. Infections that might respond include chronic forms of tuberculosis, brucellosis, leprosy, and hepatitis, So far, clinical toxicity has been found to be minimal and restricted to GI symptoms, nervousness, dysomia, metallic taste, and skin rashes (Symoens, 1977).

3.2.4. Treatment of Cancer Patients with Levamisole

In animal studies, levamisole alone has been ineffective in the treatment of experimental tumors commonly employed to screen chemotherapeutic agents (see Symoens, 1977). Chirigos *et al.* (1973, 1975) observed, however, that levamisole, if given after immunosuppressive chemotherapy but not if given alone, increased immunologic reactivity and survival of mice with transplants of virus-induced solid tumors. Spreafico *et al.* (1975) confirmed this observation in leukemic mice. Kassel (1977) and Spreafico *et al.* (1975) demonstrated that levamisole, when combined with active immunization using irradiated tumor cells, increased survival of mice bearing tumor transplants.

In cancer patients, levamisole was reported to restore impaired immune functions (Brugmans *et al.*, 1973; Tripodi *et al.*, 1973; Verhaegen *et al.*, 1973; Biniaminov and Ramot, 1975; Levo *et al.*, 1975; Rojas *et al.*, 1976). Treatment with levamisole after surgery or radiation therapy was reported to increase survival and delay recurrence in patients with breast cancer (Rojas *et al.*, 1976; Debois, 1977) and lung cancer (Study Group for Bronchogenic Carcinoma, 1975). Another encouraging observation is that restoration of bone marrow function following chemotherapy is accelerated by levamisole (Lods *et al.*, 1976).

3.3. Other Synthetic Immunopotentiators

3.3.1. Sulfur-Containing Compounds

The presence of sulfur in levamisole, and the knowledge that 2-mercaptoethanol and cysteine augment lymphocyte proliferation and antibody production *in vitro,* prompted Renoux and Renoux (1974a) to suggest that sulfur-containing substances in general may augment immune responses. They demonstrated that treatment of mice with a number of sulfur-containing compounds, including sodium thiosulfate, diethyldithiocarbamate, and thiabendazole, augments antibody production to SRBC. While these observations have not been confirmed by others, they may provide an impetus for the development of new drugs in this category.

3.3.2. Inosiplex

Another agent with immunoenhancing activity is inosiplex (isoprinosine), a complex of inosine with *p*-acetomidobenzoic acid-*n,n* dimethylamine isopropanol. It was reported to be effective in the treatment of patients and animals with viral infections, including herpes (Chang and Weinstein, 1973; Gordon *et al.*, 1974; Wickett *et al.*, 1976), influenza (Gordon and Brown, 1972; Chang and Weinstein, 1973; Longley *et al.*, 1973; Muldoon *et al.*, 1972), and rhinovirus (Pachuta *et al.*, 1974; Waldman, 1977). In addition to evidence of a direct antiviral effect, inosiplex is thought to act as an immunopotentiator (Hadden *et al.*, 1976; 1977). It enhances mitogen-induced proliferation of normal human lymphocytes when added *in vitro* (Hadden *et al.*, 1976; 1977), and increases antibody production, mitogen-induced proliferation, and lymphokine production of human lymphocytes when given to patients (Longley *et al.*, 1973; Pachuta *et al.*, 1974; Bradshaw, 1977; Waldman, 1977). Its mechanism of action appears to involve RNA metabolism (Gordon *et al.*, 1974; Ronsen and Gordon, 1976), unrelated to cyclic nucleotides (Hadden *et al.*, 1976, 1977). The limited experience with this agent suggests that it will be clinically useful.

4. Products of the Immune System

For many years, hypo- and agammaglobulinemic patients have been treated with immunoglobulin preparations, and immune serum and γ-globulin have been employed to provide passive immunity for normoglobulinemic patients with certain infections. This form of immunotherapy is well established and will not be reviewed here. We would like, however, to discuss other products of the immune system that may restore or augment cellular immune responses: transfer factor, the so-called lymphokines, interferons, and thymic hormones.

4.1. Transfer Factor

Lawrence (1955) reported in 1955 that delayed hypersensitivity to tuberculin could be transferred to a tuberculin-negative recipient with an extract prepared from leukocytes from a tuberculin-positive donor. The observation has been confirmed, and transfer factor (TF) has been used in the treatment of immunodeficiency, chronic infections, and cancer (see Lawrence, 1974; Ascher *et al.*, 1976).

TF, as defined by Lawrence, is prepared by disrupting buffy coat cells by freezing and thawing, and dialyzing the preparation against water. TF has a molecular weight of less than 10,000, and is resistant to digestion with RNAase, DNAase, and pronase. Attempts to purify TF, like those recently reported by Neidhart *et al.* (1973), Sandler *et al.* (1975), and Reymond and Grob (1975), will in the future bring us closer to a biochemical definition of what is being referred to as TF. While some studies (see Lawrence, 1974) support the view that the transfer of sensitivity with TF is specific, others indicate that TF enhances delayed hypersensitivity in a nonspecific way. Treatment with TF has been associated with induction or augmentation of DTH (even to stimuli to which the donor had not been sensitized), increased numbers of T lymphocytes in the blood, increased monocyte chemotaxis, and increased reactivity of lymphocytes *in vitro* to antigens and PHA, as measured by both proliferative response and lymphokine production (see Griscelli *et al.*, 1973; Lawrence, 1974; Ascher *et al.*, 1976; LoBuglio and Neidhart, 1976).

Ascher *et al.* (1974) reported that TF from PPD-positive donors, added to lymphocyte cultures, augmented the response of lymphocytes from PPD-negative donors to PPD. Hamblin *et al.* (1976a,b) found that TF augments both PPD- and PHA-induced lymphocyte proliferative responses *in vitro*. It is of interest that the proliferative responses were determined by the characteristics of the responder, rather than by the sensitivity of the donor, suggesting that TF under these circumstances is nonspecific.

Treatment with TF has been beneficial in immunodeficiency syndromes including Wiskott–Aldrich syndrome, ataxia telangectasia, and chronic mucocutaneous candidiasis (Kirkpatrick *et al.*, 1970; Hitzig *et al.*, 1972; Spitler *et al.*, 1972; Griscelli *et al.*, 1973), and chronic infections such as coccidiomycosis, histoplasmosis, leprosy, and hepatitis and other viral infections (Graybill *et al.*, 1973; Hastings *et al.*, 1976; Heim *et al.*, 1976; Shulman *et al.*, 1976). Therapeutic benefit has also been reported in occasional patients with melanoma (Brandes *et al.*, 1971; Spitler *et al.*, 1972; Smith *et al.*, 1973), breast cancer (Smith *et al.*, 1973; Oettgen *et al.*, 1974), and nasopharyngeal carcinoma (Goldenberg and Brandes, 1972). There were no side effects. On the whole, the investigation of TF has been hampered by the lack of a standardized product as well as a practical and precise assay. Thus, the difficulties encountered in attempting to reproduce the observed effects on immunologic functions and disease are hardly surprising.

Considerations of the mechanism of action of TF depend to a great extent on whether specificity is inherent in that action. We have no precedent on which to base speculation as to how a molecule with a molecular weight of less than 10,000 and lacking antigenic components confers an antigen-specific response on recipient lymphocytes. Lawrence (1974) suggested a derepressor effect; however, the mechanism remains obscure. It was shown that Sephadex-purified TF enhances macrophage chemotaxis (Gallin and Kirkpatrick, 1974), and that TF increases cGMP in mononuclear cells (Sandler *et al.*, 1975). TF-induced modification of macrophage functions such as chemotaxis, and perhaps proliferation and activation, might well account for the nonspecific effects of TF observed *in vivo* and *in vitro* (see Chapter 5). If indeed TF is a single- or double-stranded oligonucleotide, its mechanism of action may be comparable to that of other dsRNAs discussed in this chapter.

4.2. Lymphokines

While Tf is derived from unstimulated lymphocytes, other soluble mediators (lymphokines) are secreted by lymphocytes only after stimulation. Their biological activities are summarized in Chapters 5 and 10. Whether or not lymphokines are effective systemic immunopotentiators remains to be investigated.

Mitogen-stimulated human peripheral blood lymphocytes and established lymphoid cell lines represent easily available, rich sources of these lymphokines. Partial purification of a number of lymphokines has been achieved. Local application of crude lymphokines has been reported to induce a reaction similar to DTH reactions (see Chapter 10).

Clinically, crude preparations of lymphokines from human lymphoid cell lines have been injected into skin metastases of cancer. Regression of injected metastases was observed (Papermaster *et al.*, 1976; E. Klein *et al.*, 1976).

The mechanism of action of these crude preparations is unknown. Principal constituents of active preparations are factors that (1) attract, inhibit the migration, and induce proliferation and activation of macrophages (MCT, MIF, MMF, MAF) (reviewed in Chapters 5 and 10); and (2) have nonspecific cytotoxic and cytostatic effects on tumor cells (e.g., lymphotoxin and interferon) (see Chapter 10). Considerable effort will be required to characterize these factors and to produce them in quantities adequate for clinical use.

4.3. Interferons

The interferons represent at least two different types of substances produced by cells in response to viral infection. One is produced by cells of the immune system in response to a variety of stimuli, including viral infection; the other, by nonlymphoid cells, e.g., virus-infected fibroblasts. While the two types of interferon can be distinguished biochemically, they appear to share two principal activities: the ability to inhibit viral replication and release of virus from infected cells, and the ability to inhibit the replication of cells. The first activity justifies the use of interferon in viral infections; the second provides the rationale for its use in cancer therapy. Interferon itself is not an immunopotentiator. In fact, it may act as an immunosuppressor, since it inhibits GVH disease *in vivo* and lymphocyte proliferation and antibody production *in vitro* (Lindahl-Magnusson *et al.*, 1972; Cerottini *et al.*, 1973; Gisler *et al.*, 1974).

The mechanism of action of interferons is unknown. Its activity is potentiated by agents that increase cAMP (Friedman and Pastan, 1969; J. M. Weber and Stewart, 1975; Lopez and Hadden, unpublished observations) and antagonized by ouabain and agents that increase cGMP (Lebon *et al.*, 1975; Lopez and Hadden, unpublished observations). Two reports indicate that crude interferon preparations increase cAMP in target cells (Braun and Levy, 1972; J. M. Weber and Stewart, 1975). The antiviral action of interferon is specific, and is not shared by agents that increase cellular levels of cAMP. The cytostatic effect of interferon, however, is not specific, and is shared by agents that increase cAMP.

Although interferon can be induced by both viral and nonviral stimuli, its antiviral and antitumor activities are not separable. The antitumor activity of interferon in animals extends to virus-induced tumors as well as to tumors not demonstrably related to oncogenic viruses. In rodents, interferon has been shown to reduce the incidence and retard the development of spontaneous leukemias and mammary cancers, to retard viral induction of leukemias and solid tumors, and to inhibit growth of a variety of transplanted solid and ascitic tumors of both viral and nonviral etiology (see Gresser, 1972). Interferon also induces rapid, albeit transitory, regression of advanced spontaneous (virus-associated) leukemia in AKR mice (Kassel *et al.*, 1973).

The clinical application of human interferon (which also shows other "lymphokine" activities) has been limited to patients with viral infections and cancer (Krim and Sanders, 1977; *International Workshop on Interferon in the Treatment of Cancer*, 1974). Interferon has been reported to reduce the symptoms and duration of herpesvirus infections, and to delay the development of metastases of osteogenic sarcoma following amputation. These early reports, while encouraging, require confirmation before the clinical potential of interferon therapy can be assessed.

4.4. Thymic Hormones

The existence of a thymic hormone has long been postulated, supported by the findings that implantation of normal thymus tissue in diffusion chambers corrects the immunologic impairment of neonatally thymectomized and adult-thymectomized and -irradiated animals (Levey *et al.*, 1963; Osaba and Miller, 1963). Several groups have prepared and purified thymic extracts: thymosin (A. L. Goldstein *et al.*, 1966), thymic humoral factor (Trainin *et al.*, 1967), thymopoietin (G. Goldstein and Hoffmann, 1969), and thymic factor (originally extracted from mammalian serum) (Bach and Dardenne, 1973) (see Table 2). The molecular weights of these products differ: 12,500 for thymosin (Hooper *et al.*, 1975), 3000 for thymic humoral factor (Trainin and Small, 1970), 5700 for thymopoietin (G. Goldstein, 1975), and 1000 for thymic factor (Bach *et al.*, 1975). The amino acid composition has been determined for thymosin (Hooper *et al.*, 1975) and thymopoietin (G. Goldstein, 1975), and the complete amino acid sequence has been established for thymopoietin (Schlesinger and Goldstein, 1975). Chemically purified thymopoietin (G. Goldstein, 1975) was found to have biological activity (i.e., induction of T-cell differentiation) at concentrations as low as 20 pg/ml (Basch and G. Goldstein, 1974; G. Goldstein *et al.*, 1975). Another polypeptide termed ubiquitin, also isolated from the thymus (G. Goldstein *et al.*, 1975), was found to induce T-cell as well as B-cell differentiation. Ubiquitin has been found to be present in every tissue of every animal species, microorganism, and plant studied.

4.4.1. Effects on Cellular Immunity

Thymic factors are potentiators of cellular immunity. They have been shown to (1) promote DNA synthesis in lymphocytes *in vivo* (J. J. Klein *et al.*, 1966) and *in vitro* (A. L. Goldstein *et al.*, 1966); (2) restore the capacity of lymphocytes from neonatally thymectomized mice to reject allografts and tumor isografts *in vivo* (Trainin and Linker-Israeli, 1967), and respond to allogeneic cells and tumor cells *in vitro* (Trainin *et al.*, 1969); (3) accelerate allograft rejection in intact mice (Hardy *et al.*, 1968); (4) induce the appearance of theta and TL antigens as well as sensitivity

TABLE 2. Characteristics of Thymic Hormones

Factor	Molecular weight	Action on immune system: T-cell induction	Action on immune system: Mitogen responsiveness	Action on immune system: Augmentation of MLC or GVH	References
Thymopoietin	5,700	+	+	?	G. Goldstein (1975)
Thymosin	12,500	+	+	+	Hooper *et al.* (1975)
Thymic humoral factor	3,000	+	+	+	Trainin *et al.* (1975)
Thymic factor	1,000	+	?	?	Bach *et al.* (1975)

to azathioprine and ALS in T-cell precursors in the bone marrow of normal, congenitally athymic (nude) and adult-thymectomized mice (Bach *et al.*, 1971; Scheid *et al.*, 1973); and (5) amplify T-cell responses to mitogens, allogeneic lymphocytes, and T-cell-dependent antigens (Bach *et al.*, 1975; Cohen *et al.*, 1975; Hooper *et al.*, 1975).

Bach *et al.* (1975) observed decreased serum concentrations of thymic factor in aged persons and in patients with certain immunodeficiency diseases. A. L. Goldstein *et al.* (1976) found that thymosin reconstitutes T-cell function (measured both *in vivo* and *in vitro*) in patients with a variety of immunodeficiency diseases, and partially reconstitutes immunologic competence in patients with Hodgkin's disease.

4.4.2. Mechanism of Action

Thymopoietin and thymosin act at two levels in the thymus-dependent cell compartment: (1) at the level of the prothymocyte, inducing it to differentiate (R. S. Basch and G. Goldstein, 1974; G. Goldstein *et al.*, 1975; Scheid *et al.*, 1973), and (2) at the level of mature thymocytes and thymus-dependent lymphocytes in the blood and peripheral lymphoid tissue, promoting their proliferation (Barker and Moore, 1977; Sunshine *et al.*, unpublished observations). Most of the available evidence indicates that the effect on the prothymocyte involves cAMP (see Chapter 1). Scheid *et al.* (1975) demonstrated that cAMP and agents that induce or preserve cellular increases in cAMP simulate the action of thymosin and thymopoietin in inducing prothymocyte differentiation *in vitro*. Pharmacological data provide additional evidence that cAMP is involved. Kook and Trainin (1974, 1975) reported that thymic humoral factor increases cAMP levels and adenylate cyclase activity in mouse spleen cells and thymocytes. Of the other thymus-derived factors studied, none has been demonstrated unequivocally to increase cAMP levels in prothymocytes (Hadden and Coffey, unpublished observations; M. Bach and A. L. Goldstein, personal communication).

The action of thymosin and thymopoietin on postthymic lymphocytes, augmenting E-rosette formation, and lymphocyte proliferation in response to mitogenic stimuli (Barker and Moore, 1977; Sunshine *et al.*, unpublished observations), is very similar to actions induced by levamisole (see Section 3.2), an agent known to lower cAMP levels and to increase cGMP levels in thymus-dependent lymphocytes (Hadden *et al.*, 1975). We (Sunshine *et al.*, 1977) observed that thymopoietin increases cGMP levels in thymocytes and T-lymphocyte-rich fractions of spleen cells. The proliferative action of thymic hormones (specifically, thymopoietin) would appear to be linked to mediation by cGMP.

4.4.3. Therapeutic Applications

Of the various thymic factors described to date, only thymosin has been employed in clinical studies (A. L. Goldstein *et al.*, 1976). The thymosin used in such studies represents a relatively crude preparation, and may contain activities related to other thymic factors or to ubiquitin. When added *in vitro* to cultured lymphocytes of patients with immunodeficiency or cancer, thymosin has been reported to increase the number of E-rosette-forming cells. Responsiveness varies with the type of immunodeficiency syndrome: lymphocytes of patients having no thymus or showing depressed thymic function (Wiskott–Aldrich syndrome, ataxia telangiectasia) are particularly responsive to thymosin, while those of patients with stem cell-defects are not responsive (Wara *et al.*, 1975). Similarly, lymphocytes of patients with a variety of leukemias and lymphoid malignancies are responsive (Wara *et al.*, 1975). Interestingly, lymphocytes of some patients with acute systemic lupus erythematosis and chronic renal disease have also been shown to respond. A. L. Goldstein *et al.* (1976) interpreted *in vitro* responses of lymphocytes to thymosin as an indication of the existence of a thymus deficiency state. They therefore embarked on clinical trials with thymosin in patients with various types of immunodeficiency syndromes. Early results indicate that thymosin treatment is safe: approximately 25% of the patients show skin reactions at the site of injection, but only 6% show generalized (probably allergic) reactions requiring suspension of therapy. Although insufficient numbers of patients with any particular disease have been studied to draw conclusions, many patients have demonstrated increases in delayed hypersensitivity, circulating numbers of E-rosette-forming T cells, and lymphocyte reactivity *in vitro* to various mitogenic stimuli (A. L. Goldstein *et al.*, 1976). In view of these encouraging findings, it is hoped that as more highly purified or even synthetic thymic hormone preparations become available, allergic reactions can be controlled and therapeutic efficacy improved.

5. Conclusions

The agents discussed in this chapter offer a wide spectrum of magnitude, mode, and mechanism of action. The differences in their action provide a degree of specificity that, when better understood, may provide the basis for selective action, and ultimately for combination therapy designed to achieve a multiplicity of actions. The bacterial and plant products in general share high potency, but also high antigenicity and toxicity. The development of purified active components clearly forecasts agents with an increased efficacy/toxicity ratio. The chemical agents appear to share low toxicity, but also, in general, have a low degree of effectiveness. The biological agents show high activity with little toxicity, but as yet are not readily available in quantity or in purified form. Many of the agents discussed appear to be linked to cyclic nucleotides in their actions. A better understanding of their actions at the intracellular level will be important for developing the predictive rationale for both combination therapy and the development of other chemical substances that will potentiate or simulate their action.

Insofar as these agents have been applied to immunodeficiency disorders in which the specific immunologic defects are known, we can estimate their potential to replace, augment, or compensate for specific types of immune responses. Their application to chronic infections, in which the mechanisms of resistance are known, has provided useful information on the mode of action of these agents. Their application to autoimmune and malignant disease, in which the mechanisms of pathogenesis are less clearly understood, has been empirical. Beneficial clinical results obtained to date with these agents will surely be improved on, once their primary action (i.e., that on immune responses) becomes better documented by studies of both specific and nonspecific immune parameters. Ultimately, their employment in conjunction with specific antigens to which the subject has been sensitized (i.e., bacterial, viral, and tumor antigens) will increase the efficacy and specificity of these agents' use.

As a clearer understanding of the roles and interrelationships of lymphocytes, macrophages, and antibody in their expressive as well as in their suppressive and blocking functions develops, greater insight into the mechanism of action and potential of these agents will result. It is tempting to describe the present status of development as an early or "sulfonamide era" of immunopotentiators and to predict that in the future, a more sophisticated or "antibiotic era" will develop in which many agents with both efficacy and safety will be usefully employed in a variety of disorders ranging from immunodeficiency to cancer.

References

Adlam, C., and Scott, M. T., 1973, *J. Med. Microbiol.* **6**:261–272.

Adlam, C., Broughton, E. S., and Scott, M. T., 1972, *Nature (London) New Biol.* **235**:219–220.

Adlam, C., Reid, D. E., and Torkington, P., 1975, in: *Corynebacterium parvum: Applications in Experimental and Clinical Oncology* (B. N. Halpern, ed.), pp. 35–39, Plenum Press, New York.

Al-Askari, W., Man, G., Lawrence, H. S., and Thomas, L., 1964, *J. Immunol.* **93**:742–748.

Alexander, P., and Evans, R., 1971, *Nature (London) New Biol.* **232**:76–78.

Allison, A. C., and Davies, A. J. S., 1971, *Nature (London)* **233**:330–332.

Amiel, J. L., and Bérardet, M., 1972, *Ann. Inst. Pasteur* **122**:701–714.

Argyris, B. F., 1968, *J. Exp. Med.* **128**:459–467.

Ascher, M. S., Schneider, W. J., Valentine, F. T., and Lawrence, H. S., 1974, *Proc. Natl. Acad. Sci. U.S.A.* **71**:1178–1182.

Ascher, M. S., Gottlieb, A. A., and Kirkpatrick, C. H. (eds.), 1976, *Transfer Factor: Basic Properties and Clinical Applications,* Academic Press, New York.

Asherson, G. L., and Alwood, G. G., 1971, *Clin. Exp. Immunol.* **9**:249–258.

Bach, J.-F., and Dardenne, M., 1973, *Immunology* **25**:353–366.

Bach, J.-F., Dardenne, M., Goldstein, A. L., Guha, A., and White, A., 1971, *Proc. Natl. Acad. Sci. U.S.A.* **68**:2734–2738.

Bach, J.-F., Dardenne, M., Pleau, J.-M., and Bach, M.-A., 1975, *Ann. N.Y. Acad. Sci.* **249**:186–210.

Balner, H., Old, L. J., and Clarke, D. A., 1962, *Proc. Soc. Exp. Biol. Med.* **109**:58–62.

Band, P. R., Jao-King, C., Urtasun, R., and Haraphongse, M., 1975, *Proc. Am. Assoc. Cancer Res.* **16**:9.

Barker, A. D., and Moore, V. S., 1977, in: *Progress in Cancer Research and Therapy II* (M. A. Chirigos, ed.), pp. 289–303, Raven Press, New York.

Basch, C. M., Spitler, L. E., and Engleman, E. P., 1975, *Arthritis Rheum.* **18**:385.

Basch, R. S., and Goldstein, G., 1974, *Proc. Natl. Acad. Sci. U.S.A.* **71**:1474–1478.

Bast, R. C., Jr., Bast, B. S., and Rapp, H. J., 1976, *Ann. N.Y. Acad. Sci.* **277**:60–93.

Bekierkunst, A., 1974, *Recent Results Cancer Res.* **47**:259–261.

Bekierkunst, A., Levij, I. S., Yarkoni, E., Vilkas, E., Adam, A., and Lederer, E., 1969, *J. Bacteriol.* **100**:95–102.

Bekierkunst, A., Wang, L., Bast, B., Toubiana, R., and Lederer, E., 1974, *Infect. Immun.* **10**:1044–1050.

Benacerraf, B., and Sebestyen, M. M., 1957, *Fed. Proc. Fed. Am. Soc. Exp. Biol.* **16**:860–867.

Ben-Efraim, S., and Diamantstein, T., 1977, *Immunol. Commun.,* in press.

Bertrand, J., Renoux, G., Renoux, M., and Palat, A., 1974, *Nouv. Presse Méd.* **3**:2265.

Biniaminov, M., and Ramot, B., 1975, *Lancet* **1**:464.

Bitensky, M. W., Gorman, R. E., and Thomas, L., 1971, *Proc Soc. Exp. Biol. Med.* **138**:773–775.

Bitter-Suermann, D., Hadding, U., Schorlemmer, H. U., Limbert, M., Dierich, M., and Dukor, P., 1975, *J. Immunol.* **115**:425–430.

Bluming, A. Z., Vogel, C. L., Ziegler, J. L., Mody, N., and Kamya, G., 1972, *Ann. Intern. Med.* **76**:405–411.

Bomford, R., and Christie, G. H., 1975, *Cell. Immunol.* **17**:150–155.

Bona, C., Heuclin, C., and Chedid, L., 1974, *Recent Results Cancer Res.* **47**:196–200.

Borsos, T., and Rapp, H. J., 1973, *J. Natl. Cancer Inst.* **51**:1085–1086.

Bradner, W. T., Clarke, D. A., and Stock, C. C., 1958, *Cancer Res.* **18**:347–351.

Bradshaw, R., 1977, *Ann. N.Y. Acad. Sci.* **284**:190–196.

Brandes, L. J., Galton, D. A., and Wiltshaw, E., 1971, *Lancet* **2**:293–295.

Braun, W., 1969, *Nature (London)* **224**:1024–1025.

Braun, W., 1970, in: *Tolerance, Autoimmunity and Aging* (M. Sigel, ed.), pp. 166–180, Charles C. Thomas, Springfield, Illinois.

Braun, W., and Ishizuka, M., 1971, *Proc. Natl. Acad. Sci. U.S.A.* **68**:1114–1116.

Braun, W., and Lasky, L. J., 1967, *Fed. Proc. Fed. Am. Soc. Exp. Biol.* **26**:642.

Braun, W., and Levy, H. B., 1972, *Proc. Soc. Exp. Biol. Med.* **141**:769–773.

Braun, W., and Nakano, M., 1967, *Science* **157**:819–821.

Braun, W., Lampen, J. O., Plescia, O. J., and Pugh, L., 1963, in: *Conceptual Advances in Immunology and Oncology*, pp. 450–456, Harper and Row, New York.

Braun, W., Ishizuka, M., Yajima, Y., Webb, D., and Winchurch, R., 1971, in: *Biological Effects of Polynucleotides* (R. F. Beers, Jr., and W. Braun, eds.), pp. 139–156, Springer-Verlag, New York.

Britton, S., and Möller, G., 1968, *J. Immunol.* **100**:1326–1334.

Brugmans, J., Schuermans, V., de Cock, W., Thienpont, D., Janssen, P., Verhaegen, H., van Nimmen, L., Louwagie, A. C., and Stevens, E., 1973, *Life Sci.* **13**:1499–1504.

Bucana, C., and Hanna, M. G., Jr., 1974, *J. Natl. Cancer Inst.* **53**:1313–1323.

Bullock, W. W., and Andersson, J., 1973, *Ciba Found. Symp.* **18**:173–188.

Busch, N. N., 1866, *Berl. Klin. Wochenchschr.* **3**:245–246.

Cardenas, J. O., Gutterman, J. U., Hersh, E. M., Maviglit, G. M., Blumenschein, G. R., Livingston, R. B., Freireich, E. J., and Gottlieb, J. A., 1976, *Cancer Immunol. Immunother.* **1**:99–107.

Carswell, E. A., Old, L. J., Kassel, R. L., Green, S., Fiore, N., and Williamson, B., 1975, *Proc. Natl. Acad. Sci. U.S.A.* **72**:3666–3670.

Casavant, C. H., and Youmans, G. P., 1975, *J. Immunol.* **114**:1014–1022.

Castro, J. E., 1974, *Eur. J. Cancer* **10**:115–120.

Cerottini, J. C., Brunner, K. T., Lindahl, P., and Gresser, I., 1973, *Nature (London) New Biol.* **242**:152–153.

Champlin, R., and Hunter, R. L., 1975, *J. Immunol.* **114**:76–80.

Chan, S. H., and Simons, M. J., 1975, *Lancet* **1**:1246–1247.

Chang, T., and Weinstein, L., 1973, *Am. J. Med. Sci.* **265**:143–146.

Chedid, L., and Lamensans, A., 1974, *Recent Results Cancer Res.* **47**:166–172.

Chedid, L., Parant, M., Parant, F., Gustafson, R. H., and Berger, F. M., 1972, *Proc. Natl. Acad. Sci. U.S.A.* **69**:855–858.

Chedid, L., Lamensans, A., Parant, F., Parant, M., Adam, A., Petit, J. F., and Lederer, E., 1973, *Cancer Res.* **33**:2187–2195.

Cheers, C., and Cone, R., 1974, *J. Immunol.* **112**:1535–1539.

Chess, L., Levy, C., Schmukler, M., Smith, K., and Mardiney, M. R., Jr., 1972, *Transplantation* **14**:748–755.

Chihara, G., Hamuro, J., Maeda, Y., Arai, Y., and Fukuoka, F., 1970, *Cancer Res.* **30**:2776–2781.

Chiller, J. M., Skidmore, B. J., Morrison, D. C., and Weigle, W. D., 1973, *Proc. Natl. Acad. Sci. U.S.A.* **70**:2129–2133.

Chirigos, M. A., Pearson, J. W., and Pryor, J., 1973, *Cancer Res.* **33**:2615–2618.

Chirigos, M. A., Fuhrman, F., and Pryor, J., 1975, *Cancer Res.* **35**:927–931.

Christie, G. H., and Bomford, R., 1975, *Cell Immunol.* **17**:141–149.

Clark, A. W., and Monaco, A. P., 1974, *Immunology* **27**:887–893.

Cleveland, R., Meltzer, M., and Zbar, B., 1974, *J. Natl. Cancer Inst.* **52**:1887–1895.

Cohen, G. H., Hopper, J. A., and Goldstein, A. L., 1975, *Ann. N.Y. Acad. Sci.* **249**:145–153.

Cone, R. E., and Marchalonis, J. J., 1972, *Aust. J. Exp. Biol. Med. Sci.* **50**:69–77.

Cudkowicz, G., 1968, in: *The Proliferation and Spread of Neoplastic Disease*, pp. 661–691, The Williams and Wilkins Co., Baltimore, Maryland.

Cuttner, J., Holland, J. F., Bekesi, J. G., Ramachandar, K., and Donovan, P., 1975, *Proc. Am. Soc. Clin. Oncol.* **16**:264.

Debois, J. M., 1976, in: *Progress in Cancer Research and Therapy II* (M. A. Chirigos, ed.), pp. 175–182, Raven Press, New York.

Del Guercio, P., 1972, *Nature (London) New Biol.* **238**:213–215.
Dennert, G., and Tucker, D., 1973, *J. Natl. Cancer Inst.* **51**:1727–1729.
De Rubertis, F. R., Zenser, T. V., Adler, W. H., and Hudson, T., 1974, *J. Immunol.* **113**:151–161.
De Vita, V., Canellos, G., Carbone, P., Baron, S., Levy, H., and Gralnick, H., 1970, *Proc. Am. Assoc. Cancer Res.* **11**:21.
Di Luzio, N. R., Hoffmann, E. O., Cook, J. A., Browder, W., and Mansell, P., 1977, *Natl. Cancer Inst. Monogr.*, in press.
Dimitrov, N. V., André, S., Eliopoulos, G., and Halpern, B. N., 1975, *Proc. Soc. Exp. Biol. Med.* **148**:440–442.
Drake, W. P., Cimino, E. F., Mardiney, M. R., Jr., and Sutherland, J. C., 1974, *J. Natl. Cancer Inst.* **52**:941–944.
Dresser, D. W., and Phillips, J. M., 1973, *Ciba Found. Symp.* **18**:3–28.
Dukor, P., and Hartmann, K. U., 1973, *Cell. Immunol.* **7**:349–356.
Dukor, P., Schumann, G., Gisler, R. H., Dierich, M., König, W., Hadding, U., and Bitter-Suermann, D., 1973, *J. Exp. Med.* **139**:337–354.
Eilber, F. R., Nizze, J. A., and Morton, D. L., 1975, *Cancer* **35**:660–665.
Faanes, R. B., Dillon, P., and Choi, Y. S., 1977, *Clin. Exp. Immunol.*, in press.
Fauve, R. M., and Hévin, M. B., 1971, *Ann. Inst. Pasteur* **120**:399–411.
Fauve, R. M., Bouanchaud, D., and DeLaunay, A., 1966, *Ann. Inst. Pasteur Suppl.* **110**:106–117.
Field, A. K., Tytell, A. A., Lampson, G. P., and Hilleman, M. R., 1967, *Proc. Natl. Acad. Sci. U.S.A.* **58**:1004–1010.
Fischer, G. W., Podgore, J. K., and Bass, J. W., 1975a, *Lancet* **1**:1137.
Fischer, G. W., Podgore, J. K., Bass, J. W., Kelly, J. L., and Kobyashi, G. Y., 1975b, *J. Infect. Dis.* **132**:578–581.
Fisher, B., Wolmark, N., and Coyle, J., 1974, *J. Natl. Cancer Inst.* **53**:1793–1801.
Forbes, I. J., 1964, *J. Immunol.* **94**:37–39.
Frank, M. M., and May, J. E., 1973, *J. Infect. Dis.* **128***(Suppl.)*:176–181.
Franzl, R. E., and McMaster, P. D., 1968, *J. Exp. Med.* **127**:1087–1107.
Freund, J., and McDermott, K., 1942, *Proc. Soc. Exp. Biol. Med.* **49**:548–553.
Friedman, R. M., and Pastan, I., 1969, *Biochem. Biophys. Res. Commun.* **36**:735–740.
Gallily, R., and Ben-Ishay, Z., 1976, *Proceedings of the Seventh International Congress of the Reticuloendothelial Society,* **18**:44–52.
Gallin, J. I., and Kirkpatrick, C. H., 1974, *Proc. Natl. Acad. Sci. U.S.A.* **71**:498–502.
Gery, I., Krüger, J., and Spiesel, S. Z., 1972, *J. Immunol.* **108**:1088–1091.
Gery, I., Baer, A., Stupp, Y., and Weiss, D. W., 1974, in: *Immunological Parameters of Host–Tumor Relationships* (D. W. Weiss, ed.), Vol. 3, pp. 170–177, Academic Press, New York.
Gewurz, H., Shin, H. S., and Mergenhagen, S. E., 1968, *J. Exp. Med.* **128**:1049–1057.
Ghaffar, A., Cullen, R. T., and Woodruff, M. F. A., 1975, *Br. J. Cancer* **31**:15–24.
Gisler, R. H., Lindahl, P., and Gresser, I., 1974, *J. Immunol.* **113**:438–444.
Goldberg, N. D., Haddox, M. K., Festenstein, R., White, J. G., Lopez, C., and Hadden, J. W., 1974, in: *Cyclic AMP, Cell Growth, and the Immune Response* (W. Braun, L. Lichtenstein, and C. Parker, eds.), pp. 247–262, Springer-Verlag, New York.
Goldenberg, B. J., and Brandes, L. J., 1972, *Clin. Res.* **20**:947.
Goldstein, A. L., Slater, E. D., and White, A., 1966, *Proc. Natl. Acad. Sci. U.S.A.* **135**:485–495.
Goldstein, A. L., Cohen, G. H., Rossio, J. L., Thurman, G. B., Brown, C. N., and Ulrich, J. T., 1976, *Med. Clin. North Am.* **60**:591–606.
Goldstein, G., 1975, *Ann. N.Y. Acad. Sci.* **249**:177–185.
Goldstein, G., and Hoffman, W. W., 1969, *Clin. Exp. Immunol.* **4**:181–189.
Goldstein, G., Scheid, M., Hämmerling, U., Boyse, E. A., Schlesinger, D. H., and Niall, H. D., 1975, *Proc. Natl. Acad. Sci. U.S.A.* **72**:11–15.
Gorden, B., and Keenan, J. P., 1975, *Ann. Allergy* **35**:343–355.
Gordon, P., and Brown, E. R., 1972, *Can. J. Microbiol.* **18**:1463–1470.
Gordon, P., Ronsen, B., and Brown, E. R., 1974, *Antimicrob. Agents Chemother.* **5**:153–160.
Goyanes-Villaescusa, V., 1976, *Lancet* **1**:370.
Graybill, J. R., Silva, J., Alford, R. H., and Thor, D. E., 1973, *Cell. Immunol.* **8**:120–135.
Graziano, K. D., Levy, C. C., Schmukler, M., and Mardiney, M. R., Jr., 1974, *Cell. Immunol.* **11**:47–56.
Greaves, M., Janossy, G., and Doenhoff, M., 1974, *J. Exp. Med.* **140**:1–18.

Green, I., Benacerraf, B., and Stone, S. H., 1969, *J. Immunol.* **103**:403–412.
Gresser, I., 1972, *Adv. Cancer Res.* **16**:97–140.
Griscelli, C., Revillard, J. P., Beteul, H., Herzog, C., and Touraine, J. L., 1973, *Biomédicine* **18**:220–227.
Gutterman, J. U., Maviglit, G., McBride, C., Frei, E., III, Freireich, E. J., and Hersh, E. M., 1973, *Lancet* **1**:1208–1212.
Gutterman, J. U., Hersh, E. M., Rodriguez, V., McCredie, K. B., Maviglit, G., Reed, R., Burgess, M. A., Smith, T., Gehan, E., Bodey, G. P., Sr., and Freireich, E. J., 1974, *Lancet* **2**:1405–1409.
Haba, S., Hamaoka, T., Takatsu, K., and Kitagawa, M., 1976, *Int. J. Cancer* **18**:93–104.
Hadden, J. W., Coffey, R. G., Hadden, E. M., Lopez-Corrales, E., and Sunshine, G. H., 1975, *Cell. Immunol.* **20**:98–103.
Hadden, J. W., Hadden, E. M., and Coffey, R. G., 1976, *Infect. Immun.* **13**:382–387.
Hadden, J. W., Lopez, C., O'Reilly, R. J., and Hadden, E. M., 1977, *Ann. N.Y. Acad. Sci.* **284**:139–152.
Halpern, B. N., and Israël, L., 1971, *C. R. Acad. Sci. (Paris)* **273**:2186–2190.
Halpern, B. N., Biozzi, G., Stiffel, C., and Mouton, D., 1959, *C. R. Soc. Biol. (Paris)* **153**:919–923.
Halpern, B. N., Brévol, A. R., Biozzi, G., Stiffel, C., Mouton, D., Morard, J. C., Bouthillier, Y., and Décreusefond, C., 1964, *J. Reticuloendothel. Soc.* **1**:77–96.
Halpern, B. N., Biozzi, G. Stiffel, C., and Mouton, D., 1966, *Nature (London)* **212**:853–854.
Halpern, B. N., Fray, A., Crépin, Y., Platica, O., Lorinet, A. M., Rabourdin, A., Sparros, L., and Isac, R., 1973, *Ciba Found. Symp.* **18**:217–236.
Hamaoka, T., and Katz, D. H., 1973, *J. Immunol.* **111**:1554–1563.
Hamblin, A. S., Maini, R. N., and Dumonde, D. C., 1976a, *Clin. Exp. Immunol.* **23**:290–302.
Hamblin, A. S., Dumonde, D. C., and Maini, R. N., 1976b, *Clin. Exp. Immunol.* **23**:303–313.
Hamilton, L. D., Babcock, V. I., and Southam, C. M., 1969, *Proc. Natl. Acad. Sci. U.S.A.* **64**:878–883.
Hämmerling, U., Chin, A. F., Abbot, J., and Scheid, M. P., 1975, *J. Immunol.* **115**:1425–1430.
Hardy, M. A., Quint, J., Goldstein, A. L., State, D., and White, A., 1968, *Proc. Natl. Acad. Sci. U.S.A.* **61**:875–882.
Harmel, R. P., Jr., Zbar, B., and Rapp, H. J., 1975, *J. Natl. Cancer Inst.* **54**:515–517.
Hastings, R. C., Morales, M. J., Shannon, E. J., and Jacobson, R. R., 1976, in: *Transfer Factor: Basic Properties and Clinical Applications* (M. S. Ascher, A. A. Gottlieb, and C. H. Kirkpatrick, eds.), pp. 465–476, Academic Press, New York.
Hawrylko, E., 1975, *J. Natl. Cancer Inst.* **55**:413–423.
Heim, L. R., Bernard, G., Goldman, A. L., Dorff, G., and Rytel, M., 1976, in: *Transfer Factor: Basic Properties and Clinical Applications* (M. S. Ascher, A. A. Gottlieb, and C. H. Kirkpatrick, eds.), pp. 457–464, Academic Press, New York.
Helson, L., Green, S., Carswell, E., and Old, L. J., 1976, *Nature (London)* **258**:731–732.
Heyn, R., Borges, W., Joo, P., Karon, M., Nesbit, M., Shore, N., Breslow, N., and Hammond, D., 1973, *Proc. Am. Assoc. Cancer Res.* **14**:45.
Hibbs, J. B., Jr., Lambert, L. H., Jr., and Remington, J. S., 1972, *Nature (London) New Biol.* **235**:48–50.
Hitzig, W. H., Fontanellaz, H. P., and Muntener, V., 1972. *Schweiz. Med. Wochenchschr.* **102**:1237–1244.
Hoebeke, J., and Franchi, G., 1973, *J. Reticuloendothel. Soc.* **14**:317–323.
Hoffmann, M. K., Schmidt, D., and Oettgen, H. F., 1973, *Nature (London)* **243**:408–409.
Hoffmann, M. K., Weiss, O., Koenig, S., Hirst, J. A., and Oettgen, H. F., 1975, *J. Immunol.* **114**:738–741.
Hoffmann, M. K., Green, S., and Old, L. J., 1976, *Nature (London)* **263**:416–417.
Holmgren, I., 1935, *Schweiz. Med. Wochenchschr.* **65**:1203–1206.
Hooper, J. A., McDaniel, M. C., Thurman, G. B., Cohen, G. H., Schulof, R. S., and Goldstein, A. L., 1975, *Ann. N.Y. Acad. Sci.* **249**:125–144.
Howard, J. G., Biozzi, G., Stiffel, C., Mouton, D., and Liacopoulos, P., 1967, *Transplantation* **5**:1510–1524.
Howard, J. G., Scott, M. T., and Christie, G. H., 1973, *Ciba Found. Symp.* **18**:101–120.
Huskisson, E. C., Dieppe, P. A., Scott, J., Trapnell, J., Balme, H. W., and Willoughby, D. A., 1976, *Lancet* **1**:393–395.
International Workshop on Interferon in the Treatment of Cancer, New York, March 31–April 2, 1974 (M. Krim, A. S. Levine, R. C. Merigan, and J. Vilček, eds.), unpublished report.
Ippen, S. A., and Quadripur, H., 1975, *Dtsch. Med. Wochenschr.* **100**: 1710–1711.

Ishizuka, M., Gafni, M., and Braun, W., 1970, *Proc. Soc. Exp. Biol. Med.* **134**:963–967.
Ishizuka, M., Braun, W., and Matsumoto, T., 1971, *J. Immunol.* **107**:1027–1035.
Israël, L., 1974, *Recent Results Cancer Res.* **47**:486–487.
Israël, L., 1975, in: *Corynebacterium parvum: Application in Experimental and Clinical Oncology* (B. N. Halpern, ed.), pp. 389–401, Plenum Press, New York.
Janossy, G., Humphrey, J. H., Pepys, M. B., and Greaves, M. F., 1973, *Nature (London) New Biol.* **245**:108–112.
Jaroslow, B. N., and Ortiz-Ortiz, L., 1972, *Cell. Immunol.* **3**:123–132.
Johnson, A. G., Cone, R. E., Friedman, H. M., Han, I. H., Johnson, H. G., Schmidtke, J. R., and Stout, R. D., 1971, in: *Biological Effects of Polynucleotides* (R. F. Beers, Jr., and W. Braun, eds.), pp. 157–177, Springer-Verlag, New York.
Jones, J. M., and Kind, P. D., 1972, *J. Immunol.* **108**:1453–1455.
Juy, D., and Chedid, L., 1975, *Proc. Natl. Acad. Sci. U.S.A.* **72**:4105–4109.
Kassel, R. L., 1977, in: *Modulation of Host Immune Resistance in the Prevention or Treatment of Induced Neoplasia* (M. A. Chirigos, ed.), pp. 347–348, Fogarty International Center Proceedings No. 28, U.S. Government Printing Office, Washington, D.C.
Kassel, R. L., Old, L. J., Carswell, E. A., Fiore, N. C., and Hardy, W. D., Jr., 1973, *J. Exp. Med.* **138**:925–938.
Kearney, J. F., and Lawton, A. R., 1975, *J. Immunol.* **115**:671–681.
Kint, A., and Verlinden, L., 1974, *N. Engl. J. Med.* **291**:308.
Kirkpatrick, C. H., Chandler, J. W., and Schimke, R. N., 1970, *Clin. Exp. Immunol.* **6**:375–385.
Klein, E., and Holtermann, O. A., 1972, *Natl. Cancer Inst. Monogr.* **35**:379–402.
Klein, E., Holtermann, O., Milgrom, H., Case, R. W., Klein, D., Rosner, D., and Djerassi, I., 1976, *Med. Clin. North Am.* **60**:389–418.
Klein, J. J., Goldstein, A. L., and White, A., 1966, *Ann. N.Y. Acad. Sci.* **135**:485–495.
Kong, Y., and Capanna, S. L., 1974, *Cell. Immunol.* **11**:488–492.
Kook, A. I., and Trainin, N., 1974, *J. Exp. Med.* **139**:193–207.
Kook, A. I., and Trainin, N., 1975, *J. Immunol.* **114**:151–157.
Kouznetzova, B., Bizzini, B., Chermann, J.-C., Degrand, F., Prévot, A.-R., and Raynaud, M., 1974, *Recent Results Cancer Res.* **47**:275–293.
Krakoff, I. H., Young, C. W., and Hilleman, M. R., 1970, *Proc. Am. Assoc. Cancer Res.* **11**:45.
Krim, M., and Sanders, F. K., 1977, in: *Interferons and Their Actions* (W. E. Stewart II, ed.), CRC Press, Chicago, in press.
Kurland, J. I., Hadden, J. W., and Moore, M. A. S., 1977, *Exp. Cell Res.*, in press.
Lacour, F., Spira, A., Lacour, J., and Prade, M., 1972, *Cancer Res.* **32**:648–649.
Lacour, F., Delage, G., and Chinale, C., 1975, *Science* **187**:256–257.
Lagrange, P. H., and Mackaness, G. B., 1975, *J. Immunol.* **114**:447–451.
Lagrange, P. H., Mackaness, G. B., Miller, T. E., and Pardon, P., 1975, *J. Immunol.* **114**:442–446.
Lamensans, A., Chedid, L., Lederer, E., Rosselet, J. P., Gustafson, R. H., Spencer, H. J., Ludwig, B., and Berger, F. M., 1975, *Proc. Natl. Acad. Sci. U.S.A.* **72**:3656–3660.
Lampson, G. P., Tytell, A. A., Field, A. K., Nemes, M. M., and Hilleman, M. R., 1967, *Proc. Natl. Acad. Sci. U.S.A.* **58**:782–789.
Lawrence, H. S., 1955, *J. Clin. Invest.* **34**:219–230.
Lawrence, H. S., 1974, *The Harvey Lectures*, Series 68, pp. 239–250, Academic Press, New York.
Lebon, P., Moreau, M. C., Cohen, L., and Chany, C., 1975, *Proc. Soc. Exp. Biol. Med.* **149**:108–112.
Levey, R. H., Trainin, N., and Law, L. W., 1963, *J. Natl. Cancer Inst.* **31**:199–217.
Levo, Y., Rotter, V., and Ramot, B., 1975, *Biomédicine* **23**:198–200.
Levy, H. B., Law, L. W., and Rabson, A. S., 1969, *Proc. Natl. Acad. Sci. U.S.A.* **62**:357–361.
Lewis, P. A., and Loomis, D., 1924, *J. Exp. Med.* **40**:503–515.
Lichtenfeld, J. L., Desner, M. R., Mardiney, M. R., Jr., and Wiernik, P. H., 1974, *Fed. Proc. Fed. Am. Soc. Exp. Biol.* **58**:790.
Lichtenfield, J. L., Desner, M. R., Wiernik, P. H., and Mardinay, M. R., 1977, in: *Progress in Cancer Research and Therapy II*, pp. 135–145, Raven Press, New York.
Lindahl-Magnusson, P., Leary, P., and Gresser, I., 1972, *Nature (London) New Biol.* **237**:120–121.
LoBuglio, A. F., and Neidhart, J. A., 1976, *Med. Clin. North Am.* **60**:585–590.
Lods, J. C., Dujardin, P., and Halpern, G. M., 1976, *Lancet* **1**:548.
Longley, S., Danning, R. L., and Waldman, R. H., 1973, *Antimicrob. Agents Chemother.* **3**:506–509.

Lotzova, E., and Cudkowicz, G., 1974, *J. Immunol.* **113**:798–803.
Louis, J. A., Chiller, J. M., and Weigle, W. D., 1973, *J. Exp. Med.* **138**:1481–1495.
Lundy, J., Iritani, C. A., Wanebo, H. J., Wachtel, S. S., Tarnowski, G. S., and Old, L. J., 1973, *Proc. Am. Assoc. Cancer Res.* **14**:107.
Mackaness, G. B., 1964, *Symp. Soc. Gen. Microbiol.* **14**:213–240.
Mackaness, G. B., Auclair, D. J., and Lagrange, P. H., 1973, *J. Natl. Cancer Inst.* **51**:1655–1667.
Mackaness, G. B., Lagrange, P. H., and Ishibashi, T., 1974, *J. Exp. Med.* **139**:1540–1552.
Maeda, Y., and Chihara, G., 1973, *Int. J. Cancer* **11**:153–161.
Mankowski, Z. T., Yamashita, M., and Diller, I. C., 1957, *Proc. Soc. Exp. Biol. Med.* **96**:79–80.
Mansell, P. W. A., Ichinose, H., Reed, R. J., Krementz, E. T., McNamee, R., and Di Luzio, N. R., 1975, *J. Natl. Cancer Inst.* **54**:571–576.
Mantovani, A., and Spreafico, F., 1975, *Eur. J. Cancer* **11**:537–544.
Mastrangelo, M. J., Berd, D., and Bellet, R. E., 1976, *Ann. N.Y. Acad. Sci.* **277**:94–123.
Mathé, G., Amiel, J.-L., Schwarzenberg, L., Schneider, M., Cotton, A., Schlumberger, J. R., Hayat, M., and de Vassal, F., 1969, *Lancet* **1**:697–699.
Mathé, G., Amiel, J.-L., Schwarzenberg, L., Schneider, M., Hayat, M., de Vassal, F., Jasmin, C., Rosenfeld, C., Sakouhi, M., and Choay, J., 1970, *Eur. J. Clin. Biol. Res.* **15**:671–673.
Mathé, G., Hayat, M., Sakouhi, M., and Choay, J., 1971, *C. R. Acad. Sci. (Paris)* **272**:170–173.
Mathé, G., Kamel, M., Dezfulian, M., Halle-Pannenko, O., and Bourut, C., 1973, *Cancer Res.* **33**:1987–1997.
Maviglit, G. M., Gutterman, J. U., Burgess, M. A., Khankhanian, N., Seibert, G. B., Speer, J. F., Reed, R. C., Jubert, A. W., Martin, R. C., McBride, C. M., Copeland, E. M., Gehan, E. A., and Hersh, E. M., 1976, *Lancet* **1**:871–876.
McBride, W. H., Weir, D. M., Kay, A. B., Pearce, D., and Caldwell, J. R., 1975, *Clin. Exp. Immunol.* **19**:143–147.
Medical Research Council, 1971, *Br. Med. J.* **4**:189–194.
Melchers, F., and Andersson, J., 1974, *Eur. J. Immunol.* **4**:181–188.
Meltzer, M. S., Jones, E. E., and Boetcher, D. A., 1975, *Cell. Immunol.* **17**:268–276.
Mergenhagen, S. E., Snyderman, R., and Phillips, J. K., 1973, *J. Infect. Dis.* **128** *(Suppl.)*:86–90.
Merluzzi, V. J., Badger, A. M., Kaiser, C. W., and Cooperband, S. R., 1975, *J. Clin. Exp. Immunol.* **22**:486.
Miller, T. E., Mackaness, G. B., and Lagrange, P. H., 1973, *J. Natl. Cancer Inst.* **51**:1669–1676.
Minden, P., McClatchy, J. K., Wainberg, M., and Weiss, D. W., 1974, *J. Natl. Cancer Inst.* **53**:1325–1331.
Mitchell, M. S., Kirkpatrick, D., Mokyr, M. B., and Gery, I., 1973, *Nature (London) New Biol.* **243**:216–218.
Moertel, C. G., Ritts, R. E., Jr., Schutt, A. J., and Hahn, R. G., 1975, *Cancer Res.* **35**:3075–3083.
Möller, G., Sjöberg, O., and Andersson, J., 1973, *J. Infect. Dis.* **128***(Suppl.)*:52–56.
Morton, D. L., Eilber, F. R., Malmgren, R. A., and Wood, W. C., 1970, *Surgery* **68**:158–164.
Morton, D. L., Eilber, F. R., Holmes, E. C., Hunt, J. S., Ketcham, A. S., Silverstein, M. J., and Sparks, F. C., 1974, *Ann. Surg.* **180**:635–643.
Mozes, E., Shearer, G. M., and Sela, M., 1970, *J. Exp. Med.* **132**:613–622.
Mozes, E., Shearer, G. M., Melmon, K. L., and Bourne, H. R., 1973a, *Cell. Immunol.* **9**:226–233.
Mozes, E., Shearer, G. M., Sela, M., and Braun, W., 1973b, *J. Immunol.* **111**:439–447.
Muldoon, R. L., Mezny, L., and Jackson, G., 1972, *Antimicrob. Agents Chemother.* **2**:224–228.
Munder, P. G., and Modollel, M., 1974, *Recent Results Cancer Res.* **47**:244–250.
Nathanson, L., 1974, *Semin. Oncol.* **1**:337–350.
Nauts, H. C., Fowler, G. A., and Bogatko, F. H., 1953, *Acta Med. Scand. Suppl. 276.*
Neidhart, J. A., Schwartz, R. S., Hurtubise, P. E., Murphy, S. G., Metz, E. N., and Balcerzak, S. P., 1973, *Cell. Immunol.* **9**:319–323.
Neveu, T., Branellec, A., and Biozzi, G., 1964, *Ann. Inst. Pasteur* **106**:771–777.
Nguyen-Dang, T., Hayat, M., Chenu, E., Mayer, M., and Janot, M. M., 1973, *C. R. Acad. Sci. (Paris)* **276**:3233–3235.
Oettgen, H. F., Old, L. J., Farrow, J. H., Valentine, F. T., Lawrence, H. S., and Thomas, L., 1974, *Proc. Natl. Acad. Sci. U.S.A.* **71**:2319–2323.
Oettgen, H. F., Pinsky, C. M., and Delmonte, L., 1976, *Med. Clin. North Am.* **60**:511–538.
Old, L. J., Clarke, D. A., and Benacerraf, B., 1959, *Nature (London)* **184**:291–292.

Old, L. J., Benacerraf, B., Clarke, D. A., Carswell, E. A., and Stockert, E., 1961, *Cancer Res.* **21**:1281–1301.
Oliveira-Lima, A., Javierre, M. Q., Dias da Silva, W., and Sette Camara, D., 1974, *Experientia* **30**:945–946.
Olivotto, M., and Bomford, R., 1974, *Int. J. Cancer* **13**:478–488.
O'Neill, G. J., Henderson, D. C., and White, R. G., 1973, *Immunology* **24**:977–995.
O'Reilly, R., Chibarro, A., Wilmot, R., and Lopez, C., 1977, *Ann. N.Y. Acad. Sci.* **284**:161–170.
Ortiz-Ortiz, L., and Jaroslow, B. N., 1970, *Immunology* **19**:387–399.
Osaba, D., and Miller, J. F. A. P., 1963, *Nature (London)* **199**:653–654.
Pabst, H. F., and Crawford, J., 1975, *Clin. Exp. Immunol.* **21**:468–473.
Pachuta, O. M., Yasuhi, T., Hornick, R. B., Schwartz, A. R., and Tominaga, S., 1974, *Antimicrob. Agents Chemother.* **5**:403–408.
Papermaster, B. W., Holtermann, O. A., Klein, E., Djerassi, I., Rosner, D., Dao, T., and Costanzi, J. J., 1976, *Clin. Immunol. Immunother.* **5**:31–47.
Parant, M., and Chedid, L., 1974, *Recent Results Cancer Res.* **47**:190–255.
Peavy, D. L., Adler, W. H., and Smith, R. T., 1970, *J. Immunol.* **105**:1453–1458.
Peavy, D. L., Shands, J. W., Adler, W. H., and Smith, R. T., 1971, *Fed. Proc. Fed. Am. Soc. Exp. Biol.* **30**:396.
Peavy, D. L., Shands, J. W., Adler, W. H., and Smith, R. T., 1973, *J. Infect. Dis.* **129***(Suppl)*:91–98.
Peters, L. C., Hanna, M. G., Jr., Gutterman, J. U., Mavigilt, G. M., and Hersh, E. M., 1974, *Proc. Soc. Exp. Biol. Med.* **147**:344–349.
Pinckard, R. N., and Halonen, M., 1971, *J. Immunol.* **106**:1602–1608.
Pinckard, R. N., Weir, D. M., and McBride, W. H., 1967, *Clin. Exp. Immunol.* **2**:331–341.
Pinsky, C. M., Wanebo, H., Mike, V., and Oettgen, H. F., 1976, *Ann. N.Y. Acad. Sci.* **276**:407–410.
Powles, R. L., Crowther, D., Bateman, C. J. T., Beard, M. E. J., McElwain, T. J., Russell, T. A., Lister, J. M. A., Whitehouse, P. F. M., Wrigley, M., Pike, P., Alexander, P., and Fairley, G. H., 1973, *Br. J. Cancer* **28**:365–376.
Prévot, A.-R., and Tran Van Phi, J., 1964, *C. R. Acad. Sci. (Paris)* **258**:4619–4621.
Prévot, A.-R., Levaditti, J., Nazimov, O., and Thouvenot, H., 1958, *Ann. Inst. Pasteur* **94**:405–418.
Proctor, J. W., Auclair, B. G., and Lewis, M. G., 1976, *Eur. J. Cancer* **12**:203–210.
Pudifin, D. J., Harding, B., and MacLennan, I. C. M., 1971, *Immunology* **21**:853–860.
Quintans, J., and Lefkovits, I., 1974, *J. Immunol.* **113**:1373–1376.
Raynaud, M., Kouznetzova, B., Bizzino, B., and Chermann, J. C., 1972, *Ann. Inst. Pasteur* **122**:695–700.
Reed, R. C., Gutterman, J. U., Mavigilt, G. M., and Hersh, E. M., 1975, *Proc. Am. Soc. Clin. Oncol.* **16**:228.
Renoux, G., and Renoux, M., 1971, *C. R. Acad. Sci. (Paris)* **272**:349–350.
Renoux, G., and Renoux, M., 1972a, *C. R. Acad. Sci. (Paris)* **274D**:756–757.
Renoux, G., and Renoux, M., 1972b, *C. R. Acad. Sci. (Paris)* **274D**:3034–3035.
Renoux, G., and Renoux, M., 1972c, *C. R. Acad. Sci. (Paris)* **274D**:3149–3151.
Renoux, G., and Renoux, M., 1972d, *C. R. Acad. Sci. (Paris)* **274D**:3320–3323.
Renoux, G., and Renoux, M., 1972e, *J. Immunol.* **109**:761–765.
Renoux, G., and Renoux, M., 1974a, *C. R. Acad. Sci. (Paris)* **278D**:1139–1141.
Renoux, G., and Renoux, M., 1974b, *J. Immunol.* **113**:779–790.
Renoux, G., and Renoux, M., 1977, in: *Progress in Cancer Research and Therapy II* (M. A. Chirigos, ed.), pp. 235–237, Raven Press, New York.
Renoux, G., Renoux, M., Morand, P., and Dartigues, P., 1973, *Rev. Méd. Tours* **7**:797–801.
Renoux, G., Renoux, M., and Aycard, D., 1976, *Fed. Proc. Fed. Am. Soc. Exp. Biol.* **35**:336.
Reymond, J. F., and Grob, P. J., 1975, *Vox Sang.* **29**:338–351.
Ribi, E., Meyer, T. J., Azuma, I., and Zbar, B., 1973, *Natl. Cancer Inst. Monogr.* **39**:115–125.
Richman, S. P., 1975, *Proc. Am. Soc. Clin. Oncol.* **16**:227.
Riggi, S. J., and Di Luzio, N. R., 1961, *Am. J. Physiol.* **200**:297–300.
Robinson, E., Bartal, A., Cohen, Y., and Haasz, R., 1975, *Br. J. Cancer* **32**:1–4.
Rojas, A. F., Mickiewicz, E., Feierstein, J. N., Glait, H., and Olivari, A. J., 1976, *Lancet* **1**:211–215.
Ronsen, B., and Gordon, P., 1976, *Biochem. Pharmacol.* **25**:707–715.
Ruscetti, F. W., and Chevernick, P. A., 1974, *J. Lab. Clin. Med.* **83**:64–72.
Sampson, D., and Lui, A., 1976, *Cancer Res.* **36**:952–955.

Sandler, J. A., Smith, T. K., Manganiello, V. C., and Kirkpatrick, C. H., 1975, *J. Clin. Invest.* **56**:1271–1279.

Sarma, P. S., Shiu, G., Neubauer, R. H., Baron, S., and Huebner, R. Y., 1969, *Proc. Natl. Acad. Sci. U.S.A.* **62**:1046–1057.

Scheid, M. P., Hoffmann, M. K., Komuro, K., Hämmerling, U., Abbott, J., Boyse, E. A., Cohen, G. H., Hooper, J. A., Schulof, R. S., and Goldstein, A. L., 1973, *J. Exp. Med.* **138**:1027–1032.

Scheid, M. P., Goldstein, G., Hämmerling, U., and Boyse, E. A., 1975, *Ann. N.Y. Acad. Sci.* **249**:531–540.

Schlesinger, D. H.. and Goldstein. G.. 1975. *Nature (London)* **255**:423–424.

Schmidtke, J. R., and Dixon, F. J., 1972, *J. Exp. Med.* **136**:392–397.

Schmidtke, J. R., and Najarian, J. S., 1975, *J. Immunol.* **114**:742–746.

Schuermans, Y., 1975, *Lancet* **1**:111.

Scott. M. T.. 1972. *Cell. Immunol.* **5**:459–479.

Scott. M. T.. 1974. *Semin. Oncol.* **1**:367–378.

Seigler, H. F., Shingleton, W. W., and Pickrell, K. L., 1975, *Plast. Reconstr. Surg.* **55**:294–298.

Shear, M. J., Turner, F. C., Perrault, A., and Shovelton, T., 1943, *J. Natl. Cancer Inst.* **4**:81–97.

Shulman, S. T., Hutto, J. H., Scott, B., Ayoub, E. M., and McGuigan, J. E., 1976, in: *Transfer Factor: Basic Properties and Clinical Applications* (M. S. Ascher, A. A. Gottlieb, and H. C. Kirkpatrick, eds.), pp. 439–448, Academic Press, New York.

Sjöberg, O., Andersson, J., and Möller, G., 1972, *Eur. J. Immunol.* **2**:326–331.

Skopinska, E., 1972, *Transplantation* **14**:432–437.

Smith, G. V., Morse, P. A., Deraps, G. D., Raju, S., and Hardy, J. D., 1973, *Surgery* **74**:59–68.

Sokal, J. E., Aungst, C. W., and Grace, J. T., Jr., 1973, *Natl. Cancer Inst. Monogr.* **39**:195–198.

Spitler, L. E., Levin, A. S., Stites, D. P., Fudenberg, H. H., Pirofsky, B., August, C. S., Stiehm, E. R., Hitzig, W. H., and Gatti, R. A., 1972, *J. Clin. Invest.* **51**:3216–3224.

Spitler, L. E., Glogan, R., Nelms, D., Basch, K., Olson, J., Silverman, S., and Engleman, L., 1977, in: *Progress in Cancer Research and Therapy II* (M. A. Chirigos, ed.), pp. 217–226, Raven Press, New York.

Spitznagel, J. K., and Allison, A. C., 1970, *J. Immunol.* **104**:128–139.

Spreafico, F., Vecchi, A., Mantovani, A., Poggi, A., Franchi, G., Anaclerio, A., and Garattini, S., 1975, *Eur. J. Cancer* **11**:555–563.

Steinkuller, C. B., Krigbaum, L. G., and Weiss, D. W., 1969, *Immunology* **16**:255–275.

Stjernswärd, J., 1966, *Cancer Res.* **26**:1591–1594.

Strausser, H. R., Bober, L. A., Bucsi, R. A., Shillcock, J. A., and Goldstein, A. L., 1971, *Exp. Gerontol.* **6**:373–375.

Study Group for Bronchogenic Carcinoma, 1975, *Br. Med. J.* **3**:461–464.

Stupp, Y., Navok, T., and Gery, I., 1975, *Israel J. Med. Ser.* **11**:1387–1395.

Stupp, Y., Manny, N., Weiss, D. W., and Izak, G., 1977, *Proceedings of the International Society of Hematology,* European and African Division, Third Meeting, London, in press.

Sunshine, G., Corrales-Lopez, E., Hadden, E. M., Coffey, R. G., Wanebo, H., Hadden, J. W., and Rojas, A., 1977, in: *Modulation of Host Immune Resistance in the Prevention or Treatment of Induced Neoplasia* (M. A. Chirigos, ed.), pp. 31–38, Fogarty International Center Proceedings No. 28, U.S. Government Printing Office, Washington, D.C.

Symoens, J., 1977, in: *Progress in Cancer Research and Therapy II* (M. A. Chirigos, ed.), pp. 1–24, Raven Press, New York.

Symoens, J., and Brugmans, J., 1976, *Br. Med. J.* **4**:529.

Taniyama, T., Azuma, I., Aladin, A. A., and Yamamura, Y., 1975, *Gann* **66**:705–709.

Thorbecke, G. J., Old, L. J., Benacerraf, B., and Clarke, D. A., 1961, *J. Histochem. Cytochem.* **9**:392–399.

Tizard, I. R., 1971, *Infect. Immun.* **4**:402–406.

Toujas, L., Dazord, L., Martin, A., and Guelfi, J., 1973, *Bioméd. Express* **19**:503–505.

Trabert, U., Rosenthal, M., Müller, W., Müller, S., and Wurm, K., 1975, *Dtsch. Med. Wochenschr.* **100**:2297–2298.

Trainin, N., and Linker-Israeli, M., 1967, *Cancer Res.* **27**:309–313.

Trainin, N., and Small, M., 1970, *J. Exp. Med.* **132**:885–897.

Trainin, N., Burger, M., and Kaye, A., 1967, *Biochem. Pharmacol.* **16**:711–720.

Trainin, N., Small, M., and Globerson, A., 1969, *J. Exp. Med.* **130**:765–776.

Trainin, N., Kook, A., Umiel, T., and Abala, M, 1975, *Ann. N.Y. Acad. Sci.* **249**:349–361.
Tripodi, D., Parks, L. C., and Brugmans, J. N., 1973, *N. Engl. J. Med.* **289**:354–357.
Vandeputte, M., Datta, S. V., Billiau, A., and de Sommer, P., 1970, *Eur. J. Cancer* **6**:323–327.
Van Eygen, M., Znamensky, P. Y., Heck, E., and Raymaekers, I., 1976, *Lancet* **1**:382–385.
Verhaegen, H., de Cree, J., Verbruggen, F., Hoebeke, J., de Brabander, M., and Brugmans, J., 1973, *Verh. Dtsch. Ges. Inn. Med.* **79**:623–628.
Versijp, G., van Zwet, T. L., and van Furth, R., 1975, *Lancet* **1**:798.
Vitale, B., and Allegretti, N., 1963, *Nature (London)* **199**:507–508.
Vogler, W. R., and Chan, Y.-K., 1974, *Lancet* **2**:128–131.
Wagner, H., and Cone, R. E., 1974, *Cell. Immunol.* **10**:394–403.
Waldman, R. H., 1977, *Ann. N.Y. Acad. Sci.* **284**:153–160.
Waldman, R. H., and Lackmann, P. J. 1975, *Eur. J. Immunol.* **5**:185–193.
Wanebo, H. J., Oettgen, H. F., Lundy, J., Stock, C. C., and Old, L. J., 1975, *Proc. Am. Assoc. Cancer Res.* **16**:274.
Wara, D. W., Goldstein, A. L., Doyle, W., and Ammann, A. J., 1975, *N. Engl. J. Med.* **292**:70–74.
Warr, G. W., and Sljivic, V. S., 1974, *Clin. Exp. Immunol.* **17**:519–532.
Watson, J., 1975, *J. Exp. Med.* **141**:97–111.
Watson, J., Trenker, E., and Cohn, M., 1973, *J. Exp. Med.* **138**:699–714.
Weber, J. M., and Stewart, R. B., 1975, *J. Gen. Virol.* **28**:363–372.
Weber, W. T., 1973, *J. Immunol.* **111**:1277–1280.
Weinstein, Y., Chambers, D. A., Bourne, H. R., and Melmon, K. L., 1974, *Nature (London)* **251**:352–353.
Weiss, D. W., 1976, *Med. Clin. North Am.* **60**:473–497.
Weiss, D. W., and Wells, A. Q., 1960, *Am. Rev. Respir. Dis.* **82**:339–357.
Weiss, D. W., and Yashpe, D. J., 1973, in: *Dynamic Aspects of Host–Parasite Relationships* (A. Zuckerman and D. W. Weiss, eds.), pp. 163–223, Academic Press, New York.
Weiss, D. W., Bonhag, R. S., and Parks, J. A., 1964, *J. Exp. Med.* **119**:53–70.
Whitcomb, M. E., Merluzzi, V. J., and Cooperband, S. R., 1976, *Cell. Immunol.* **21**:272–277.
Wickett, W. H., Bradshaw, L. J., Wilson, J., and Glasky, A. J., 1976, *Proc. 76th Ann. Meet. Am. Soc. Microbiol.*, p. 78.
Wiener, E., 1975, in: *Corynebacterium parvum: Applications in Experimental and Clinical Oncology* (B. N. Halpern, ed.), pp. 59–73, Plenum Press, New York.
Wiener, E., and Bandieri, A., 1975, *Immunology* **29**:265–274.
Wiener, E., and Levanon, D., 1968, *Lab. Invest.* **19**:584–590.
Wilkinson, P. C., O'Neill, G. J., McInroy, R. J., Cater, J. C., and Roberts, J. A., 1973, *Ciba Found. Symp.* **18**:121–140.
Wilton, J. M., Rosenstreich, D. L., and Oppenheim, J. J., 1975, *J. Immunol.* **114**:388–393.
Winchurch, R., and Braun, W., 1969, *Nature (London)* **223**:843–844.
Winchurch, R., Ishizuka, M., Webb, D., and Braun, W., 1971, *J. Immunol.* **106**:1399–1400.
Wolmark, N., Levine, M., and Fisher, B., 1974, *J. Reticuloendothel. Soc.* **16**:252–257.
Wood, D. D., and Cameron, P. M., 1976, *Cell. Immunol.* **21**:133–145.
Woodruff, M. F. A., and Boak, J. L., 1966, *Br. J. Cancer* **20**:345–355.
Woods, W. A., Siegal, M. J., and Chirigos, M. A., 1974, *Cell. Immunol.* **14**:327–331.
Woods, W. A., Fliegelman, M. J., and Chirigos, M. A., 1975, *Proc. Soc. Exp. Biol. Med.* **148**:1048–1050.
Wright, D. G., Kirkpatrick, C. H., and Gallin, J. F., 1977, in: *Progress in Cancer Research and Therapy II* (M. A. Chirigos, ed.), pp. 227–234, Raven Press, New York.
Yagel, S., Gallily, R., and Weiss, D. W., 1975, *Cell. Immunol.* **19**:381–386.
Yamamoto, I., and Webb, D. R., 1975, *Proc. Natl. Acad. Sci. U.S.A.* **72**:2320–2324.
Yamamura, T., Azuma, I., Taniyama, T., Ribi, E., and Zbar, B., 1974, *Gann* **65**:179–181.
Yamamura, Y., Azuma, I., Taniyama, T., and Hirao, F., 1975, in: *Host Defense Against Cancer and Its Potentiation* (D. Mizuo, G. Chihara, F. Fukuoka, T. Yamamoto, and Y. Yamamura, eds.), pp. 421–433, University of Tokyo Press, Tokyo.
Youn, J. K., Barski, G., and Huppert, J., 1968, *C. R. Acad. Sci. (Paris)* **267**:816–819.
Zbar, B., Rapp, H. J., and Ribi, E., 1972a, *J. Natl. Cancer Inst.* **48**:831–835.
Zbar, B., Bernstein, I. D., Bartlett, G. L., Hanna, M. G., Jr., and Rapp, H. J., 1972b, *J. Natl. Cancer Inst.* **49**:119–130.

15

Immunoassay of Drugs and the Biological Use of Antidrug Antibodies

VINCENT P. BUTLER, JR.

1. Introduction

Clinically useful drugs are usually of relatively small molecular size, generally with molecular weights less than 1000, and hence they are not ordinarily antigenic. It is of course known from the classic studies of Landsteiner (1945) with what he called "artificial conjugated antigens" that low-molecular-weight compounds, when chemically coupled as haptens to protein or polypeptide carriers, will elicit the production of antibodies capable of binding the specific hapten used. In the past decade, many investigators have made use of this principle to elicit antibodies specific for drugs or for other small molecules of pharmacological interest (Butler and Beiser, 1973; Beiser *et al.*, 1976). Drug-specific antibodies have been utilized extensively in the development of sensitive, specific, precise, and convenient immunologic assay methods for the measurement of drug concentrations in serum and in other biological fluids; these immunoassay methods have been used extensively in studies of the bioavailability, absorption, pharmacokinetics, metabolism, and excretion of many drugs, as well as in the clinical monitoring of drug therapy (Butler 1973, 1975; Spector, 1973; Marks *et al.*, 1974; Langone *et al.*, 1975; Cleeland *et al.*, 1976; Landon and Moffat, 1976; Broughton and Strong, 1976). In some instances, hapten-specific antibodies have been used to neutralize the biological activities of drugs and of other small molecules of pharmacological importance (Butler *et al.*, 1973, 1974). It is the purpose of this chapter to describe the production of antibodies to drugs and to other small molecules of pharmacological importance, the detection and immunologic characterization of such antibodies,

VINCENT P. BUTLER, JR., • Department of Medicine, Columbia University College of Physicians and Surgeons, New York, New York 10032.

their use in the development of specific immunoassays, and, finally, the applications of these antibodies in clinical and experimental studies.

2. Production of Antidrug Antibodies

2.1. Choice of a Carrier

Virtually any immunogenic protein or synthetic polypeptide may be employed as a carrier for a haptenically conjugated drug. The serum albumins of various species have been most commonly used as such carriers because of their ready availability in large quantity at low cost, their excellent solubility, their high degree of immunogenicity, and their relative resistance to denaturation by the organic solvents and rigorous chemical conditions employed in some conjugation procedures. Other frequently used carriers include the γ-globulins, fibrinogens, and thyroglobulins of various species, hen ovalbumin, hemocyanin, and several synthetic polypeptides (Butler and Beiser, 1973).

The functional groups in protein and polypeptide carriers to which haptenic drugs or drug derivatives may be coupled include free amino groups (lysine and NH_2-terminal amino acids), free carboxyl groups (aspartic acid, glutamic acid, and COOH-terminal amino acids), phenolic groups (tyrosine), sulfhydryl groups (cysteine), imidazo groups (histidine), and guanidino groups (arginine). Drugs and drug derivatives have been most frequently coupled to the amino, carboxyl, or phenolic groups of protein carriers (Butler and Beiser, 1973; Erlanger, 1973; Beiser *et al.*, 1976).

2.2. Choice of a Conjugation Method

The functional groups of the hapten govern the choice of the method used to conjugate the hapten to the functional groups of the protein carrier. A number of methods have been described that enable the coupling of drugs or drug derivatives to protein carriers under chemical conditions that do not cause significant structural alterations of the hapten and that do not produce sufficient denaturation of the carrier protein to render it insoluble. For example, drugs or drug derivatives with free carboxyl groups can be coupled to amino groups of proteins either by the mixed anhydride (Erlanger *et al.*, 1957) or water-soluble carbodiimide (Goodfriend *et al.*, 1964) method. Drugs or drug derivatives with aliphatic amino groups can be coupled to the carboxyl groups of carriers by the water-soluble carbodiimide method (Goodfriend *et al.*, 1964), or to the amino groups of carriers, using bifunctional diisocyanates (Haber *et al.*, 1965a). Aromatic amines can be diazotized and then coupled to the tyrosine groups of carriers (Hamburger, 1966). Drugs with vicinal hydroxyl groups can conveniently be conjugated to amino groups of protein carriers by the periodate oxidation method (Erlanger and Beiser, 1964; Butler and Chen, 1967). The hydroxyl groups of steroids react with succinic anhydride to form the hemisuccinate, which can then be coupled to amino groups of protein carriers via its carboxyl group, using the mixed anhydride or carbodiimide method (Erlanger *et al.*, 1957; Oliver *et al.*, 1968; Dumasia *et al.*, 1973). Phenols have been converted to active reagents by reaction with diazotized *p*-aminobenzoic acid (Weliky and Weetall, 1965); such *p*-aminobenzoate derivatives, like hemisuccinate derivatives, can then be conjugated to the amino groups of carriers via their functional carboxyl group. These and other conjugation methods have been reviewed in detail recently (Parker, 1972; Butler and Beiser, 1973; Erlanger, 1973; Marks *et al.*, 1974; Beiser *et al.*, 1976).

2.3. Characterization of Conjugates

Landsteiner (1945) and Erlanger (1973) stated that the incorporation of too many, as well as of too few, haptenic groups into a hapten–carrier conjugate may result in a poor antibody response; in their experience, ten haptenic groups per molecule of carrier seemed optimal when serum albumin was used as the carrier. Thus, prior to immunization, it is desirable to determine the average number of hapten molecules one has conjugated to the carrier employed. If the haptenic group has a suitable absorption spectrum, one can make a reasonably accurate estimate of the molar incorporation of hapten by determining the difference in molar extinction coefficients between conjugate and carrier at a given wavelength, and then comparing this difference with the molar extinction coefficient of the hapten at the same wavelength (Erlanger *et al.*, 1957; Little and Donahue, 1968; Smith *et al.*, 1970; Erlanger, 1973; Butler, 1975). The extent of haptenic incorporation into a hapten–protein conjugate can also be determined by various chemical analyses of conjugates (Goodfriend *et al.*, 1964; Dumasia *et al.*, 1973), by the extent of incorporation of radiolabeled drug into conjugates (Butler, 1975), or by the decrease in free amino groups of carrier following conjugation of a hapten to carrier by a method that utilizes the amino groups of the carrier (Erlanger *et al.*, 1957; Erlanger, 1973).

2.4. Immunization

Hapten–protein conjugates are ordinarily suspended in complete Freund's adjuvant mixture (Freund *et al.*, 1948) at a final concentration of 1 mg/ml or less; usually, less than 1 mg is injected into experimental animals, most frequently rabbits or guinea pigs, at intervals of 1 week or more. Longer periods of time (8–16 months, in some instances) than are employed for protein antigens may be required to obtain antihapten antibody of satisfactory titer, specificity, and affinity (Smith *et al.*, 1970; Jaffe *et al.*, 1971). Vaitukaitis *et al.* (1971) described a method that employs a small, divided primary immunizing dose together with *Bordetella pertussis* vaccine and that may be useful when the supply of hapten or conjugate is limited. These and other practical considerations connected with raising antibodies for use in immunoassays have been reviewed recently (Chase, 1967; Hurn and Landon, 1971; Parker, 1972; Hurn, 1974).

3. Characterization of Antidrug Antibodies

3.1. Detection of Antibodies

Inasmuch as most animals immunized with drug–protein conjugates form antibodies with specificity for the carrier protein, the method used for detection of antidrug antibodies must be one in which antibodies specific for the carrier will not also interact. The simplest and most direct methods for the detection of drug-specific antibodies without interference by antibodies to carrier involve the direct demonstration of the binding of radioactively labeled drugs or drug derivatives by antibody. Such binding can be demonstrated directly by equilibrium dialysis (Eisen, 1964), or by one of the many methods now available to separate antibody-bound drug from unbound drug (Daughaday and Jacobs, 1971; Hunter and Ganguli, 1971; Parker, 1972; Hunter, 1973; Ratcliffe, 1974); currently popular methods include the dextran-coated charcoal technique (Herbert *et al.,* 1965), gel or membrane filtration (Haber *et al.,* 1965b; VanVunakis and Levine, 1974), electrophoretic methods (Yalow and Berson, 1964), coprecipitation of radiolabeled drug with antibody on additon of an antiimmunoglobulin antibody in the "double antibody" technique (VanVunakis and Levine, 1974), and coprecipitation of radiolabeled drug with antibody following the addition of an appropriate amount of ammonium sulfate (Minden and Farr, 1973). Since many drugs are normally bound to a significant degree by nonimmunoglobulin serum proteins (especially in undiluted serum), it is important to ascertain that binding of radiolabeled drug is not observed with appropriate dilutions of control sera from nonimmunized animals and from animals immunized with unrelated antigens.

The most useful methods for radiolabeling of drugs for use in the detection of drug-specific antibodies involve the incorporation of either tritium (^{3}H) or radioiodine (^{125}I) into drugs or drug derivatives. ^{14}C-labeled drugs can also be used, but the specific activities achieved by ^{14}C-labeling are low when compared with ^{3}H- or ^{125}I-labeling; because of these low specific activities, methods employing ^{14}C labels are relatively insensitive both in the detection of antibodies and in the development of radioimmunoassays.

Tritium can readily be introduced into most drugs by the Wilzbach (1957) technique, followed by chromatographic purification. It has a long half-life of 12.3 years, and it represents no major external radiation hazard. However, it is not ideal. First, since tritium emits only β particles, liquid scintillation counting of radioisotopic disintegration must be employed. This technique can be cumbersome, time-consuming, and costly; quench corrections with the addition of internal standards may be necessary, and chemiluminescence can cause delays or misleading results unless proper control procedures are carried out (Butler, 1971). Second, in the cases of certain drugs, sufficient specific activity cannot be achieved to provide the sensitivity needed for the subsequent development of radioimmunoassay procedures.

^{125}I-labeled drugs have certain advantages over ^{3}H-labeled drugs. ^{125}I is a γ emitter, and γ counting is more rapid, more convenient, and less expensive than liquid scintillation counting. In addition, higher specific activities can be achieved with ^{125}I than with ^{3}H, with resultant increases in sensitivity, both in antibody detection and in the subsequent development of radioimmunoassay methods. To label with ^{125}I, however, one must first introduce a tyrosine or other phenolic group to which the iodine has been attached (Bolton and Hunter, 1973; Broughton and Strong, 1976) or can subsequently be attached (Hunter, 1973). Such coupling of a phenolic group to a drug may be chemically difficult; moreover, the resultant change in drug structure may alter its immunologic behavior. Other disadvantages of ^{125}I include a relatively short half-life of 60 days, possible chemical damage to the drug caused by radioiodine, and the need for frequent iodination with purification and immunologic assessment of each newly iodinated batch.

In the absence of radiolabeled drug, antibodies to drugs can be demonstrated by other methods, including inactivation of drug–enzyme conjugates (Scharpé *et al.,* 1976) or of drug–bacteriophage conjugates (Andrieu *et al.,* 1974). It is also possible to employ classic precipitin, complement fixation, or passive hemagglutination methods to demonstrate the interaction of antidrug antibody with conjugates in which the hapten is attached to a carrier antigenically unrelated to the carrier used for immunization; in this latter instance, it is particularly important to ascertain that the interaction with antiserum is specifically inhibited by free, unconjugated drug (Butler and Beiser, 1973).

3.2. Assessment of Antibody Specificity

Once it has been demonstrated that a radiolabeled drug or drug derivative is bound by an antiserum, it must be shown that this binding is specific. First, one must demonstrate that nonradioactive drug is an effective inhibitor of the binding. Then one must proceed to assess the degree of inhibition caused by metabolic products of the drug and by other structurally related molecules. To indicate the degree of specificity that can be achieved in selected antidrug antisera, the structural formula of digoxin is compared in Figure 1 with the structural formulas of digitoxin, a closely related cardiac glycoside, and of dihydrodigoxin, a pharmacologically ineffective metabolic breakdown product of digoxin. Despite the minimal

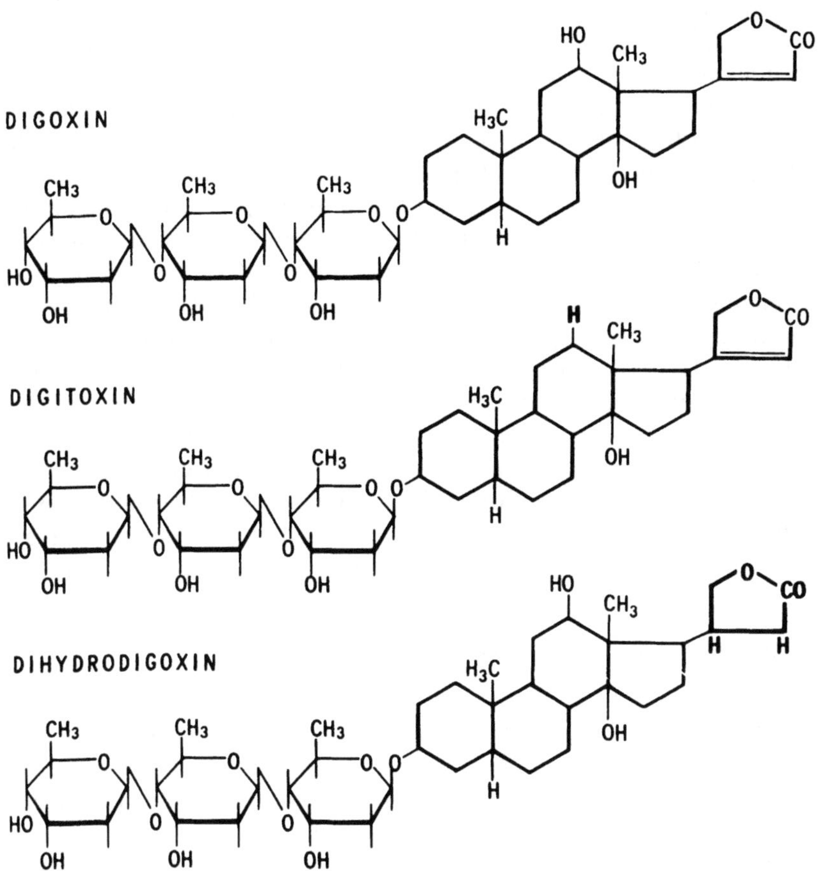

Figure 1. Structural formulas of digoxin, digitoxin, and dihydrodigoxin. The portions of the digitoxin and dihydrodigoxin molecules that differ structurally from digoxin are depicted in boldface. Reprinted with permission from Butler *et al.* (1974).

chemical differences between digoxin and these two closely related glycosides, it is possible to elicit antidigoxin antibodies that bind digoxin 20–30 times more effectively than they bind either digitoxin or dihydrodigoxin (Butler and Chen, 1967; Smith *et al.*, 1970; Butler *et al.*, 1974). Finally, it is also necessary to demonstrate that structurally more distant compounds, notably other drugs or substances normally present in human plasma, do not inhibit the binding of drug by antibody. For example, antibodies to digitalis glycosides react with steroid hormones (Butler and Chen, 1967); therefore, it was necessary to demonstrate that concentrations of steroid hormones encountered in human sera did not inhibit the binding of [^{3}H]digoxin by antidigoxin antibodies before the radioimmunoassay method could be used clinically to measure serum digoxin concentrations (Smith *et al.*, 1969, 1970).

In connection with studies of antibody specificity, it is important to recognize that antibodies to a given drug will usually react with metabolites of that drug. It may occasionally be possible to remove some of the antibodies that cross-react in this manner. It should be remembered, however, that absolute specificity of antibodies for a given molecule will rarely, if ever, be observed (Beiser *et al.*, 1976). Cross-reactivity with drug metabolites may not represent a major disadvantage if, in practice, serum concentrations of "immunoreactive" drug correlate well with values obtained by other methods and with the clinical state of the patients studied. For example, such a correlation does exist in the case of digoxin; this correlation, however, does not necessarily apply to other drugs, because digoxin is somewhat unusual in that it is not extensively degraded in man, and in that several of its major metabolites are both pharmacologically and immunologically active (Butler, 1972).

Antibodies to a given drug will often react with related drugs of the same class, but this cross-reactivity should not constitute a major problem clinically if it can be established with certainty that the patient is receiving a given drug and has not recently received a chemically related agent (Butler, 1972).

If problems are encountered in obtaining antibodies of satisfactory specificity for use in an immunoassay procedure, it is important to remember that different individual animals may produce antibodies that vary greatly in specificity; one should therefore examine several antisera before selecting the one with optimum specificity. It also may be useful to recall that the specificity of antihapten antibodies appears to be directed primarily against that portion of the hapten molecule furthest from the site of conjugation to the carrier; antibodies of different specificity can usually be obtained if the hapten is coupled to the carrier via a different functional group (Parker, 1972; Butler and Beiser, 1973; Erlanger, 1973).

3.3. Assessment of Antibody Affinity

Antiserum to a given drug usually contains a heterogeneous population of antidrug antibodies with different avidities or association constants. In general, the greater the affinity of antibody for drug, the more sensitive will be the immunoassay that can be developed, and the simpler it will be to make assay behavior constant and reproducible. In view of these considerations, the determination of association constants is useful in the selection of antisera for use in immunoassay work; it is not essential, however, since the avidity of antibodies may be inferred from a variety of measurements of hapten–antibody interactions (Hunter, 1973).

Recent studies have also called attention to the fact that dissociation constants of drug–antibody complexes may be important when the adsorbent used to separate free from antibody-bound drug in an immunoassay procedure competes with antibody for drug molecules that dissociate from antibody during the separation step of the immunoassay (Smith and Haber, 1973).

It should be pointed out that no two antisera to any antigen may ever be considered to be identical either in specificity or in affinity. Even in antisera obtained at different times from a single animal, striking changes in the affinity and specificity of antidrug antibodies have been observed with time (Smith *et al.*, 1970). Thus, published results regarding the specificity or affinity of antidrug antibodies should never be extrapolated to one's own antisera; furthermore, it would seem reasonable to require commercial suppliers of drug antisera or of drug immunoassay kits to provide data concerning specificity and affinity with every sample sold.

3.4. Assessment of Antibody Titer

By antibody titer is meant the greatest dilution of antibody that will produce a given degree of binding of a stated amount of a drug (Hunter, 1973). The higher the titer, the more determinations one can perform with a given volume of antiserum; e.g., antidigoxin sera can frequently be used at dilutions theoretically great enough to allow for the performance of 200,000 digoxin determinations with 1 ml antiserum. A high-titered antiserum is useless, however, unless both specificity and affinity are satisfactory.

4. Use of Antibodies in Immunoassays

4.1. Immunoassay Methods

Immunoassay methods for the measurement of drugs are based on the ability of drugs to inhibit the reaction between drug-specific antibodies and the corresponding drug–carrier conjugate or the corresponding labeled hapten. Using principles delineated by Berson and Yalow (1966), increasing concentrations of a known standard solution of the drug are incubated with constant predetermined amounts of drug-specific antibody and of drug–carrier conjugate, or of labeled drug, under conditions of antigen excess. A standard curve is then constructed, on which decreasing amounts of interaction between labeled drug and antibody can be shown to correspond with increasing concentrations of unlabeled drug. If the biological fluid to be assayed (1) does not interfere with the drug–antibody reaction, (2) does not degrade the drug, and (3) does not contain substances that cross-react significantly with the drug antibody, the concentration of the drug in that biological fluid can be determined from the degree to which it inhibits the reaction between antibody and drug–carrier conjugate or labeled drug, when compared with a simultaneously performed standard curve (Yalow and Berson, 1964; Parker, 1972; Ekins, 1974; Ratcliffe, 1974). The standard curve employed in a representative serum digoxin radioimmunoassay procedure is illustrated in Figure 2.

Inhibition of complement fixation (Hamburger, 1966) or of passive hemagglutination (Adler, 1974) has been used to measure drugs. However, because of their greater sensitivity, precision, rapidity, and convenience, greater experience has been obtained with immunoassay methods that employ radioactively or physicochemically labeled drugs or drug derivatives.

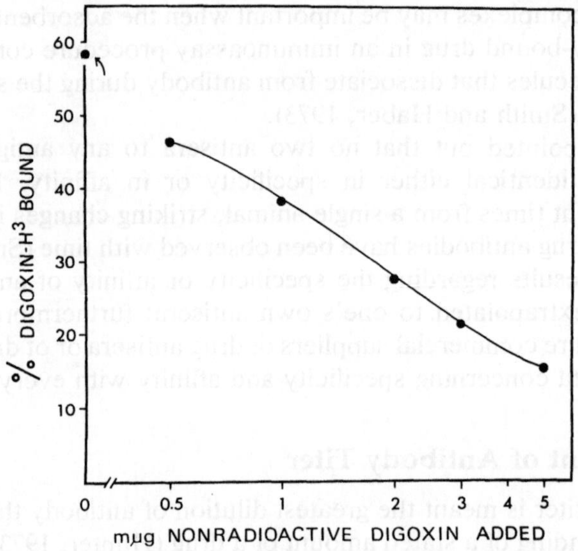

Figure 2. Representative standard curve for serum digoxin radioimmunoassay procedure. In the presence of increasing concentrations of nonradioactive digoxin (in known reference standard solutions), the percentage of [^{3}H]digoxin (3 ng) bound by a constant amount of rabbit antidigoxin serum (50 μl of a 1:2500 dilution) decreases from 59% in the absence of unlabeled digoxin to 16% in the presence of 5 ng (mμg) unlabeled digoxin. If, under identical conditions, a patient's serum reduces binding of [^{3}H]digoxin to 29%, that serum contains 2 ng digoxin/ml. Reprinted with permission from Butler (1970).

Until recently, most of the studies with labeled haptens employed radioactively labeled drugs or drug derivatives. Many methods are now available for the separation of free, unbound radiolabeled drug from antibody-bound radioactivity in the development of radioimmunoassay procedures (Hunter and Ganguli, 1971; Daughaday and Jacobs, 1971; Parker, 1972; Hunter, 1973). These methods include electrophoresis, gel filtration, adsorption systems (e.g., dextran-coated charcoal, membrane filtration), solvent and salt precipitation systems, solid-phase antibody procedures, and the double antibody method (Table 1). Because of its convenience and rapidity, the dextran-coated charcoal method of Herbert *et al.* (1965) has been widely used in drug radioimmunoassay procedures. It involves the almost instantaneous adsorption of non-antibody-bound drug onto charcoal particles and its rapid centrifugal separation from antibody-bound radioactivity; thus, it is not useful in instances in which radiolabeled drugs or drug derivatives are not effectively adsorbed to the charcoal, nor in instances in which the dissociation constant of a drug–antibody complex is great enough to cause a temporally related variability in results as dissociated drug is progressively adsorbed to charcoal as a function of the duration of the charcoal incubation step in the immunoassay procedure (Smith and Haber, 1973). Because of such problems with adsorption methods, many newly developed radioimmunoassay procedures have employed either the double antibody method or a solid-phase antibody procedure. Theoretically, "immunoradiometric" assay procedures employing radioiodinated antibody (Woodhead *et al.*, 1974) can also be used, but extensive experience has not yet been obtained with such procedures in the assay of drugs.

To eliminate some of the technical problems associated with the use of radiolabeled drugs in clinical laboratories or in automated equipment, physicochemically labeled drugs have recently been employed in the development of nonisotopic immunoassay procedures. For example, spin-labeled drugs have been used in an immunoassay procedure that takes advantage of the fact that the mobility of free radicals of spin-labeled drugs in the free, unbound state differs from their mobility when bound to specific antibody, as measured in an electron spin resonance spectrometer. This technique has proved useful in screening biological fluids for the detection of opiates and other drugs of abuse (Schneider *et al.*, 1974). Most recently, another perhaps more useful method has been introduced into clinical use. This method is based on the fact that antidrug antibodies will inactivate drug–enzyme conjugates in a reproducible manner that is readily quantifiable by simple spectrophotometric assays of enzymatic activity; increasing quantities of drug will reduce the degree of enzyme inactivation in a reproducible and predictable manner that can be used as the basis for a simple immunoassay procedure (Scharpé *et al.*, 1976).

4.2. Limitations and Problems

It is most convenient when an immunoassay procedure can be carried out with untreated serum, plasma, or other biological fluid. In some instances, however, prior treatment or separatory procedures may be necessary to inactivate substances that degrade the drug being studied. In other cases, prior extractions or separatory procedures may be necessary to concentrate a drug, to remove it from a normal binding site on a plasma protein in the test serum, or to separate it from certain of its metabolites or from other structurally related compounds also capable of inhibiting the drug–antibody interaction (Parker, 1972; Butler and Beiser, 1973). In radioimmunoassay procedures, the presence of a radioisotope (administered for diagnostic or therapeutic purposes) in a patient's serum constitutes a potential source of error, if the presence of the isotope is not known to the laboratory; in radioimmunoassay procedures employing liquid scintillation counting methods, chemiluminescence

TABLE 1. Separation of Unbound from Antibody-Bound Radiolabeled Drug in Radioimmunoassay Procedures

	Mode of separation	
Method	Antibody and antibody-bound radioactivity	Unbound (free) radioactivity
Equilibrium dialysis	Retained inside sac.	Equal concentration inside and outside sac.
Dextran-coated charcoal	Not adsorbed to charcoal; in supernatant after centrifugation.	Adsorbed to charcoal; in precipitate after centrifugation.
Gel filtration	Eluted early.	Eluted late.
Membrane filtration	Bound to nitrocellulose membrane.	Washed through membrane.
Electrophoresis and chromatoelectrophoresis	In γ-globulin electrophoretic fraction.	Migrates with its own electrophoretic mobility.
Double antibody method	Precipitated by antibody to animal γ-globulin.	In supernatant after centrifugation.
Solid-phase antibody methods	Bound to insoluble supporting matrix.	Remains in soluble phase after incubation period.

produced by urine and certain sera (especially from azotemic patients) may also interfere with assay results. Neither of these latter sources of error in radioimmunoassay procedures, however, should cause a problem if proper control procedures are carried out (Butler, 1971; Smith and Haber, 1973).

Although antibodies are stable for many years if properly stored in concentrated form, deterioration of antisera may occur if appropriate precautions are not taken. Deterioration of radiolabeled drugs or drug derivatives may also occur with time, particularly in the case of radioiodinated derivatives of drugs (Kirkham and Hunter, 1971). Similarly, great care must be exercised in the preparation and storage of the drug standards used in the construction of standard immunoassay curves, because results in unknown specimens will be calculated on the basis of values obtained with these standards of predetermined, known concentration (Bangham and Cotes, 1974).

As with all drug assay procedures, drug immunoassay methods will yield useful information only if it can be established, experimentally or clinically, that the drug concentrations in the specimens being assayed bear some relationship to a pharmacological effect of, or the clinical response to, that drug (Koch-Weser, 1972). In this latter connection, the time at which the specimen is best obtained with respect to the last dose of the drug is quite important, and must be established before the immunoassay procedure can be used properly (Butler, 1972; Koch-Weser, 1972; Gibaldi and Levy, 1976).

4.3. Applications

The introduction of drug immunoassay methods into clinical and investigative medicine has added a new dimension to the identification and measurement of pharmacologically active substances in the plasma and tissues of man and experimental animals (Butler, 1973, 1975; Spector, 1973; Marks *et al.*, 1974; Langone *et al.*, 1975; Landon and Moffat, 1976; Cleeland *et al.*, 1976; Broughton and Strong, 1976). Immunoassay methods often provide the sensitivity, specificity, precision, rapidity, and convenience needed for the daily performance of large numbers of drug analyses on small volumes of serum in clinical laboratories. The convenience and rapidity of many of these methods are such that it is easily possible for one technician to perform blood drug level determinations on microliter volumes of unextracted serum from 40 patients within a few hours; automated equipment is now available that can increase the number of analyses performed daily to 200 or more. Thus, the convenience and rapidity of immunoassay methods are major advantages in the clinical laboratory where the rapid analysis of large numbers of specimens is highly desirable in the evaluation of drug therapy and in the prompt determination of appropriate dosage schedules for individual patients being treated with a given drug. The simplicity and convenience of immunoassay methods also render them highly suitable for large-scale studies of drug bioavailability (Lindenbaum *et al.*, 1971; Wagner *et al.*, 1973; Preibisz *et al.*, 1974), pharmacokinetics (Selden and Smith, 1972), compliance (Weintraub *et al.*, 1973), and abuse (Mulé *et al.*, 1974; Cleeland *et al.*, 1976).

To illustrate the broad pharmacological applicability of immunoassay methods, Table 2 contains a list of some drugs and toxins for which immunoassay methods have already been developed. These compounds include a variety of narcotic and analgesic agents, several antibiotics, certain anticonvulsants, antiinflammatory

TABLE 2. Immunoassays for Drugs and Toxins

- Analgesics and narcotics
  - Anileridine
  - Antipyrine
  - Codeine
  - Etorphine
  - Fentanyl
  - Meperidine
  - Methadone
  - Morphine
  - Pentazocine
- Antibiotics
  - Amikacin
  - Chloramphenicol
  - Clindamycin
  - Gentamicin
  - Isoniazid
  - Penicillin
  - Sisomycin
  - Tobramycin
- Anticonvulsants
  - Clonazepam
  - Phenytoin
  - Primidone
- Antiinflammatory agents
  - Colchicine
  - Indomethacin
  - Phenylbutazone
- Antineoplastic agents
  - Adriamycin
  - Bleomycin
  - Daunomycin
  - Methotrexate
- Bronchodilators
  - Theophylline
- Cardiovascular drugs
  - Cardiac glycosides
    - Acetylstrophanthidin
    - Cedilanid
    - Deslanoside
    - Digitoxin
    - Digoxin
    - Gitoxin
    - Methyl digoxin
    - Ouabain
    - Proscillaridin
  - Dihydroergotamine
  - Propranolol
  - Quinidine
- CNS stimulants
  - Amphetamine
  - Benzoyl ecgonine (cocaine metabolite)
  - Methamphetamine
  - Pimozide
- Diuretics
  - Bumetanide
- Hallucinogenic drugs
  - Lysergic acid diethylamide (LSD)

- Hallucinogenic drugs (*cont'd*)
  - Mescaline
  - Tetrahydrocannabinol
- Hypoglycemic agents
  - Butylbiguanide
  - Glibenclamid
- Insecticides
  - Aldrin
  - DDT
  - Dieldrin
  - Malathion
- Narcotic antagonists
  - Cyclazocine
  - Naloxone
- Sedatives and tranquilizers
  - Barbiturates
    - Barbital
    - Pentobarbital
    - Phenobarbital
  - Chlordiazepoxide
  - Chlorpromazine
  - Desmethylimipramine
  - Diazepam and *N*-desmethyldiazepam
  - Glutethimide
  - Methaqualone
- Skeletal muscle relaxants
  - *d*-Tubocurarine
- Synthetic peptides
  - DDAVP
  - Saralasin
- Synthetic steroids
  - Anabolic steroids
    - Trienbolone acetate
  - Androgens
    - Fluoxymesterone
  - Estrogens
    - Diethylstilbestrol
    - Ethinylestradiol
    - Mestranol
  - Glucocorticoids
    - Dexamethasone
    - Methylprednisolone
    - Prednisolone
    - Prednisone
  - Metyrapone
  - Progestins
    - Medroxyprogesterone acetate
    - Norethindrone
    - Norethisterone
    - Norgestrel
- Toxins
  - Aflatoxin B_1
  - Genistein
  - Nicotine and metabolites
  - Ochratoxin A
  - Paralytic shellfish poison
  - Tartrazine

TABLE 3. **Other Immunoassays of Pharmacological Interest**

Bile acid conjugates	Peptide hormones
Cholylglycine	Angiotensin
Cholyltaurine	Anterior pituitary
Catecholamines	Bradykinin
Epinephrine	Gastric
Norepinephrine	Hypothalamic
Tyramine	Intestinal
Fibrinopeptides	Pancreatic
Fibrinopeptide A	Parathyroid
Fibrinopeptide B	Posterior pituitary
Indolealkylamines	Thyroid (calcitonin)
Melatonin	Plant hormones
Serotonin	Indole-3-acetic acid
Insect hormones	Gibberellic acid
Ecdysone	Polyamines
Nucleosides and nucleotides	Spermine
Cyclic AMP	Prostaglandins
Cyclic GMP	Steroid hormones
N^2-Dimethylguanosine	Thyroid hormones
7-Methylguanosine	Thyroxine
Pseudouridine	Triiodothyronine
Thymidine	Vitamins
	Vitamin B_{12}
	Vitamin D

drugs, antineoplastic agents, a large number of cardiovascular drugs (including at least nine different cardiac glycosides), CNS stimulants, diuretics, hallucinogenic drugs, oral hypoglycemic agents, several insecticides, various sedatives and tranquilizers (most notably, the barbiturates), D-tubocurarine, more than a dozen synthetic steroid drugs (including androgens, estrogens, glucocorticoids, metyrapone, and oral progestins), and finally, several toxins, including nicotine and paralytic shellfish poison. Table 3 lists other immunoassays of pharmacological interest, including assays for conjugated bile acids, catecholamines, serotonin and melatonin, insect and plant hormones, nucleosides and nucleotides, numerous mammalian peptide hormones, spermine, prostaglandins, numerous steroid hormones, thyroid hormones, and vitamin B_{12}.

5. Biological Properties of Antibodies to Drugs and to Other Compounds of Pharmacological Importance

Until the past decade, there has been relatively little physiologic or pharmacological application of antibodies as specific antagonists of drugs and other biologically active low-molecular-weight substances. There is now a considerable body of evidence that antibodies specific for cardiac glycosides, carcinogens, chloramphenicol, histamine, morphine, pyridoxal phosphate, serotonin, and various peptide and steroid hormones are capable, by virtue of their capacity to bind these substances, of inhibiting certain physiologic effects of these compounds on cells, either *in vivo* or *in vitro* (Butler *et al.*, 1973). Table 4 lists the biological properties of antibodies to the cardiac glycoside digoxin that have been demonstrated to date. In this instance, not only do antibodies (and their Fab fragments) neutralize the drug, but they are also capable of removing digoxin from cells, thereby reversing its cellular effects. In the case of human erythrocytes, studies have revealed that antibody removes membrane-bound digoxin more slowly then it removes intracellular digoxin, and that the reversal of the inhibitory action of digoxin on red cell cation influx is correlated temporally with the removal of the membrane-bound fraction of digoxin. These studies with digoxin-specific antibodies lend strong support to other pharmacological data suggesting that there are at least two fractions of erythrocyte digoxin, but that only one of these fractions, namely, the membrane-bound fraction, contains the digoxin molecules that are responsible for the inhibitory effect of the glycoside on monovalent cation transport. Antidigoxin antibodies also exert their effects *in vivo;* both they and their Fab fragments (which are smaller in molecular size, less immunogenic, and more rapidly eliminated than intact antibodies) were shown to be capable of rapidly reversing advanced digoxin intoxication in experimental animals and in man (Butler *et al.,* 1973, 1974; Smith *et al.,* 1977).

It would appear that antibodies to other drugs may also be useful as specific antagonists of drug action at the cellular level. In some instances, antibodies (or their Fab fragments) may also be useful *in vivo* as specific drug antidotes; however, the utility of such specific immunotherapy will be limited to those instances in which it is possible to accumulate and to administer sufficient antibody to achieve an appreciable therapeutic effect. In the case of a hypothetical model drug with a molecular weight of 500, 1 g of specific Fab fragments (or 1.6 g of specific antibody) would be required to neutralize 10 mg (20 μmol) of drug. Thus, unless smaller active fragments of specific antibodies can be isolated or synthesized, the potential therapeutic use of drug-specific antibodies would appear to be limited at present to the antagonism of substances that exert toxic effects at the milligram, rather than the gram, level in man.

TABLE 4. Biological Properties of Digoxin-Specific Antibodies[a]

1. Prevention of uptake of digoxin by cells *in vitro*
   - Rat renal cortical cells
   - Human erythrocytes
2. Prevention of pharmacological effects of digoxin *in vitro*
   - Prevention of inhibitory effect of digoxin on potassium influx in human erythrocytes
   - Prevention of digoxin-induced inhibition of myocardial Na^+, K^+-ATPase
   - Prevention of positive inotropic effect of digoxin on isolated myocardial preparations
3. Prevention of digoxin intoxication in digoxin-immunized rabbits
4. Removal of digoxin from cells *in vitro*
   - Rat renal cortical cells
   - Human erythrocytes
5. Reversal of pharmacological and toxic effects of digoxin *in vitro*
   - Reversal of inhibitory effect of digoxin on potassium influx in human erythrocytes
   - Reversal of digoxin-induced inhibition of myocardial Na^+, K^+-ATPase
   - Reversal of positive inotropic and toxic electrophysiologic effects of digoxin on isolated myocardial preparations
6. Reversal of established digoxin intoxication in nonimmunized dogs
7. Alteration of digoxin metabolism in rabbits and dogs
   - Inceased serum concentrations
   - Decreased urinary excretion

[a]Reprinted with permission from Butler *et al.* (1974).

Acknowledgments

This work was supported by grants from the National Institutes of Health (HL-10608) and the New York Heart Association. Dr. Butler is the recipient of an Irma T. Hirschl Career Scientist Award.

References

Adler, F. L., 1974, in: *Immunoassays for Drugs Subject to Abuse* (S. J. Mulé, I. Sunshine, M. Braude, and R. E. Willette, eds.), pp. 37–43, CRC Press, Cleveland.

Andrieu, J. M., Mamas, S., and Dray, F., 1974, *Prostaglandins* **6**:15–22.

Bangham, D., and Cotes, P. M., 1974, *Br. Med. Bull.* **30**:12–17.

Beiser, S. M., Butler, V. P., Jr., and Erlanger, B. F., 1976, in: *Textbook of Immunopathology*, 2nd Ed. (P. A. Miescher and H. J. Müller-Eberhard, eds.), pp. 15–29, Grune and Stratton, New York.

Berson, S. A., and Yalow, R. A., 1966, *Harvey Lect.* **62**:107–163.

Bolton, A. E., and Hunter, W. M., 1973, *Biochem. J.* **133**:529–539.

Broughton, A., and Strong, J. E., 1976, *Clin. Chem.* **22**:726–732.

Butler, V. P., Jr., 1970, *N. Engl. J. Med.* **283**:1150–1156.

Butler, V. P., Jr., 1971, *Lancet* **1**:186.

Butler, V. P., Jr., 1972, *Prog. Cardiovasc. Dis.* **14**:571–600.

Butler, V. P., Jr., 1973, *Metabolism* **22**:1145–1153.

Butler, V. P., Jr., 1975, *J. Immunol. Methods* **7**:1–24.

Butler, V. P., Jr., and Beiser, S. M., 1973, *Adv. Immunol.* **17**:255–310.

Butler, V. P., Jr., and Chen, J. P., 1967, *Proc. Natl. Acad. Sci. U.S.A.* **57**:71–78.

Butler, V. P., Jr., Watson, J. F., Schmidt, D. H., Gardner, J. D., Mandel, W. J., and Skelton, C. L., 1973, *Pharmacol. Rev.* **25**:239–248.

Butler, V. P., Jr., Schmidt, D. H., Watson, J. F., and Gardner, J. D., 1974, *Ann. N.Y. Acad. Sci.* **242**:717–730.

Chase, M. W., 1967, in: *Methods in Immunology and Immunochemistry,* Vol. 1 (C. A. Williams and M. W. Chase, eds.), pp. 197–224, 237–306, Academic Press, New York.

Cleeland, R., Christenson, J., Usategui-Gomez, M., Heveran, J., Davis, R., and Grunberg, E., 1976, *Clin. Chem.* **22**:712–725.

Daughaday, W. H., and Jacobs, L. S., 1971, in: *Principles of Competitive Protein-Binding Assays* (W. D. Odell and W. H. Daughaday, eds.), pp. 303–324, J. B. Lippincott Co., Philadelphia.

Dumasia, M. D., Chapman, D. I., Moss, M. S., and O'Connor, C., 1973, *Biochem. J.* **133**:401–404.

Eisen, H. N., 1964, *Methods Med. Res.* **10**:106–114.

Ekins, R. P., 1974, *Br. Med. Bull.* **30**:3–11.

Erlanger, B. F., 1973, *Pharmacol. Rev.* **25**:271–280.

Erlanger, B. F., and Beiser, S. M., 1964, *Proc. Natl. Acad. Sci. U.S.A.* **52**:68–74.

Erlanger, B. F., Borek, F., Beiser, S. M., and Lieberman, S., 1957, *J. Biol. Chem.* **228**:713–727.

Freund, J., Thomson, K. J., Hough, H. B., Sommer, H. E., and Pisani, T. M., 1948, *J. Immunol.* **60**:383–398.

Gibaldi, M., and Levy, G., 1976, *J. Am. Med. Assoc.* **235**:1987–1992.

Goodfriend, T. L., Levine, L., and Fasman, G. D., 1964, *Science* **144**:1344–1346.

Haber, E., Page, L. B., and Jacoby, G. A., 1965a, *Biochemistry* **4**:693–698.

Haber, E., Page, L. B., and Richards, F. F., 1965b, *Anal. Biochem.* **12**:163–172.

Hamburger, R. N., 1966, *Science* **152**:203–205.

Herbert, V., Lau, K.-S., Gottlieb, C. W., and Bleicher, S. J., 1965, *J. Clin. Endocrinol. Metab.* **25**:1375–1384.

Hunter, W. M., 1973, in: *Handbook of Experimental Immunology* (D. M. Weir, ed.), 2nd Ed., pp. 17.1–17.36, Blackwell Scientific Publications, Oxford.

Hunter, W. M., and Ganguli, P. C., 1971, in: *Radioimmunoassay Methods* (K. E. Kirkham and W. M. Hunter, eds.), pp. 243–257, Churchill Livingstone, Edinburgh.

Hurn, B. A. L., 1974, *Br. Med. Bull.* **30**:26–28.

Hurn, B. A. L., and Landon, J., 1971, in: *Radioimmunoassay Methods* (K. E. Kirkham and W. M. Hunter, eds.), pp. 121–142, Churchill Livingstone, Edinburgh.
Jaffe, B. M., Smith, J. W., Newton, W. T., and Parker, C. W., 1971, *Science* **171**:494–496.
Kirkham, K. E., and Hunter, W. M. (eds.), 1971, *Radioimmunoassay Methods*, pp. 100–104, 189–193, Churchill Livingstone, Edinburgh.
Koch-Weser, J., 1972, *N. Engl. J. Med.* **287**:227–231.
Landon, J., and Moffat, A. C., 1976, *Analyst* **101**:225–243.
Landsteiner, K., 1945, *The Specificity of Serological Reactions*, Revised Ed., pp. 156–210, Dover Publications, New York.
Langone, J. J., Van Vunakis, H., and Levine, L., 1975, *Acc. Chem. Res.* **8**:335–342.
Lindenbaum, J., Mellow, M. H., Blackstone, M. O., and Butler, V. P., Jr., 1971, *N. Engl. J. Med.* **285**:1344–1347.
Little, J. R., and Donahue, H., 1968, in: *Methods in Immunology and Immunochemistry*, Vol. 2 (C. A. Williams and M. W. Chase, eds), pp. 163–174, Academic Press, New York.
Marks, V., Morris, B. A., and Teale, J. D., 1974, *Br. Med. Bull.* **30**:80–86.
Minden, P., and Farr, R. S., 1973, in: *Handbook of Experimental Immunology* (D. M. Weir, ed.), 2nd Ed., pp. 15.1–15.21, Blackwell Scientific Publications, Oxford.
Mulé, S. J., Sunshine, I., Braude, M., and Willette, R. E., 1974, *Immunoassays for Drugs Subject to Abuse*, CRC Press, Cleveland.
Oliver, G. C., Parker, B. M., Brasfield, D. L., and Parker, C. W., 1968, *J. Clin Invest.* **47**:1035–1042.
Parker, C. W., 1972, *Prog. Clin. Pathol.* **4**:103–141.
Preibisz, J. J., Butler, V. P., Jr., and Lindenbaum, J., 1974, *Ann. Intern. Med.* **81**:469–474.
Ratcliffe, J. G., 1974, *Br. Med. Bull.* **30**:32–37.
Scharpé, S. L., Cooreman, W. M., Blomme, W. J., and Laekeman, G. M., 1976, *Clin. Chem.* **22**: 733–738.
Schneider, R. S., Bastiani, R. J., Leute, R. K., Rubenstein, K. E., and Ullman, E. F., 1974, in: *Immunoassays for Drugs Subject to Abuse* (S. J. Mulé, I. Sunshine, M. Braude, and R. E. Willette, eds.), pp. 45–72, CRC Press, Cleveland.
Selden, R., and Smith, T. W., 1972, *Circulation* **45**:1176–1182.
Smith, T. W., and Haber, E., 1973, *Pharmacol. Rev.* **25**:219–228.
Smith, T. W., Butler, V. P., Jr., and Haber, E., 1969, *N. Engl. J. Med.* **281**:1212–1216.
Smith, T. W., Butler, V. P., Jr., and Haber, E., 1970, *Biochemistry* **9**:331–337.
Smith, T. W., Butler, V. P., Jr., and Haber, E., 1977, in: *Antibodies in Human Diagnosis and Therapy* (E. Haber and R. M. Krause, eds.), pp. 365–389, Raven Press, New York.
Spector, S., 1973, *Annu. Rev. Pharmacol.* **13**:359–370.
Vaitukaitis, J., Robbins, J. B., Nieschlag, E., and Ross, G. T., 1971, *J. Clin. Endocrinol. Metab.* **33**:988–991.
VanVunakis, H., and Levine, L., 1974, in: *Immunoassays for Drugs Subject to Abuse* (S. J. Mulé, I. Sunshine, M. Braude, and R. E. Willette, eds.), pp. 23–35, CRC Press, Cleveland.
Wagner, J. G., Christensen, M., Sakmar, E., Blair, D., Yates, D., Willis, P. W., III, Sedman, A. J., and Stoll, R. G., 1973, *J. Am. Med. Assoc.* **224**:199–204.
Weintraub, M., Au, W. Y. W., and Lasagna, L., 1973, *J. Am. Med. Assoc.* **224**:481–485.
Weliky, N., and Weetall, H. H., 1965, *Immunochemistry* **2**:293–322.
Wilzbach, K. E., 1957, *J. Am. Chem. Soc.* **79**:1013.
Woodhead, J. S., Addison, G. M., and Hales, C. N., 1974, *Br. Med. Bull.* **30**:44–49.
Yalow, R. S., and Berson, S. A., 1964, *Methods Biochem. Anal.* **12**:69–96.

16

Receptors for Low-Molecular-Weight Hormones on Lymphocytes

KENNETH L. MELMON, YACOB WEINSTEIN, TAK C. POON, HENRY R. BOURNE, G. M. SHEARER, PHILIP COFFINO, and PAUL A. INSEL

1. Introduction

Receptors for vasoactive amines have been detected by pharmacologic techniques in or on mixed leukocytes from human peripheral blood and mouse spleens (Bourne and Melmon, 1971; Bourne *et al.*, 1971a, 1972). The evidence for the existence of receptors for small amines and lipids was at first scanty, and initially their function was totally unknown. The receptors were defined primarily by dose–response curves to histamine, the β-mimetic catecholamines, and the prostaglandins of the E and A series. Human and murine leukocytes responded to these agonists by elevation of their intracellular cyclic AMP (cAMP) concentrations (Bourne and Melmon, 1971; Bourne *et al.*, 1971a, 1972). The specificity of the responses was demonstrated by the selective and competitive antagonism of the effects of each agonist. The effect of histamine was specifically and competitively antagonized by four classes of antihistamines. The effects of β-adrenergic catecholamines were blocked by propranolol, a β-adrenergic antagonist, but were not affected by phentolamine (an α-adrenergic antagonist) or antihistamines. Neither the antihistamines

KENNETH L. MELMON, YACOB WEINSTEIN, TAK C. POON, HENRY R. BOURNE, and PAUL A. INSEL • Division of Clinical Pharmacology, Departments of Medicine, Pharmacology, and the Cardiovascular Research Institute, University of California, San Francisco, California 94143 **PHILIP COFFINO** • Division of Clinical Pharmacology, Departments of Medicine and Microbiology, University of California, San Francisco, California 94143 **G. M. SHEARER** • Immunology Branch, National Cancer Institute, National Institutes of Health, Bethesda, Maryland 20014. **Dr. Weinstein's present address is:** Department of Hormone Research, Weizmann Institute of Science, Rehovot, Israel.

nor the adrenergic antagonists affected the action of prostaglandin (PG) (Bourne and Melmon, 1971; Bourne *et al.*, 1971b, 1974). These data suggest that at least some of the leukocytes of mouse and man possess specific pharmacological receptors for vasoactive amines and PGs. In this chapter, we will not discuss leukocyte receptors for polypeptide hormones, antigens, or steroids, which are covered in other chapters and volumes of this series.

At the time that pharmacological specificity for the response of leukocytes to vasoactive amines and lipids was established, many questions arose, of which the four most pressing were: (1) Which cells in the heterogenous mixtures were responding to the agonists? (2) Were single cells selectively endowed with receptors, or could most cells respond to most agonists? (3) What was the location of the receptor on the cell? (4) What was the function(s) of such receptors, if any, on these cells? It seemed likely, because one pharmacological response being measured was activation of adenylate cyclase, that at least part of the receptors would be membrane-bound. This hypothesis was both tested and used to advantage in the separation of cells with and without receptors. The other three questions have been the subject of intensive investigation. The investigations have helped to consolidate the scientific interests between pharmacologists, who are concerned with inflammation and its mediators, and immunologists, who are interested in cells that appear to have receptors for some mediators of inflammation (i.e., histamine, β-mimetic amines, and selected PGs).

2. Determination of the 'Physiologic' Importance of Leukocyte Receptors

2.1. General Actions on Inflammatory and Immunologic Processes

Table 1 summarizes the multiple leukocytic functions that can be modulated by the various hormones that we are discussing. In each instance, where the data are adequate, we conclude that stimulation of these receptors inhibits a variety of cellular functions. Thus, a consistent panoply of endogenous hormones can modulate the functions of leukocytes involved in: (1) the inflammatory process [inhibition of histamine, slow-reaching substance of anaphylaxis (SRS-A), and lysosomal enzyme release (Bourne *et al.*, 1974)]; (2) T-cell lymphocyte responses: (a) suppressor T cell functions—inhibition, and subsequent modulation of the ultimate degree of response to either a cell-mediated or a humorally mediated event (Bourne *et al.*, 1974; Mozes *et al.*, 1973, 1974), (b) inhibition of T effector cell cytolytic functions (Plaut *et al.*, 1975) (In the latter instance the histamine effects are time dependent, which suggests that the receptors for histamine develop as a function of T effector cell commitment to cytolysis.), and (*c*) inhibition of T effector cell production or release of the lymphokines interferon (human) and migration-inhibitory factor (MIF) (guinea pig) (Bourne *et al.*, 1974); and (3) inhibition of B-cell production or release of antigen-specific antibody by any agonist that increases lymphocyte adenylate cyclase activity (Melmon *et al.*, 1974a). (The precursers of antibody forming cells do not seem responsive to histamine—see below.)

In the vast majority of instances, the inhibition of each function is accompanied by an appropriate elevation in cAMP production (Bourne *et al.*, 1974). Temporally, the inhibitory event occurs as augmentation of the intracellular cAMP concentration begins; the extent of the inhibition correlates with the extent of cAMP accumulation. The inhibitory events are augmented by agents that enhance accumulation of cAMP

TABLE 1. Hormonal Control of Effector Cell Function[a]

Function	Effector cell	Effect[b]	Inhibitory effects of: Histamine	β-Catechol-amines	PGs[b]	Cholera toxin	Correlation with cAMP[c]
Immediate hypersensitivity	Human basophil	Histamine release	+	+	+	+	+
	Human and monkey lung (mast cell)	Histamine, SRS-A, and ECF release	?	+	+	?	+
Acute inflammation	Human neutrophil	Release of lysosomal hydrolases	+	+	+	−	?
Cell-mediated immunity	T lymphocyte of:						
	guinea pig	MIF release	+	?	?	?	?
	mouse and rat	Immune cytolysis	+	+	+	+	+
	man	Interferon production	?	+	+	+	+
Humoral immunity	B lymphocyte/plasma cell (mouse)	Plaque formation on SRBC	+	+	+	+	+

[a] Data derived from Bourne *et al.* (1974).
[b] Abbreviations: (PGs) prostaglandins; (cAMP) cyclic AMP; (SRBC) sheep red blood cells; (MIF) migration-inhibitory factor; (SRS-A) slow-reacting substance of anaphylaxis; (ECF) eosinophilic chemotactic factor.
[c] (+) Indicates that all pharmacological agents that inhibited the leukocyte function also caused increased accumulation of cAMP in cells; (−) indicates that the agent did not cause inhibition.

by inhibiting its degradation. The events caused by agonists are mimicked by adding dibutyryl cAMP (DB-cAMP) to cell cultures or by administration to animals. Last, a "nonspecific" agonist that is a very potent stimulator of adenylate cyclase, cholera toxin, can reproduce all the inhibitory activities in relation to its ability to augment cAMP production.

2.2. Cyclic AMP Actions on Mitogenesis*

We are beginning to gain some insight into the actual mechanisms by which the cAMP may be producing its effects. Two lines of experimentation appear promising. One approach has been to study the effects of a cyclic nucleotide produced endogenously or of the pharmacologically active congener DB-cAMP on the effects of mitogens on leukocytes (Weinstein *et al.*, 1974, 1975a, 1976). The mitogens used in these studies included concanavalin A (Con A), phytohemagglutinin (PHA) (mitogens for T cells), and lipopolysaccharide (LPS) (a mitogen for B cells). If the additions of nucleotides were made within 6 hr of adding the mitogen, eventual production of DNA and RNA synthesis was inhibited. That is, when added with or up to 6 hr after mitogen, DB-cAMP or agonists able to stimulate production of cAMP inhibited thymidine incorporation into DNA by 80–90%. But when the DB-cAMP or the agonists were added more than 6 hr after the cells were exposed to mitogen, the inhibitory effects gradually diminished. When the drugs were added just prior to a pulse of [^{3}H]thymidine at 40 hr after the mitogen was added, they had no inhibitory effects on DNA synthesis *per se*. The data suggested that cAMP indirectly inhibits mitogen-stimulated incorporation of precursors into nucleic acids, and acts at a critical regulatory stage prior to the actual synthesis of these macromolecules.

The reports of other investigators make it appear unlikely that the cyclic nucleotide directly antagonizes certain very early sequelae of mitogen activation, because the inhibitory effects were seen when cAMP was elevated as late as 4 hr into the reaction. These early events, which include changes in membrane permeability and metabolism (Peters and Hausen, 1971; Kay, 1968; Fisher and Mueller, 1968; Resch *et al.*, 1972), accumulation of cyclic GMP (cGMP) (Hadden *et al.*, 1972) and cAMP (Smith *et al.*, 1971), and metabolism of histones (Pogo *et al.*, 1966; Kleinsmith *et al.*, 1966), have been shown to be well established, maximal, or (in the case of cGMP elevation) to have ended by 4 hr after exposure of the cells to mitogen (Hadden *et al.*, 1972).

3. Somatic Genetic Analysis of Cyclic AMP Action as a Means of Assessing Receptor Function

The study of the perturbation of fundamental biosynthetic pathways by endogenously produced or exogenous cAMP added to heterogeneous cell mixtures has helped to define both its mechanism of action and the probable function of receptors that are fundamental to its production. In addition, somatic genetic analysis provides a promising and particularly relevant experimental means of studying the functions of receptors on leukocytes. We have developed techniques for a somatic genetic analysis of cAMP action in a cultured cell line of S49 mouse lymphoma cells.

*See Chapters 1 and 2 for background.

We have isolated and characterized mutants of these animal cells that are deficient in their responses to cAMP. These studies are frankly imitative of work done over the last three decades with microorganisms. Such mutant microorganisms have contributed significantly to the considerable progress of molecular biology. Isolation of a relevant mutant in bacterial or bacteriophage investigation is frequently the first means of defining a basic biological phenomenon (Cairns *et al.*, 1966). In some cases, the mere existence of a mutant may allow clear-cut conclusions to be drawn. For instance, the proposed role of *Escherichia coli* polymerase I as the DNA replicase was ruled out definitively when mutant organisms lacking the enzyme were found to replicate their DNA normally (DeLucia and Cairns, 1969). The technical problems with genetic manipulation of animal cells are substantial, and we lack basic knowledge of the organization and regulation of the animal cell genome. Nonetheless, animal cell biologists are now adopting the sophisticated approaches previously used only in work with microorganisms, and are generating and isolating mutants of mammalian cells.

Our studies on animal cell genetics and the basic mechanisms of hormone action of S49 mouse lymphoma cells (Horibata and Harris, 1970) have been initiated and are detailed elsewhere (Coffino *et al.*, 1976). The cells are grown in liquid suspension culture, and they double in number about every 16 hr. Like many mouse lymphoid lines, the cultures are "immortal" in the sense that they have grown continuously for several years without showing signs of senescence. S49 has an active adenylate cyclase and accumulates cAMP in response to β-adrenergic agonists, cholera toxin, and PGE_1 in the same manner as the leukocytes we have been discussing. Any of these agents or DB-cAMP can cause arrest of cell growth and, several days later, cell death (Daniels *et al.*, 1973a,b). We have exploited these effects to select mutants resistant to the killing action of cAMP. Thus far, three broad classes of mutants have been obtained and characterized (Coffino *et al.*, 1976). One group is deficient in adenylate cyclase, another has abnormalities or complete absence of cAMP-dependent protein kinase, and a third group lacks a function required for cAMP-dependent cell death. These cells are being used to characterize the requirements for and mechanisms of action of cAMP within cells. Perhaps this approach will be useful in defining specific mechanisms that occur in lymphocytes when cAMP modulates the aspects of inflammation and immune response listed above.

3.1. General Scheme for Selection of Mutants

There are two prerequisites for obtaining clones of mutant cells: (1) Either the mutants should exist as a result of spontaneous events or they should be created by treatment of the wild-type cells with mutagenic agents. Of course, a cell that is fully deficient in some function required for viability cannot be isolated. Because of its ubiquitous nature, cAMP might be considered essential to the cellular economy; therefore, mutants defective in the metabolism of, or response to, cAMP should not be viable. However, this is not the case. (2) A technique to isolate these mutants must be available. In our case, we kill the wild-type cells with activators of adenylate cyclase or with DB-cAMP. Briefly, the procedure is as follows: S49 cells are grown in a medium made semisolid by adding agarose. The cells are in proximity to a feeder layer of mouse embryo fibroblasts that are required to maintain proliferation of the S49 cells at low densities. Each individual lymphoma cell divides and forms a separate colony. After 8–10 days, the colonies can be counted and removed from agar to be grown in mass suspension culture in sufficient number for biochemical analysis. Wild-type cells form colonies with an efficiency that approaches 100% (i.e., if 100 cells are seeded in a petri dish, approximately 100 colonies form). If 100 wild-type cells are plated but DB-cAMP is added at a concentration of 1 mM, colony formation is completely suppressed. However, when 10^6 cells are plated per dish with the drug, the rare resistant cells survive. They form colonies, and they can be recovered for further characterization.

The frequency of these rare cells in a given culture depends on the history of that culture; it is typically a few to several score per 10^6 cells. By performing fluctuation analysis as described for bacteria (Luria and Delbrück, 1943), we showed that this mutation occurs at a rate of about 2×10^{-7}/cell per generation. The mutation is spontaneous, and is inherited by the progeny of the mutant cell (Coffino *et al.*, 1975a,b). The frequency of cells resistant to DB-cAMP is greatly enhanced by treating the wild-type cells with chemicals known to be mutagenic for bacteria. These chemicals include nitrosoguanidine, ethyl methyl sulfonate, and ICR 191, a frame-shift mutagen (Coffino *et al.*, 1975a,b; Creech *et al.*, 1972; Ames and Whitfield, 1966). We have found that maintenance of the mutant phenotype does not require continued exposure to the selective agent (i.e., DB-cAMP); resistant mutants have been cultured continuously in normal nutritional medium for more than 1 year without reversion of phenotype.

The findings that resistant cells arise at a frequency consistent with mutation in microbial systems, that they are spontaneous and clonally inherited, that their frequency is increased by known bacterial mutagens, and that the phenotype is stable are important in determining whether a variant phenotype is the result of a mutation, i.e., a structural alteration in DNA (Chu, 1974). In fact, whether such mutation can account for any phenotypic variation in animal cell cultures is a subject of controversy (Harris, 1971; Chasin, 1973). If structural alteration of a gene product could be demonstrated, this would constitute a rigorous criterion for mutation. Such demonstration has been achieved for some somatic cell markers (Beaudet *et al.*, 1973; Thompson *et al.*, 1973; Chasin, 1974). Some of the cAMP-resistant mutants fulfill this criterion (Coffino *et al.*, 1976). Many of the conclusions that we propose regarding the mode of action of cAMP depend on the specificity of the mutation. For example, we have reached certain conclusions regarding the role of cAMP-dependent protein kinase (PK) by examining a variety of biological functions in a mutant with altered PK activity (Coffino *et al.*, 1976). These conclusions can be valid only if the mutation in question affects PK specifically, rather than being a pleiotropic mutation affecting multiple cellular functions. Persuasive evidence of a structural mutation in the PK would assure the validity of our conclusions, and such evidence has been obtained demonstrating that cAMP-dependent PK mediates the functions of cAMP in S49 cells. The functions of PK include regulation of the induction of phosphodiesterase (PDE) activity, arrest of the cell at the G_1 phase of the growth cycle, and killing of the cells.

3.2. Potential Value of the Adenylate-Cyclase-Negative S49 Cell

One mechanism for applying selective pressure to isolate mutants resistant to the cell-killing effects of cAMP has been to incubate wild-type cells with DB-cAMP.

Another method that may have more interesting use, *vis-à-vis* definition of receptor function and composition, is to use isoproterenol (in combination with an inhibitor of cyclic nucleotide PDE) to isolate mutant clones. The majority of clones selected in this fashion exhibit a consistent phenotype, termed AC^- (Bourne *et al.*, 1975). While AC^- cells possess normal cAMP-dependent PK and are as responsive to DB-cAMP as wild-type (WT) cells, they fail to show induction of PDE or inhibition of growth in response to isoproterenol, cholera enterotoxin, and PGE_1. The β-adrenergic amine, the bacterial toxin, and the PG all stimulate cAMP accumulation in WT cells, but not in AC^- cells. Clones of identical phenotype can be isolated when cholera enterotoxin, rather than isoproterenol, is used as the selective agent (unpublished results).

The biochemical lesion of AC^- cells appears to reside in the particulate fraction, and probably in the plasma membrane. Unlike WT cells, particulate fractions of AC^- cells do not synthesize detectable amounts of cAMP from ATP in the presence of compounds that stimulate adenylate cyclase in WT cell particulates, such as isoproterenol, PGE_1, and fluoride ion (Bourne *et al.*, 1975).

Current models of hormone-sensitive adenylate cyclase (Perkins, 1973) are being used to seek the explanation of how cAMP synthesis in many cells can be controlled by more than one kind of receptor. It is not clear whether each receptor is associated with its own distinctive class of adenylate cyclase molecule in intact cells, or whether one type of cyclase molecule can be regulated by several kinds of receptors. These alternatives must ultimately be resolved by standard biochemical techniques, involving purification of adenylate cyclase(s), receptors, and other membrane components, followed by their functional recombination *in vitro*.

The AC^- phenotype is probably caused by a mutation affecting a single gene product. If this gene codes for the catalytic component of adenylate cyclase itself, the AC^- mutant supports the notion of a common type of adenylate cyclase molecule, controlled by more than one receptor. Preliminary studies, in collaboration with M. Maguire and A. G. Gilman, indicate similar β-adrenergic receptors in both the WT and the AC^- cells (as determined by binding of a radioactive β-adrenergic antagonist). Thus, the β-receptor appears to be a gene product distinct from the adenylate cyclase molecule.

If the β-adrenergic receptor of WT S49 cells is a gene product distinct from adenylate cyclase, another class of mutants might be expected to survive selection with isoproterenol. These mutants should be unresponsive to isoproterenol, presumably because of a deficient β-receptor, but normally responsive to other stimulators of adenylate cyclase. We are actively searching for such mutants, which could prove to be useful tools for investigating the functional relationship between hormone receptors and adenylate cyclase.

3.3. Receptors and Cell Regulation

A major difficulty in many investigations of receptors is to assign the functions of a receptor to discrete chemical structures within a cell. The genetic approach described here has defined the biochemical nature of the cAMP receptor of S49 cells. It is the cAMP-dependent PK. We can now begin to ask the next question: How does this model receptor transduce a chemical signal (cAMP concentration) into biological effects?

It is attractive to imagine that, for example, the PK regulates cell functions by virtue of its catalytic component, which could phosphorylate specific substrate proteins critical in growth control or enzyme induction. Our results do not rule out an alternative possibility, that the cAMP–R complex mediates the actions of cAMP directly, by analogy with *E. coli* (Pastan and Perlman, 1970). This question could be resolved by discovery of other mutant phenotypes such as clones resistant to the action of cAMP in which either the R or the C subunit of the kinase holoenzyme is absent or completely inactive.

A related problem is to determine biochemical branch points, distal to cAMP-dependent kinase, at which the multiple actions of cAMP diverge. For example, if the kinase does act by phosphorylating specific cell proteins, is the substrate protein critical for induction of PDE identical with the protein involved in regulation of growth? We are seeking new classes of mutant S49 cells that could help us to unravel such problems. A mutant clone recently isolated is resistant to DB-cAMP cytolysis, but has an intact cAMP receptor (including both R and C subunits of the holoenzyme). It could prove useful in defining physiologically important substrates of the cAMP-dependent kinase.

Similarly, one theory suggests that cell growth is regulated by modulation of cellular uptake of nutrient substances such as glucose (Holley, 1972). Uptake of radiolabeled glucose, amino acids, and uridine is inhibited by DB-cAMP in WT, but not in cAMP-resistant S49 cells (Daniel *et al.,* 1973b). This finding suggests that membrane transport of these substances, like growth arrest, is mediated by the cAMP-dependent PK. Inhibition of membrane transport, however, may not be necessary for the regulation of growth by cAMP. In fact, it appears that DB-cAMP-induced G_1 growth arrest in S49 cells is almost immediate in onset (Coffino *et al.,* 1975b) and precedes the inhibition of 2-deoxyglucose uptake, which may require 24 hr or more to develop (Jones and Tomkins, personal communication).

Finally, the mutant phenotypes described here bear on the interesting question of whether cAMP itself is essential for cell viability or for the internal timing of cell functions. Since cAMP is virtually ubiquitous in eukaryotes, and since cAMP content of synchronized cells rises and falls reproducibly during certain phases of the cell cycle (Burger *et al.,* 1972), it is possible that cAMP is an integral component of an internal clock that regulates repetitive cell functions. However, the cell cycle of cells that lack the cAMP receptor activity, i.e., cAMP-dependent PK, is similar to that of WT cells (Coffino *et al.,* 1975b). In addition, by sequential selection with isoproterenol and DB-cAMP, we have isolated a double mutant deficient in both adenylate cyclase and PK activities. This cell proliferates normally in culture, although it can neither synthesize nor respond to cAMP. Thus, it appears that no vital function of S49 cells requires cAMP. While cAMP may regulate the cell cycle clock, it is unlikely that cAMP is an essential part of the clock's mechanism. cAMP may be necessary for survival of a multicellular organism as in functions related to immune response, but is probably unnecessary for the survival of each individual cell.

3.4. Probing the Receptor

Finally, the tool available to us for probing receptor function on lymphocytes is the actual measurement of the receptors for vasoactive amines. Although the measurement is difficult, a number of laboratories, including our own, have now been able to label ligands that bind specifically to the β-adrenergic receptor, and displace active agonists appropriately. The markers include radiolabeled alprenolol, propranolol, and, more recently, iodinated hydroxypindolol (Maguire *et al.*, 1976; Lefkowitz, 1975). The use of these markers has established the plasma membrane as a major if not exclusive site of the receptor for β-mimetic amines. Measurements of the β-adrenergic receptors indicate 200–400 sites/cell, and selective loss of receptor sites occurs as a function of receptor occupancy by the agonist. Preliminary experiments using tritiated PGs have been done by at least one group, and have indicated specific pharmacologically active membrane receptor sites for the lipids (Bruton *et al.*, 1976). Approaches to the histamine receptors are much more tentative.

In summary, the tools that we have discussed so far can be used to probe the presence and biological importance of receptors for histamine, β-mimetic catecholamines, and selected PGs by determining the effects of the agonists in both *in vivo* and *in vitro* models of inflammation and immunity. The measurement of receptors on cells is also an important advance, because it may eventually allow distinguishing of one cell from another on the basis of its ability to respond to a single agonist.

The major drawback to all these approaches is that they demand study of a heterogeneous group of cells or a homogeneous group of highly abnormal lymphocytes in culture, i.e., the S49 mouse lymphoma cell. There is no way, by the techniques so far described, to distinguish specific cells within a complex mixture of leukocytes that are responsible for a given event. To define the exact sequence of cells that must be stimulated before a given event is completed requires an ability to separate cells on the basis of their receptors before the experiments begin. Exposure of given segments of cells to various stimuli (antigen or pharmacolical agents or both) becomes feasible. Then the true function of a given cell (based on its physiologic and not necessarily its physical characteristics) might be illustrated. One approach to being able to work with cells that have physiologic rather than physical homology is to separate them on the basis of their physiologic receptors. We have attempted to do this as described in the following section.

4. Separation of Cells on the Basis of a Physiologic Function

The models used to study the biological function of amines in the processes summarized in Table 1 involve a mixture of various cell types. To date, cells could not be separated on the basis of their complement of receptors to vasoactive amines; i.e., morphologically similar cells that may differ in biological function could not be separated on the basis of whether or not they responded to specific endogenous hormones.

The importance of separating cell types became apparent several years ago. Investigators took advantage of the fact that recognition of antigen by lymphocytes required only extremely small chemical determinants of synthetic antigens, almost comparable to the molecular weight of the vasoactive amines (Sela, 1969; Segal *et al.*, 1969). Wigzell and others found that lymphocytes specifically adhered to columns of insolubilized antigens (Wigzell and Andersson, 1969; Truffa-Bachi and Wofsy, 1970). Cells that passed through the columns were not responsive to the free antigens. In addition, Hertzenberg and his group found that fluoresceinated antigen could be specifically bound to lymphocytes with receptors for the nonfluoresceinated antigen (Hulett *et al.*, 1973; Julius *et al.*, 1975) and used the flow microfluorometer to separate lymphocytes on the basis of their affinity for the fluorescent markers.

We imagined that a similar approach could be used to separate cells on the basis of their receptors for amines. Conjugates of amines on monovalent or polyvalent carriers were linked to Sepharose beads, or they were fluoresceinated, thus constructing insoluble or soluble conjugates, respectively. We used both preparations to separate cells.

Two techniques for construction of conjugates were used. Histamine conjugation to a protein via carbodiimide (ECDI) establishes a peptide bond between the amine and the carboxyl group of the carrier protein or peptide. The conjugate can then be insolubilized by linking it to cyanogen-bromide-activated Sepharose beads (Melmon *et al.*, 1972). We were concerned that a linking process that resulted in a peptide bond between the amino function of the amine and the carboxyl group of the carrier could substantially modify the critical chemical structures for the pharmacological effects of the amine, as well as the binding of amine to receptor. We therefore considered an additional process for linking amines to carriers. When glutaraldehyde was used as a conjugating agent, an alkyl chain was placed between the amino group of the amine and the carboxyl group of the carrier (Figure 1). This procedure converted a primary amine to a secondary amine. Soluble conjugates were also used to attach a fluorescein label. We attempted to separate cells with the use of the flow microfluorometer.

The results of these approaches are described below; we feel that they have enabled us to separate cells on the basis of their receptors for the amines that were

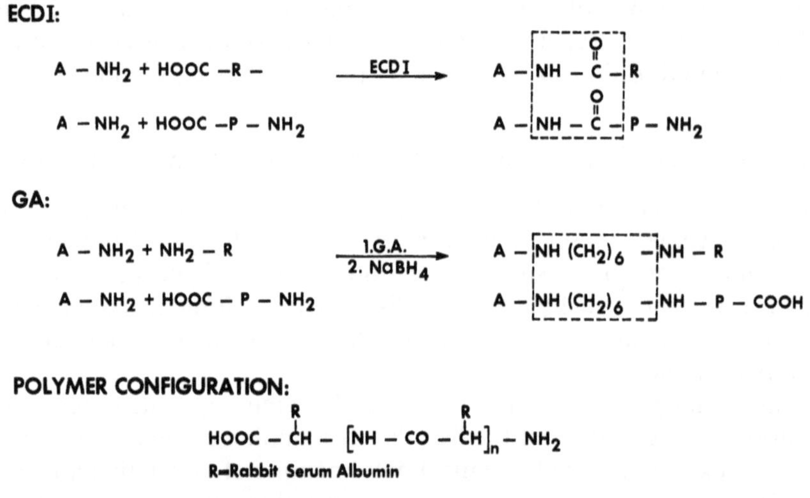

Figure 1. Schematic chemical reactions between an amine (A-NH_2) and polymer carrier (DL-alanine–L-tyrosine random copolymer) or molecule of rabbit serum albumin (R). (ECDI) 1-Ethyl-3,3-dimethyl aminopropyl carbodiimide; (G.A.) glutaraldehyde. Details of the method are described by Weinstein *et al.* (1973).

used to make conjugates. We also include examples of cell testing that illustrate the type of biological information that our approaches can generate.

4.1. Evidence That Cell Separation Is Related to Cell Receptors

In our first group of experiments, we used suspensions of human peripheral leukocytes and histamine conjugated to rabbit serum albumin (HRSA). The conjugates were insolubilized by linking them to Sepharose beads (HRS) (Melmon *et al.*, 1972; Weinstein *et al.*, 1973). Beads (termed RS) carrying only rabbit serum albumin (RSA) without histamine did not bind cells. Those that carried conjugates of histamine (HRS) bound leukocytes, but did not bind red blood cells or platelets (Melmon *et al.*, 1972; Weinstein *et al.*, 1973). Differential counts of residual unbound leukocytes showed no particular preferences of binding of the various types of leukocytes.

A series of experiments was designed to determine whether the selective binding of leukocytes was related to their histamine receptors. Pharmacological antagonists of histamine prevented leukocyte binding to histamine–rabbit serum albumin–Sepharose. Antihistamines did not interfere with the binding of cells to insolubilized conjugates of norepinephrine that were linked to RSA via glutaraldehyde [NE–R–S-(GA)] (Table 2). β-Adrenergic antagonists displaced cells from NE–R–S–(GA), but not from HRS. High concentrations of free amines produced partially specific inhibition of binding (Bourne *et al.*, 1971b).

We gained further information about the subpopulations of leukocytes that bind to various conjugates by studying the cAMP responses of the cells that passed through various columns (i.e., nonadherent cells) to corresponding free amines. Responsiveness to both amines and cholera toxin was tested (Melmon *et al.*, 1974b; Poon *et al.*, 1977).

Cells that passed through HRS columns responded less to histamine and epinephrine than did nonchromatographed cells (Figure 2). The column did not nonspecifically change the ability of the cells to respond to every stimulant; cholera toxin effectively stimulated the accumulation of cAMP in nonadherent cells from HRS columns as well as in nonchromatographed cells. After cells were chromatographed over NE–R–S–(GA), the nonadherent cells responded poorly to epinephrine and histamine, relative to those that were not chromatographed or to cells chromatographed on a control column of rabbit serum albumin–Sepharose (data not shown). The responses of cells that did not adhere to control columns of RS or normetanephrine–RSA–Sepharose or *o*-methyl histidine–R–S were no different from unchromatographed cells. Normetanephrine, like other congeners of catecholamines that are pharmacologically inactive and are not competitive inhibitors of the active catecholamines, did not retain cells better than the control column of RS. This also is true for *o*-methyl histidine.

In summary, it appears that leukocytes can be separated on the basis of their amine receptors. If insolubilized conjugates are made from pharmacologically inactive amines, nonadherent cells behave the same as control suspensions of cells. If insolubilized conjugates are made from pharmacologically active histamine (bound to carrier via ECDI or glutaraldehyde) or norepinephrine (bound to carrier via glutaraldehyde), the nonadherent cells respond less actively to histamine,

TABLE 2. Characteristics of Binding of Human Leukocytes by Drug–RSA–Sepharose[a]

Drug in preincubation[c]	Concentration (M)	Beads binding > 20 cells (%)[b] HRS[d]	NE–R–S-(GA)[d]
Control		87 ± 7	86 ± 6
Antihistamines			
Diphenhydramine	10^{-3}	28 ± 22[e]	52 ± 6
	10^{-4}	33 ± 7[e]	85 ± 7
Antazoline	10^{-3}	21 ± 13[f]	79 ± 5
	10^{-4}	57	—
Tripelennamine	10^{-3}	31 ± 7[f]	85 ± 10
	10^{-4}	38	—
Pyrilamine	10^{-3}	24 ± 4[f]	69 ± 7
	10^{-4}	44	87
Adrenergic blocking agents			
Propranolol	10^{-3}	84 ± 7	11 ± 8[e]
	10^{-4}	—	37 ± 6[e]
Phentolamine	10^{-3}	45	53 ± 38
	10^{-4}	95 ± 1	71 ± 10
Agonists			
Histamine	10^{-3}	64 ± 29[f]	86 ± 5
	10^{-5}	91 ± 2	—
Epinephrine	10^{-3}	84 ± 13	60 ± 27
D,L-Isoproterenol	10^{-3}	86 ± 16	56 ± 19[f]
D-Isoproterenol	10^{-3}	87	39 ± 6[e]
L-Isoproterenol	10^{-3}	81	23 ± 12[e]
Norepinephrine	10^{-3}	82 ± 21	84 ± 6
Phenylephrine	10^{-3}	87 ± 6	75 ± 12
Prostaglandin E_2	10^{-3}	85 ± 12	90 ± 7

[a]Data derived from Melmon *et al.* (1974c).
[b]Data are expressed as means or means + S.D. Standard deviation was calculated only when 7 or more points were obtained. Means without SD are from 3 points. Each point represents the mean of triplicates. Variance between duplicate samples is <6%. Statistical comparisons were determined only between controls and groups with more than 7 points.
[c]5×10^6 cells were preincubated for 10 min at 37°C with drug as indicated in 0.45 ml minimal essential media, pH 7.4. Then 0.05 ml 25% vol/vol mixture of drug–Sepharose was added, and the cells were then incubated for 10 min with gentle shaking.
[d]Abbreviations—HRS: Histamine–RSA conjugates produced by ECDI and insolubilized on Sepharose beads; NE–R–S-(GA): norepinephrine conjugated to RSA via glutaraldehyde and insolubilized Sepharose beads. The methods are described by Weinstein *et al.* (1973).
[e]$P < 0.001$ compared with control (paired test).
[f]$P < 0.01$ compared with control (paired test).

norepinephrine, epinephrine, and PGs than would unchromatographed cells or cells that had not adhered to a control column of RS. Columns of highly charged substances, such as Sepharose–polylysine, Sepharose–ethanolamine, or *o*-methyl histidine–R–S, do bind cells, but not in relation to their amine receptors. Columns that do attract cells with receptors do not damage the nonadherent cells, nor do they attract cells solely because of the presence of membrane adenylate cyclase, because the nonadherent cells respond as well as control cells to cholera toxin.

We do not know to what extent this phenomenon can be generalized. The utility of using conjugates of pharmacologically active amines to separate cells will have to be tested for each new tissue source of suspended cells. In two preparations, cells that responded to histamine were not attracted by insolubilized histamine (Plaut *et al.*, 1975; Melmon *et al.*, 1974a,b). These experiments are discussed below.

We do not know the mechanism by which cells adhere to the conjugates. Although binding of cells seems to correlate with their complement of receptors for the amines used to construct the conjugate, we do not know the actual extent of binding created by the interaction of the amine moiety with its cell receptor site. Some binding may be dependent on the microenvironment of the cell receptor and its relationship to the secondary and tertiary configurations of the carrier–amine conjugate. Characteristics of the conjugates that are distinct from the active amine *per se* may also be critical to cell binding.

After we determined the specificity of cell separation, we were surprised to find that the insolubilized conjugates of amines had no detectable pharmacological effects. cAMP did not accumulate in cells that adhered to hormone–Sepharose beads (Melmon *et al.*, 1974b; Shearer *et al.*, 1974a). We initially thought that this meant that binding was unrelated to receptors. We knew that the amines are active only in molar concentrations 1000-fold higher than the peptide hormones (e.g.,

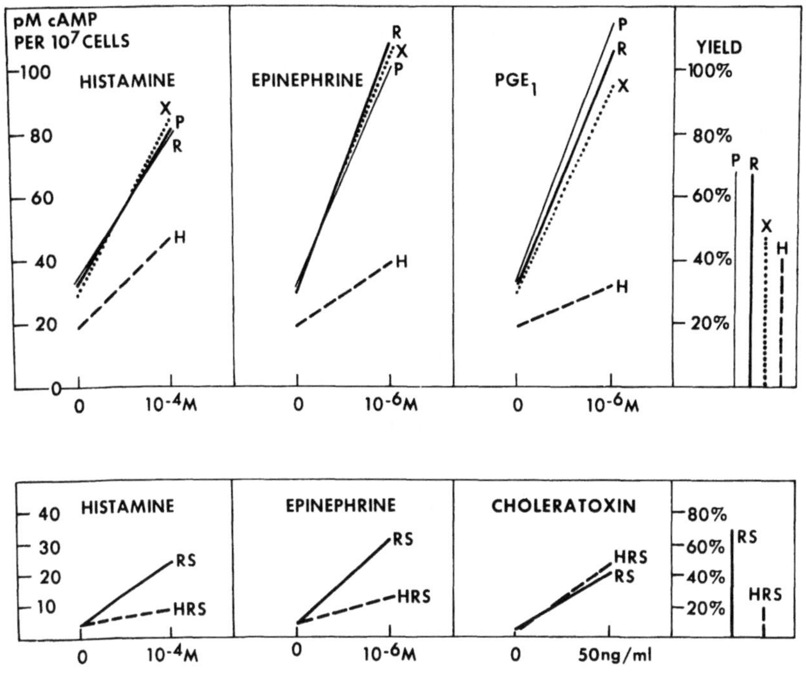

Figure 2. Illustrations of two separate experiments (top and bottom panels), showing baseline (0) and drug-stimulated increases in cellular cAMP. Cells stimulated were those that did not adhere to RS (R in top panel, RS in bottom panel), the *o*-methyl ester of histidine (X), or HRS (H in top panel, HRS in bottom panel). P designates cells that were not chromatographed. Note that the cells nonadherent to HRS responded significantly less to all agonists except choleratoxin. The column of *o*-methyl ester of histidine retained as many cells as HRS, but did not concentrate cells that were responsive to vasoactive amines, PGE_1, or choleratoxin. The *o*-methyl ester of histadine is pharmacologically inactive.

insulin), and that only small portions of the cell membranes were attached to the bead. We therefore tested the effects of soluble conjugates to determine whether the lack of pharmacological effect of insolubilized conjugates was due to: (1) inadequate contact of conjugated hormone with a sufficient number of cell receptors to effect changes in cAMP, or (2) no contact at all between the conjugates and cell receptors.

Selected soluble conjugates of histamine–RSA and NE–polymer–(GA) did produce pharmacological effects (Weinstein *et al.*, 1975b) (Figure 3), which were blocked by appropriate amine antagonists (Table 3). The pharmacological effects of the conjugates were not produced by amines released from the conjugate.

Studies of the pharmacology of other conjugates have indicated that the conjugating process clearly creates a new class of drugs (Weinstein *et al.*, 1975b). Thus, the conjugated amines, at least in the soluble form, can interact with leukocyte receptor sites. These results, combined with the fact that columns of insolubilized conjugates specifically remove cells with hormone receptors, provide evidence that the chromatographic procedures separate at least some types of cells on the basis of receptors.

Such separation may help to establish physiologic roles for the respective amines.

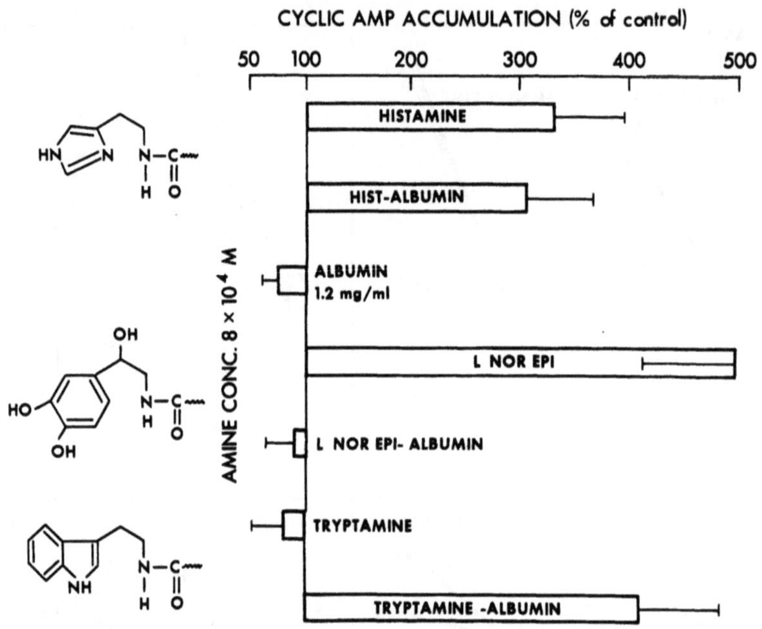

Figure 3. Effects of free histamine, norepinephrine, tryptamine, and rabbit serum albumin (RSA) on intracellular cAMP concentrations compared with conjugates of hormone with RSA. These conjugates are made with ECDI. The pharmacological effects of conjugated histamine were appropriately blocked by antihistamines; norepinephrine had no pharmacological effects when conjugated via ECDI, but appeared to have the effects of epinephrine when conjugated to RSA or a copolymer via glutaraldehyde. Such conjugates of L- and *o*-norepinephrine maintained their stereospecificity (data not shown). When tryptamine was conjugated to RSA via ECDI, an entirely "new drug" appeared. The effects of conjugated tryptamine were not antagonized by adrenergic blocking agents, antihistamines, or peripheral antagonists of indoleamines (data not shown).

TABLE 3. **Effects of Blocking Agents on Conjugated Amines (Histamine–RSA 50:1)**

Chemical	Concentration (M)	% Control ± S.D. Cellular	cAMP
Histamine (H)	10^{-4}		246 ± 62
Diphenhydramine (D)	4×10^{-4}	97 ± 6	
H (10^{-4}) + D	4×10^{-4}		97 ± 7
H (10^{-4}) + D	10^{-4}		132 ± 60
H (10^{-4}) + D	10^{-5}		274 ± 61
Burimimide (B)	4×10^{-4}	97 ± 5	
H (8×10^{-4}) + B	4×10^{-4}		83 ± 21
H (8×10^{-4}) + B	10^{-4}		109 ± 17
H (8×10^{-4}) + B	10^{-5}		98 ± 21
Propranolol (P)	4×10^{-4}	96 ± 10	
H (8×10^{-4}) + P	4×10^{-4}		224 ± 44
Histamine–RSA(HRSA)	8×10^{-4}		209 ± 61
HRSA + D	10^{-3}		101 ± 28
HRSA + D	4×10^{-4}		127 ± 50
HRSA + D	10^{-5}		174 ± 19
HRSA + B	4×10^{-4}		107 ± 25
HRSA + B	10^{-4}		110 ± 29
HRSA + B	10^{-5}		183 ± 13
HRSA + P	4×10^{-4}		217 ± 24

4.2. A Discussion of Apparently Conflicting Data Related to the Specificity of Cell Adherence to Insolubilized Conjugates of Amines

Two groups recently examined the effects of both insolubilized conjugates of amines and their carriers and separation of cells by insolubilized conjugates (Plaut *et al.*, 1975; Matthyssens *et al.*, 1975). We would like to put their results into the perspective of this chapter. Matthyssens *et al.*, (1975), working with soluble conjugates of histamine, ethylamine, valine, and others to RSA or a polymer {poly (Tyr,Glu)–poly DL-Ala–poly Lys [(T,G)–A–L]}, came to the conclusion that binding of the conjugates to murine splenic lymphocytes was not unique for the histamine conjugates. They believe that the binding was not as dependent on the ligand as on the general properties of the cell membrane, such as its lipophilic character or charge distribution that may have attracted portions of the carrier modified by the conjugation process. The primary basis of their conclusions was that conjugates of histamine with either carrier were not displaced from cells by high concentrations of histamine, and did not displace tritiated histamine from cells. They also indicated that although carriers themselves did not displace conjugates of histamine, conjugates of histamine, ethylamine, or valine with either carrier could partially displace HRSA from cells. Our published results characterized insolubilized conjugates only. Our results also indicated that cells could be bound by a variety of insolubilized conjugates of amines with RSA or bovine serum albumin, but that displacement of cells from the Sepharose beads coated with HRSA or prevention of cell binding could be accomplished by incubation of the beads plus cells with antagonists of histamine. Antagonists of amines other than histamine were not able to displace cells.

The antagonists of histamine were effective only on the insolubilized conjugates of histamine, not on other conjugates of alternative agonists that were able to bind cells. We share the conclusions that a variety of substances may bind cells, that the conjugates of a spectrum of amines with carriers can all appear quantitatively similar, and that the carrier may contribute to the binding process. If all conjugates were binding cells by analogous mechanisms, however, the antagonist of specific amines would not have worked selectively for their respective amine–carrier conjugate. High concentrations of free histamine did not readily displace cells from insolubilized multivalent HRSA in our experiments, nor did they displace solubilized HRSA at all in the experiments done by Matthyssens *et al.* (1975) that used soluble conjugates. These data do not argue for or against the specificity of the binding of the conjugates by the ligand. As was stated above, Wigzell and Andersson (1969) separated lymphocytes on the basis of their adherence to insolubilized antigen. In studies to which our studies are analogous, the authors found that high concentrations of free antigen did not displace cells bound to the column. Their results could have been consistent with nonspecific cell adherence, but they carried the experiments beyond this point. They eventually concluded that the polyvalency of the antigen-coated beads increased the chances of cell adherence to insolubilized vs. soluble antigen. The binding was specific, since only the cells able to respond to the free antigen were adherent to the insolubilized antigen; other cells without such receptors passed through the columns unaffected. The polyvalency of conjugates of histamine may make it difficult for the free ligand to displace cells from the insoluble conjugates, and it is even more unlikely that the ligand or its antagonists could displace cells from soluble conjugates that may have an even better chance of allowing coaptation of the histamine moiety with its binding sites on cell membranes. Thus, the lack of inhibition of amine-conjugate binding by free ligand does not speak for or against the specificity of conjugated ligand binding to cells. That polymer–histamine vs. RSA–histamine conjugates were mutually inhibitory to the other's binding property does support specificity.

Matthyssens *et al.* (1975) interpreted the lack of displacement of tritiated histamine by conjugates of histamine as evidence for nonspecific binding of the conjugates. Unfortunately, their experiments did not record the percentage of viable cells or the distribution of histamine on the cell or within it. The authors did not correlate the binding of histamine with their pharmacological effects, determine what portion of free ligand binding was specific, or try to displace the tritiated histamine with antagonists of histamine. These procedures have now become standard in trying to ascertain the specificity of binding of other amine ligands (Melmon *et al.*, 1975). Considerable nonspecific binding and intracellular transport of amines such as β-catecholamines by living and dead cells have been detected, even though there is unequivocal evidence that amine receptors are definitely located on the cell membrane (Sutherland and Robison, 1966). Interpretation of the lack of displacement of tritiated histamine by the histamine conjugates might have been anticipated in the studies cited. In fact, the results of Matthyssens *et al.* (1975) again cannot be used to conclude that amine receptors do not exist on the membrane, or that conjugate binding does not take place in part via the amine receptor.

The two types of data obtained in our laboratories that most strongly indicate that the conjugates can bind to native amine receptors are summarized as follows:

(1) The pharmacological effect of soluble conjugates of HRSA is to stimulate the adenylate cyclase of human and murine spleen leukocytes (Melmon *et al.*, 1975). The stimulation is almost equal to the stimulation that would be produced by the free ligand, although less than 0.5% of the ligand is released from the conjugate. (2) Furthermore, and most convincing of the type of specificity by which the conjugates are bound, is the fact that antagonists of histamine, but not of other amines (e.g., β-adrenergic blockers), inhibit the pharmacological effects of the conjugates of histamine. Conjugates of carriers that may bind to cells, such as ethylamine, have no detectable pharmacological effects on the same cells. Thus, there seems to be a dependency on multiple factors on or within the cell membrane that are responsible for binding of any given conjugate. In the case of the histamine conjugate, one of the determinants appears to be the histamine receptor.

There are a few interesting additional points to be made about the results using insolubilized conjugates of histamine to separate cells. In the article by Matthyssens *et al.* (1975), the transfer to irradiated syngeneic recipients of cells that were nonadherent to histamine–RSA or ethylamine–RSA resulted in minor, equivalent enhancement of production of plaque-forming cells in the recipients challenged with SRBC. The magnitude of response in these results was considered insignificant in the experiments of Shearer *et al.* (1974a,b). The latter group showed a 6- to 20-fold enhancement of the responses from cells nonadherent to insolubilized HRSA, but no significant alterations in response to SRBC by leukocytes excluded from insolubilized ethylamine–RSA or poly Lys–RSA (see below). These latter experiments illustrate that the selectivity of different insolubilized conjugates is quite different in relation to the functional qualities of the cells that are adherent to each. Furthermore, when the response (accumulation of intracellular cAMP) of human leukocytes to free histamine was compared in equal numbers of cells either unchromatographed or chromatographed and excluded from insolubilized RSA or excluded from insolubilized HRSA, only the cells nonadherent to HRSA had lower or almost absent response to histamine (see above; Melmon *et al.*, 1975). All cell preparations responded equally to cholera toxin, indicating that cells were not damaged in their passage through the columns, and that the basis of separation was not some nonspecific quality of the cell membrane related to its adenylate cyclase content. Thus, cell chromatography that uses insolubilized conjugates of histamine can separate cells in part on the basis of their receptor complement.

That cell chromatography via insolubilized conjugates of HRSA can separate cells on the basis of their complement of receptors to histamine does not imply that all cells with such receptors will be separated by this procedure. We have shown that the spleen cells with histamine receptors taken from the F_1 and one parent can be readily separated from other cells, but those from the other parent could not (Melmon *et al.*, 1974a). Yet mixed spleen cells from all three strains had their adenylate cyclase stimulated by free histamine. There must be other determinants on the cell membrane besides the receptor itself that are critical to eventual binding of cells to the insolubilized hormones. We do not yet know what these determinants are. The inconsistency of binding of cells with histamine receptors by insolubilized conjugates of HRSA may account for the inability of Plaut *et al.* (1975) to remove effector cells that responded to histamine and participated in immune cytolysis by such chromatographic procedures. These authors did not determine whether such insolubilized conjugates could attract the precursor cells that might modulate the production of effector cells.

4.3. Immunologic Implications of Cell Binding to Amine Conjugates

It has been suggested that suppressor cells may actively inhibit immune responses *in vivo* (Diener and Feldman, 1970; Gershon, 1974). Our laboratories showed that a type of suppressor T cell can be selectively bound to HRS (Shearer *et al.*, 1974b). Histamine and other drugs that stimulate cAMP accumulation or mimic its effects (e.g., DB-cAMP) may alter suppressor cell activity, as suggested by experiments in which cell populations that do not adhere to HRS behave functionally like unchromatographed cell populations in which cAMP is elevated.

Suppressor cells have been removed from suspensions of murine spleen cells by trapping the suppressor cells on HRS. Nonadherent cells transferred to lethally radiated syngeneic recipients, susbsequently challenged with SRBC, produce an augmented humoral antibody response (Figure 4). Similar results were obtained in experiments that used *in vitro* models of antibody response (Figure 5).

The same results can be achieved without cell chromatography. If drugs that elevate cAMP are introduced *in vivo* at the same time as antigen challenge, the humoral antibody response to such a challenge is enhanced over control conditions (Figure 6). Thus, in both types of experiments (the first type uses cell chromatography to remove suppressor cell physically; the second type pharmacologically alters the function of unchromatographed cells), the net results are qualitatively the same. These types of experiments have led us to postulate that vasoactive amines might substantially modulate the early phases of a humoral antibody response to antigen.

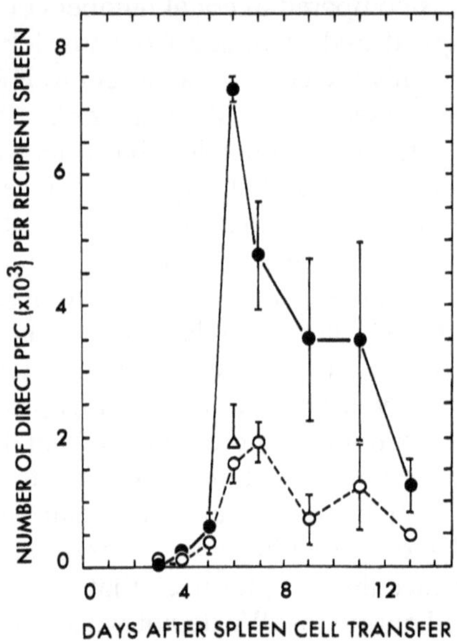

Figure 4. Mean number of direct PFC per recipient spleen in irradiated mice injected with 5×10^6 unfiltered spleen cells (○) or 5×10^6 spleen cells that did not adhere to R–S (△) or to HRS (●), and immunized with 3×10^8 SRBC, as a function of time after cell transfer. The vertical brackets denote S.D. Probability values: days 6 and 7, < 0.001; day 9, < 0.05. Reprinted with permission from Shearer *et al.* (1974b).

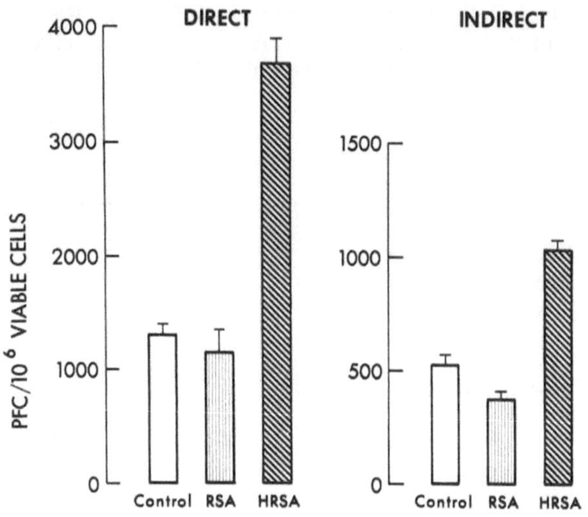

Figure 5. A primary culture (Mishell–Dutton) *in vitro* of BALB/c spleen cells and SRBC. Control cells are unchromatographed, RSA are cells nonadherent to R–S. HRSA are cells nonadherent to HRS. Augmentation of both direct and indirect plaque-forming cells parallels the *in vivo* results demonstrated in Figure 4. Unpublished work of B. Brodeur, Y. Weinstein, K. L. Melmon, and T. Merigan, with the permission of the authors.

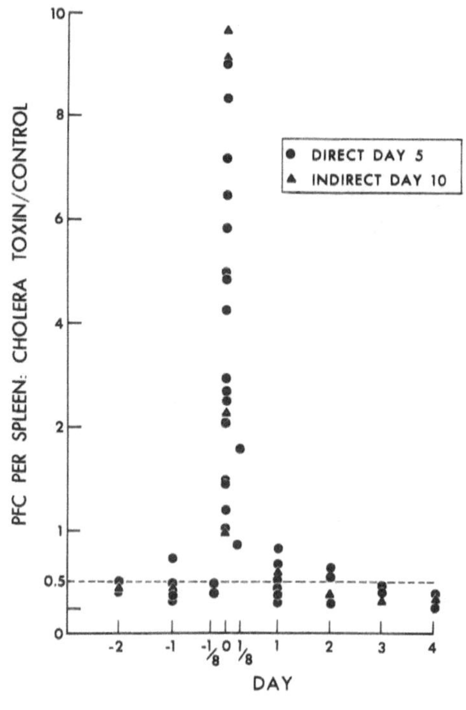

Figure 6. Effects of choleratoxin on IgM (●) and IgG (▲) plaque-forming cells. C57BL/6 and BALB/c mice were injected intraperitoneally with SRBC on day O, and with 2 μg cholera toxin on the day indicated. Spleens were removed on the 5th day after the injection of SRBC to determine IgM levels, or on the 12th day to determine IgG levels. Plaque formation was assayed by a modification (Shearer *et al.*, 1968) of the Jerne technique (Jerne *et al.*, 1963).

TABLE 4. Effect of Cell Chromatography with Control RS or HRS Columns and Elimination of θ-Sensitive Cells on Suppressor Capacity of Spleen Cells from Mice Tolerant to SRBC[a]

Group	Manipulation of spleen cells from tolerant mice before transfer to radiated recipient	Hemagglutinin titer at day 7[b]	
		−2ME (IgM)	+2ME (IgG)
1	Nonchromatographed	2^6	2^2
2	Depleted of cells adherent to RS	2^6	2^4
3	Depleted of cells adherent to HRS	2^9	2^7
4	Depleted of cells adherent to HRS plus 2.5 × 10^6 cells eluted from HRS	2^9	2^0
5	Group 4, but eluted cells treated with normal mouse serum plus complement	2^8	2^3
6	Group 4, but eluted cells treated with anti-θ serum plus complement	2^8	s^7

[a]Reprinted, with permission, from Melmon *et al.* (1975).
[b]Sera pooled from 5 mice in each group; 10^7 splenic cells were transferred unless otherwise indicated. Data from S. Segal, Y. Weinstein, H. McDevitt, and K. L. Melmon.

4.4. 'Histamine Receptors' and Immunotolerance or Immunosuppression

Immunotolerance might provide a useful model for studying cells that suppress immune reactions to antigens. If tolerance results from active suppression of cells, rather than elimination of clones (Dresser and Mitchison, 1968), then immune responses should be restored when suppressor cells are removed. Mice become tolerant to SRBC when they are repeatedly injected with lysates of SRBC (Anderson *et al.*, 1972). Transfer of spleen cells from tolerant mice to lethally irradiated syngeneic recipients suppresses the IgG response (i.e., tolerance can be transferred) (Table 4). When the spleen cells from tolerant mice were chromatographed over an HRS column and the nonadherent cells were transferred, the IgG response was restored. Part of the cells that were bound to the HRS column were recovered by mechanical shaking. When these cells were added to the HRS nonadherent cells (in a ratio of 1:5), the IgG response was suppressed (Table 4). The suppressor activity of the cells that adhered to HRS was abolished after they had been treated with a specific anti-θ serum plus complement to remove T cells.

In a different experimental setting, we demonstrated that cAMP can abolish the immune suppression that is caused by normal spleen cells that have been transferred to lethally irradiated syngeneic recipients. In these experiments, a synthetic antigen, poly(L-Tyr,L-Glu)–poly-L-Pro–poly-L-Lys [(T,G)–Pro–L], was incubated for 15–30 min with spleen cells from a normal donor. The cells were then washed and transferred to a syngeneic recipient, and 24 hr later, the recipient was challenged with additional (T,G)–Pro–L. Control recipients received donor cells that had been incubated without antigen or incubated with antigen but without drugs. At 14 days after the antigen challenge, the serum antibody titers were assayed by passive

TABLE 5. Effect of Dibutyryl Cyclic AMP and Cholera Enterotoxin on Antigen-Induced Immune Suppression[a,b]

Drug	Titers (% of positive responding sera)[c]	cAMP accumulation (% of control)[d]
Control (no drug)	64 ± 7[e] (52)[f]	100
(T,G)–Pro–L	32 ± 7 (41)	104
Dibutyryl cAMP (10^{-4} M)	60 ± 15 (10)	NT[g]
Dibutyryl cAMP (10^{-4} M) + (T,G)–Pro–L	59 ± 14 (12)	NT
Cholera enterotoxin	60 ± 13 (15)	298
Cholera enterotoxin + (T,G)–Pro–L	60 ± 13 (15)	NT
Antitoxin (1:1000)	70 ± 14 (10)	125
Antitoxin (1:1000) + (T,G)–Pro–L	30 ± 13 (12)	118
Cholera enterotoxin + antitoxin (1:1000)	60 ± 12 (15)	85
Cholera enterotoxin + antitoxin (1:1000) + (T,G)–Pro–L	40 ± 14 (12)	NT

[a]Reprinted, with permission, from Mozes *et al.* (1974).
[b]Spleen cells were injected into irradiated (750 rad) syngeneic recipients immediately after *in vitro* incubation of cell suspensions. Recipients were immunized intraperitoneally with 10 μ (T,G)–Pro–L 24 hr after cell transfer and bled 2 weeks later.
[c]Donor-derived responses showing anti-(T,G)–Pro–L hemagglutination titers at recipient sera dilutions greater than 1:4.
[d]Percentage of control (14 pmol cAMP/10^7 cells). On different days, basal cAMP varied from 10 to 25 pmol/10^7 cells.
[e]Data are expressed as means ± standard error of percent.
[f]The numbers in parentheses are the numbers of recipients tested.
[g]NT: Not tested.

TABLE 6. Effect of Histamine and Prostaglandin on Antigen-Induced Immune Suppression[a,b]

Drug	Titers (% of positive responding sera)[c]	cAMP accumulation (% of control)[d]
Control (no drug)	64 ± 7[e] (52)[f]	100
(T,G)–Pro–L	32 ± 7 (41)	104
Histamine (10^{-4} M)	58 ± 14 (12)	190
Histamine (10^{-4} M) + (T,G)–Pro–L	67 ± 16 (9)	NT[g]
Diphenhydramine (10^{-4} M)	50 ± 16 (10)	NT
Diphenhydramine (10^{-4} M) + (T,G)–Pro–L	33 ± 19 (6)	NT
Histamine (10^{-4} M) + diphenhydramine (10^{-4} M)	67 (3)	157
Histamine (10^{-4} M) + diphenhydramine (10^{-4} M) + (T,G)–Pro–L	47 ± 11 (19)	147
Histamine (10^{-4} M) + diphenhydramine (10^{-3} M) + (T,G)–Pro–L	27 ± 13 (11)	98
Prostaglandin E_1 (10^{-4} M)	63 (11)	400
Prostaglandin E_1 (10^{-4} M) + (T,G)–Pro–L	69 (13)	403
Prostaglandin $F_2\alpha$ (10^{-4} M)	60 (10)	267
Prostaglandin $F_2\alpha$ (10^{-4} M) + (T,G)–Pro–L	57 (14)	253

[a]Reprinted, with permission, from Mozes *et al.* (1974).
[b–g]See footnotes to Table 5.

hemagglutination (Mozes *et al.*, 1973, 1974). Those who received cells preincubated with antigen had significantly lower titers of antibody than did the control group (Tables 5 and 6). This antigen-induced immunosuppression was reversed when drugs such as DB-cAMP (Table 5), or agents such as histamine, β-adrenergic catecholamines, cholera toxin, and selected PGs, were incubated with cells plus antigen (Tables 5 and 6). These experiments are similar to the experiments that used chromatography. The suppressor cells that produce IgG tolerance were physically removed by binding to HRS; immunosuppression, probably IgG, was reversed when mixed cell populations were stimulated by histamine or other agents that increased cAMP. Although we do not know the specific cell types that are responsible for the two phenomena, they may be identical and should be identified.

4.5. Use of Fluorescent Hormone Conjugates to Separate Cells

To estimate the number of cells that might be involved in these kinds of immune suppression, and to minimize the effects of nonspecific cell trapping, which is produced by Sepharose columns, we used a cell sorter developed by Hertzenberg's group that separates cells on the basis of the amount of fluorescent label that they carry (Hulett *et al.*, 1973; Julius *et al.*, 1975). We synthesized fluoresceinated histamine RSA (FHR). To do this, we first linked fluorescein to RSA by standard techniques. We then linked histamine to the fluorescein–RSA via ECDI to form FHR. With this technique, only 3–5 mol histamine was coupled to 1 mol F-RSA (the conjugates linked to Sepharose had 50 mol histamine to 1 mol RSA). Low substitution of hormone on carrier eliminated clumping caused by high-substituted RSA. After the cells were incubated with FHR, they were sorted, according to their fluorescence, in the cell sorter. The cells with the most intense fluorescence (which represented 20% of the total cell population) were removed from the heterogeneous mixture. The control cells and cells with lower fluorescence were injected, with SRBC, into irradiated syngeneic mice in the same way that the previous adoptive transfer experiments were performed. At 7 days later, we assayed for the number of splenic plaque-forming cells (PFC) (Table 7). The cells that were left after the 20%

TABLE 7. Direct PFC to SRBC in Irradiated Mice Injected with 6×10^6 Spleen Cells and 3×10^8 SRBC[a]

	Plaque/spleen			
Cells[b]	Expt. 1		Expt. 2	
Control cells	1355		420	
	725		1030	
		M 1315		M 760
	2300		1010	
	800		380	
			960	
Cells + FR	1090		1000	
	2250		1860	
		M 1480		M 1214
	1780		1570	
	820		910	
			730	
Cells + FRH less 20% brightest	3970		2970	
	9490		3270	
		M 5513		M 2507
	3080		2660	
			1190	

[a]Reprinted, with permission, from Melmon *et al.* (1975).
[b]FR: Fluoresceinated rabbit serum albumin; FRH: fluoresceinated rabbit serum albumin–histamine conjugate. Cells were incubated 15 min with fluoresceinated derivation before sorting began. M: Mean of 2 experiments, each with duplicates. See the text for details. Data from L. Hertzenberg, S. Segal, Y. Weinstein, and K. L. Melmon.

highly fluorescent cells had been removed produced a 3-fold enhancement of PFC. In essence, the cell sorter had accomplished what the HRS columns had accomplished, but far fewer cells were subtracted from the population (HRS columns removed about 80% human and 75% murine cells).

We do not yet know whether intensely fluoresceinated cells will respond to histamine or the other drugs that we are interested in, whether they represent precisely the same population that is responsible for the immunologic enhancement produced by HRS, or whether the cells that are not highly fluoresceinated bind to HRS. We do know that the fluoresceinated RSA did not bind to suppressor cells. Removal of cells that bound fluoresceinated RSA did not alter the transfer experiments produced by the unsorted control cells.

Finally, a novel approach that demonstrates that lymphocytes have HRSA binding sites has recently been described. The use of a rosette technique in which SRBC are coated with HRSA showed nonrandom binding to selected lymphocytes (Kedar and Bonavida, 1974). The formation of rosettes was inhibited by antihistamine, but no information is currently available on the function of these cells or on their ability to respond to pharmacological agents such as histamine.

4.6. Use of HRS Column Cell Separation in Other Immunologic Systems

4.6.1. Antibody-Producing Cells

A substantial portion of antibody-producing cells (PFC) was substracted from spleen cells of mice that had been immunized with SRBC by chromatography over HRS columns, or columns of NE–R–S-(GA) and PGE_1–R–S (Melmon *et al.*, 1974b). In similar observations, the corresponding drugs (histamine, PGE, norepinephrine) inhibited the release (or synthesis) of antibodies from unchromatographed spleen cells (Melmon *et al.*, 1974a). Although the drugs inhibited plaque formation in every mouse strain tested, the HRS column subtracted PFC only from BALB/c and BALB/BL, and not from the C57BL strain (Melmon *et al.*, 1974b). These data indicate (as we discussed above) that some cells that do respond to histamine may not be attracted to the HRSA columns sufficiently to separate them from cells that do not respond to the amine.

4.6.2. Precursors to Cytotoxic Cells

HRS columns appear to separate precursors of cytotoxic cells in *in vitro* allogeneic systems (Simpson *et al.*, 1973); the precursor cells can be recovered from the column. In similar experiments, drugs that elevated cAMP inhibited the generation of those cytotoxic cells.

5. Conclusions

In several immunologic model systems, the removal of cells that bind to HRS produces effects parallel to those seen when nonchromatographed cells are treated with histamine and other drugs that elevate cAMP. Although we have not demonstrated the precise mechanisms by which cells are bound to insolubilized conjugated hormones, we have shown that binding relies in some way on the receptor complement of the adherent cells. Even if HRS does not bind directly to the native receptor, the membrane environment of the receptor may be a determinant of cell binding to conjugated insolubilized hormone. The binding of soluble conjugates clearly makes some of the hormone available to native receptor sites. If it had not, the characteristic pharmacological effects of the amine moiety would not have been seen.

The mechanism by which cells bind to insolubilized and soluble conjugates of hormone warrants further study. In the meantime, the techniques that use insolubilized conjugates and fluoresceinated conjugates are clearly able to separate some types of cells on the basis of their hormone receptors. This fact seemed most convincingly demonstrated in a series of experiments in which physical separation of cells could yield biological data similar to pharmacological stimulation by the same free amines used in the conjugation and insolubilization processes.

Perhaps these experiments can be used to characterize cells with and without receptors, to determine biological stimuli that result in alteration of the receptor complements of cells, and possibly to determine the physiologic and pathologic function of amines or other substances in various organs the cells of which may be dispersed without damage to their membranes.

ACKNOWLEDGMENTS

This work was supported by N.I.H. grants HL-06285, GM-16496, GM-01791, and GM-00001.

References

Ames, B. N., and Whitfield, H. J., Jr., 1966, *Symp. Quant. Biol.* **31**:221–225.
Anderson, T.-H., Roethle, J., and Auerbach, R., 1972, *J. Exp. Med.* **136**:1666–1671.
Beaudet, A. C., Roufa, D. J., and Caskey, C. T., 1973, *Proc. Natl. Acad. Sci. U.S.A.* **70**:320–324.
Bourne, H. R., and Melmon, K. L., 1971, *J. Pharmacol. Exp. Ther.* **178**:1–7.
Bourne, H. R., Melmon, K. L., and Lichtenstein, L. M., 1971a, *Science* **173**:743–745.
Bourne, H. R., Lehrer, R. I., Cline, M. J., and Melmon, K. L., 1971b, *J. Clin. Invest.* **50**:920–929.
Bourne, H. R., and Lichtenstein, L. M., and Melmon, K. L., 1972, *J. Immunol.* **108**:695–705.
Bourne, H. R., Lichtenstein, L. M., Melmon, K. L., Henney, C. S., Weinstein, Y., and Shearer, G. M., 1974, *Science* **184**:19–28.
Bourne, H. R., Coffino, P., and Tomkins, G. M., 1975, *Science* **187**:750–752.
Bruton, L., Wiklund, R. A., Van Arsdale, P. M., and Gilman, A. G., 1976, *J. Biol. Chem.* **251**:3037–3044.
Burger, M. M., Bombik, B. M., Breckenridge, B. M., and Sheppard, J. R., 1972, *Nature (London) New Biol.* **239**:161–163.
Cairns, J., Stent, G. S., and Watson, J. D. (eds.), 1966, *Phage and the Origin of Molecular Biology,* Cold Spring Harbor Laboratory of Quantitative Biology, Cold Spring Harbor, New York.
Chasin, L. A., 1973, *J. Cell. Physiol.* **82**:299–308.
Chasin, L. A., 1974, *Cell* **2**:37–41.
Chu, E. H. Y., 1974, *Genetics* **78**:115–132.
Coffino, P., Bourne, H. R., and Tomkins, G. M., 1975a, *J. Cell. Physiol.* **85**:603–610.
Coffino, P., Gray, J. W., and Tomkins, G. M., 1975b, *Proc. Natl. Acad. Sci. U.S.A.* **72**:878–882.
Coffino, P., Bourne, H. R., Friedrich, U., Hochman, Y., Insel, P., LeMaire, I., Melmon, K. L., and Tomkins, G. M., 1976, *Recent Prog. Horm. Res.* Vol. 32, pp. 669–684, Academic Press, New York.
Creech, H. J., Preston, R. K., Peck, R. M., and O'Connell, A. P., 1972, *J. Med. Chem.* **15**:739–746.
Daniel, V., Litwack, G., and Tomkins, G. M., 1973a, *Proc. Natl. Acad. Sci. U.S.A.* **70**:76–79.
Daniel, V., Bourne, H. R., and Tomkins, G. M., 1973b, *Nature (London) New Biol.* **244**:167–169.

DeLucia, P., and Cairns, J., 1969, *Nature (London)* **224**:1164–1166.

Diener, E., and Feldman, M., 1970, *J. Exp. Med.* **132**:31–43.

Dresser, D. W., and Mitchison, N. A., 1968, *Adv. Immunol.* **8**:129–181.

Fisher, D. B., and Mueller, G. C., 1968, *Proc. Natl. Acad. Sci. U.S.A.* **60**:1396–1402.

Gershon, R. K., 1974, *Contemp. Top. Immunobiol.* **3**:1–40.

Hadden, J. W., Hadden, E. M., Haddox, M. K., and Goldberg, N. D., 1972, *Proc. Natl. Acad. Sci. U.S.A.* **69**:3024–3027.

Harris, M., 1971, *J. Cell. Physiol.* **78**:177–184.

Holley, R. W., 1972, *Proc. Natl. Acad. Sci. U.S.A.* **69**:2840–2845.

Horibata, K., and Harris, A. W., 1970, *Exp. Cell Res.* **60**:61–70.

Hulett, H. R., Bonner, W. A., Sweet, R. G., and Herzenberg, L. A., 1973, *Clin. Chem.* **19**:813–816.

Jerne, N. K., Nordin, A. A., and Henry, C., 1963, in: *Cell-Bound Antibodies* (B. Amos and H. Kaprowski, eds.), pp. 109–121, Wistar Inst. Press, Philadelphia.

Julius, M. H., Sweet, R. G., Fathman, C. G., and Hery, L. A., 1975, *AEC Symp. Ser. (CONS 73-1007)*, in press.

Kay, J. E., 1968, *Nature (London)* **219**:172–173.

Kedar, E., and Bonavida, B., 1974, *J. Immunol.* **113**:1544–1552.

Kleinsmith, L. S., Allfrey, V. G., and Mirsky, A. E., 1966, *Science* **154**:780–781.

Lefkowitz, R. K., 1975, *Biochem. Pharmacol.* **24**:1651–1658.

Luria, S. E., and Delbrück, N., 1943, *Genetics* **28**:491–511.

Maguire, M. E., Wiklund, R. A., Anderson, H. J., and Gilman, A. G., 1976, *J. Biol. Chem.* **251**:1221–1231.

Matthyssens, G. E., Hurwitz, E., Givol, D., and Sela, M., 1975, *Mol. Cell. Biochem.* **7**:119–126.

Melmon, K. L., Bourne, H. R., Weinstein, Y., and Sela, M., 1972, *Science* **177**:707–709.

Melmon, K. L., Bourne, H. R., Weinstein, Y., Shearer, G. M., Kram, J., and Bauminger, S., 1974a, *J. Clin. Invest.* **53**:13–21.

Melmon, K. L., Weinstein, Y., Shearer, G. M., Bourne, H. R., and Bauminger, S., 1974b, *J. Clin. Invest.* **53**:22–30.

Melmon, K. L., Weinstein, Y., Shearer, G. M., and Bourne, H. R., 1974c, *in: Cyclic AMP, Cell Growth, and the Immune Response* (W. Braun, L. M. Lichtenstein, and C. W. Parker, eds.), pp. 114–134, Springer-Verlag, New York.

Melmon, K. L., Weinstein, Y., Bourne, H. R., Shearer, G. M., Poon, T., Krasny, L., and Segal, S., 1975, *in: Cell Membrane Receptors for Viruses, Antigens, and Antibodies, Polypeptide Hormones and Small Molecules* (R. F. Beers and E. G. Bassett, eds.), pp. 117–133, Raven Press, New York.

Mozes, E., Shearer, G. M., and Sela, M., 1970, *J. Exp. Med.* **132**:613.

Mozes, E., Shearer, G. M., Melmon, K. L., and Bourne, H. R., 1973, *Cell. Immunol.* **9**:226–233.

Mozes, E., Weinstein, Y., Bourne, H. R., Melmon, K. L., and Shearer, G. M., 1974, *Cell. Immunol.* **11**:57–63.

Pastan, I., and Perlman, R., 1970, *Science* **169**:339–344.

Perkins, J. P., 1973, in: *Advances in Cyclic Nucleotide Research* (P. Greengard and G. A. Robison, eds.), Vol. 3, pp. 1–64, Raven Press, New York.

Peters, J. H., and Hausen, P., 1971, *Eur. J. Biochem.* **19**:502–508, 509–513.

Plaut, M., Lichtenstein, L. M., and Henney, C. S., 1975, *J. Clin. Invest.* **55**:856–874.

Pogo, B. G. T., Allfrey, V. G., and Mirsky, A. E., 1966, *Proc. Natl. Acad. Sci. U.S.A.* **55**:805–812.

Poon, T., Melmon, K. L., Weinstein, Y., Insel, P. A., and Krasny, L. T., 1977, *Mol. Pharmacol.*, in press.

Resch, K., Gelfand, E. W., Hansen, K., and Ferber, E., 1972, *Eur. J. Immunol.* **2**:598–601.

Segal, S., Globerson, A., Feldman, M., Haimovich, J., and Givol, D., 1969, *Nature (London)* **223**:1374–1375.

Sela, M., 1969, *Science* **166**:1365–1374.

Shearer, G. M., Cudkowicz, G., Connell, M. J., and Priore, R. L., 1968, *J. Exp. Med.* **128**:437–457.

Shearer, G. M., Weinstein, Y., Melmon, K. L., and Bourne, H. R., 1974a, in: *Cyclic AMP, Cell Growth, and the Immune Response* (W. Braun, L. M. Lichtenstein, and C. W. Parker, eds.), pp. 135–146, Springer-Verlag, New York.

Shearer, G. M., Weinstein, Y., and Melmon, K. L., 1974b, *J. Immunol.* **113**:597–607.

Simpson, E., Shearer, G. M., Weinstein, Y., and Melmon, K. L., 1973, *Fed. Proc. Fed. Am. Soc. Exp. Biol.* **32**:877 (abstract).

Smith, J. W., Steiner, A. L., and Parker, C. W., 1971, *J. Clin. Invest.* **50**:442–448.

Sutherland, E. W., and Robison, G. A., 1966, *Pharm. Rev.* **18**:145–161.
Thompson, L. H., Harkins, J. L., and Stanners, C. P., 1973, *Proc. Natl. Acad. Sci. U.S.A.* **70**:3094–3098.
Truffa-Bachi, P., and Wofsy, L., 1970, *Proc. Natl. Acad. Sci. U.S.A.* **66**:685–692.
Weinstein, Y., Melmon, K. L., Bourne, H. R., and Sela, M., 1973, *J. Clin. Invest.* **52**:1349–1361.
Weinstein, Y., Chambers, D. A., Bourne, H. R., and Melmon, K. L., 1974, *Nature (London)* **251**:352–353.
Weinstein, Y., Segal, S., and Melmon, K. L., 1975a, *J. Immunol.* **115**:112–117.
Weinstein, Y., Poon, T., Bourne, H. R., and Melmon, K. L., 1975b, *Clin. Res.* **23**:385a (abstract).
Weinstein, Y., Melmon, K. L., and Segal, S., 1976, in: *The Role of Mitogens in Immunobiology,* (U. U. Oppenheim and D. L. Rosenstreich, eds.), pp. 119–134, Academic Press, New York.
Wigzell, H., and Andersson, B., 1969, *J. Exp. Med.* **129**:23–36.

17

Polypeptide Hormone Receptors on Lymphoid Cells

Application to the Study of Receptor Alterations and Radioreceptor Assay of Polypeptide Hormones

JAMES R. GAVIN, III

1. Introduction

There is a large and impressive body of evidence to suggest that the initial event in polypeptide-hormone- and catecholamine-mediated cellular actions is the specific interaction of the hormone with recognition sites, i.e., receptors on the cell surface. Although the complex scheme of biochemical events ultimately seen in response to hormone administration may be affected by alterations at different points in the metabolic pathways involved, the binding of the hormone is prerequisite to all subsequent biological phenomena. Thus, the understanding of this key interaction assumes great importance. That it is of great importance becomes especially true in light of evidence that in some instances, the receptor itself, by alterations of affinity and concentration, may be an important determinant of the sensitivity of a cell to the action of hormones (Roth *et al.*, 1975).

For certain polypeptide hormones, such as insulin and growth hormone, a variety of tissues show responses that differ both in their biological manifestations and in their sensitivity to similar concentrations of hormone. However, these various hormone-sensitive tissues have at least one biochemical mechanism in

JAMES R. GAVIN III • Department of Internal Medicine, Barnes Hospital, Washington University School of Medicine, St. Louis, Missouri 63110.

common: the initial interaction of the hormone with cellular recognition sites. For example, a great deal of evidence is available to show that receptors from a variety of insulin-responsive tissues are identical in several physicochemical parameters and in their recognition of insulin and insulinlike polypeptides. In view of this common denominator among various target tissues for the same hormone, it becomes possible to study the effects of alterations in the *in vivo* or *in vitro* milieu on the interaction of a hormone with its receptor, and to correlate changes in hormone–receptor interactions in a readily accessible tissue with changes occurring at tissue sites not available for direct study. It also becomes possible to quantitatively assay the biopotency of circulating hormones using such biologically specific receptors as the binding protein. Thus, one can use accessible tissue for such direct investigations, and use these systems as mirrors of more general phenomena. This observation holds whether one is studying the effect of pH or Ca^{2+} on hormone–receptor binding, the effects of serum factors that directly alter the concentration of receptors available for specific interaction with a hormone, or altered metabolism of biologically important circulating polypeptide hormones.

1.1. Early Developments

It has been during the last decade that refinements in techniques have made possible the sensitive and specific direct study of polypeptide hormone–receptor interaction. Prior to this time, there was indirect evidence that polypeptide hormones reacted with specific recognition sites on the cell surface as the initial event in triggering biological responses. Investigators in early studies proposed that a rapid chemical reaction occurred between insulin and the outer surface of the membrane (Stadie *et al.*, 1949). These workers showed that only brief exposure of rat diaphragm was necessary for significant and prolonged biological effects. Later studies (Pastan *et al.*, 1966) showed that thyroid-stimulating hormone (TSH) and insulin had persistent effects in rat thyroid and skeletal muscle preincubated with hormone followed by washing in hormone-free buffer. These investigators also demonstrated substantial reduction in the magnitude of the persistent hormonal effects on the later addition of antibodies to TSH and insulin or trypsin. Other investigators demonstrated the uptake of native insulin by intact fat cells (Crofford, 1968), and the abolition of biological effects of insulin by incubation of adipocytes with trypsin (Kono, 1969).

Additional indirect evidence for the presence of cell-surface receptors has been derived from studies with polypeptide hormones linked to high-molecular-weight polymers. Recent reports have seriously questioned the validity of some of the studies using these agents, but these investigations are still generally regarded as supportive of the concept of cell-surface receptors (Katzen and Vlahakes, 1973). These bulky, insoluble derivatives were shown to be biologically active in preparations of ACTH linked to cellulose (Schimmer *et al.*, 1968), insulin (Cuatrecasas, 1969), prolactin (Turkington, 1970) and nerve growth factor (Frazier *et al.*, 1973) linked to Sepharose, and glucagon linked to agarose (Johnson *et al.*, 1972). Thus, a large body of indirect evidence has been amassed in support of the interaction of polypeptide hormones and surface receptors.

Although some early attempts at direct study of hormone–receptor interaction had been made (Stadie *et al.*, 1953; Haugaard and Stadie, 1954), it was not until 1969 that the direct study of such interactions was made possible by refinements in radioactive labeling techniques that preserved the biological activity of the peptide hormones. It was at this time that the binding of biologically active monoiodinated ACTH to adrenal tissue showed evidence of saturability, reversibility, and biological specificity (Lefkowitz *et al.*, 1969, 1970a). Simultaneously, similar findings were made in the interaction of monoiodinated angiotensin with a variety of tissues (Lin and Goodfriend, 1970). The principles and techniques demonstrated by these studies have achieved widespread application in the study of many polypeptide hormones (Roth, 1973).

1.2. Later Developments

The availability of techniques for direct study of hormone–receptor interaction achieves great impact when the techniques are for study of readily accessible tissue preparations that may serve as models of systemic events. An important development in this regard was the demonstration of specific hormone receptors on freshly isolated circulating white blood cells (Lin and Goodfriend, 1970; Gavin *et al.*, 1972a; Archer *et al.*, 1973; Olefsky and Reaven, 1974; Schwartz *et al.*, 1975; Fussganger *et al.*, 1976), and the demonstration of similar receptors in white blood cells maintained in culture (Gavin *et al.*, 1972a, 1973; Marx *et al.*, 1974). These intact cell preparations offer many advantages in the study of receptors. They are metabolically active and may be used to correlate hormone–receptor interactions with biological events. They are obtained without the use of rigorous isolation techniques or enzymic digestions, and therefore most closely approximate the state of the receptor *in vivo* under appropriate conditions. These cell preparations permit assessment of the effect of specific metabolic agonists and antagonists on hormone–receptor binding. Moreover, it is possible to correlate actual morphological alterations with changes in receptor binding. Preparations may be obtained from subjects with a variety of metabolic conditions. Under certain conditions of experimentation, these cells are known to degrade appreciably less hormone than broken cell preparations (Gavin *et al.*, 1973; Kahn *et al.*, 1974). Finally, cultured lymphoid cells offer a homogeneous, readily available cell preparation for receptor studies, and these cells can be maintained in culture for long periods without alterations in properties (Moore and Minowada, 1973; Gavin *et al.*, 1973). Cultured cells also provide a source of tissue that can be prepared in quantities suitable for the isolation of receptor (Gavin *et al.*, 1972b,c, 1973). Disadvantages of intact cell preparations include the inability to store this tissue with maintenance of stability, the restriction on types of chemical agents in which receptor interactions may be studied, and the need to provide experimental incubation conditions that will most effectively preserve viability.

Other intact cell preparations have been used in polypeptide hormone receptor studies, and these preparations have their own advantages and disadvantages unique to the tissues and dependent on the goal of the study. Preparations of this type include fibroblasts grown in monolayer culture (Gavin *et al.*, 1972a; Thomopoulos *et al.*, 1976; Rechler *et al.*, 1974), gonadal cells (Dufau *et al.*, 1971; Kammerman and Canfield, 1972; Leidenberger and Reichert, 1972), isolated fat cells (Freychet *et al.*, 1971; Cuatrecasas, 1971; Hammond *et al.*, 1972; Thompson *et al.*, 1972), hepatocytes (Kahn *et al.*, 1973), and avian erythrocytes (Ginsberg *et al.*, 1976).

It must be emphasized that the techniques and principles that have directed the study of receptors in intact cells are derived from the elegant work using purified plasma membranes (House and Weidemann, 1970; Freychet *et al.*, 1971; Finn *et al.*, 1972; Marx *et al.*, 1972; Rodbell *et al.*, 1971; Rao *et al.*, 1972; Cuatrecasas, 1972; Kahn *et al.*, 1972). These preparations have been of inestimable value in broadening our understanding of polypeptide hormone receptor mechanisms. However, the advantages mentioned previously for intact cell preparations indicate the limitations of plasma membrane preparations for certain kinds of studies. In this chapter, we shall focus on the existence and characteristics of polypeptide hormone receptors in lymphoid cells, and explore the applicability and implications of these observations. Chapter 16 is devoted to the nonpolypeptide hormone receptors, and no duplication of that effort will follow in this study.

2. Existence of Insulin Receptors on Circulating Cells

The original studies of insulin receptors on circulating cells were inspired by the need to devise means of studying hormone–receptor interactions in man. The binding of insulin to its specific receptors in rat liver and fat cell or purified plasma membrane preparations had been clearly demonstrated (House and Weidemann, 1970; Freychet *et al.*, 1971). Moreover, Freychet *et al.* (1971) had shown that the ability of insulin analogues to bind to specific receptors varied directly with the ability of the peptide to stimulate oxidation of glucose in isolated rodent adipocytes. With the use of the techniques described by Freychet *et al.* (1971), the binding of biologically active monoiodinated insulin to a variety of human circulating cells was studied.

2.1. Presence of Insulin Receptors on Erythrocytes

Binding of insulin to mature erythrocytes was reported by several groups (Haugaard and Stadie, 1954; Cuatrecasas, 1971; Gavin *et al.*, 1972a). The latter two groups of investigators reported that radioiodinated insulin bound to erythrocytes is inhibited by as little as 10^{-8} M insulin. However, the "specific" binding to the cells was uniformly small, requiring large numbers of cells and relatively high concentrations of insulin or insulin analogues for binding studies. Moreover, it was not determined to what extent the binding observed in erythrocyte preparations may be due to contaminating white blood cell elements. Thus, despite its extreme appeal as an easily obtained, plentiful tissue of human and animal origin, the mature erythrocyte has proved unsuitable to date for the study of polypeptide hormone receptors in intact cells.

It is of interest that the nucleated avian erythrocyte was shown by Ginsberg *et al.* (1976) to contain insulin receptors with binding properties identical to those of the well-characterized mammalian receptors. These workers point out that these cells, because of their biochemical simplicity, provide a convenient way of studying membrane–receptor interactions, a simple means of purifying plasma membrane and insulin receptor, and a means of studying the relationship between the insulin receptor and the well-characterized catecholamine receptor in these cells (Bilezikian and Aurbach, 1973). The biological significance of the receptor in avian erythrocytes remains unclear, but is currently under investigation.

2.2. Presence of Insulin Receptors on Granulocytes

Granulocytes were shown to contain specific binding sites for insulin (Gavin *et al.,* 1972a; Fussganger *et al.,* 1976). The study of receptors on granulocytes is complicated by the small number of receptors present and the extensive degradation of insulin by these cells (Fussganger *et al.,* 1976; Chandler and Varandani, 1974). These factors place limitations on the usefulness of granulocytes as a routine tissue preparation in the study of receptor mechanisms. Fussganger *et al.* (1976) showed, however, that in the presence of specific inhibitors of insulin degradation, it is possible to study the insulin receptors of granulocytes and to demonstrate their similarity to those described in other tissues. It would be of interest to determine the role of insulin in granulocyte function. For example, insulin administration *in vitro* corrects the chemotactic defect in leukocytes from diabetic subjects (Mowat and Baum, 1971). Other clinical disorders such as the "lazy leukocyte" syndrome, the Chediak–Higashi syndrome, and several acquired conditions characterized by impairment of chemotaxis (e.g., terminal shock, ethanol ingestion) have been described (Baehner, 1973). The demonstration of insulin receptors on granulocytes makes it possible to determine what role, if any, alterations in insulin–receptor interaction play in these conditions.

2.3. Presence of Insulin Receptors on Lymphoid Cells

2.3.1. Studies in Peripheral Blood Mononuclear Cells

Peripheral blood mononuclear leukocytes from normal volunteer blood donors, purified by ficoll–hypaque gradient centrifugation, were shown to contain insulin receptors of the same biological specificity as those described for receptors in liver and fat (Gavin, *et al.,* 1972a,b; Olefsky and Reaven, 1974). Since lymphocytes constitute by far the greatest fraction of cells prepared by this technique, we assumed that they were responsible for the specific binding observed, especially since a direct correlation could be observed in the amount of insulin bound and the number of lymphocytes in a number of different experiments (Gavin *et al.,* 1973). Krug *et al.* (1972) failed, however, to detect any specific insulin binding to peripheral lymphocytes purified by passage of leukocyte suspensions over nylon wool columns. This technique is known to remove B lymphocytes (Eisen *et al.,* 1972; Greaves and Brown, 1974). Therefore, Olefsky and Reaven (1974) suggested that the discrepancy in findings could be explained on the basis of differences in techniques used for cell purification. They suggested that the binding observed in our studies was due to B lymphocytes, a population that would have been depleted in the purified preparations of Krug *et al.* (1972). These various observations were clarified when Schwartz *et al.* (1975) restudied the problem and determined that ficoll–hypaque-gradient-purified preparations of lymphocytes contained monocytes that were the principal insulin-binding cells of the mononuclear cell fraction. They found a high correlation between the specific insulin binding in mononuclear cell preparations and the number of monocytes. These workers used phagocytosis of latex particles to identify monocytes, and then localized [^{125}I]insulin binding to these cells by autoradiography. Using these and other techniques, they showed that 85–90% of the insulin bound to mononuclear cells was accounted for by binding to monocytes, while the remaining 10–15% was due to binding to large, nonphagocytic mononuclear cells. The latter cells may represent circulating large lymphocytes, or a nonphagocytic subpopulation of monocytes (Schwartz *et al.*, 1975). Alternatively, these cells could represent a subpopulation of B lymphocytes in a state of activation. In this regard, Krug *et al.* (1972) reported the emergence of insulin receptors in lectin-activated peripheral lymphocytes. In contrast, however, Rabinowitz *et al.* (1974) found that concanavalin A (Con A) transformation of peripheral lymphocytes does not lead to the appearance of insulin receptors. Rabinowitz *et al.* (1974) further pointed out that their results are in agreement with the observation that lymphocytes of the T-cell variety in culture fail to demonstrate specific insulin binding. It is generally agreed that the predominant responders to Con A stimulation are T lymphocytes (Stobo and Paul, 1972; Rawson and Huang, 1975). Therefore, it seems reasonable that mitogen stimulation would not cause the emergence of specific receptors unless the respondent population was a subpopulation of B lymphocytes. In fact, recent studies suggest that there may be some response to Con A by B lymphocytes (Chess *et al.*, 1974). Thus, the differences between the results of Krug *et al.* (1972) and those of Rabinowitz *et al.* (1974) could be explained on this basis. In light of these studies, the contribution of the small, unstimulated lymphocyte to the specific binding of insulin in mononuclear cell preparations is not clear at this time. Of interest is the report of insulin-induced augmentation of lymphocyte-mediated cytotoxicity (Strom *et al.*, 1975), which is generally felt to be a T-lymphocyte function. It is possible that T-cell subpopulations exist that contain specific receptors of sufficient quantity to trigger a biological response, but inadequate for detection in routine binding assays.

The insulin receptors in monocytes were found to be indistinguishable from those described in liver, fat, and other cell preparations (Bianco *et al.*, 1974). These cells constitute a direct means of studying changes in the insulin–receptor interaction in disease states characterized by altered levels of sensitivity to the hormone.

2.3.2. Studies in Cultured Mononuclear Cell Lines

(a) Insulin Receptors on Cultured B Lymphocytes. The detection of insulin receptors in peripheral blood mononuclear cells prompted the investigation of hormone binding to lymphoid cells in culture (Gavin *et al.*, 1972a). These cells represented a very convenient source of tissue for insulin-specific binding sites. Moreover, a great variety of cell lines are available, and many of these lines have been well characterized (Moore and Minowada, 1973). The major features of the lymphoid cell cultures were reviewed by Fahey *et al.* (1971). The first cell line we studied was No. 4265, which was originally obtained in 1965 from a 42-year-old male with chronic myelogenous leukemia (Moore *et al.*, 1966). These cells were shown to possess a normal distribution of chromosomes, except for several small "marker" chromosomes that probably represented broken tetraploid metaphases. This cell line contained insulin receptors with specificity for binding that was identical to that observed in liver membranes or isolated fat cells (Table 1).

Moreover, these cells have at least 10 times greater numbers of receptors per cell than the peripheral blood mononuclear cells (Gavin *et al.*, 1972a). These findings prompted examination of a number of lymphoid cell lines that had been established in various laboratories from healthy volunteers and from patients with a wide variety of diseases. The cell lines revealed a wide range in the concentration of specific insulin receptors per cell (Table 2). With a few notable exceptions, lines of B-cell (bone-marrow- or "bursal"-derived) lymphocytes consistently bound more insulin than T-cell (thymus-derived) lymphocytes, and this difference could not be explained on the basis of cell volumes or total surface areas (Table 3).

Table 2 provides a summary of our results in screening cultured cell lines for insulin and human growth hormone (hGH) receptors. Insulin-binding to B-cell lines showed distinct patterns. To facilitate discussion of results, arbitrary categories were assigned to groups of cells according to their apparent binding capacities under the conditions of assay. For insulin binding, cell line IM-9 was used as a reference, and the maximum binding achieved with a tracer of [^{125}I]insulin with this cell line was considered to be 100%. This cell line was tested frequently in our laboratory for over 2 years, and consistently showed the same binding pattern under standard assay conditions. Other cells were compared with IM-9 under identical conditions. Those cells that bound a maximum of 75–100% as much insulin as IM-9 constitute insulin receptor class I (IRC-I); those that bound 25–75% as much hormone, class II (IRC-II); those that bound 5–25% as much hormone, class III (IRC-III); and those cells that demonstrated no competitive insulin binding, class IV (IRC-IV). Results of insulin-binding to human B-cell lines are summarized in Figure 1. IRC-I cell lines (represented by JQ, Figure 1, inset) demonstrated the highest levels of insulin binding on a per-cell basis. Of the 7 cell lines in this group, 4 were derived from normal subjects (Table 2), 2 were obtained from patients with acute myelogenous leukemia, and 1 was obtained from a patient with multiple myeloma. IRC-II cells are represented by 4265 (Figure 1, inset). Cells from a variety of sources are found in this group, including several cultures derived from normal subjects (Table 2). Within the IRC-II cell population are several lines established from patients with infectious mononucleosis, represented by cell line Noland (Figure 1, inset). Cells that bound little insulin are represented by Daudi (Figure 1, inset). This cell line was derived from a patient with Burkitt's lymphoma.

TABLE 1. Potency of Preparation (%) Relative to Porcine Insulin[a]

Preparation	Fat cells (glucose oxide)	Liver membranes	Lymphocytes	Immunoassay
Porcine insulin	100	100	100	100
Human insulin	100	100	100	70
Fish insulin	50	53	48	0.2
Porcine proinsulin	4.5	4.0	3.7	47
Bovine des Ala des Asp	1.4	1.7	1.0	15
Bovine desoctapeptide	1.5	1.9	1.2	
Guinea pig insulin	1.0	1.1	1.7	0.001
NSILA-s[b]	0.3	0.4	0.4	0.0005

[a]Adapted from Freychet *et al.* (1971) and Gavin *et al.* (1973, 1975).
[b]Nonsuppressible insulinlike activity in plasma (soluble).

TABLE 2. **Insulin- and hGH-Binding to Cultured Lymphoid Cells**

Cell line	Source	Insulin bound (ng/1.5×10^7 cells)	hGH bound (ng/2×10^7 cells)[a]
IRC-I			
8866	Acute myelogenous leukemia	0.71	0.59
6410	Acute myelogenous leukemia	0.74	NT
JQ	Normal	0.66	NT
Connor	Normal	0.72	NT
1788	Normal	0.74	NT
1120	Normal	0.76	NT
IM-9	Multiple myeloma	0.78	0.58
IRC-II			
IM-10	Multiple myeloma	0.43	0.32
4265	Chronic myelogenous leukemia	0.37	0.41
IM-4	American Burkitt's lymphoma	0.20	NT
Ly46	Burkitt's lymphoma	0.50	0.27
IM-1	Lymphoblastic sarcoma	0.19	0.42
8057	Normal	0.19	NT
446	Hodgkin's disease	0.23	NT
NK-9	Burkitt's lymphoma	0.17	NT
8205	Chronic myelogenous leukemia	0.18	0.27
Levins	Infectious mononucleosis	0.45	0.26
Erlanger	Infectious mononucleosis	0.20	0.28
Kaplan	Infectious mononucleosis	0.38	0.27
Lyzensky	Infectious mononucleosis	0.30	0.25
Baldus	Infectious mononucleosis	0.49	0.26
Noland	Infectious mononucleosis	0.44	0.27
B 46 M	Burkitt's lymphoma	0.22	0.000
B 35 M	Burkitt's lymphoma	0.20	0.000
IRC-III			
Raji-K	Burkitt's lymphoma	0.12	0.000
Maku	Burkitt's lymphoma	0.12	0.000
Onesmus	Burkitt's lymphoma	0.07	0.000
Daudi	Burkitt's lymphoma	0.06	0.003
Molt-4	Lymphoblastic leukemia	0.06	0.000
IRC-IV			
Namalwa	Burkitt's lymphoma	0.02	0.000
Akuba	Burkitt's lymphoma	0.00	0.000
AL-I	Burkitt's lymphoma	0.00	0.000
Naliaka	Burkitt's lymphoma	0.00	0.000
EB-3	Burkitt's lymphoma	0.00	0.000
P_3HRIK	Burkitt's lymphoma	0.00	0.000
P_3BU	BUDR treated—P_3HRIK	0.01	0.000
8226	Myeloma	0.02	NT
CEM	Acute lymphocytic leukemia	0.00	0.000
HSB-2	Acute lymphocytic leukemia	0.00	0.000

[a]Not tested.

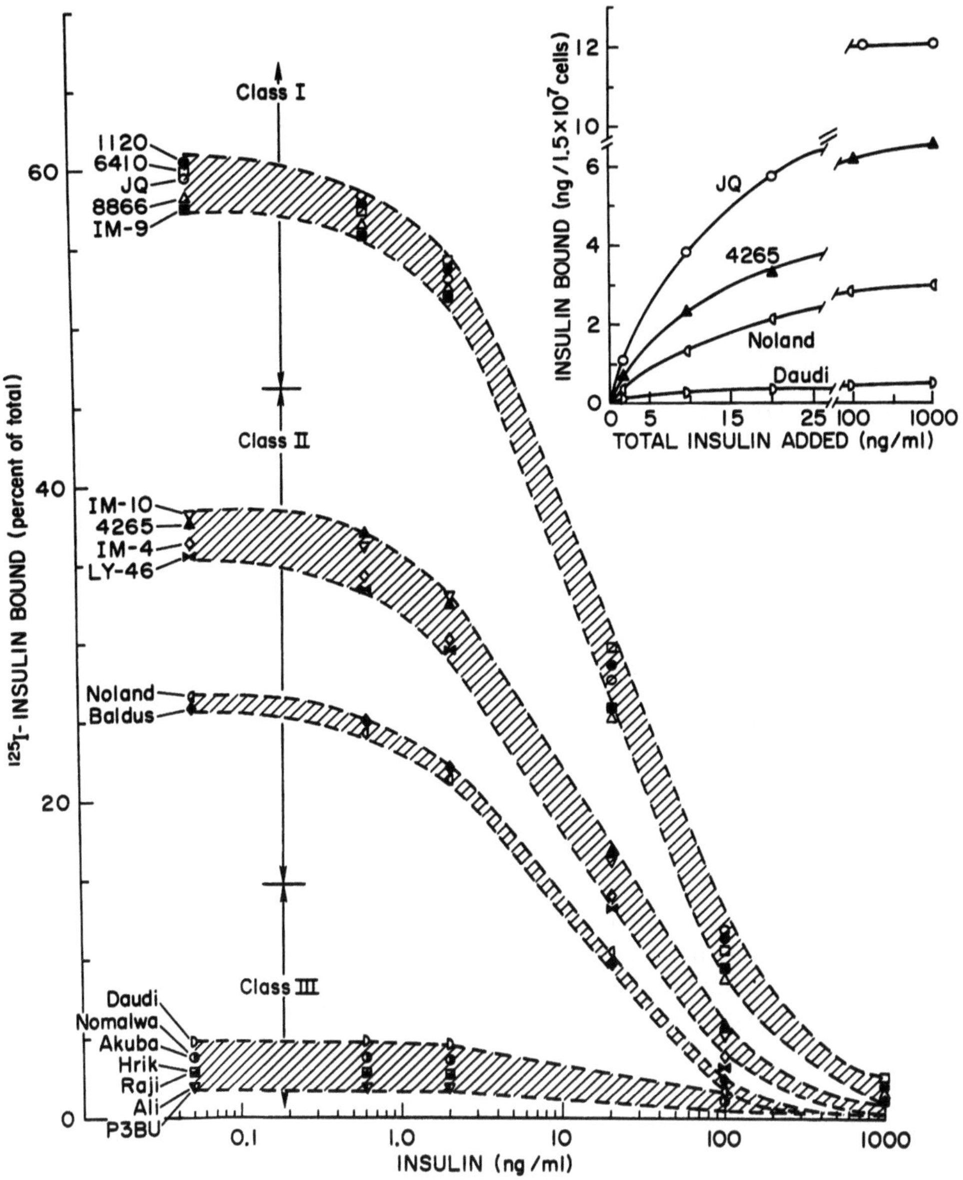

Figure 1. Insulin-binding to a variety of cultured B lymphoid cells. *Inset:* Quantitative insulin-binding to representative cell lines as a function of total insulin in assay.

TABLE 3. **Cell Volumes and Surface Areas of B- and T-Cell Lines**

Cell line	Type	Average volume (μm^3)[a]	Average surface area (μm^2)[b]	Relative insulin binding (%)	Relative hGH binding (%)[c]
IM-9[d]	B	1478	628	100	100
8866	B	1575	655	91	100
4265	B	1444	618	41	71
SB	B	3138	1037	69	NT
8392	B	1508	630	52	NT
Raji	B	1420	611	15	0
Naliaka	B	1513	637	0	0
Molt-4	T	1408	608	7	0
CEM	T	645	361	0	0
HSB-2	T	894	449	0	0
8402	T	798	416	0	0

[a]Determined from Coulter counter volume plot.
[b]Calculated from *(a)* using formulas for volume and surface of a sphere.
[c]Not tested.
[d]Cell line IM-9 taken as 100% standard.

As a group, the African-Burkitt's-lymphoma-derived cell lines showed little or no capacity to bind insulin. Of the 10 cell lines in our IRC-IV category, 7 were obtained from patients with this disorder (Table 2). We have extended these observations to show the relative absence of insulin receptors in cells derived from fresh tissue biopsy specimens from patients with the disease (Buell and Gavin, 1977). There is strong evidence that most Burkitt's-lymphoma-derived cell lines represent the malignant lymphoma cell in culture (Fialkow *et al.*, 1970, 1971). The striking loss of hormone receptors may be a significant characteristic of these malignant cells. It seems reasonable to propose that the loss of receptors is accompanied by a loss of regulatory effects of hormones in these cells. While no specific effects of insulin (or hGH) are known for these cells at this time,* it is possible that a mechanism of receptor disappearance exists that enables the transformed malignant cells to "escape" the control mechanisms triggered by hormones or other molecules that initiate their actions by a process involving specific receptor binding as the first step. If indeed a marked receptor deficit is characteristic of Burkitt's lymphoma (and perhaps other) malignant cells, it is of interest that not all the Burkitt's cells in culture studied by us fall into the IRC-IV category (Table 2). In contrast, all the biopsy specimens of Burkitt's lymphoma tissue studied to date have demonstrated virtually complete absence of receptors. In this regard, contamination of Burkitt's-lymphoma-derived cells in culture by non-Burkitt's cells was reported by Fialkow *et al.* (1971). This contamination is a possible explanation for

*Recently, Bar *et al.* (1976b) showed that insulin receptors are present on macrophage cells—mouse tumor cell line $P388D_1$, and the mixed macrophage–lymphoid population from normal mouse spleen—that are indistinguishable from receptors on human monocytes. In addition, insulin (10^{-10} M) alters the specific immunologic function; i.e., insulin can inhibit macrophage-induced antibody-dependent cytotoxicity. In another recent study, Leroux *et al.* (1975) demonstrated that insulin (4×10^{-10} M) increased glucose consumption by polymorphonuclear leukocytes without influencing the permeability of membranes to glucose.

the discrepancies observed, and suggests that a more careful characterization of those Burkitt's cells with receptor binding capacity is warranted. Thus, it is possible that B-cell lymphocytes of "malignant" origin undergo loss of hormone (and other) receptors concomitant with malignant transformation. Also in this category is cell line 8226, which has minimum insulin-binding and represents a malignant myeloma cell in culture (Matsuoka *et al.*, 1969). The two remaining cell lines in this category, which had no insulin-binding, were obtained from patients with acute lymphocytic leukemia.

(b) Insulin Receptors on Cultured T Lymphocytes. T cells have consistently shown a marked deficiency in insulin receptor concentration. Table 3 shows that the difference between B-cell and T-cell binding is intrinsic to the cell, rather than due to surface area, viability, or similar parameters. In other studies, we further demonstrated that this difference is not accounted for by increased degradation of hormone by T cells (unpublished observations). Cell lines Molt-4, CEM, HSB-2, and 8402 are T-cell lines established from patients with active lymphoblastic leukemia. Lines CEM, HSB-2, and 8402 appear to represent neoplastic T lymphocytes of the poorly differentiated childhood lymphoma of convoluted type (Kaplan *et al.*, 1974; Smith *et al.*, 1973), which usually undergoes leukemic transformation. Molt-4 was also derived from a patient with a T-cell leukemia (Royston *et al.*, 1974). Wherever possible, we performed direct comparisons between T cells and B cells from the same host. Cell lines SB and 8392 (Table 3) represent B-cell lines derived

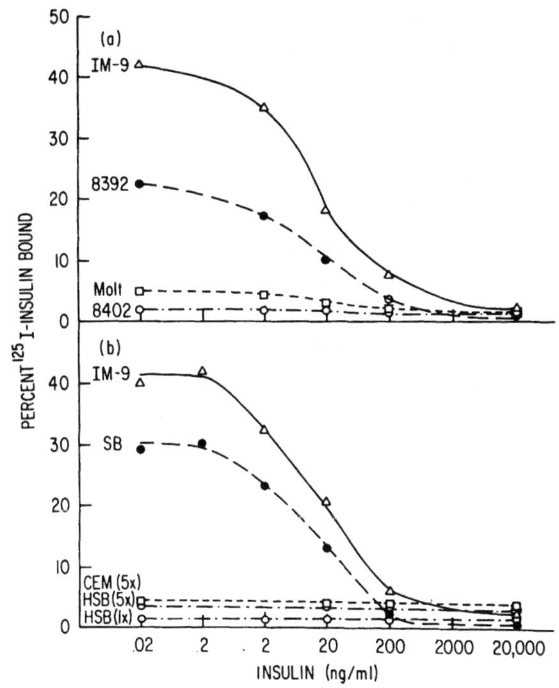

Figure 2. Insulin-binding to B-cell and T-cell lines from the same host, with IM-9 as a B-cell standard. Lines 8392 and 8402(a) are a B-cell/T-cell pair, as are SB and HSB(b). Lines Molt and CEM are other T-cell lines. (5×) = 5 × 10^7 cells/ml.

from the same patients as HSB-2 (Kaplan *et al.*, 1974) and 8402 (Minowada and Moore, 1975), respectively. Figure 2a shows the increased binding of 8392 over its T-cell counterpart, 8402; Figure 2b shows similar differences for the B-cell/T-cell pair of SB and HSB. Since SB cells were found to have 4 times the volume of HSB-2, the latter cells were tested at 5 times the usual cell concentration used for assay, yet no specific (competitive) insulin-binding was seen (Figure 2b). Cell line CEM likewise showed no binding at 5 times the usual cell concentration. Molt (Molt-4) is the only one of the T-cell lines that shows any competitive insulin-binding, albeit low (Figure 2a).

T-cell lines have been derived from patients with acute lymphoblastic T-cell leukemia or the leukemic phase of lymphosarcoma, and probably represent the malignant cells. The absence or relative lack of receptors in human T cells may be an intrinsic property of the cell. Alternatively, these studies may indicate that lymphoid lines of malignant-cell origin are characterized in part by few or no hormone receptors in the membrane.

(c) Summary of Insulin Receptor Studies in Cultured B Cells and T Cells. A wide variety of cell lines have been studied and found to have enormous differences in hormone-binding capacity. B cells consistently bound more hormone than T cells, except for the B-cell lines derived from patients with Burkitt's lymphoma.

Cell lines demonstrating significant binding have been derived from normal subjects and from patients with infectious mononucleosis. There is a well-known association between Epstein–Barr virus (EBV) and Burkitt's lymphoma cells (Epstein *et al.*, 1964) and infectious mononucleosis (Henle and Henle, 1973). Thus, the lack of receptors in lymphoid lines of proved or strongly suggestive malignant-cell origin appears to be a concomitant of malignant-cell transformation distinct from the EB-viral "transformation" necessary for normal B lymphocytes to become established as permanent lines (Gerber *et al.*, 1969), and from the "transformation" resulting in infectious mononucleosis.

The findings made available from the screening of numerous cell lines for insulin receptors may be useful for future investigations. For example, to study insulin–receptor interaction using human lymphoid cells, a line from IRC-I should be selected. In this regard, it is of interest that Hadden *et al.* (1972) demonstrated a direct effect of insulin on cell line 1788, one of our IRC-I lines. Conversely, in studying hormone-mediated membrane alterations or metabolic effects in cells of this type, cell lines from IRC-IV, which lack receptors, can serve as elegant controls. Manipulations designed to induce receptor appearance may likewise be studied using cells from category IRC-IV in the same fashion that manipulations designed to reduce receptor concentrations were studied in cells of the IRC-I category (Gavin *et al.*, 1974).

2.3.3. Studies in Mononuclear Cells of Animal Origin

Goldfine *et al.* (1972) demonstrated the presence of specific binding sites for insulin in thymocytes from suckling rats. These receptors share the same biological specificity as those described in liver, fat, and peripheral or cultured human mononuclear cells. These investigators further demonstrated the direct correlation between insulin-binding and insulin-stimulated uptake of aminoisobutyric acid (AIB) (Goldfine and Sherline, 1972). Similarly, insulin receptors were described in thymic lymphocytes from genetically obese *(ob/ob)* mice (Soll *et al.*, 1974). These investigators showed that the insulin receptor in the thymic lymphocyte mirrors the defect in receptor concentration described in liver and fat cells from these animals (Soll *et al.*, 1975).

3. Characteristics of the Insulin Receptor on Lymphoid Cells

The binding of polypeptide hormones to specific receptors is proportional to hormone and receptor concentrations, and is time-dependent. (Roth, 1973). The binding of insulin to its receptor is rapid and reaches steady-state levels within minutes (Figure 3). The increased binding at lower temperatures and the maintenance of a more stable plateau are accounted for in part by loss of receptor into the medium at higher temperatures (Gavin *et al.*, 1973), and by a marked temperature dependence of the dissociation rate.

The binding of insulin to lymphoid cells is a saturable and readily reversible process. Our initial studies revealed a kinetic analysis consistent with binding sites for insulin of varying affinities (Gavin *et al.*, 1973). Further studies by De Meyts *et al.* (1973) demonstrated that the insulin receptor in lymphoid cells shows negative cooperativity in its interaction with hormone. Furthermore, insulin-binding shows pH dependence, with an optimum of approximately pH 7.8 (Gavin *et al.*, 1973). Ca^{2+}, Mg^{2+}, and $EDTA^{2+}$ were shown to have no effect on insulin-binding to cultured lymphoid cells over a 10-fold range of concentration (1–10 mM) (Gavin *et al.*, 1973).

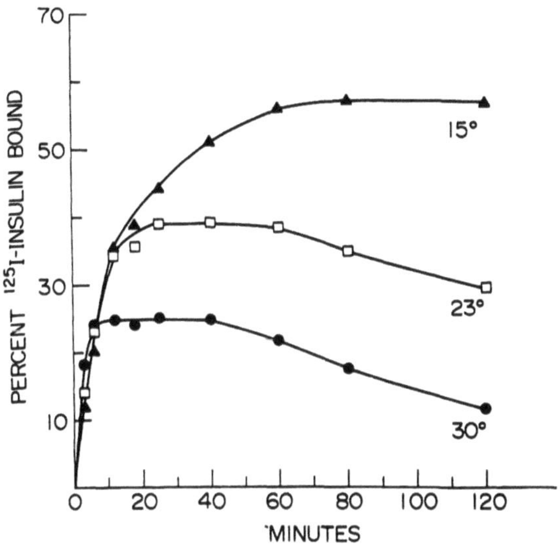

Figure 3. Time course of binding of insulin to lymphoid cells at various temperatures. Reproduced from Gavin *et al.* (1973) with permission.

There is no significant degradation of radiolabeled insulin by peripheral or cultured mononuclear cells. At 30°C, less than 15% degradation of labeled hormone is observed, while at 15°C, no degradation is seen (Gavin *et al.*, 1973).

Digestion of cultured lymphoid cells with DNase, RNase, or neuraminidase had no effect on the binding of insulin to its specific receptors (Gavin *et al.*, 1973). In contrast, digestion of these cells with varying concentrations of trypsin results in loss of hormone-binding (Figure 4). Studies with trypsin digestion suggest that the receptor is an accessible membrane protein (Gavin *et al.*, 1973). The concept was strengthened by the finding that insulin receptors are shed spontaneously from cultured lymphoid cell membranes into the aqueous medium under appropriate conditions of temperature and ionic strength (Gavin *et al.*, 1972b; Buell and Gavin, 1973). We extended these studies to show that the loss of binding is due to actual release of receptors, not to loss of cell viability or degradation of labeled hormone (Figure 5). The shed receptors were recovered in the medium as water-solubilized receptors with binding specificity similar to that of the intact cell (Gavin *et al.*, 1972b,c).

4. Effects of Insulin on Lymphoid Cells

The biological significance of specific receptors for insulin on lymphoid cells is a recurrent and unsettled question. While it is agreed that mononuclear cells are not

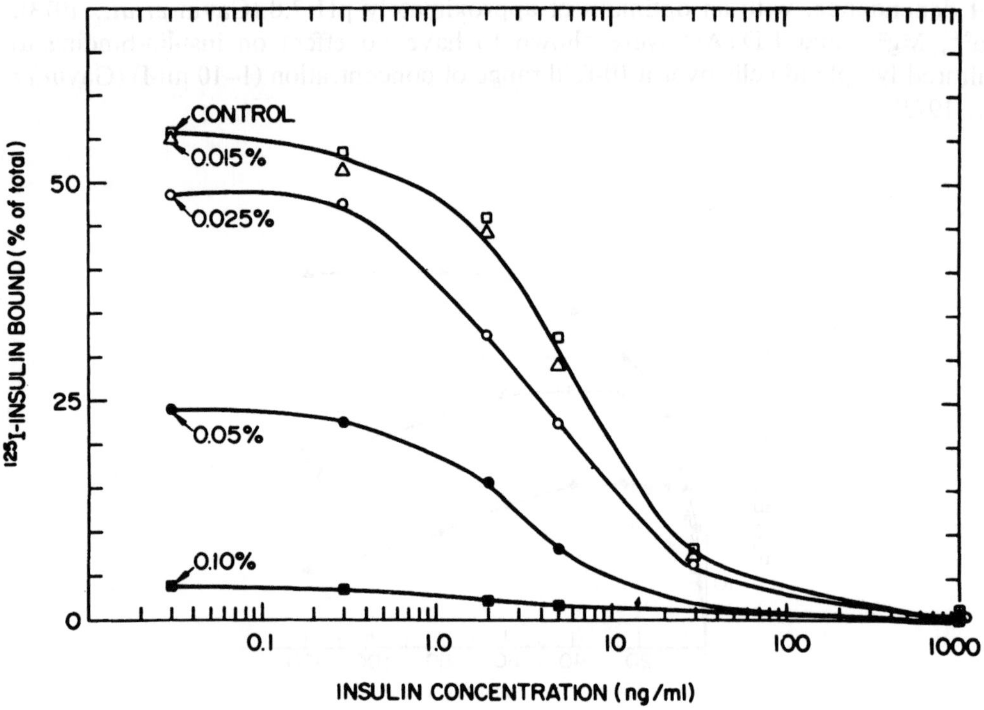

Figure 4. Effect of tryptic digestion on lymphoid insulin receptors using increasing concentrations of enzyme. Residual binding determined immediately after digestion.

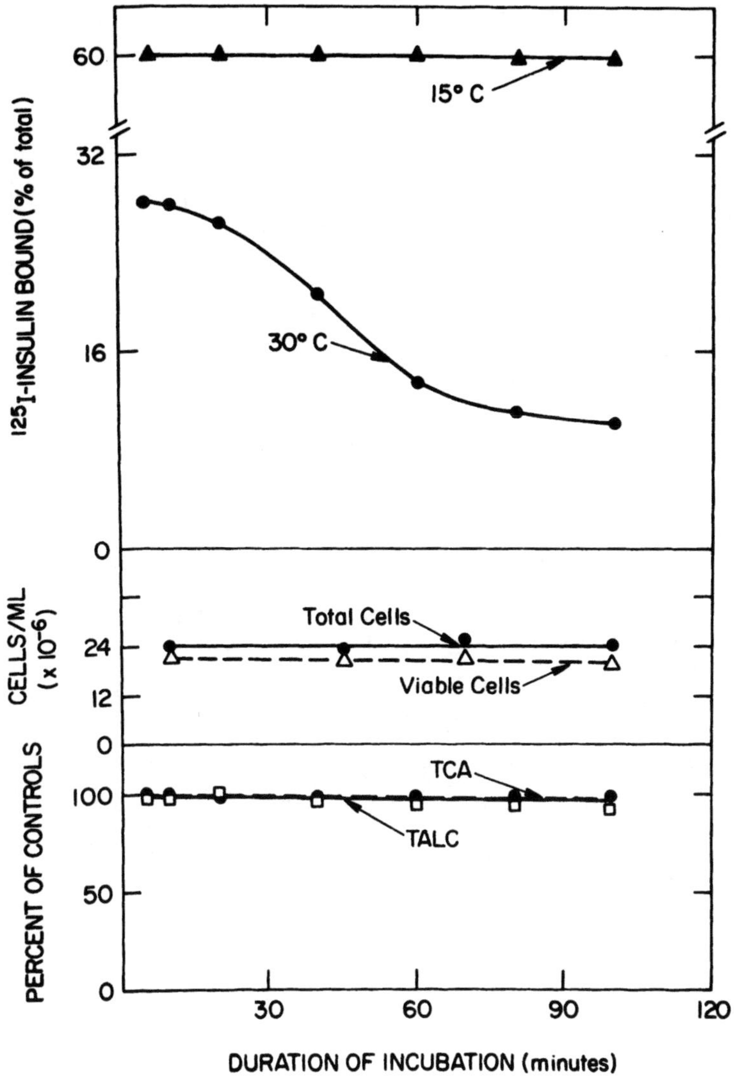

Figure 5. Spontaneous release of insulin receptors into aqueous medium at 15° and 30°C as a function of time. The observed loss of binding at 30°C was not due to cell death, loss of cells, or degradation of hormone. (TCA) Trichloroacetic-acid-precipitable insulin in the medium; (TALC) binding of talc.

major target tissues for insulin, there have been several reports describing effects of this hormone on these cells (Table 4). To date, the interplay between the well-characterized polypeptide hormones and immune response has not been subjected to systematic investigation. It was demonstrated, however, that insulin is involved in inflammatory and hypersensitivity reactions (Koltai *et al.*, 1974, 1975). It is possible that the regulatory contribution of insulin, including its effects on lymphocyte activation and mitogenesis (Pallavicini and Nichols, 1976) is a function of the ability of insulin to inhibit the action of cyclic AMP (cAMP) (Bourne *et al.*, 1974). It is of interest that the insulin-induced augmentation of lymphocyte-mediated cyto-

TABLE 4. Insulin Effects on Lymphoid Cells

Tissue	Source	Response observed	References
Leukocytes	Normal humans	Increased glucose utilization *in vitro;* increased glycogen synthesis	Weinberg and Field (1959)
	Diabetic humans	Increased glucose utilization, lactate production, and glycogen synthesis *in vivo*	Esmann (1963)
Peripheral lymphocytes and cultured human lymphocytes (RPMI 1788)	Humans	Increased membrane ATPase activity and increased glucose and rubidium uptake *in vitro*	Hadden *et al.* (1972)
Cultured leukemic cells	Humans	Increased growth with insulin in chemically defined or unsupplemented growth media	Moore *et al.* (1966)
Thymus-derived lymphocytes	Rat	Increased AIB influx	Goldfine and Sherline (1972)
		Increased glucose uptake	Boyett and Hofert (1972)
Lymphoid tissue	Rat	Growth increase	Lundin and Angerwall (1970)
Spleen and lymph nodes	Rat	Increased DNA synthesis with	
		insulin + antigenic stimulation	Maor *et al.* (1974)
		+ mitogenic stimulation	Pallavicini and Nichols (1976)
Lymph nodes	Rats, rabbits, pigs, calves	Production of anaphylactoid-inflammation-promoting factor	Koltai *et al.* (1975)
		No effects with thymus cells	
Splenic lymphocytes	Rats	Augmentation of lymphocyte-mediated cytotoxicity	Strom *et al.* (1975)

toxicity (Strom *et al.*, 1975) closely resembles the effect of cGMP in cytotoxic reactions. It will also be of interest to determine the effects of insulin on immunoglobulin and lymphokine synthesis in lymphoid cells in light of the demonstration of an insulin-induced anaphylactoid-inflammation-promoting factor by Koltai *et al.* (1975). Additional areas of investigation in this regard include determining effects of insulin on interferon and macrophage-inhibiting factor production in lymphoid cells (see Chapters 1 and 3 for further discussion).

5. Existence of Human Growth Hormone (hGH) Receptors on Lymphoid Cells

Using the techniques previously discussed, Lesniak *et al.* (1973) described the presence of specific binding sites for hGH in cultured lymphoid cells. These sites show remarkable biological specificity and demonstrate the physicochemical features characteristic of a specific receptor. In contrast to the insulin system, no hGH receptors have been demonstrated in peripheral mononuclear cells to date (Lesniak *et al.*, 1974).

5.1. Presence of hGH Receptors on Cultured Human Lymphoid Cells

Many of the cell lines screened for insulin receptors have likewise been studied for hGH receptors. The results of these studies are summarized in Table 2. Similar to the results obtained with insulin, various cell lines showed distinct patterns of binding (Figure 6). Although these cells bound less hGH than insulin on a per-cell basis, relative patterns of hGH-binding were very similar to those observed for insulin. Thus, it is possible in these studies to assign various lines to arbitrary classes I–IV (Figure 6). Typically, cells from IRC-I bound the most hGH, while cells from patients with infectious mononucleosis consistently bound somewhat less hGH than 4265 and fall in class II, a finding consistent with the pattern observed in the insulin studies. In addition, there was a group of cells that demonstrated no specific binding of hGH, and that constitute class IV (Table 2 and Figure 6). The great majority of African-Burkitt's-lymphoma-derived cells fall in this group. This striking deficiency of hGH receptors in cultured Burkitt's lymphoma cells was also observed in tissue biopsy specimens, and may represent a characteristic lesion in these cells (Buell and Gavin, 1977). We have not detected specific hGH-binding to T lymphocytes.

5.2. Characteristics of the hGH Receptor on Lymphoid Cells

Binding of hGH to lymphoid cells is rapid, saturable, and reversible. In contrast to the insulin receptor, there is a less marked pH dependence, with virtually no change in binding noted between pH 6.4 and 8.8 (Lesniak *et al.*, 1974). As with the insulin receptor, Mg^{2+}, Ca^{2+}, and $EDTA^{2+}$ showed no effect on binding over a wide range of concentrations. Optimum binding of hGH occurs at higher temperatures than required for insulin (Lesniak *et al.*, 1974). There was minimum degradation of labeled hGH or of the receptor under test conditions (Lesniak *et al.*, 1974). The hGH receptor was shown to be much more susceptible to trypsin than

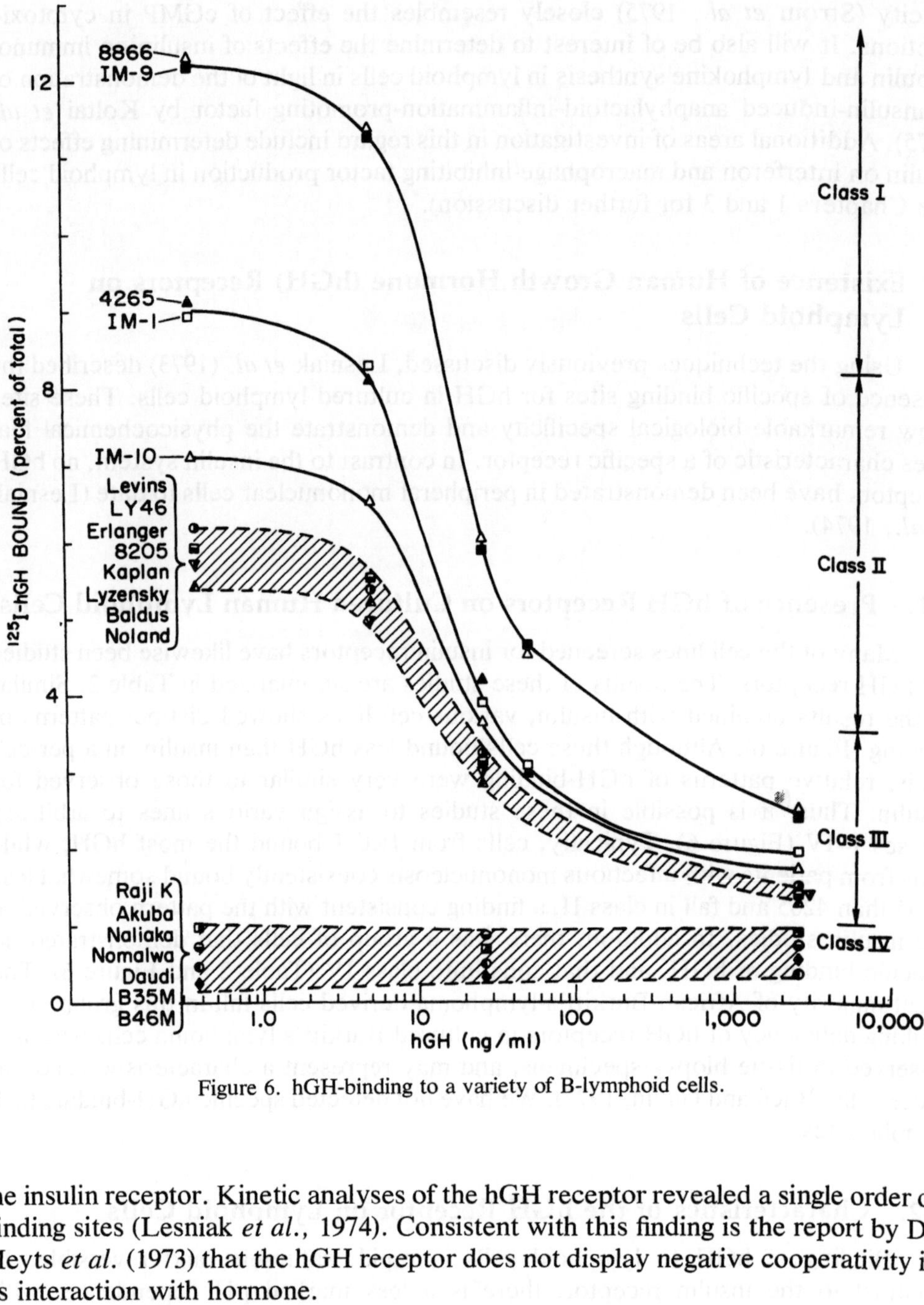

Figure 6. hGH-binding to a variety of B-lymphoid cells.

the insulin receptor. Kinetic analyses of the hGH receptor revealed a single order of binding sites (Lesniak *et al.*, 1974). Consistent with this finding is the report by De Meyts *et al.* (1973) that the hGH receptor does not display negative cooperativity in its interaction with hormone.

5.3. Effects of hGH on Lymphoid Cells

The exact mechanism of action through which hGH exerts a biological effect in tissues is unknown. Lymphoid cells have not traditionally been considered major target tissues for this hormone, but as with insulin, effects of hGH have been reported. A role for hGH in the stimulation of lymphoblasts was suggested by

Astaldi *et al.* (1972). These workers also demonstrated a reversal of the defect in proliferation of thymic lymphocytes in genetically dwarf mice. In similar studies using antigen-stimulated rats, Maor *et al.* (1974) proposed hormone-augmented DNA synthesis in lymphocytes from spleen or lymph nodes. We have not directly studied biological effects of hGH in lymphoid cells. It is possible that hGH exerts a direct effect on the immune response, or it may mediate effects through complex interplay with other humoral factors.

6. Existence of Calcitonin Receptors on Human Lymphoid Cells

The detection of specific receptors for insulin and hGH on cultured lymphoid cells led to investigation for other polypeptide hormone receptors in these tissues. Marx *et al.* (1974) described calcitonin receptors on cultured lymphocytes that have striking similarities to receptors from kidney and bone (Marx *et al.*, 1972). These receptors bind hormone with high affinity and show time and temperature dependence. A considerably longer time of incubation is required for binding, and there exists a requirement for $EDTA^{2+}$ that is not present for insulin- or hGH-binding to these cells (Marx *et al.*, 1974). Kinetic studies revealed findings compatible with a single order of binding sites, similar to results obtained for hGH. These observations were shown by De Meyts *et al.* (1973) to represent absence of negative cooperativity in the hormone–receptor interaction. Earlier studies by Marx *et al.* (1973) reported findings in renal and skeletal membranes consistent with at least two "orders" of binding sites for calcitonin. This discrepancy was explained in part by a mechanism causing appearance of multiple sites following freezing and thawing of the membrane preparations (Glossman *et al.*, 1974; Marx *et al.*, 1974).

Marx *et al.* (1974) also described affinity purification of labeled calcitonin using cultured lymphoid cell receptors. The hormone that was eluted from the cells showed marked enhancement of its ability to bind to fresh cells. This observation confirms the findings of Freychet *et al.* (1972), who reported that binding of insulin to its receptor protected it from degradation, and that the eluted hormone showed enhanced specificity in binding to fresh receptor. These studies suggest that the receptors bind or "select" those molecules of hormone that have greatest preservation of that conformation with maximum biological specificity. Indeed, the use of a physiologically specific receptor site with minimum nonspecific interactions represents an optimum means of purifying a hormone preparation.

Binding sites for calcitonin were detected in lymphoid cell lines of T-cell and B-cell types, in contrast to insulin and hGH receptors, which could be demonstrated only in B cells. However, there is a striking lack of receptors for calcitonin in cells derived from patients with Burkitt's lymphoma, similar to the findings demonstrated for insulin and hGH receptors (Marx *et al.*, 1974). There was wide variation in the specific binding of calcitonin to the cell lines, but the striking parallelism observed in patterns of binding between insulin and hGH did not hold for calcitonin receptors. Thus, the relative densities of insulin, hGH, and calcitonin receptors vary independently across numerous cell lines, with calcitonin showing the widest differences.

The biological significance of receptors for calcitonin on lymphoid cells remains unclear. Whitfield *et al.* (1970) reported that porcine calcitonin inhibited the cAMP-mediated mitogenesis in rat thymocytes. In later studies, these investigators showed that low concentrations of salmon calcitonin decrease the ability of PGE_1 to increase cAMP in thymic lymphoblasts, with a resultant decrease of cAMP-mediated DNA synthesis (Whitfield *et al.*, 1972). These effects were dose-dependent, and highly sensitive, entirely consistent with the presence of high-affinity receptors in these cells. The mechanisms responsible for the observed effects remain unclear, however, since calcitonin was shown to either promote or inhibit the progression of stimulated lymphoblasts into mitosis, depending on the extracellular calcium concentration and the magnitude of the hormone-induced initial increment in intracellular cAMP (Whitfield *et al.*, 1972).

7. Radioreceptor Assay of Polypeptide Hormones Using Lymphoid Cell Receptors

Up to this point, we have described how radioactivity labeled and native polypeptide hormones have served as a probe for the study of receptors. We will now focus on the use of well-characterized receptors and labeled hormones to detect the presence of native hormones and their derivatives. This concept was first applied by Korenman (1968) using tritiated estradiol-19β and a soluble binding protein from rabbit uterus supernatant in the study of estrogen binding. This concept was first applied to the study of polypeptide hormones by Lefkowitz *et al.* (1970b) using labeled ACTH and extracts from ACTH-sensitive adrenal tumors. Since then, the concept of radioreceptor assay for polypeptide hormones has experienced wide application (Schulster, 1974; Labrosse and Lakatua, 1975; Herington *et al.*, 1974; Korenman and Sherman, 1975; Gorden *et al.*, 1974; Landesman and Saxena, 1974; Turkington, 1971; Gavin *et al.* 1975).

Development of highly specific and sensitive radioreceptor assays has proceeded from the pioneering work of Berson and Yalow (1959), who introduced radioimmunoassay methodology in 1959 for the measurement of plasma insulin (see Chapter 15). This was the first assay generally applicable to all peptide hormones, and it served to promote the concept of "unity among the peptide hormones" (Roth, 1973). Furthermore, radioimmunoassay methods have recently been extended to a number of classes of compounds (e.g., steroids, cyclic nucleotides, antibiotics, prostaglandins, thyroid hormones), and this extension has had far-reaching biological consequences. Immunoassay affords great sensitivity in the measurement of polypeptide hormones in biological fluids and other media. This assay measures immunologic specificity, however, which is more often than not different from biological specificity. Antigenic determinants on a polypeptide may show tremendous variation from species to species; in fact, polypeptides may contain within the same molecule multiple regions varying appreciably in "antigenic potency." On the other hand, biologically active sites are felt to be less variable from species to species.

The radioimmunoassay and the radioreceptor assay are powerful complementary tools in the measurement of polypeptide hormones. Each technique has unique advantages as well as limitations. Radioimmunoassay affords a highly sensitive, widely applicable means of detecting determinants related to the antigen eliciting the test antibody. Assays can be routinely conducted on a large scale (in fact, they are sometimes automated), and are usually performed with no difficulty on plasma samples. Antisera and other agents can be easily stored for long-term use, and relatively small quantities of material are needed per individual determination. The assay is limited by its measurement of immunologic specificity, and there may be variability in the sensitivity of antisera directed at the same peptide (Berson and Yalow, 1968a,b; Herington *et al.*, 1974). The assays generally require a number of days before results are obtained. There have been reports of overnight immunoassays (Brown *et al.*, 1974), but such assays have not been generally applied.

Radioreceptor assay affords similar sensitivity, and further offers biological specificity. In general, the assays are rapid; results are obtained within hours. The assay is limited by the lack of receptor preparations amenable to long-term storage or to repetitive freezings and thawings. In receptor preparations, the contributions of hormone and receptor degradation must be assessed (Kahn *et al.*, 1974).

Immunoassay and receptor assays are *in vitro* assays, and are therefore subject to discrepancies in cases in which metabolism of hormone or hormone products plays a significant role. For example, antisera directed at different immunologic specificities in parathyroid hormone (PTH) give discrepant estimations of the level of circulating hormone in cases in which hormone fragments containing those specificities vary significantly in their biological turnover (Silverman and Yalow, 1973; Reiss and Canterbury, 1974). Hypothetically, in the case of receptor assays, underestimation of biological activity may occur in those cases in which hormone precursors, which show little bioactivity *in vitro,* are converted to more active forms at the target tissue or other peripheral sites.

The presence of highly sensitive, specific, well-characterized receptor sites on cultured lymphoid cells has been exploited in the development of radioreceptor assays applicable to insulin, hGH, calcitonin, and nonsuppressible insulinlike activity in plasma (NSILA). In this section, we shall discuss the development and applications of these assays.

7.1. Radioreceptor Assay for Insulin and Insulin-Related Peptides

The insulin receptors in cultured lymphoid cells have been thoroughly described. Radioactivity labeled insulin of high specific activity and the population of receptors available in a number of cultured lymphoid cells satisfy the essential requirements for a receptor assay. The stimulation of glucose oxidation in fat cells is a widely used standard method to determine the biopotency of insulin and related peptides. The ability of a given insulin preparation to inhibit binding of labeled insulin to lymphocytes or to purified liver membrane receptors is directly proportional to the potency of that preparation in stimulating glucose oxidation in fat cells *in vitro* (see Table 1). In contrast, radioimmunoassay may distinguish insulins of equal biopotency (Table 1), whereas preparations of very different biopotencies are poorly distinguished. For example, proinsulin, which is readily distinguished by receptor assay and bioassay, is poorly distinguished by standard immunoassay, and requires for such distinction antiserum directed against the connecting peptide (Melani *et al.*, 1970). The correlation between *in vitro* biopotency and radioreceptor activity for insulin and its analogues was extended to proinsulin and its related intermediates (Gavin *et al.*, 1975). The increased biopotency of these peptides *in vivo* is almost certainly due to their prolonged half-lives in the circulation (Chance,

1970). Radioreceptor assay in combination with immunoassay of insulin and proinsulin has provided useful information on the nature of the circulating forms of these hormones.

Gel filtration of plasma reveals at least two readily distinguished immunoreactive insulin components. The major, insulinlike component (ILC) elutes with labeled insulin and is indistinguishable from pancreatic insulin (Gavin *et al.*, 1975), while the less retarded component is proinsulinlike (PLC). The PLC usually constitutes 10–30% of the total immunoreactive insulin. Greater proportions may be seen in hypoinsulinemic subjects and in patients with islet cell tumors, in whom the PLC may constitute virtually all the immunoreactive insulin activity (Gorden *et al.*, 1971; Gutman *et al.*, 1971). When the ILC and PLC are completely separated by gel filtration, the ILC has the same activity as native insulin by radioreceptor assay. The PLC shows significantly less activity. When purified pancreatic proinsulins and proinsulin intermediates (Chance, 1970) are studied by receptor assay, considerable variation in biopotency is seen (Gavin *et al.*, 1975). When PLCs from a variety of plasmas were studied in the receptor assay, these components were more active than native or split proinsulin, but less active than desdipeptide or desnonapeptide proinsulin. These findings support the concept that the PLC is a heterogeneous substance comprising two or more closely related components (Gordon *et al.*, 1972; Gutman *et al.*, 1972). Furthermore, one form or another may predominate in different disease states (Berson and Yalow, 1971; Gorden *et al.*, 1971). Gorden *et al.* (1971) reported that the PLC of a patient with islet cell tumor showed greater biopotency (by fat cell bioassay) than a similar preparation from an obese patient. Subsequent comparison of PLCs from these patients in the radioreceptor assay revealed no difference in potency (Gavin *et al.*, 1975). However, the PLC from the islet cell tumor patient used for bioassay was collected and assayed at a different time from the preparation used for receptor assay. Because of the immunologic nonidentity of the islet cell tumor material (Gorden *et al.*, 1971), precise quantitation of the concentrations of material used for each assay could not be assured. Conclusions concerning differences in biopotency of the PLCs from patients with islet cell tumors compared with those from patients with other disorders must await simultaneous bioassay and receptor assay of a single lot of material.

The radioreceptor studies we have reported for insulin and related peptides were performed with isolated individual plasma components and purified pancreatic components. We have found in other studies that the assay can be performed with dilute unextracted plasma. However, the potency estimates for insulin activity derived from such studies reflect contributions from insulin and its derivatives, proinsulin and its derivatives, and the insulinlike activity in plasma that is measured by bioassay, but not by immunoassay, a preparation referred to as nonsuppressible insulinlike activity (NSILA). One component of this fraction, NSILA-s (soluble), was shown to have activity in the receptor assay commensurate with its biopotency in fat cells (see Table 1). It should be pointed out that NSILA-s may represent only a small portion of the total plasma NSILA, so comparisons of bioassay, receptor assay, and immunoassay results of unextracted plasma are subject to grossly imprecise quantitation.

In the lymphocyte receptor assay, serially purified NSILA-s preparations inhibit [^{125}I]insulin-binding to lymphocytes in direct proportion to their bioactivity in fat cells (Figure 7), although potency estimates of less-purified preparations are somewhat spurious in the lymphocyte assay. Of extreme interest are the elegant studies of Megyesi *et al.* (1974a,b, 1975) showing that although NSILA-s binds to the insulin receptor in a variety of tissues, there are unique receptors for this peptide in liver membranes. These receptors have been characterized and show striking differences from the insulin receptors of liver membranes or lymphocytes in optimum temperature for binding, in association and dissociation rates, in pH optima, and in their enormously greater affinity for purified NSILA-s than for purified insulin (Megyesi *et al.*, 1975). These receptors in liver membranes have been used to develop a specific radioreceptor assay for NSILA-s. Studies with this assay showed that in some patients with non-islet-cell tumors and hypoglycemia, there are 5- to 10-fold increases in levels of NSILA-s, while immunoreactive insulin levels are low or undetectable (Megyesi *et al.*, 1975). Thus, while the specific receptor assay for NSILA-s was developed in liver membranes, the lymphocyte insulin assay has been an important and useful tool in furthering these interesting and significant investigations.

In summary, the lymphocyte receptor assay enjoys the same sensitivity and ease of application as radioimmunoassay for insulin, and is simpler in design and execution than *in vitro* bioassay using isolated fat cells. All the cell lines in IRC-I

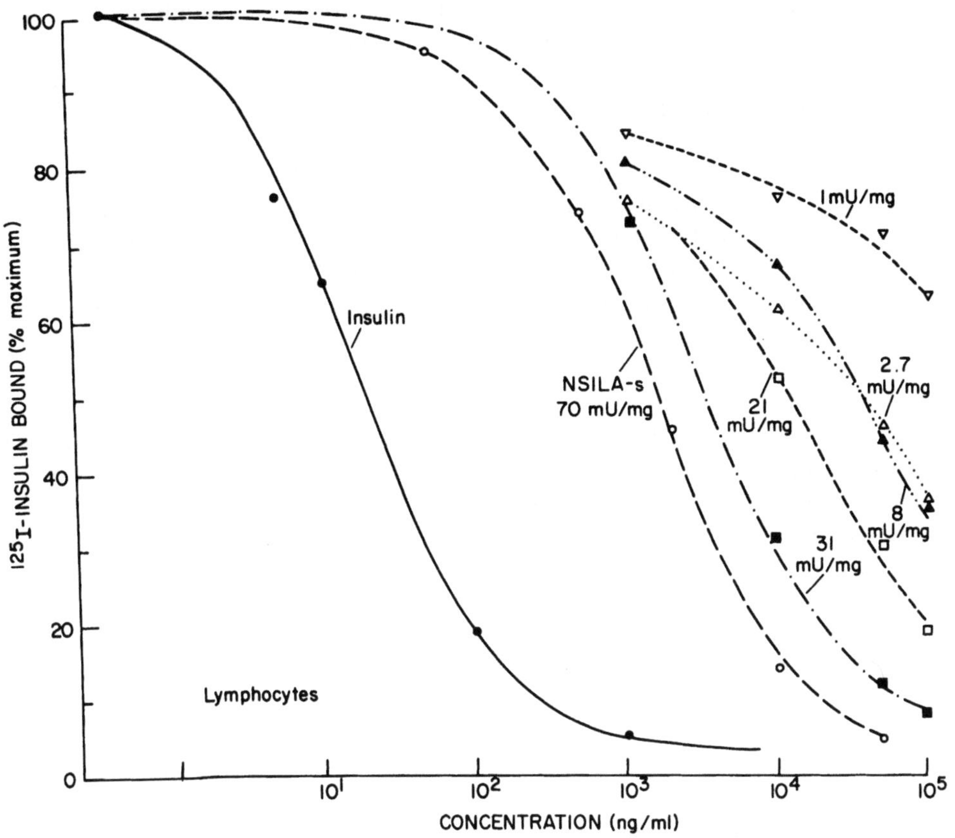

Figure 7. Effect of serially purified preparations of NSILA-s on labeled insulin-binding to its receptors in cultured human lymphocytes. Reproduced from Megyesi *et al.* (1975) with permission.

and many of those in IRC-II (see Table 2) have been found suitable as receptor preparations in our assays. The homogeneous nature of this receptor population would sharply limit interlaboratory variability that might be introduced into bioassay determinations by the use of enzymic digestion and other vigorous isolation techniques.

7.2. Radioreceptor Assay for hGH

Similar to the studies described for insulin, the specific receptors for hGH in cultured lymphoid cells were used to develop a sensitive receptor assay (Lesniak *et al.*, 1973). Since hGH is active only in humans, these cells offer the additional advantage of human origin. Development of this assay represents a significant advancement in the study of hGH, inasmuch as there has not been a simplified, sensitive, specific, quantitative *in vitro* assay for hGH. An additional GH receptor assay has been described by Tsushima and Friesen (1973), using liver membranes from pregnant rabbits. This assay was shown to be highly sensitive and capable of binding human, monkey, bovine, and ovine GH. The latter assay reflects the capacity of rodent membrane preparations to bind GH from a variety of species with comparable sensitivity. This finding parallels the well-known observation that the hypophysectomized rat is a suitable test animal for bioassay of multiple species of GH. No explanation for this difference has been found, although the homology among the various species has given much credence to the concept of an "active core" in all GH molecules (Kostyo, 1974). The availability of an hGH-specific radioreceptor assay combined with an assay with multiple specificities should allow more precise study of structure–function relationships. This combination should prove especially useful in the study of GH fragments, in which *in vivo* assays are complicated by problems of compartment distribution and turnover. Previous *in vitro* assays measuring [^{14}C]leucine incorporation in rat diaphragm (Nutting *et al.*, 1970), glucose oxidation in fat cells (H. M. Goodman, 1965), or lipolysis in isolated fat cells (Fain *et al.*, 1965) were generally limited by requirements of relatively high concentrations of hormone, cumbersome preparative techniques for the tissues, and imprecise quantitation.

Labeled hGH binds to cultured lymphocytes and is inhibited by physiologic concentrations of unlabeled hormone. Other species of GH have no activity even at high concentrations (Lesniak *et al.*, 1974). Assays of multiple GH fractions of variable purity reveal that with purification of the hormone, the radioreceptor potency increases relatively more than the bioassay potency (Lesniak *et al.*, 1974). Correlation between radioreceptor assay and radioimmunoassay is not so close as correlation between the receptor assay and the *in vivo* bioassays (Lesniak *et al.*, 1974). This disparity is especially marked during early stages of purification, in which immunologic potency increases more rapidly than receptor potency. This difference is explained by the presence of multiple forms of hGH in pituitary and plasma extracts (Bala *et al.*, 1970; Berson and Yalow, 1971; H. D. Goodman *et al.*, 1972; Gorden *et al.*, 1973). The major component corresponds to native ("little") hGH, while the larger component ("big" hGH) has roughly twice the apparent molecular weight of native hGH (Gorden *et al.*, 1973). An even larger immunoreactive species of hGH was described by Berson and Yalow (1971), although the significance of these differences in apparent size is not clear. The plasma or pituitary fraction corresponding to native hGH has approximately the same activity in the receptor assay as in the radioimmunoassay. On the other hand, the "big" hGH component has only 20% the potency in the receptor assay as in the radioimmunoassay (Gorden *et al.*, 1974). The radioreceptor assay represents at present the only available means of measuring the biological potency of the small quantities of high-molecular-weight GH components. The utility of cultured lymphoid cells in the study of hGH is further emphasized by the fact that the proposed mediator for much of the biological action of GH, somatomedin, can also be assayed by lymphocyte receptor assay using labeled insulin or labeled NSILA-s (Gavin *et al.*, 1973; Megyesi *et al.*, 1975).

7.3. Radioreceptor Assay for Calcitonin

Receptors for calcitonin on cultured lymphoid cells were used to develop a sensitive receptor assay similar in design to those described for insulin and hGH (Marx *et al.*, 1974). The potency estimates for calcitonin analogues are similar in this assay to those obtained using membranes from kidney or bone (Marx *et al.*, 1972). To date, no data have been presented on application of this assay to plasma components or related peptides.

8. Further Applications of Polypeptide Hormone Receptors on Lymphoid Cells

Since the initial description of insulin receptors on human circulating and cultured blood cells (Gavin *et al.*, 1972a), a tremendous wealth of information has accumulated concerning hormone–receptor interactions in a number of species and in a variety of *in vivo* and *in vitro* settings. The peripheral mononuclear cell has provided a means of directly studying alterations of insulin–receptor interactions in man (Archer *et al.*, 1973, 1975; Bar *et al.*, 1976a; Kahn *et al.*, 1976; Olefsky and Reaven, 1975; Amatruda *et al.*, 1975; Flier *et al.*, 1975) and in rodents (Mahler and Szabo, 1971; Kahn *et al.*, 1972, 1973; Kahn and Roth, 1975; Soll *et al.*, 1974, 1975). In addition to their usefulness in development of radioreceptor assays, cultured lymphoid cells have been especially useful for studying directly *in vitro* the ways in which hormone receptor concentrations and affinities are regulated by interaction with homologous hormone. In this section, we shall focus briefly on some of the significant developments in which receptors of lymphoid cells have played an important role.

8.1. Receptor Alterations in Metabolic Disorders

Of the insulin-resistant states in man, obesity is the most common. It was shown that the elevated concentrations of circulating insulin found in this condition are associated with decreased binding to peripheral mononuclear cells; calorie restriction was shown to return the receptors toward normal (Archer *et al.*, 1975; Bar *et al.*, 1976a). This pattern of decreased insulin receptors exactly parallels the observations in rodents with acquired or genetic forms of obesity (Kahn *et al.*, 1972, 1973; Soll *et al.*, 1975). Soll *et al.* (1974) further demonstrated that thymic lymphocytes of the genetically obese mice reflect the receptor deficiency demonstrated in liver and fat. These studies and others indicate that mechanisms exist whereby the hormone sensitivity of target tissues may be regulated by hormone-induced alterations in the available receptors. Another important development in this regard is the demonstration by Flier *et al.* (1975) of antibodies to insulin receptors in some diabetic patients with severe insulin resistence. This is a new concept in hormone resistance, and raises the possibility that spontaneous release of hormone receptors (Gavin *et al.*, 1972b; McGuffin *et al.*, 1976) may stimulate specific antibodies to the receptor. We await with extreme interest further developments along this line, since the functional significance of spontaneous release is at present unknown. Kahn and Roth (1975) provided an excellent summary of the studies in this area.

8.2. 'Down Regulation' of Hormone Receptors on Lymphoid Cells

The demonstration of decreased receptors in obese patients and animals with elevated hormone levels prompted investigation of an appropriate *in vitro* model for more detailed study of this phenomenon. The cultured human lymphocyte provided such a model. We demonstrated that chronic exposure of cultured lymphocytes to levels of insulin comparable to those attained in the *ob/ob* mouse (Figure 8) resulted in time- and temperature-dependent loss of insulin receptors from the cells (Gavin

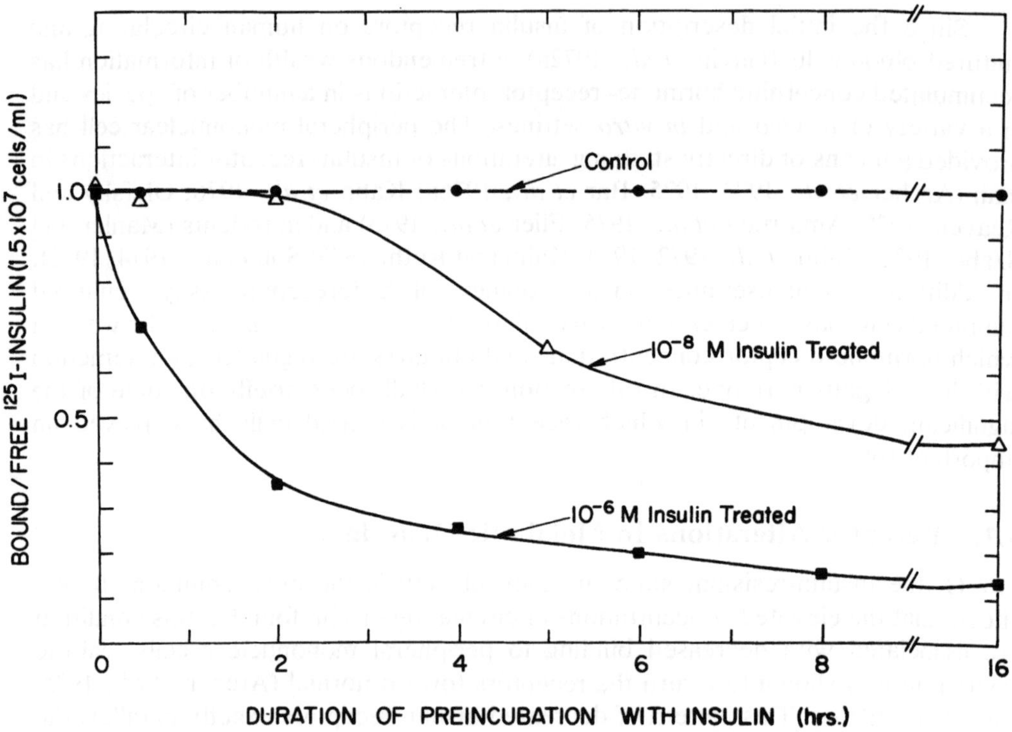

Figure 8. Effect of duration of exposure to unlabeled insulin on [^{125}I]insulin-binding to cultured human lymphocytes. Cells were tested for binding following indicated preincubation periods and thorough washings. Reproduced from Gavin *et al.* (1974) with permission.

et al., 1974). The remaining receptors remain unchanged in their binding properties. When insulin is removed from the medium, full restoration of receptor concentration is achieved in 16–18 hr. The reappearance is blocked by inhibitors of protein synthesis (Kosmakos, personal communication). A further demonstration of "down regulation" of surface receptors was achieved when Lesniak and Roth (1976) showed that hGH-binding to receptors in cultured cells could be reduced by as little as 2×10^{-10} M hGH. This effect was clearly distinct from receptor occupancy, and was due to loss of receptors, not to reduced affinity or loss of cells. The effect produced by exposure to hGH was clearly different from the effects of cycloheximide administration. Exposure to hGH resulted in no change in insulin-receptor concentration and vice versa. These and other studies suggest that hormone-induced loss of homologous receptors may be a widespread phenomenon and probably an important regulatory mechanism in the actions of many peptides. The exact mechanism(s) by which the receptor loss occurs remains obscure, although Huang and Cuatrecasas (1975) suggested the possibility that insulin-receptor loss is due to weak intrinsic proteolytic activity of insulin. No similar suggestions have been made to account for the effects of hGH or the numerous other peptides for which this phenomenon has been described. Further studies of "down regulation" of insulin receptors in cultured cells by Kosmakos and Roth (personal communication) indicate that insulin causes an acceleration of the rate of receptor degradation, although the overall process is complex.

8.3. Negative Cooperativity of Polypeptide Hormone Receptors on Lymphoid Cells

One of the most exciting developments in receptor methodology was the demonstration by De Meyts *et al.* (1973) that insulin-binding induces site–site interactions among the receptor sites wherein increased fractional occupancy results in decreased affinity of receptors for hormone (negative cooperativity). This phenomenon adds yet another means through which insulin receptors (and receptors for numerous other polypeptide hormones) are responsive to fluctuations in hormone concentration. Insulin induces the negative cooperativity under conditions under which insulin exists in monomeric form. The proposed model is one in which the insulin-receptor sites switch from a "slow-dissociating" state to a "fast-dissociating" state when their occupancy increases; the proportion of sites in each state is a function of occupancy of the receptor sites by the insulin monomer, as well as of the physicochemical environment (De Meyts *et al.*, 1976). The switch of the receptors to a low-affinity state is favored by decreases in pH and by increases in temperature, but these factors have a greater effect at low receptor occupancy (De Meyts *et al.*, 1976). These investigators suggest that insulin receptors may exist as oligomeric structures or clusters in the plasma membrane. Such models of conformational and topological alterations in the membrane on binding of hormone to specific receptors represent an extension of a phenomenon that has been observed for a variety of cell-surface markers. Surface rearrangements of this sort have been most extensively studied in lymphoid cells (Raff, 1976). The cultured lymphocyte is particularly suitable for study of morphological correlates of functional perturbations in the dynamic fluid membrane. The large number of well-characterized surface markers in these cells makes it possible to study interrelationships between surface molecules linked to metabolic responses and those linked to immune response mechanisms.

9. Conclusions

Lymphoid cells offer a versatile approach to the study of numerous surface molecules, including polypeptide hormone receptors. Peripheral and cultured lymphoid cell preparations have been used to characterize alterations of hormone-receptor interactions, and receptors in cultured cells constitute the basis for a powerful new biological assay. These cells have provided a means of examining the topological alterations in membrane structure subsequent to binding of numerous ligands, and these observations may now be extended to polypeptide hormones and their receptors.

Specific receptors on these cells make it possible to study relationships between hormone effects and immune response. Although receptors have been described only for insulin, hGH, and calcitonin, it is very likely that others exist. The availability of a large variety of lymphoid cells makes such screening a convenient endeavor. This report has touched only briefly on the myriad possibilities for future investigations made possible by the studies to date on polypeptide hormone receptors in lymphoid cells.

References

Amatruda, J. M., Livingston, J. N., and Lockwood, D. H., 1975, *Science* **188**:264–266.

Archer, J. A., Gorden, P., Gavin, J. R., III, Lesniak, M. A., and Roth, J., 1973, *J. Clin. Endocrinol. Metab.* **36**:627–633.

Archer, J. A., Gordon, P., and Roth, J., 1975, *J. Clin. Invest.* **55**:166–174.

Astaldi, G., Bargia, G. R., Astaldi, A., Jr., Yolcin, B., Meardi, G., and Gotti, G., 1972. *Lancet* **2**:709.

Baehner, R. L., 1973, *Adv. Pediatr.* **20**:323–351.

Bala, R. M., Ferguson, K. A., and Beck, J. C., 1970, *Endocrinology* **87**:506–516.

Bar, R. S., Gorden, P., Roth, J., Kahn, C. R., and De Meyts, P., 1976a, *J. Clin. Invest.* **58**(5):1123–1135.

Bar, R. S., Koren, H., and Roth, J., 1976b, *Diabetes, Suppl. 1*, p. 348.

Berson, S. A., and Yalow, R. S., 1959, *J. Clin. Invest.* **38**:1996–2016.

Berson, S. A. and Yalow, R. S., 1968a, *J. Clin. Endocrinol. Metab.* **28**:1037–1047.

Berson, S. A. and Yalow, R. S., 1968b, in: *Protein and Polypeptide Hormones*, Part I (M. Margoulies, ed.), *Int. Congr. Ser.* No. 161, pp. 36–44, Excerpta Medica, Amsterdam.

Berson, S. A. and Yalow, R. S. 1971, in: *Proceedings of the Eleventh Reunion of French Speaking Endocrinologists*, pp. 239–269, Masson and Cie, Paris.

Bianco, A. R., Schwartz, R. H., and Handwerger, B. S., 1974, *Diabetologia* **10**:359.

Bilezikian, J. and Aurbach, G. D., 1973, *J. Biol. Chem.* **248**:5577–5583.

Bourne, H. R., Lichlenstein, L. M., Melmon, K. L., Henney, C. S., Weinstein, Y., and Shearer, G. M., 1974, *Science* **184**:19–28.

Boyett, J. B. and Hofert, J. F., 1972, *Horm. Metab. Res.* **4**:163–167.

Brown, L. P., Besch, P. K., Buttram, V. C., Jr., Fleischer, N. S., and Skelley, D. S., 1974, *J. Lab. Clin. Med.* **84**:129–133.

Buell, D. N., and Gavin, J. R., III, 1973, *In Vitro* **8**:439.

Buell, D. N., and Gavin, J. R., III, 1977, *J. Natl. Cancer Inst.*, in press.

Chance, R. E., 1970, in: *Proceedings of the Seventh Congress of the International Diabetes Federation*, Buenos Aires, pp. 292–305, Excerpta Medica; Amsterdam.

Chandler, M. L., and Varandani, P. T., 1974, *Diabetes* **23**:232–239.

Chess, L., MacDermott, R. P., and Schlossman, S. F., 1974, *J. Immunol.* **113**:1113–1121.

Crofford, O. B., 1968, *J. Biol. Chem.* **243**:362–369.

Cuatrecasas, P., 1969, *Proc. Natl. Acad. Sci. U.S.A.* **63**:450–457.

Cuatrecasas, P., 1971, *Proc. Natl. Acad. Sci. U.S.A.* **68**:1264–1269.

Cuatrecasas, P., 1972, *J. Biol. Chem.* **247**:1980–1991.
De Meyts, P., Roth, J., Neville, D. M., Jr., Gavin, J. R., III, and Lesniak, M. A., 1973, *Biochem. Biophys. Res. Commun.* **55**:154–161.
De Meyts, P., Bianco, A. R., and Roth, J., 1976, *J. Biol. Chem.* **251**:1877–1888.
Dufau, M. L., Catt, K. J., and Tsuruhara, T., 1971, *Biochem. Biophys. Res. Commun.* **44**:1022–1029.
Eisen, S. A., Wedner, H. J., and Parker, C. W., 1972, *Immunol. Commun.* **1**:571–574.
Epstein, M. A., Achong, B. G., and Barr, Y. M., 1964, *Lancet* **1**:702–703.
Esmann, V., 1963, *Diabetes* **12**:545–549.
Fahey, J. L., Buell, D. N., and Sox, H. C., 1971, *Ann. N. Y. Acad. Sci.* **190**:221–234.
Fain, J. N., Scow, R. O., Urgoiti, E. J., and Chernick, S. S., 1965, *Endocrinology* **77**:137–149.
Fialkow, P. J., Klein, G., Gartler, S. M., and Clifford, P., 1970, *Lancet* **1**:384–386.
Fialkow, P. J., Klein, G., Giblett, E. R., Gothoskar, B., and Clifford, P., 1971, *Lancet* **1**:883–886.
Finn, F. M., Widnell, C. C., and Hofmann, K., 1972, *J. Biol. Chem.* **247**:5695–5702.
Flier, J. S., Kahn, C. R., Roth, J., and Bar, R. S., 1975, *Science* **190**:63–65.
Frazier, W. A., Boyd, L. F., and Bradshaw, R. A., 1973, *Proc. Natl. Acad. Sci. U.S.A.* **70**:2931–2935.
Freychet, P., Roth, J., and Neville, D. M., Jr., 1971, *Biochem. Biophys. Res. Commun.* **43**:400–408.
Freychet, P., Kahn, C. R., Roth, J., and Neville, D. M., Jr., 1972, *J. Biol. Chem.* **247**:3953–3961.
Fussganger, R., Kahn, C. R., Roth, J., and De Meyts, P., 1976, *J. Biol. Chem.* **251**:2761–2769.
Gavin, J. R., III, Roth, J., Jen, P., and Freychet, P., 1972a, *Proc. Natl. Acad. Sci. U.S.A.* **69**:747–751.
Gavin, J. R., III, Buell, D. N., and Roth, J., 1972b, *Science* **178**:168–170.
Gavin, J. R., III, Mann, D. L., and Roth, J., 1972c, *Biochem. Biophys. Res. Commun.* **49**:870–875.
Gavin, J. R., III, Gorden, P., Roth, J., Archer, J. A., and Buell, D. N., 1973, *J. Biol. Chem.* **248**:2202–2207.
Gavin, J. R., III, Roth, J., Neville, D. M., Jr., De Meyts, P., and Buell, D. N., 1974, *Proc. Natl. Acad. Sci. U.S.A.* **71**:84–88.
Gavin, J. R., III, Kahn, C. R., Gorden, P., Roth, J., and Neville, D. M., Jr., 1975, *J. Clin. Endocrinol. Metab.* **41**:438–445.
Gerber, P., Whang-Peng, J., and Monroe, J. H., 1969, *Bibl. Haematol. (Basel)* **36**:739–750.
Ginsberg, B. H., Kahn, C. R., and Roth, J., 1976, *Biochem. Biophys. Act.* **443**(2):227–240.
Glossman, H., Baukal, A., and Catt, K. J., 1974, *J. Biol. Chem.* **249**:664–666.
Goldfine, I. D., and Sherline, P., 1972, *J. Biol. Chem.* **247**:6927–6931.
Goldfine, I. D., Gardner, J. D., and Neville, D. M., Jr., 1972, *J. Biol. Chem.* **247**:6919–6926.
Goodman, H. M., 1965, *Endocrinology* **76**:216–225.
Goodman, H. D., Tanenbaum, R., and Rabinowitz, D., 1972, *J. Clin. Endocrinol. Metab.* **35**:868–878.
Gorden, P., Freychet, P., and Nankin, H., 1971, *J. Clin. Endocrinol. Metab.* **33**:983–987.
Gorden, P., Roth, J., Freychet, P., and Kahn, C. R., 1972, *Diabetes* **21***(Suppl. 2)*:673–677.
Gorden, P., Lesniak, M. A., Hendricks, C., and Roth, J., 1973, *Science* **182**:829–831.
Gorden, P., Lesniak, M. A., Hendricks, C. M., Roth, J., McGuffin, W., and Gavin, J. R., III, 1974, *Isr. J. Med. Sci.* **10**:1239–1246.
Greaves, M. F., and Brown, G., 1974, *J. Immunol.* **112**:420–423.
Gutman, R. A., Lazarus, N. R., Penhos, J. C., Fajans, S., and Recant, L., 1971, *N. Engl. J. Med.* **284**:1003–1008.
Gutman, R. A., Lazarus, N. R., and Recant, L., 1972, *Diabetologia* **8**:136–140.
Hadden, J. W., Hadden, E. M., Wilson, E. E., Good, R. A., and Coffey, R. G., 1972, *Nature (London) New Biol.* **235**:174–176.
Hammond, J. M., Jarrett, L., Mariz, I. K., and Daughaday, W. H., 1972, *Biochem. Biophys. Res. Commun.* **49**:1122–1128.
Haugaard, N. E., and Stadie, W. C., 1954, *J. Biol. Chem.* **211**:289–295.
Henle, W., and Henle, G., 1973, *N. Engl. J. Med.* **288**:264–168.
Herington, A. C., Jacobs, L. S., and Daughaday, W. J., 1974, *J. Clin. Endocrinol. Metab.* **39**:257–262.
House, P. D. R., and Wiedemann, M. J., 1970, *Biochem. Biophys. Res. Commun.* **41**:541–548.
Huang, D., and Cuatrecasas, P., 1975, *J. Biol. Chem.* **250**:8251–8259.
Johnson, C. B., Blecher, M., and Giorgio, N. A., Jr., 1972, *Biochem. Biophys. Res. Commun.* **46**:1035–1041.
Kahn, C. R., and Roth, J., 1975, *Am. J. Clin. Pathol.* **63**:656–668.
Kahn, C. R., Neville, D. M., Jr., Gorden, P., and Roth, J., 1972, *Biochem. Biophys. Res. Commun.* **48**:135–142.
Kahn, C. R., Neville, D. M., Jr., and Roth, J., 1973, *J. Biol. Chem.* **248**:244–250.

Kahn, C. R., Freychet, P., Roth, J., and Neville, D. M., Jr., 1974, *J. Biol. Chem.* **249**:2249–2257.
Kahn, C. R., Archer, J. A., Bar, R. S., Flier, J. S., Gorden, P., Martin, M. M., and Roth, J., 1976, *N. Engl. J. Med.* **294**:739–745.
Kammerman, S., and Canfield, R. E., 1972, *Endocrinology* **90**:384–389.
Kaplan, J., Mastrangelo, R., and Peterson, W. D., Jr., 1974, *Cancer Res.* **34**:521–525.
Katzen, H. M., and Vlahakes, G. J., 1973, *Science* **179**:1142–1143.
Koltai, M., Ottlecz, A., Minker, E., and Blazsó, G., 1974, *Int. Arch. Allergy* **46**:261–274.
Koltai, M., Blazsó, G., Minker, E., Lonovics, J., and Ottlecz, 1975, *Int. Arch. Allergy* **46**:261–274.
Kono, T., 1969, *J. Biol. Chem.* **244**:5777–5784.
Korenman, S. G., 1968, *J. Clin. Endocrinol.* **28**:127–130.
Korenman, S. G., and Sherman, B. M., 1975, *Semin. Nucl. Med.* **5**:263–272.
Kostyo, J. L., 1974, *Metabolism* **23**:885–899.
Krug, U., Krug, F., and Cuatrecasas, P., 1972, *Proc. Natl. Acad. Sci. U.S.A.* **69**:2604–2608.
Labrosse, M. S., and Lakatua, D., 1975, *Am. J. Clin. Pathol.* **63**:285–286.
Landesman, R., and Saxena, B. B., 1974, *Fertil. Steril.* **25**:1022–1029.
Lefkowitz, R. J., Pastan, I., and Roth, J., 1969, in: *The Role of Adenyl Cyclase and Cyclic 3′,5′-AMP in Biological Systems* (T. W. Rall, M. Rodbell, and P. Condliffe, eds), pp. 88–95, NIH Fogarty International Center Proceedings No. 4, Bethesda, Maryland, National Institutes of Health.
Lefkowitz, R. J., Roth, J., Pricer, W., and Pastan, I., 1970a, *Proc. Natl. Acad. Sci. U.S.A.* **65**:745–752.
Lefkowitz, R. J., Roth, J., and Pastan, I., 1970b, *Science* **170**:633–635.
Leidenberger, F., and Reichert, L. E., Jr., 1972, *Endocrinology* **91**:135–143.
Leroux, J. P., Marchand, J. C., Hong, R., and Cartier, P., 1975, *Eur. J. Biochem.* **58**:367–373.
Lesniak, M. A. and Roth, J., 1976, *J. Biol. Chem.* **251**:3720–3729.
Lesniak, M. A., Roth, J., Gorden, P., and Gavin, J. R., III, 1973, *Nature (London) New Biol.* **105**:20–22.
Lesniak, M. A., Gorden, P., Roth, J., and Gavin, J. R., III, 1974, *J. Biol. Chem.* **249**:1661–1667.
Lin, S.-Y. and Goodfriend, T. L., 1970, *Am. J. Physiol.* **218**:1319–1328.
Lundin, P. M. and Angerwall, L., 1970, *Pathol. Eur.* **5**:273–278.
Mahler, R. J., and Szabo, O., 1971, *Am. J. Physiol.* **221**:980–893.
Maor, D., Englander, T., Eylan, E., and Alexander, P., 1974, *Acta Endocrinol.* **75**:205–208.
Marx, S. J., Fedak, S. A., and Aurbach, G. D., 1972, *J. Biol. Chem.* **247**:6913–6918.
Marx, S. J., Woodard, C., Aurbach, G. D., Glossman, J., and Keutmann, H. T., 1973, *J. Biol. Chem.* **248**:4797–4802.
Marx, S. J., Gavin, J. R., III, Aurbach, G. D., and Buell, D. N., 1974, *J. Biol. Chem.* **249**:6812–6816.
Matsuoka, Y., Yagi, Y., Moore, G. E., and Pressman, D., 1969, *J. Immunol.* **102**:1136–1143.
McGuffin, W. L., Jr., Gavin, J. R., III, Lesniak, M. A., Gorden, P., and Roth, J., 1976, *J. Clin. Endocrinol. Metab.* **98**:1401–1407.
Megyesi, K., Kahn, C. R., Roth, J., Froesch, E. R., Humbel, R. E., Zapf, J., and Neville, D. M., Jr., 1974a, *Biochem. Biophys, Res. Commun.* **57**:307–315.
Megyesi, K., Kahn, C. R., Roth, J., and Gorden, P., 1974b, *J. Clin. Endocrinol. Metab.* **38**:931–934.
Megyesi, K., Kahn, C. R., Roth, J., Neville, D. M., Jr., Nissley, S. P., Humbel, R. E., and Froesch, E. R., 1975, *J. Biol. Chem.* **250**:8990–8996.
Melani, E., Rubenstein, A. H., Oyer, P. E., and Steiner, D. F., 1970, *Proc. Natl. Acad. Sci. U.S.A.* **67**:148–155.
Minowada, J., and Moore, G. E., 1975, *Bibl. Haematol. (Basel)* **40**:251–261.
Moore, G. E., and Minowada, J., 1973, *N. Engl. J. Med.* **288**:106.
Moore, G. E., Ito, E., Ulrich, K., and Sandberg, A. A., 1966, *Cancer* **19**:713–723.
Mowat, A. G., and Baum, J., 1971, *N. Engl. J. Med.* **284**:621–627.
Nutting, D. F., Kostyo, J. L., Goodman, H. M., and Fellows, R. E., Jr., 1970, *Endocrinology* **86**:416–419.
Olefsky, J. and Reaven, G. M., 1974, *J. Clin. Endocrinol. Metab.* **38**:554–560.
Olefsky, J. M., and Reaven, G. M., 1975, *J. Clin. Invest.* **54**:1323–1328.
Pallavicini, M. G., and Nichols, W. K., 1976, *Diabetes,* **25**(7):614–622.
Pastan, I., Roth, J., and Macchia, V., 1966, *Proc. Natl. Acad. Sci. U.S.A.* **71**:2407–2410.
Rabinowitz, D., Fowlkes, B. J., and Buell, D. N., 1974, presented at the Ninth Leukocyte Culture Conference.
Raff, M., 1976, *Nature (London)* **259**:265–266.

Rao, C. V., Saxena, B. B., and Gandy, H. M., 1972, *Excerpta Med. Int. Congr. Ser.*, No. 246, *Fourth International Congress of Endocrinology*, abstract No. 500.
Rawson, A. J., and Huang, T. C., 1975, *Cell. Immunol.* **17**:310–314.
Rechler, M. M., Podskalny, J. M., Goldfine, I. D., and Wells, C. A., 1974, *J. Clin. Endocrinol. Metab.* **39**:512–521.
Reiss, E., and Canterbury, J. M., 1974, *Recent Prog. Horm. Res.* **30**:391–429.
Rodbell, M., Krans, H. M. J., Pohl, S. L., and Birnbaumer, L., 1971, *J. Biol. Chem.* **246**:1861–1871.
Roth, J., 1973, *Metabolism* **22**:1059–1073.
Roth, J., Kahn, C. R., Lesniak, M. A., Gorden, P., De Meyts, P., Megyesi, K., Neville, D. M., Jr., Gavin, J. R. III, Soll, A. H., Freychet, P., Goldfine, I. D., Bar, R. S., and Archer, J. A., 1975, *Recent Prog. Horm. Res.* **31**:95–139.
Royston, I., Graze, P. R., and Pitts, R. B., 1974, *J. Natl. Cancer Inst.* **53**:361–367.
Schimmer, B. P., Ueda, K., and Sato, G. H., 1968, *Biochem. Biophys. Res. Commun.* **32**:806–810.
Schulster, D., 1974, *Br. Med. Bull.* **30**:28–31.
Schwartz, R. H., Bianco, A. R., Kahn, C. R., and Handwerger, B. S., 1975, *Proc. Natl. Acad. Sci. U.S.A.* **72**:474–478.
Silverman, R., and Yalow, R. S., 1973, *J. Clin. Invest.* **52**:1958–1971.
Smith, J. L., Klein, G. P., Barker, C. R., and Collins, R. D., 1973, *Lancet* **1**:74–77.
Soll, A. H., Goldfine, I. D., Roth, J., Kahn, C. R., and Neville, D. M., Jr., 1974, *J. Biol. Chem.* **249**:4127–4131.
Soll, A. H., Kahn, C. R., and Neville, D. M., Jr., 1975, *J. Biol. Chem.* **250**:4702–4707.
Stadie, W. C., Haugaard, N., Marsh, J. B., and Hills, A. G., 1949, *Am. J. Med. Sci.* **218**:265–274.
Stadie, W. C., Haugaard, N., and Vaughn, M., 1953, *J. Biol. Chem.* **200**:745–752.
Stobo, J. D., and Paul, W. E., 1972, *Cell. Immunol.* **4**:367–380.
Strom, T. B., Bear, R. A., and Carpenter, C. B., 1975, *Science* **187**:1206–1208.
Thomopoulos, P., Roth, J., Lovelace, E., and Pastan, I., 1976, *Cell,* **8**(3):417–423.
Thompson, E. E., Freychet, P., and Roth, J., 1972, *Endocrinology* **91**:1199–1205.
Tsushima, T., and Friesen, H. G., 1973, *J. Clin. Endocrinol. Metab.* **37**:334–337.
Turkington, R. W., 1970, *Biochem. Biophys. Res. Commun.* **41**:1362–1367.
Turkington, R. W., 1971, *J. Clin. Invest.* **50**:94A.
Weinberg, A. N., and Field, J., 1959, *Clin. Res.* **7**:247.
Whitfield, J. F., MacManus, J. P., and Gillan, D. J., 1970, *J. Cell Physiol.* **76**:65–76.
Whitfield, J. F., MacManus, J. D., Franks, D. J., Braceland, B. M., and Gillan, D. J., 1972, *J. Cell. Physiol.* **79**:353–362.

18

Assays for Cyclic Nucleotides Including Clinical Applications

RONALD G. COFFEY

1. Introduction

Biological regulation by cyclic nucleotides occurs in various forms in most, if not all, living cells. The effects of nearly all hormones and many drugs are mediated in part by changes in cellular levels of cyclic 3′,5′-adenosine monophosphate (cAMP) and cyclic 3′,5′-guanosine monophosphate (cGMP) (Sutherland and Robison, 1969; Robison *et al.*, 1971; N. D. Goldberg *et al.*, 1973a,b). Alterations of normal or resting as well as hormone-stimulated levels of both nucleotides have been discovered in human tissues, plasma, and urine in association with an impressive number of disease states. In clinical and experimental investigation, therefore, it is of the utmost importance that reliable and sensitive techniques for measurement of the cyclic nucleotides be employed.

The most commonly used methods were collected and published in Volume 2 of *Advances in Cyclic Nucleotide Research* (Greengard *et al.*, 1972). Included in this volume are refinements and theoretical discussions of the previously published protein-binding method of Gilman (1970) for measuring cAMP, now adopted for cGMP; the modification of this method by Brown *et al.* (1971); the protein kinase activation method of Kuo and Greengard for cAMP (Kuo and Greengard, 1970) and cGMP (Kuo and Greengard, 1972); the radioimmunoassay methods of Steiner *et al.* (1969) for both nucleotides; the enzyme recycling techniques of Goldberg and co-workers for cAMP (N. D. Goldberg *et al.*, 1969a) and cGMP (N. D. Goldberg *et al.*, 1969b); luminescence methods for cAMP (R. A. Johnson *et al.*, 1970; Ebadi *et al.*, 1971); the enzymatic displacement method of Brooker *et al.* (1968) for cAMP; and

RONALD G. COFFEY • Laboratory of Immunopharmacology, Memorial Sloan-Kettering Cancer Center, New York, New York 10021.

the high-pressure chromatography techniques of Brooker (1970), now adapted for both nucleotides. Finally, the radioactive adenine prelabeling methods of Kuo and DeRenzo (1969) and Humes *et al.* (1969) are discussed by Kebabian *et al.* (1972). The sensitivities of these methods are compared in Table 1.

Despite the various advantages offered by many of these methods, and several more recently published variations, the original procedures of Gilman (1970) for cAMP and of Steiner *et al.* (1969) for cGMP have remained the most popular and are used with certain modifications in our laboratory. The details of the other assays will not be repeated or reviewed here. Instead, we will present a brief outline of our current procedures for the extraction, purification, and assay of cAMP and cGMP, together with some insights regarding common pitfalls that may result in spurious measurements or interpretations. This essay will conclude with a discussion of some clinical applications of cyclic nucleotide measurements utilizing accessible body fluids and blood cells. Emphasis is placed on the dualism of regulation by cAMP and cGMP in lymphocyte biology in relation to the immune response as well as cell proliferation.

2. Extraction, Purification, and Measurement of Cyclic Nucleotides

2.1. Extraction

Glass-distilled water and the cleanest possible glassware are used throughout. Tissue samples are processed by the method of N. D. Goldberg *et al.* (1972). We employ the following method for extraction of cyclic nucleotides from cells in suspension:

1. A small volume of ice-cold 50% trichloroacetic acid (TCA) is added to the cell suspension, so that a final concentration of 10% TCA is achieved. Samples are vortexed immediately and stored frozen.
2. Samples are thawed, and a small volume of [^{3}H]cGMP (containing 2000 cpm, which is equivalent to 0.1–0.5 pmol, depending on specific activity) is added to each sample for estimation of cGMP recovery. One tube containing 10 pmol cAMP and 10,000 cpm [^{3}H]cAMP is included with each set of samples for estimation of cAMP recovery.
3. Protein is removed by centrifugation (3,000–10,000 rpm, 15 min, 0°C).
4. TCA is removed from the supernatants by five extractions with 2–3 vol water-saturated ether. Residual ether is removed by heating the tubes at 60–70°C with agitation for 5 min. Samples can be frozen at this step.

2.2. Purification

1. Samples are added to 0.5×3.5 cm columns of Dowex-1 formate (Murad *et al.*, 1971) (AG 1-X8, 100–200 mesh, Bio-Rad Laboratories, Richmond, California, converted from the chloride form by several washings with 0.5 N formic acid) and washed with 10 ml H_2O. cAMP is eluted with 10 ml redistilled 1 M formic acid, collected in a 15-ml conical tip glass tube, and dried in a rotary evaporator (Buchler Vortex-Evaporator, Fort Lee, New Jersey). cGMP is then eluted with 10 ml 4 M formic acid and similarly dried.

TABLE 1. Cyclic Nucleotide Assay Methods

Procedure	Purification[a]	Sensitivity (pmol)		References
		cAMP	cGMP	
Enzymatic displacement	Dowex-1 column, $BaSO_4$	25		Brooker *et al.* (1968)
High-pressure chromatography	As above + TLC	5	5	Brooker (1970)
Protein kinase activation	Dowex-50, alumina columns	0.3	0.5	Kuo and Greengard (1972)
Protein kinase activation	Dowex-1 column		0.5	Murad *et al.* (1971)
Luminescence	Dowex-50, QAE columns	0.1		R. A. Johnson *et al.* (1970)
Luminescence	Dowex-50 column	0.05		Ebadi *et al.* (1971)
Protein-binding	Dowex-1 column[b]	0.1	0.5	Gilman (1972)
Protein-binding	Alumina column		0.2	Kobayashi and Fang (1975)
Protein-binding		0.03		Brown *et al.* (1971)
Enzyme-cycling	TLC: Avicel (cAMP), silica (cGMP)	0.1	0.01	N. D. Goldberg *et al.* (1972)
Enzymic conversion to [^{32}P]GDP	QAE columns		0.1	G. Schultz *et al.* (1973a)
Radioimmunoassay (RIA)		0.05	0.1	Steiner *et al.* (1972)
RIA after succinylation		0.005	0.005	Cailla *et al.* (1973, 1976)
RIA after succinylation	Alumina, Dowex-1 columns		0.005	Asakawa *et al.* (1976)
RIA after succinylation or acetylation		0.005	0.005	Frandsen and Krishna (1976)
RIA after acetylation		0.005	0.005	Harper and Brooker (1975)

[a]Abbreviations: (TLC) thin-layer chromatography; (QAE) quaternary amino ethyl Sephadex A-25.
[b]Purification is recommended for cAMP and cGMP in liver and for all samples containing less than 2 pmol cAMP/mg protein.

2. cGMP is further purified using QAE-Sephadex A-25 formate (G. Schultz *et al.*, 1973a) (Pharmacia Fine Chemicals, Piscataway, New Jersey, converted from the chloride form by successively washing with 0.1 N NaOH, H_2O, 0.1 N formic acid, and H_2O). Samples are suspended in 2 ml H_2O and added to 0.8×4 cm disposable columns (Kontes Glass Company No. K-420160, Vineland, New Jersey) of QAE-Sephadex A-25 formate and washed successively with 10 ml H_2O and 10 ml 0.1 M ammonium formate, pH 9.0. cGMP is then eluted with 0.1 M ammonium formate, pH 6.0, discarding the predetermined eluate preceding the peak (usually 6–8 ml), and eluting the peak volume directly into a 0.8×4.5 cm column of Dowex-50^+ (AG 50W-X8, 100–200 mesh, Bio-Rad Laboratories, Richmond, California, prewashed with 1 N HC1 and H_2O). The eluates from the Dowex-50 columns and a final 2-ml H_2O wash are collected and dried as before.

2.3. Measurement

cAMP samples are suspended in a small volume of 10 mM Tris·HCl, pH 7.5, containing 2 mM $MgCl_2$. Aliquots are incubated 40 min at room temperature with 1–2 μl phosphodiesterase (Boehringer-Mannheim, New York, 10 mg/ml solution), then boiled 3 min. Treated and untreated samples are then assayed by the protein-binding method of Gilman (1970), using either the 50 or the 300-μl volume, depending on whether the aliquots are expected to possess less or more than 0.5 pmol, respectively (Gilman, 1972). The only modifications we have made in this procedure are: (1) addition of premixed sodium acetate buffer and [^{3}H]cAMP simultaneously and (2) counting the air-dried filters directly in toluene-based scintillation mixture without prior solvation with ethoxyethanol.

cGMP samples are similarly suspended and aliquots are treated with phosphodiesterase. They are then assayed essentially by the radioimmunoassay method of Steiner *et al.* (1972), using the reagents supplied by Collaborative Research, Inc., Waltham, Massachusetts. The second antibody may be omitted; the mixture of primary antibody, antigen ([^{125}I]2′-O-succinyl cGMP–tyrosine methyl ester), and unknown or standard in 50 mM NaOAc, pH 6.2, final volume 400 μl, is filtered as in the cAMP procedure. The membranes may be counted in a γ counter or suspended in toluene-based scintillation fluid and counted in a liquid scintillation counter using the channel setting for ^{3}H + ^{14}C.

Calculations of the cGMP levels in the original samples involve: (1) estimating picomoles of cGMP from the standard curve, usually plotted as percentage cGMP bound vs. log picomoles; (2) subtracting picomoles of cGMP found in the reagent blank; (3) subtracting the immunoinhibitory "cGMP-equivalent" picomoles found in the phosphodiesterase-treated aliquots; and (4) correcting the final value for recovery of tracer [^{3}H]cGMP. Until recently, the highest specific activity of [^{3}H]cGMP available was only 5 Ci/mmol, or 2000 cpm/0.45 pmol. Thus, if the sample appears to contain 1.0 pmol (equivalent to 10^6–10^7 cells of most origins), one must subtract half of this due to tracer! This fact placed one in the position of choosing very large sample sizes or omitting tracer. Currently available sources of [^{3}H]cGMP, specific activity 15 Ci/mmol, have reduced this correction by a factor of 3. The lower limit of sensitivity is correspondingly reduced, but remains at approximately 0.1 pmol if tracer is to be added. A final correction must be made if liquid scintillation counting under ideal (^{3}H + ^{14}C energy gates) conditions are used: the counts per minute of the tracer must be subtracted from the counts per minute of the ^{125}I prior to step 1 above.

Micromodifications of this procedure involving succinylation (Frandsen and Krishna, 1976) or acetylation (Harper and Brooker, 1975) of cGMP in the 2′-O position permit assay of as little as 5–10 fmol (10^{-14} mol) cGMP. Both procedures avoid the high concentration of succinate left in solution by the original procedure of Cailla *et al.* (1973), and employ ethanol or charcoal addition and centrifugation to separate bound from free cGMP. Cailla *et al.* (1976) recently stated that succinate did not interfere, while Asakawa *et al.* (1976) found it necessary to remove succinate prior to assay. Assays performed simultaneously by three methods are compared in Figure 1. The claim by Harper and Brooker (1975) that the extreme sensitivity of their method obviates the need to purify samples may depend on the nature of the samples; we have found it necessary to purify lymphocyte extracts as discussed below.

2.4. Strategic and Tactical Errors

The extensive literature on cAMP indicates that many investigators have measured effects of agents on this nucleotide alone. Since cGMP is now known to modulate several biological events, it is apparent that any serious effort to evaluate the mode of a hormone, drug, or other effector substance must include simultaneous measurements of both nucleotides. For example, it was thought that α-adrenergic vasoconstriction and smooth muscle contraction were caused by a lowering of cAMP, but new evidence indicates that increased cGMP is the more probable signal (Dunham *et al.*, 1974; G. Schultz and Hardman, 1975). Other examples include the mode of action of (1) secretin and pancreozymin, which were once thought to act through cAMP (Case *et al.*, 1969), and were recently shown by Thompson *et al.* (1974) and Haymovitz and Scheele (1976) to stimulate guanylate cyclase and cGMP levels in pancreas; (2) estrogen, which may indirectly stimulate adenylate cyclase (Szego and Davis, 1969), but which has a primary effect of stimulating cGMP levels

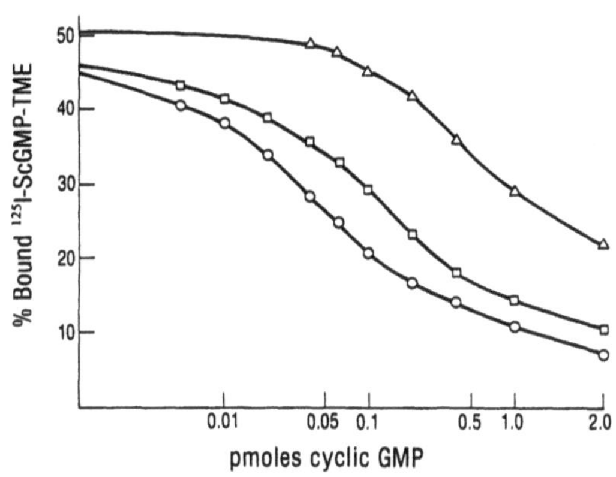

Figure 1. Assay of cGMP using the cGMP antibody and [^{125}I]2′-O-succinyl–cGMP tyrosine methyl ester antigen ([^{125}I]ScGMP–TME) provided by Collaborative Research. Except for the modification of separating antibody bound from free nucleotide by millipore filtration as described in the text, the procedures were as described by Steiner *et al.* (1972) for native cGMP (Δ——Δ), by Harper and Brooker (1975) for acetylated cGMP (□——□), and by Frandsen and Krishna (1976) for succinylated cGMP (○——○).

in the uterus (Kuehl *et al.*, 1974; Ham *et al.*, 1975); and (3) catecholamines, which were long thought to stimulate DNA synthesis in the parotid through elevation of cAMP (Guidotti *et al.*, 1972), but are now suspected to exert this effect by the α-adrenergic stimulation of cGMP levels (Durham *et al.*, 1974). However, even simultaneous assays of both cyclic nucleotides often go unrewarded because of specific errors in methodology.

Strategic errors are those involving incorrect concentrations of stimulants, sample size, incubation medium, time, temperature, and the method for ending the reaction. Each of these variables was examined briefly for lymphocyte cultures, and the accumulated data (Hadden *et al.*, 1975a, 1976; Coffey *et al.*, 1975; Coffey and Hadden, unpublished observations) are able to account for some discrepancies reported by various laboratories regarding lymphocyte cGMP stimulation by mitogens, acetylcholine (ACh), and other agents.

We noted an inverse relationship between basal cGMP levels and concentration of lymphocytes (Hadden *et al.*, 1975a). Between 1×10^6 and 5×10^6 cells/ml provide 0.05–0.2 pmol/10^6 cells, while progressively lower concentrations are measured when higher cell densities are used (Table 2). This difference may reflect difficulties in extracting cGMP from the larger cell masses, but we now believe this not to be true, since (1) recovery of added [^{3}H]cGMP is the same regardless of the cell number and (2) repeated extractions with TCA or other agents do not yield more cGMP from the larger cell samples. The differences may be due to a cell contact mechanism for reducing the resting level of cGMP, similar to that reported for confluent cell monolayers (N. D. Goldberg *et al.*, 1974a; Seifert and Rudland, 1974). Another aspect of cell density is the degree of response to mitogens. Schumm *et al.* (1974) obtained 70-fold increases with 1.5×10^6 cells/ml, while others found no increases with $10–100 \times 10^6$ cells/ml (see Table 3).

Incubation media vary with respect to divalent cation concentrations, serum content, presence of phosphodiesterase inhibitors, glucose, and other nutrients, type of buffer, and pH indicator. We have not investigated each of these, but suspect several effects, since Gillespie *et al.* (1974) reported large differences in leukocyte cAMP levels, depending on the nature of the buffer and the level of calcium ion, and since Ca^{2+} is essential to maintain basal levels of cGMP as well as to observe stimulation of cGMP levels by most agents (N. D. Goldberg *et al.*, 1973b; G. Schultz *et al.*, 1973b; G. Schultz and Hardman, 1975). The pH should be carefully regulated (Murad, 1973); additions such as aminophylline (10 mM) can increase the pH and correspondingly increase basal levels of cAMP (Logsdon *et al.*, 1973), thus masking a large fraction of the stimulation by catecholamines and other agents observed in the presence of theophylline at pH 7.4. Theophylline itself often confers unwanted side effects, including inhibition of basal activity (Pohl *et al.*, 1969; Rosen and Rosen, 1969) and catecholamine stimulation (H. Sheppard, 1970) of adenylate cyclase. While potentiation of a hormone effect with theophylline was once considered presumptive evidence for the participation of cAMP, it is now recognized that theophylline inhibits both cGMP and cAMP phosphodiesterases (N. D. Goldberg *et al.*, 1973a; N. D. Goldberg and Hadden, 1975), and can be expected to maintain stimulated levels of both nucleotides. Phenol red is a commonly used pH indicator, and yet interferes with the purification and assay of cGMP (N. D. Goldberg and Coffey, unpublished observations). Serum constituents have pro-

TABLE 2. Cyclic Nucleotide Variation with Leukocyte Concentration[a]

Cells[b]	Number of experiments	Cyclic GMP				Cyclic AMP			
		1	3	5	10	1	3	5	10
		(cells/ml × 10^6)				(cells/ml × 10^6)			
HPBL[c] (15)	1	0.60	0.47	0.42	0.35	39	33	29	29
ALL (2)	2	4.3	2.9	1.9	0.8	82	85	78	73
AML (1)	1	—	1.6	1.2	0.9	22	12	8	6
CLL (5)	5	8.7	4.0	3.7	1.9	40	32	29	26
CML (1)	1	7.2	2.3	1.4	0.6	173	37	26	10
L1210 (1)	1	9.2	3.1	2.0	1.0	7.5	3.6	3.0	2.1
Sezary (1)	1	3.3	1.7	1.0	0.5	131	110	87	61

[a]Data are given as picomoles nucleotide per milligram protein, representing the average of duplicate or triplicate assays for the number of experiments indicated in parentheses.

[b]Abbreviations: (HPBL) Human peripheral blood lymphocytes; (ALL) acute lymphocytic leukemia cells; (AML) acute myelogenous leukemia; (CLL) chronic lymphocytic leukemia; (CML) chronic myelogenous leukemia. Cells were suspended in Hank's buffer and inactivated with trichloroacetic acid, and the cyclic nucleotides were determined as described in the text.

[c]Human peripheral blood lymphocyte cyclic nucleotide levels in these experiments may be altered greatly by changing the constituents in the medium or the time of equilibration at temperature, and may vary approximately 4-fold depending on the donor.

TABLE 3. Effect of Proliferative Stimuli on Cyclic Nucleotide Levels

Cells[a]	Stimulus[a]	cGMP[a]	cAMP[a]	Notes[b]	References
Human					
PBL	PHA	ND	↑	A	J. W. Smith *et al.* (1971)
PBL	PHA, Con A	ND	0		DeRubertis *et al.* (1974)
PBL	PHA	ND	0		Glasgow *et al.* (1975)
PBL	Con A	0	↑	B	Lyle and Parker (1974)
PBL	PHA	0	↑	B	Wedner *et al.* (1975)
PBL	PHA, Con A	↑	0		Hadden *et al.* (1972, 1974)
PBL	PHA, Con A	↑	0		N. D. Goldberg *et al.* (1973b, 1974a,b)
PBL	PMA	↑	0		Estensen *et al.* (1974)
PBL	A23187	↑	0		Hadden *et al.* (1975a)
PBL	Con A, S-Con A	↑	↑	C	Hadden *et al.* (1976)
LNL	PWM	ND	0		R. S. Smith *et al.* (1974)
LNL	PHA	0	0	B	Weber and Goldberg (1976)
Mouse					
SL	Several	ND	0		DeRubertis *et al.* (1974)
SL	Several	0	0	D	DeRubertis and Zenser (1976)
SL	LPS	↑	0		Watson (1975)
SL	Con A	↑	0		Heidrick (1973)
SL	Con A	↑	0		Katagiri *et al.* (1976)
SL	SRBC	↑	↑	E	Yamamoto and Webb (1975)
SL	Periodate	↑	0		Haddox *et al.* (1976)

Rat					
PBL	PHA	↑	0		Schumm *et al.* (1974)
LNL	PHA	ND	0		Novogrodsky and Katchalski (1970)
TL	PHA	ND	0		Makman (1971)
TL	Con A	↑	↑	E	Whitfield *et al.* (1974)
Guinea pig					
LNL	Several	0	0	F	Burleson and Sage (1976)
SL	Periodate	↑	0		Haddox *et al.* (1976)
Mouse embryo					
Fibroblasts	Insulin	↑	0		N. D. Goldberg *et al.* (1974a,b)
Fibroblasts	Insulin, serum	↑	↓		Rudland *et al.* (1974a,b)
Fibroblasts	PMA	↑	↓		Estensen *et al.* (1974)
Fibroblasts	FGF	↑	0		Rudland *et al.* (1974a)
Fibroblasts	Virus	↑	↓		Moens *et al.* (1975)
Fibroblasts	FGF, virus, serum	↓	↓ or 0	G	Nesbitt *et al.* (1976)
Chick embryo					
Fibroblasts	Insulin, serum	0	0		Hovi *et al.* (1974)
Sea urchin					
Ova	Sperm	↑	0		N. D. Goldberg *et al.* (1973a, 1974a)

[a]Abbreviations and symbols: (↑) increase; (↓) decrease; (ND) not done; (Con A) concanavalin A; (FGF) fibroblast growth factor; (LNL) lymph node lymphocytes; (LPS) lipopolysaccharide; (PBL) peripheral blood lymphocytes; (PHA) phytohemagglutinin; (PMA) phorbol myristate acetate; (PWM) pokeweed mitogen; (S-Con A) succinylated Con A; (SL) splenic lymphocytes; (SRBC) sheep red blood cells; (TL) thymic lymphocytes.

[b]Notes: (A) Small increases in cAMP were attributed by others to leukogglutinating PHA; (B) lack of measured increase in cGMP may be due to failure to measure levels in the medium, poor purification procedures, and high cell densities; (C) agglutinating Con A increased cAMP at high doses that inhibit proliferation; S-Con did not; (D) lack of measured increase in cGMP may be due to heterogenous cell populations; (E) only the cGMP increases were correlated with proliferation by the authors; (F) lack of measured increases in cGMP may be due to timing, since this system requires macrophage processing of mitogen (Lipsky *et al.*, 1976); (G) rat kidney cells were also investigated, with similar results.

found influences on both cAMP and cGMP (Murad, 1973; N. D. Goldberg *et al.*, 1974a; Seifert and Rudland, 1974; Rudland *et al.*, 1974b; Astaldi *et al.*, 1976).

The time of incubation is critical for registering maximum increases in both cAMP and cGMP. Peak changes induced by catecholamines and ACh require only seconds to a few minutes in most cells, while lymphocytes develop maximum levels in 2–20 min. The rapid decline in peak levels of cAMP following catecholamine stimulation may be due to activation of phosphodiesterase (J. Schultz, 1975), a situation that apparently does not occur when prostaglandins of the E series are used. Rapid increases in cGMP are seen in most cells, and mitogens induce peak levels in lymphocytes at 1–20 min (Hadden *et al.*, 1972, 1975a; Estensen *et al.*, 1974; Schumm *et al.*, 1974; Haddox *et al.*, 1976). Neutrophil cGMP levels may reach a peak as early as 2 sec following stimulation (see Chapter 4). It is suspected that cGMP may be a signal for mast cell degranulation (Coffey and Middleton, 1973; W. A. Taylor and Sheldon, 1974), and if this proves to be true, one would expect increases within 1 sec following addition of compound 48/80, which induces release within this period of time. Gillespie (1973) reported a lowering of cAMP levels at 30 sec, but whether this decrease is actually a signal causing degranulation (Lichtenstein, 1973) or is a delayed consequence of increased cGMP levels often observed in other systems (N. D. Goldberg *et al.*, 1974a,b, 1975) remains to be tested. In any event, careful timing of the reaction must be employed to interpret the data properly. Preincubation times may also be critical, since agents such as sodium diatrizoate, used in preparing the cells, can temporarily alter cyclic nucleotide levels (Patrick *et al.*, 1975).

Physiologic temperatures must also be used to avoid artifacts involving different profiles of enzyme and receptor responses at various temperatures: (1) Apparent interconversion of both adrenergic (Amer and Byrne, 1975) and histamine (Kenakin *et al.*, 1974) receptors occurs between room temperature and 37°C. (2) Activation energies and transition point changes vary widely among regulatory enzymes; one consequence is a relatively greater activity at low temperatures for cyclic nucleotide phosphodiesterases than for the cyclases (N. D. Goldberg *et al.*, 1973a). Another consequence is the perturbation of intracellular cation levels so vital to both cyclases caused by inactivation of the cation pump ATPase activities at low temperature.

The method for ending the reaction should be swift for the time and temperature reasons cited above (see also Kimura *et al.*, 1974). Centrifuging cells and discarding the medium eliminates many substances that interfere with both the Gilman and the Steiner method, thus reducing the necessity for purifying the nucleotides. However, the time required to centrifuge produces ambiguity in placing the peak time of nucleotide production, adds the cell-crowding artifact discussed above, and probably alters the relative and absolute concentrations of the nucleotides due to temperature changes during centrifugation. In addition, we found a greater leak of cGMP than of cAMP from cells to the medium, accounting for over half the mitogen-stimulated increases (Hadden *et al.*, 1975a; Coffey *et al.*, 1975). Burleson and Sage (1976) also reported significant levels of cGMP but not cAMP in the medium following lymphocyte incubations. Other cells undoubtedly leak proportionately greater amounts of cGMP than cAMP, since the ratio of cGMP to cAMP in most tissues is 0.01–0.1, while the ratio in urine is 0.2–0.3 (N. D. Goldberg *et al.*, 1973a; Ball *et al.*, 1972). Boiling may produce high levels of nonenzymatically formed cGMP (Kimura and Murad, 1974), and should be avoided unless samples are first acidified. For these reasons, we have elected to end the reaction by adding an agent such as TCA to the entire cell incubation mixture, rather than to subsequently isolated cells.

Tactical errors are those involved in purification and assay. For example, insufficient ether extraction leaves traces of TCA, which interfere with the protein-binding assay for cAMP (Wright and Price, 1975). Many investigators employ at least one purification step, but some do not, citing the linearity of graphs of nucleotide level vs. sample size. Several investigators documented the importance of purifying cGMP (Murad *et al.*, 1971; N. D. Goldberg *et al.*, 1972, 1974a; Stoner *et al.*, 1974; Yamamoto and Webb, 1975), and Gilman (1972) showed that cAMP must also be purified if its level is less than 2 pmol/mg protein. While the assay methods are sufficiently specific for nucleotides, it is our experience that other components of the reaction mixtures interfere with both assays, and most of these components are conveniently removed by the Dowex-1 formate column (Murad *et al.*, 1971). The column also removes theophylline, which may interfere with the radioimmunoassay for cGMP (Wedner *et al.*, 1975). Lymphocyte cultures, however, contain unknown interferents that must be removed by a second purification step (Burleson and Sage, 1976; N. D. Goldberg *et al.*, unpublished observations). We have found the QAE-Sephadex columns (G. Schultz *et al.*, 1973a) satisfactory for this purpose; other methods such as silica thin-layer chromatography (N. D. Goldberg *et al.*, 1972) or alumina columns (Ham *et al.*, 1975) may work equally well. One method of establishing the degree of purification needed is simply to compare the results obtained before and after each step, including reagent blanks and phosphodiesterase-treated aliquots of the samples. In addition, we recommend adding a known amount of standard to aliquots of samples to test whether this increment is accurately measured. Using the latter test, we found that even the succinylation (Frandsen and Krishna, 1976) or acetylation (Harper and Brooker, 1975) modifications of the method of Steiner *et al.* (1969), while producing excellent standard curves from 5 to 100 fmol, are not adequate for measuring cGMP levels in lymphocyte cultures unless the second purification step has been used.

While a description of all the substances that interfere with the radioimmunoassay of cGMP is not yet available, serious attempts (Burleson and Sage, 1976; Coffey and Hadden, in preparation; Webb, personal communication; N. D. Goldberg and Haddox, personal communication) have yielded the following information:

1. Components of Hank's buffer and other culture media inhibit the assay of known amounts of cGMP while producing a high "blank" value that is not destroyed by phosphodiesterase. These components are mostly (but not entirely) removed by the Dowex-1 column. The subsequent Sephadex column completely removes them.
2. Phenol red interferes with the assay of cGMP and is not removed by the Dowex-1 column, but can be removed by the Sephadex column. However, cGMP yields are lower when purified from phenol-red-containing mixtures.
3. Materials present in lymphocytes are both immunoinhibitory and immunoenhancing, and may produce a net result that involves both an underestimation of the stimulated level of cGMP and an under- or overestimation of the resting or control level. Preliminary experiments in our laboratory

indicate that mitogen-stimulated lymphocytes contain a substance that binds cGMP, obscuring its measurement prior to the Sephadex step. All these materials are removed by the three-step procedure outlined above, while the Dowex-1 column removes only the immunoenhancing substances.
4. Impurities in formic acid, used to develop the Dowex-1 columns, are immunoinhibitory and not destroyed by phosphodiesterase. These impurities can be avoided by using freshly redistilled formic acid or removed by the subsequent Sephadex columns.

Applying the considerations outlined above to the problem of demonstrating cGMP increases in cells following the addition of proliferative stimuli, it is possible to understand why some experiments have failed (see Table 3). The disparity in experimental data can be attributed in most cases to the overlooking of one or two simple but vital precautions, and yet it is unfortunate that so much labor has been expended on the attempt to demonstrate a single concept. Difficulties are being circumvented by use of other approaches, however, and three laboratories have succeeded in measuring increased guanylate cyclase activity following exposure of lymphocytes (Deviller *et al.*, 1975; Katagiri *et al.*, 1976) or adipocytes (Hollenberg and Cuatrecasas, 1975) to mitogens.

Human urinary excretion of cAMP and cGMP normally ranges from 2.2 to 4.2 and 0.16 to 1.38 μmol/day, respectively (Murad, 1973), so both assays can be readily performed on 0.5- to 5-μl samples with no prior treatment other than protein removal and neutralization. Plasma concentrations are considerably lower and require some purification prior to assay.

2.5. Application of Sutherland's Criteria to Cyclic GMP

If the precautions discussed in the preceding section are observed, the investigator should be able to register appropriate increases in cyclic nucleotide levels following addition of a hormone or other agent to cells, thus satisfying the first of the four criteria for the second messenger hypothesis of Sutherland (Sutherland and Robison, 1969; Robison *et al.*, 1971). One final strategic error may result, however, from attempts to satisfy the second criterion—that exogenously added cyclic nucleotides or their more lipophilic butyrated derivatives should mimic the action of an effector substance (Robison *et al.*, 1971). One may properly question puzzling results ensuing from this approach for the following reasons:

1. Dibutyryl cAMP quickly decomposes to monobutyryl cAMP in mildly aqueous buffers (Swislocki, 1970).
2. The free butyrate is then able to stimulate adenylate cyclase in some systems (Ryan and Heidrick, 1974).
3. Dibutyryl cAMP does not penetrate all cells as well as cAMP (Ryan and Durrick, 1972).
4. Dibutyryl cAMP and cAMP may bind to different intracellular proteins (Filler and Litwack, 1973), resulting in opposite biological effects in some tissues (Hilz and Tarnowski, 1970; Solomon *et al.*, 1970; Ryan and Heidrick, 1974).
5. Exogenously added cAMP may cause increased intracellular cGMP (Ide, 1969).

The third criterion—that the agent, when added to broken cells, should stimulate the cyclase enzyme—has usually failed for cGMP-related agents (N. D. Goldberg *et al.*, 1973b; N. D. Goldberg and Hadden, 1975). This failure may be attributed mostly to the loss of intact membrane receptor and calcium transport systems.

The fourth criterion—that the action of the agent should be potentiated by phosphodiesterase inhibitors—has not been rigorously applied for cGMP-related agents because most such inhibitors block both cAMP and cGMP phosphodiesterases, producing elevations in both nucleotides and mimicking cAMP predominant effects (N. D. Goldberg and Hadden, 1975). The use of imidazole as a selective inhibitor of cGMP phosphodiesterase has been of value in satisfying this requirement for cGMP as a second messenger.

3. Clinical Applications

3.1. Diseases with Cyclic Nucleotide Abnormalities

Excellent reviews of this subject have been written by Murad (1973), N. D. Goldberg and Hadden (1975), and Hadden (1975b), and prior to the completion of this chapter, a book totally devoted to this subject has appeared (Weiss, 1975a), eliminating the need to present here anything more than a brief outline.

Considering the numerous effects in which cAMP and cGMP are known to play roles, it is obvious that abnormalities in either formation, function (e.g., protein kinase activation), or degradation of the nucleotides may contribute to a variety of abnormal clinical states. Over 40 such states are listed in Table 4, which includes some drug-induced disorders, and this list is by no means complete. Many more certainly await discovery as research into hormone receptors and cyclic-nucleotide-binding proteins continues to expand. Among the various abnormalities now partially understood, the following categories of possibilities emerge: (1) abnormal basal activities of the generating enzymes, adenylate cyclase and guanylate cyclase; (2) abnormal responsiveness of the generating enzymes to hormones, drugs, and other agents; (3) abnormal phosphodiesterase activities or subcellular locations; (4) abnormal phosphodiesterase regulator protein activities; (5) abnormal levels or functioning of protein kinases and other cyclic-nucleotide-binding proteins; (6) abnormal levels of protein kinase inhibitory and modulator proteins; and (7) abnormal degrees of leakage or secretion of cyclic nucleotides from cells.

Subcategories may appear involving abnormal subcellular distribution of the enzymes enumerated above, abnormal phospholipid environments of membrane-bound enzymes, and altered levels of bound or free cations. Thus, diseased tissue may respond abnormally to a hormone, while cell-free preparations may show an apparent normal response due to the removal of an inhibitory constituent. Almost all endocrine and exocrine disorders are expected to involve cyclic nucleotide abnormalities, either in the hormone-generating tissue or in receptors of the target tissues. In the former case, a dual abnormality would result, as discussed below for diabetes. Similar two-tissue defects can readily be envisioned for pituitary and the trophic hormone target tissues. A variety of disorders associated with growth and development may be related to defects in the two cyclic nucleotide-dependent

TABLE 4. Disorders Involving Cyclic Nucleotide Abnormalities

Disorder	Observation[a]	References
Heart failure	↓ Cardiac a.c.	Sobel *et al.* (1969)
Heart failure	↓ Cardiac a.c. response to glucagon	Gold *et al.* (1970)
Hypertension	↑ Arterial g.c.	Amer *et al.* (1974)
Cancer (nonendocrine)	↑ Urinary cGMP	Murad *et al.* (1975b)
Hypoparathyroidism	↓ Urinary cAMP	A. L. Taylor *et al.* (1970)
Hyperparathyroidism	↑ Urinary cAMP	A. L. Taylor *et al.* (1970)
Parathyroid adenoma	↑ Urinary cAMP	A. L. Taylor *et al.* (1970)
Renal disease	↓ Urinary cAMP	A. L. Taylor *et al.* (1970)
Renal failure	↓ Urinary cAMP and cGMP	Hamet *et al.* (1975)
Renal failure	↑ Plasma cAMP and cGMP	Hamet *et al.* (1975)
Pseudohypoparathyroidism	↓ Urinary cAMP response to PTH	Chase *et al.* (1969)
Hyperthyroidism	↑ Urinary and thyroid cAMP	Rosen (1972), Levey *et al.* (1969)
Hypercalcemia	↓ Urinary cAMP, ↑ cGMP	Chase and Aurbach (1967), Murad (1973)
Basal cell nevus syndrome	↓ Urinary cAMP, ↓ response to PTH	Aurbach *et al.* (1970)
Gardner's syndrome	↑ Urinary cAMP, ↓ response to PTH	Aurbach *et al.* (1970)
Vit.-D-resistant osteomalacia	↑ Urinary cAMP, ↓ response to PTH	Aurbach *et al.* (1970)
Basal ganglia calcification	↑ Urinary cAMP, ↓ response to PTH	Aurbach *et al.* (1970)
Hepatoma	↑ Particulate g.c.	Kimura and Murad (1975)
Grave's disease	↑ Thyroid cAMP due to ↑ LATS	Levey and Pastan (1970)
Osteogenesis imperfecta	↑ Platelet (and bone?) cAMP	Solomons and Millar (1972)
Cystic fibrosis	↓ Urinary cAMP, ↑ cGMP	Murad *et al.* (1975a)
Diabetes mellitus	↑ cAMP in fat, liver, etc.	Tucci *et al.* (1973)
Diabetes mellitus	↓ cAMP-PDE, pancreas	Das (1973)
Diabetes (alloxan)	Altered pancreatic and adipose modulator of cAMP- and cGMP-dependent PK	Kuo (1975a)

Nephrogenic diabetes insipidus	↓ Urinary cAMP, ↓ response to ADH, PTH, glucagon	cf. Murad (1973)
Idiopathic edema	↑ Plasma cAMP	Kuchel *et al.* (1975)
Cholera	↑ Intestinal a.c.	Sharp *et al.* (1971)
E. coli infection	↑ Intestinal a.c.	Evans *et al.* (1972)
Depression	↓ Urinary cAMP	Abdulla and Hamadah (1970)
Mania	↑ Urinary cAMP	Paul *et al.* (1970)
Grand mal seizures	↑ Forebrain cAMP	Sattin (1971)
Schizophrenia	↑ Dopamine-stimulated cAMP, brain	Iversen (1975)
Parkinson's disease	↓ Dopamine-stimulated cAMP, brain	Iversen (1975)
Myasthenia gravis	↓ Neuromuscular responses to acetylcholine	Goldstein (1975)
Psoriasis	↓ Epidermal cAMP, ↑ cGMP	Voorhees *et al.* (1973)
Asthma	↓ β-Adrenergic cAMP responses	Chapt. 11, Sect. 3.3
Starvation	↓ Heart modulator of cAMP-PK	Walsh and Ashby (1973)
Drug-induced		
Sulfonylurea		
Cardiovascular death	↑ Heart a.c.	Levey *et al.* (1971)
Other dysfunctions	↑ Kidney, pancreas cAMP-PDE	Brooker and Fichman (1971)
Ouabain toxicity	↓ Thyroid cAMP response to TSH	Burke (1970)
Lithium		
Thyroid dysfunction	↓ Thyroid cAMP response to TSH	Forrest (1975)
Kidney dysfunction	↓ Kidney cAMP response to ADH	Forrest (1975)
Morphine		
CNS depression	↑ Neural cell cGMP	Gullis *et al.* (1975)
Dependence	↓ Neural cell a.c., then ↑ basal a.c.	Sharma *et al.* (1975)
Isoniazid: convulsion	↑ Cerebellar cGMP	Mao *et al.* (1975)
Diazepam: anticonvulsant	↓ Cerebellar cGMP	Mao *et al.* (1975)

[a]Abbreviations: (a.c.) Adenylate cyclase; (g.c.) guanylate cyclase; (PTH) parathyroid hormone; (PDE) phosphodiesterase; (PK) protein kinase; (ADH) antidiuretic hormone; (TSH) thyroid-stimulating hormone.

protein kinases, the levels of which change notably (and reciprocally) in lung, heart, and brain of experimental animals during development and aging (Kuo, 1975b).

In most cases, it cannot be assumed that the first cause of these abnormal states is the abnormal functioning of the cyclic nucleotide system. On the other hand, it is obvious that a severely abnormal functioning of the system, due to whatever cause, may aggravate or actually mediate the process that results in clinical symptoms. That it may is particularly well documented for certain bacterial infections. A *Bordetella pertussis* product causes reduced basal cAMP levels as well as β-adrenergic subresponsiveness (Parker and Morse, 1973) and heightened cGMP responses to histamine (Polson *et al.*, 1974). An exotoxin of *Bacillus thurigensis* also inhibits adenylate cyclase (Graham-Smith *et al.*, 1975). Enterotoxins of *Vibrio cholerae* (Sharp *et al.*, 1971; Schafer *et al.*, 1971) and *Escherichia coli* (Evans *et al.*, 1972) cause enormous stimulation of adenylate cyclase activity of intestine and all other tissues tested to date, and inhibit guanylate cyclase and cGMP phosphodiesterase (Kiefer *et al.*, 1975). The lipopolysaccharide of bacterial endotoxins stimulates cGMP levels of bone-marrow-derived lymphocytes (Watson, 1975).

The simplest clinical applications of cyclic nucleotide assays involve plasma and urine. These fluids normally show prompt increases in cAMP levels following infusion of epinephrine and glucagon, while increases primarily in the urine result from administration of PTH (Chase and Aurbach, 1967; Murad, 1973). cGMP increases are seen following administration of Ca^{2+}, ACh, calcitonin (N. D. Goldberg *et al.*, 1974a), or epinephrine plus a β-adrenergic blocking drug (Ball *et al.*, 1972). Since the kidney is the source of about one-third of urine cAMP, some renal diseases are accompanied by greatly reduced urine cAMP (Taylor *et al.*, 1970; Hamet *et al.*, 1975). Hypoparathyroidism is also associated with reduced cAMP excretion, which can be normalized by PTH administration, while hyperparathyroidism and parathyroid adenoma cause greatly elevated cAMP excretion (Taylor *et al.*, 1970). Among parathyroid-refractory syndromes, Aurbach *et al.* (1970) found reduced cAMP excretion in basal cell nevus syndrome and increased levels in Gardner's syndrome, vitamin-D-resistant osteomalacia, and basal ganglia calcification. Diabetes mellitus, which may involve reduced cAMP production in the pancreas, as postulated by Sutherland and Robison (1969) and Sutherland (1970), is associated with increased urinary cAMP, which probably originates in liver, adipose, and other peripheral tissues due to unregulated epinephrine stimulation, and is reversed by insulin administration (Tucci *et al.*, 1973). An intriguing correlation between these levels and the protein kinase modulator protein (inhibitor of cAMP and stimulator of cGMP protein kinase) was recently found in pancreas and adipose tissues of alloxan-diabetic rats (Kuo, 1975a).

Asthma involves reduced β-adrenergic responsiveness in several cells besides the lung, as demonstrated by the urinary studies of Bernstein *et al.* (1972). Glucocorticosteroid therapy causes increased cAMP excretion in asthmatics, possibly by restoring responsiveness to endogenous catecholamines (Chapter 11), and probably decreases cGMP (N. D. Goldberg *et al.*, 1973b) (see also Chapter 4). Depression and mania are associated with, respectively, greatly reduced and elevated levels of urinary cAMP (Abdulla and Hamadah, 1970; Paul *et al.*, 1970), which may not be assumed to originate entirely from the affected tissue, since the CNS regulates so many bodily functions. It will be of great interest to test whether antipsychotic treatments are associated with restoration to normal of these levels as suggested by some results: (1) tricyclic antidepressants, such as imipramine, increased cAMP levels in brain (Kodama *et al.*, 1971); and (2) dopamine antagonists in use for schizophrenia blocked the dopamine-induced stimulation of brain adenylate cyclase (Iversen, 1975). On the other hand, lithium treatment for affective disorders blocks stimulation of adenylate cyclase in the thyroid by TSH and in the kidney by vasopressin, and incautious use of this agent leads to diabetes insipidus (Forrest, 1975).

Unfortunately, cGMP was not measured in the studies cited above. Due to the frequently observed reciprocal responses of cGMP and cAMP to many hormones (N. D. Goldberg *et al.*, 1973b, 1974a,b, 1975; N. D. Goldberg and Hadden, 1975), one might expect diabetes to be associated with reduced cGMP excretion, while asthma attacks would correlate with increases. The latter possibility is supported by PGF2α-provocation tests (Alston and Coffey, unpublished observations). By simultaneously measuring both cGMP and cAMP excretion, Murad *et al.* (1975a) were able to measure marginal abnormalities of each in cystic fibrosis, but a significant reduction in the cAMP:cGMP ratio.

Cyclic nucleotide assays will certainly be of diagnostic value for many conditions in which only one abnormality involving the cyclic nucleotide system is apparent, and in which urine or plasma levels can be shown to accurately reflect the clinical condition. One must exercise caution in interpreting data from such tests, since natural fluctuations due to diurnal rhythms, menstrual cycle, and pregnancy are notable, and vary from subject to subject (A. L. Taylor *et al.*, 1970; Murad, 1973). Exercise and methyl xanthines do not appear to affect cAMP, but caffeine may increase cGMP excretion by 25–40% (Murad, 1973). The future of clinical usefulness of cyclic nucleotide assays in diseases that involve significant alterations in tissue but not plasma or urine levels will depend primarily on the availability of biopsied material and specific catheterization techniques. However, saliva, CSF, milk, and seminal fluids contain cyclic nucleotides and may prove to be useful sources for clinical testing (Murad, 1973).

3.2. Cyclic Nucleotide Regulation of the Immune System

This area, which was recently reviewed by Parker *et al.* (1974), Hadden (1975a,b), and others (cf. Braun *et al.*, 1974), warrants special attention because of its primary involvement in all pathogen-mediated diseases, and also because of the ease with which appropriate cells may be examined *in vitro*. Early work by Bourne *et al.* (1971) showed that cAMP and agents that stimulate cAMP levels in neutrophils inhibit the bactericidal capacity of these cells. Furthermore, recent work by Hill *et al.* (1975) demonstrated inhibition of leukotaxis by cAMP and augmentation by cGMP. Phagocytic release of lysosomal enzymes, but not phagocytosis itself, is also inhibited by cAMP with accompanying increased levels of cGMP (Ignarro and George, 1974; Weissman *et al.*, 1975) (see also Chapter 4). Similarly, cAMP inhibits while cGMP augments and, together with Ca^{2+}, possibly mediates antigen-induced mast cell histamine release (Kaliner and Austen, 1974) and the platelet aggregation and release reactions (White *et al.*, 1973; Haslam and McClenaghan, 1974; N. D. Goldberg *et al.*, 1975), which play important roles in many physiologic as well as abnormal immune responses (H. J. Weiss, 1975). Finally, several aspects of lymphocyte immune functions including clonal proliferation of thymus-dependent

(Hadden *et al.*, 1972, 1974, 1975a; Hadden 1975a) and bone-marrow-derived lymphocytes (Watson, 1975), release of soluble mediators or lymphokines (Hadden, 1975a,b), and lymphocyte-mediated cytotoxicity (Strom *et al.*, 1973; Henney and Lichtenstein, 1971) are all inhibited by cAMP while being augmented—and possibly mediated—by increases in intracellular levels of cGMP and Ca^{2+}.

A justified but perhaps oversimplified expectation, therefore, is that repeated and severe infections would be associated with and aggravated by naturally occurring as well as drug-induced increases in cAMP or decreases in cGMP. This expectation may not be valid, of course, for immunodeficiencies that result from absent or reduced subpopulations of lymphocytes (Kersey *et al.*, 1974), but may apply to other cases such as adenosine deaminase deficiency, in which excessive cAMP levels may be involved (Hadden, 1975b). Several laboratories are now comparing cyclic nucleotide responses in human neutrophils, platelets, and lymphocytes to a myriad of agents. From this flurry of activity, correlations between the ability to stimulate lymphocyte cGMP levels and the biological effects of some known immunopotentiators (Hadden *et al.*, 1975a,b) are emerging. Applications of such agents in the immunotherapy of cancer are discussed in Chapter 14 of this volume.

3.3. Cyclic Nucleotides and Cancer

Reduced adenylate cyclase activity in virus-transformed cell cultures (Burk, 1968) and inhibition of cell growth by cAMP (Ryan and Heidrick, 1968) provided the first clues to cAMP regulation of somatic cell growth. Others (Hadden *et al.*, 1970; Hirschhorn *et al.*, 1970) showed that cAMP and agents that stimulate cAMP increase intracellularly were able to inhibit human lymphocyte proliferation *in vitro*, and Otten *et al.* (1971) and J. R. Sheppard (1971) confirmed this effect in several types of cell cultures. Shortly afterward, Hadden *et al.* (1972) provided the first evidence that cGMP might constitute a positive signal for lymphocytes to proliferate. This concept was strengthened and generalized to other systems by the findings that mitogenic concentrations of insulin (N. D. Goldberg *et al.*, 1974a,b; Rudland *et al.*, 1974a,b), and the tumor promoter phorbol myristate acetate, which lowers cAMP (Belman and Troll, 1974), caused large increases in cultured mouse fibroblast cGMP levels and subsequent cell proliferation (N. D. Goldberg *et al.*, 1974b; Estensen *et al.*, 1974). Virus-induced transformation of these cells causes a 2-fold increase in cGMP and a reduction in cAMP (Moens *et al.*, 1975). In addition, N. D. Goldberg *et al.* (1973a, 1974a) showed that sperm contact increases cGMP in ova.

The concept of a dual regulatory system involving the two cyclic nucleotides exerting opposing signals, formulated by N. D. Goldberg, Hadden, and co-workers (N. D. Goldberg *et al.*, 1973b, 1974a, 1975; N. D. Goldberg and Hadden, 1975), is thus particularly applicable to the study of proliferative disorders (Hadden *et al.*, 1972). The first successful application of the concept resulted in the discovery of elevated cGMP and reduced cAMP in the rapidly growing cells of psoriasis (Voorhees *et al.*, 1973). In many studies, the prediction, based on the early cell culture studies, that malignancy would be associated with reduced cAMP and elevated cGMP concentrations was verified. These studies were reviewed by Abell and Monahan (1973), Ryan and Heidrick (1974), Pastan and Johnson (1974), B. Weiss (1975), Perkins *et al.* (1975), Anderson and Pastan (1975), and Chlapowski *et al.*

(1975). All leukemic samples tested to date have higher cGMP levels than normal human lymphocytes, and some, but not all, have lower cAMP levels (see Table 2). Whether this situation is due to abnormal levels of the cyclases or the phosphodiesterases is under investigation. Abnormal levels of both phosphodiesterases and the calcium-dependent regulator protein were recently found in human mammary tissue, producing an estimated net effect of increased cGMP:cAMP ratio (Singer *et al.*, 1976). The most provocative data thus far are those of Murad *et al.* (1975b), who reported greatly elevated amounts of urinary cGMP in animals with tumors, and suggested that such measurements will be of great utility in detecting a recurrence of the tumor following surgical removal. It is not yet known whether the increments in cGMP arise from the tumor itself or from the lymphocytes responding to tumor antigens or secretory products. The latter possibility must be examined, since other studies (DeRubertis *et al.*, 1976) did not find elevated cGMP levels in malignant human colon tissue, while lymphocyte cGMP metabolism was significantly altered in animals bearing nonlymphocytic tumors (Schumm *et al.*, 1974). In studies with hepatoma cell lines, the degree of malignancy did not correlate inversely with cyclic AMP levels (Thomas *et al.*, 1973), but this apparent paradox was resolved by the workers in the same laboratory (M. L. Goldberg *et al.*, 1975), who found the inverse correlation with cAMP-binding proteins. Similarly, Prasad *et al.* (1975) showed that cAMP-induced differentiation of neuroblastoma cells is associated with increased cAMP-binding proteins. It remains to be seen whether a positive correlation between degree of malignancy and cGMP-binding proteins will also be found, as suggested by the data of M. L. Goldberg *et al.* (1975). Of special interest will be the analysis of nuclear acidic nonhistone chromatin proteins with high affinity for cGMP (E. M. Johnson and Hadden, 1975).

3.4. Summary

In summary, it would appear that a potentially limitless number of disease states will be found with abnormalities involving one or more aspects of the cyclic nucleotide regulatory system. Some of these abnormalities will prove to be causative, while more will probably be found to mediate or aggravate the disorder. While we have given emphasis to cyclic nucleotide measurements, it is obvious that phosphodiesterases and protein kinases merit extensive study as well, if the underlying molecular defects are to be completely understood. Defective cell-surface receptors for hormones may also account for certain states, some of which are listed in Table 4. Nevertheless, we believe that with the exception of blood cell disorders, the convenience of plasma and urine specimens will result in their predominant use in future clinical testing. Indeed, such assays have already formed an integral part of large research programs devoted entirely to the design of drugs that selectively alter cAMP or cGMP levels in appropriate tissues (Amer and McKinney, 1973; C. G. Smith, 1974).

References

Abdulla, Y. H., and Hamadah, K. H., 1970, *Lancet* **1**:378–381.
Abell, C. W., and Monahan, T. M., 1973, *J. Cell Biol.* **59**:549–558.
Amer, M. S., and Byrne, J. E., 1975, *Nature (London)* **250**:421–424.

Amer, M. S., and McKinney, G. R., 1973, *Life Sci.* **13**:753–767.
Amer, M. S., Gomoll, A. W., Perhach, J. L., Jr., Ferguson, H. C., and McKinney, G. R., 1974, *Proc. Natl. Acad. Sci. U.S.A.* **71**:4930–4934.
Anderson, W. B., and Pastan, I., 1975, *Adv. Cyclic Nucleotide Res.* **5**:681–698.
Asakawa, T., Russell, T. R., and Ho, R.-J., 1976, *Biochem. Biophys. Res. Commun.* **68**:682–690.
Astaldi, A., Astaldi, G. C. B., Schellekens, P. T. A., and Eijsvoogel, V. P., 1976, *Nature (London)* **260**:713–715.
Aurbach, G. D., Marcus, R., Winickoff, R. N., Epstein, E. H., Jr., and Nigra, T. P., 1970, *Metab. Clin. Exp.* **19**:799–808.
Ball, J. H., Kaminsky, N. I., Hardman, J. G., Broadus, A. E., Sutherland, E. W., and Liddle, G. W., 1972, *J. Clin. Invest.* **51**:2124–2129.
Belman, S., and Troll, W., 1974, *Cancer Res.* **34**:3446–3455.
Bernstein, R. A., Linarelli, L., Facktor, M. A., Friday, G. A., Drash, A., and Fireman, P., 1972, *J. Lab. Clin. Med.* **80**:772–779.
Bourne, H. R., Lehrer, R. I., Cline, M. J., and Melmon, K. L., 1971, *J. Clin. Invest.* **50**:920–929.
Braun, W., Lichtenstein, L. M., and Parker, C. W., 1974, in: *Cyclic AMP, Cell Growth, and the Immune Response,* pp. 1–413, Springer-Verlag, New York.
Brooker, G., 1970, *Anal. Chem.* **42**:1108–1110.
Brooker, G., and Fichman, M., 1971, *Biochem. Biophys. Res. Commun.* **42**:824–828.
Brooker, G., Thomas, L. J., Jr., and Appleman, M. M., 1968, *Biochemistry* **7**:4177–4181.
Brown, B. L., Albano, J. D. M., Ekins, R. P., Sgherzi, A. M., and Tampion, W., 1971, *Biochem. J.* **121**:561–562.
Burk, R. R., 1968, *Nature (London)* **219**:1272–1275.
Burke, G., 1970, *Biochim. Biophys. Acta* **220**:30–41.
Burleson, D. G., and Sage, H. T., 1976, *J. Immunol.* **116**:696–703.
Cailla, H. L., Racine-Weisbuch, M. S., and DeLaage, M. A., 1973, *Anal. Biochem.* **56**:394–407.
Cailla, H. L., Vannier, C. J., and DeLaage, M. A., 1976, *Anal. Biochem.* **70**:195–202.
Case, R. M., Laundy, T. J., and Scratcherd, T., 1969, *J. Physiol.* **204**:45p–47p.
Chase, L. R., and Aurbach, G. D., 1967, *Proc. Natl. Acad. Sci. U.S.A.* **58**:518–525.
Chase, L. R., Melson, G. L., and Aurbach, G. D., 1969, *J. Clin. Invest.* **48**:1832–1844.
Chlapowski, F. J., Kelly, L. A., and Butcher, R. W., 1975, *Adv. Cyclic Nucleotide Res.* **6**:245–338.
Coffey, R. G., and Middleton, E., Jr., 1973, *Int. Arch. Allergy Appl. Immunol.* **45**:593–611.
Coffey, R. G., Hadden, J. W., and Hadden, E. M., 1975, *Fed. Proc. Fed. Am. Soc. Exp. Biol.* **34**:1029.
Das, I., 1973, *Horm. Metab. Res.* **5**:330–332.
DeRubertis, F. R., and Zenser, T., 1976, *Biochim. Biophys. Acta* **428**:91–103.
DeRubertis, F. R., Zenser, T. V., Adler, W. H., and Hudson, T., 1974, *J. Immunol.* **113**:151–161.
DeRubertis, F. R., Chayoth, R., and Field, J. B., 1976, *J. Clin. Invest.* **57**:641–649.
Deviller, P., Cille, Y., and Betuel, H., 1975, *Enzyme* **19**:300–313.
Dunham, E. W., Haddox, M. K., and Goldberg, N. D., 1974, *Proc. Natl. Acad. Sci. U.S.A.* **71**:815–819.
Durham, J. P., Baserga, R., and Butcher, F. R., 1974, *Biochim. Biophys. Acta* **372**:196–217.
Ebadi, M. S., Weiss, B., and Costa, E., 1971, *J. Neurochem.* **18**:183–192.
Estensen, R. D., Hadden, J. W., Hadden, E. M., Touraine, F., Touraine, J. L., Haddox, M. K., and Goldberg, N. D., 1974, in: *Control of Proliferation in Animal Cells* (B. Clarkson and R. Baserga, eds.), pp. 627–634, Cold Spring Harbor Press, New York.
Evans, D. J., Jr., Chen, L. C., Curlin, G. T., and Evans, D. G., 1972, *Nature (London) New Biol.* **236**:137–138.
Filler, R., and Litwack, G., 1973, *Biochem. Biophys. Res. Commun.* **52**:159–167.
Forrest, J. N., Jr., 1975, *N. Engl. J. Med.* **292**:423–424.
Frandsen, E. K., and Krishna, G., 1976, *Life Sci.* **18**:529–542.
Gillespie, E., 1973, *Experientia* **29**:447–448.
Gillespie, E., Valentine, M., and Lichtenstein, L. M., 1974, *J. Allergy Clin. Immunol.* **53**:27–33.
Gilman, A. G., 1970, *Proc. Natl. Acad. Sci. U.S.A.* **67**:305–312.
Gilman, A. G., 1972, *Adv. Cyclic Nucleotide Res.* **2**:9–24.
Glasgow, A., Polgar, P., Saporoschetz, I., Kim, H., Rutenburg, M., and Mannick, J. A., 1975, *Clin. Immunol. Immunopathol.* **3**:353–362.
Gold, H. K., Prindle, K. H., Levey, G. S., and Epstein, S. E., 1970, *J. Clin. Invest.* **49**:999–1006.
Goldberg, M. L., Burke, G. C., and Morris, H. P., 1975, *Biochem. Biophys. Res. Commun.* **62**:320–327.

Goldberg, N. D., and Hadden, J. W., 1975, in: *Molecular Pathology* (R. A. Good, S. B. Day, and J. J. Yunis, eds.), pp. 417–439, Charles C. Thomas, Springfield, Illinois.
Goldberg, N. D., Dietz, S. B., and O'Toole, A. G., 1969a, *J. Biol. Chem.* **244**:4458–4466.
Goldberg, N. D., Larner, J., Sasko, H., and O'Toole, A. G., 1969b, *Anal. Biochem.* **28**:523–544.
Goldberg, N. D., O'Toole, A. G., and Haddox, M. K., 1972, *Adv. Cyclic Nucleotide Res.* **2**:63–80.
Goldberg, N. D., O'Dea, R. F., and Haddox, M. K., 1973a, *Adv. Cyclic Nucleotide Res.* **3**:155–223.
Goldberg, N. D., Haddox, M. K., Hartle, D. K., and Hadden, J. W., 1973b, in: *Proceedings of the Fifth International Congress of Pharmacology: Pharmacology and the Future of Man,* Vol. 5, pp. 146–169, S. Karger, Basel.
Goldberg, N. D., Haddox, M. K., Dunham, E., Lopez, C., and Hadden, J. W., 1974a, in: *Control of Proliferation in Animal Cells* (B. Clarkson, and R. Baserga, eds.), pp. 609–626, Cold Spring Harbor Press, New York.
Goldberg, N. D., Haddox, M. K., Estensen, R., White, J. G., Lopez, C., and Hadden, J. W., 1974b, in: *Cyclic AMP, Cell Growth, and the Immune Response* (W. Braun, L. M. Lichtenstein, and C. W. Parker, eds.), pp. 247–262, Springer-Verlag, New York.
Goldberg, N. D., Haddox, M. K., Nicol, S. E., Glass, D. B., Sanford, C. H., Kuehl, F. A., and Estenson, R., 1975, *Adv. Cyclic Nucleotide Res.* **5**:307–330.
Goldstein, G., 1975, *Ann. N. Y. Acad. Sci.* **249**:177–185.
Graham-Smith, D. G., Isaac, P., Heal, D. J., and Bond, R. P. M., 1975, *Nature (London)* **253**:58–60.
Greengard, P., Paoletti, R., and Robison, G. A. (eds.), 1972, in: *Advances in Cyclic Nucleotide Research,* Vol. 2, pp. 1–144, Raven Press, New York.
Guidotti, A., Weiss, B., and Costa, E., 1972, *Mol. Pharmacol.* **8**:521–530.
Gullis, R., Traber, J., and Hamprecht, B., 1975, *Nature (London)* **256**:57–59.
Hadden, J. W., 1975a, in: *Combined Immunodeficiency Disease and Adenosine Deaminase Deficiency: A Molecular Defect* (H. J. Meuwissen, R. J. Pickering, E. B. Hook, B. Pollara, I. H. Porter, and S. Kelly, eds.), pp. 173–186, Academic Press, New York.
Hadden, J. W., 1975b, in: *Molecular Pathology* (R. A. Good, S. B. Day, and J. J. Yunis, eds.), pp. 90–114, Charles C. Thomas, Springfield, Illinois.
Hadden, J. W., Hadden, E. M., and Middleton, E., Jr., 1970, *J. Cell. Immunol.* **1**:583–595.
Hadden, J. W., Hadden, E., Haddox, M., and Goldberg, N., 1972, *Proc. Natl. Acad. Sci. U.S.A.* **60**:3024–3027.
Hadden, J. W., Hadden, E. M., and Goldberg, N. D., 1974, in: *Cyclic AMP, Cell Growth, and the Immune Response* (W. Braun, L. M. Lichtenstein, and C. W. Parker, eds.), pp. 237–247, Springer-Verlag, New York.
Hadden, J. W., Johnson, E. M., Hadden, E. M., Coffey, R. G., and Johnson, L. D., 1975a, in: *Immune Recognition* (A. Rosenthal, ed.), pp. 359–389, Academic Press, New York.
Hadden, J. W., Coffey, R. G., Hadden, E. M., Lopes-Corrales, E., and Sunshine, G. A., 1975b, *Cell. Immunol.* **20**:98–103.
Hadden, J. W., Hadden, E. M., Sadlik, J. R., and Coffey, R. G., 1976, *Proc. Natl. Acad. Sci. U.S.A.* **73**:1717–1721.
Haddox, M. K., Furcht, L. T., Gentry, S. R., Moser, M. E., Stephenson, J. H., and Goldberg, N. D., 1976, *Nature (London)* **262**:146–148.
Ham, E. A., Cirillo, V. J., Zanetti, M. E., and Kuehl, F. A., Jr., 1975, *Proc. Natl. Acad. Sci. U.S.A.* **72**:1420–1424.
Hamet, P., Stouder, D. A., Ginn, H. E., Hardman, J. G., and Liddle, G. W., 1975, *J. Clin. Invest.* **56**:339–345.
Harper, J. F., and Brooker, G., 1975, *J. Cyclic Nucleotide Res.* **1**:207–218.
Haslam, R. J. and McClenaghan, M. D., 1974, *Biochem. J.* **138**:317–320.
Haymovitz, A., and Scheele, G. A., 1976, *Proc. Natl. Acad. Sci. U.S.A.* **73**:156–160.
Heidrick, M. L., 1973, *J. Cell Biol.* **59**:139a.
Henney, C. S., and Lichtenstein, L. M., 1971, *J. Immunol.* **107**:610–612.
Hill, H. R., Estensen, R. D., Quie, P. G., Hogan, N. A., and Goldberg, N. D., 1975, *Metabolism* **24**:447–456.
Hilz, H., and Tarnowski, W., 1970, *Biochem. Biophys. Res. Commun.* **40**:973–981.
Hirschhorn, R., Grossman, J., and Weissmann, G., 1970, *Proc. Soc. Exp. Biol. Med.* **133**:1361–1365.
Hollenberg, M. D., and Cuatrecasas, P., 1975, *Fed. Proc. Fed. Am. Soc. Exp. Biol.* **34**:1556–1563.
Hovi, T., Keski-Oja, J., and Vaheri, A., 1974, *Cell* **2**:235–240.

Humes, J. L., Roundbehler, M., and Kuehl, F. A., Jr., 1969, *Anal. Biochem.* **32**:210–217.
Ide, M., 1969, *Biochem. Biophys. Res. Commun.* **36**:42–46.
Ignarro, L. J., and George, W. J., 1974, *Proc. Natl. Acad. Sci. U.S.A.* **71**:2027–2031.
Iversen, L. L., 1975, *Science* **188**:1084–1089.
Johnson, E. M., and Hadden, J. W., 1975, *Science* **187**:1198–1200.
Johnson, R. A., Hardman, J. G., Broadus, A. E., and Sutherland, E. W., 1970, *Anal. Biochem.* **35**:91–97.
Kaliner, M., and Austen, K. F., 1974, in: *Cyclic AMP, Cell Growth, and the Immune Response* (W. Braun, L. M. Lichtenstein, and C. W. Parker, eds.), pp. 163–175, Springer-Verlag, New York.
Katagiri, T., Terao, T., and Osawa, T., 1976, *J. Biochem.* **79**:849–852.
Kebabian, J. W., Kuo, J. F., and Greengard, P., 1972, *Adv. Cyclic Nucleotide Res.* **2**:131–137.
Kenakin, T. P., Krueger, C. A., and Cook, D. A., 1974, *Nature (London)* **252**:54–55.
Kersey, J. H., Gajl-Peczalska, K. J., and Nesbit, M. E., 1974, *J. Pediatr.* **84**:789–796.
Kiefer, H. C., Atlas, R., Moldan, D., and Kantor, S., 1975, *Biochem. Biophys. Res. Commun.* **66**:1017–1023.
Kimura, H., and Murad, F., 1974, *J. Biol. Chem.* **249**:329–331.
Kimura, H., and Murad, F., 1975, *Proc. Natl. Acad. Sci. U.S.A.* **72**:1965–1969.
Kimura, H., Thomas, E., and Murad, F., 1974, *Biochim. Biophys. Acta* **343**:519–528.
Kobayashi, R., and Fang, V. S., 1975, *Biochem. Biophys. Res. Commun.* **67**:493–500.
Kodama, T., Matsukado, Y., Suzaki, T., Tanaka, S., and Shimizu, H., 1971, *Biochim. Biophys. Acta* **252**:165–170.
Kuchel, O., Hamet, P., Cuche, J. L., Tolis, G., Fraysse, J., and Genest, J., 1975, *J. Clin. Endocrinol. Metab.* **41**:282–289.
Kuehl, F. A., Jr., Ham, E. A., Zanetti, M. E., Sanford, C. H., Nicol, S. E., and Goldberg, N. D., 1974, *Proc. Natl. Acad. Sci. U.S.A.* **71**:1866–1870.
Kuo, J. F., 1975a, *Biochem. Biophys. Res. Commun.* **65**:1214–1220.
Kuo, J. F., 1975b, *Proc. Natl. Acad. Sci. U.S.A.* **72**:2256–2259.
Kuo, J. F., and DeRenzo, E. C., 1969, *J. Biol. Chem.* **244**:2252–2260.
Kuo, J. F., and Greengard, P., 1970, *J. Biol. Chem.* **245**:4067–4073.
Kuo, J. F., and Greengard, P., 1972, *Adv. Cyclic Nucleotide Res.* **2**:41–50.
Levey, G. S., and Pastan, I., 1970, *Life Sci.* **9**:67–73.
Levey, G. S., Skelton, C. L., and Epstein, S. E., 1969, *Endocrinology* **85**:1004–1009.
Levey, G. S., Palmer, R. F., Lasseter, K. C., and McCarthy, J., 1971, *J. Clin. Endocrinol. Metab.* **33**:371–374.
Lichtenstein, L. M., 1973, in: *Asthma: Physiology, Immunopharmacology, and Treatment* (K. F. Austen and L. M. Lichtenstein, eds.), pp. 91–104, Academic Press, New York.
Lipsky, P. E., Ellner, J. J., and Rosenthal, A. S., 1976, *J. Immunol.* **116**:868–875.
Logsdon, P. J., Carnright, D. V., Middleton, E., Jr., and Coffey, R. G., 1973, *J. Allergy Clin. Immunol.* **52**:148–157.
Lyle, L. R., and Parker, C. W., 1974, *Biochemistry* **13**:5415–5420.
Makman, M. H., 1971, *Proc. Natl. Acad. Sci. U.S.A.* **68**:885–889.
Mao, C. C., Guidotti, A., and Costa, E., 1975, *Naunyn-Schmiedebergs Arch. Pharmakol.* **289**:369–378.
Moens, W., Vokaer, A., and Kram, R., 1975, *Proc. Natl. Acad. Sci. U.S.A.* **72**:1063–1067.
Murad, F., 1973, *Adv. Cyclic Nucleotide Res.* **3**:355–383.
Murad, F., Manganiello, V., and Vaughan, M., 1971, *Proc. Natl. Acad. Sci. U.S.A.* **68**:736–739.
Murad, F., Moss, W. W., Johanson, A. J., and Selden, R. F., 1975a, *J. Clin. Endocrinol. Metab.* **40**:552–559.
Murad, F., Kimura, H., Hopkins, H. A., Looney, W. B., and Kovacs, C. J., 1975b, *Science* **190**:58–60.
Nesbitt, J. A., III, Anderson, W. B., Miller, Z., Pastan, I., Russell, T. R., and Gospodarowicz, D., 1976, *J. Biol. Chem.* **251**:2344–2352.
Novogrodsky, A., and Katchalski, E., 1970, *Biochim. Biophys. Acta* **215**:291–296.
Otten, J., Johnson, G. S., and Pastan, I., 1971, *Biochem. Biophys. Res. Commun.* **44**:1192–1198.
Parker, C. W., and Morse, S. I., 1973, *J. Exp. Med.* **137**:1078–1091.
Parker, C. W., Sullivan, T. J., and Wedner, H. J., 1974, *Adv. Cyclic Nucleotide Res.* **4**:1–80.
Pastan, I., and Johnson, G. S., 1974, *Adv. Cancer Res.* **19**:303–329.
Patrick, J. C., Jr., Rengachary, S., and Melnykovych, G., 1975, *In Vitro* **11**:404–408.
Paul, M. I., Ditzion, B. R., Pauk, G. L., and Janowsky, D. S., 1970, *Am. J. Psychiatry* **126**:1493–1497.

Perkins, J. P., Moore, M. M., Kalisker, A., and Su, Y. F., 1975, *Adv. Cyclic Nucleotide Res.* **5**:641–660.
Pohl, S. L., Birnbaumer, L., and Rodbell, M., 1969, *Science* **164**:566–567.
Polson, J. B., Krzanowski, J. J., and Szentivanyi, A., 1974, *J. Allergy Clin. Immunol.* **53**:100.
Prasad, K. N., Sinha, P. K., Sahu, S. K., and Brown, J. L., 1975, *Biochem. Biophys. Res. Commun.* **66**:131–138.
Robison, G. A., Butcher, R. W., and Sutherland, E. W., 1971, in: *Cyclic AMP,* pp. 1–531, Academic Press, New York.
Rosen, O. M., 1972, *N. Engl. J. Med.* **287**:670, 671.
Rosen, O. M., and Rosen, S. M., 1969, *Arch. Biochem. Biophys.* **131**:449–456.
Rudland, P. S., Gospodarowicz, D., and Seifert, W., 1974a, *Nature (London)* **250**:741–744.
Rudland, P. S., Seeley, M., and Seifert, W., 1974b, *Nature (London)* **251**:417–419.
Ryan, W. L., and Durrick, M. A., 1972, *Science* **177**:1002–1003.
Ryan, W. L., and Heidrick, M. L., 1968, *Science* **162**:1484–1485.
Ryan, W. L., and Heidrick, M. L., 1974, *Adv. Cyclic Nucleotide Res.* **4**:81–116.
Sattin, A., 1971, *J. Neurochem.* **18**:1087–1096.
Schafer, D. E., Lust, W. D., Polson, J. B., Hedtke, J., Sircar, B., Thakur, A. K., and Goldberg, N. D., 1971, *Ann. N. Y. Acad. Sci.* **185**:376–385.
Schultz, G., and Hardman, J. G., 1975, *Adv. Cyclic Nucleotide Res.* **5**:339–352.
Schultz, G., Hardman, J. G., Schultz, K., Davis, J. W., and Sutherland, E. W., 1973a, *Proc. Natl. Acad. Sci. U.S.A.* **70**:1721–1725.
Schultz, G., Hardman, J. G., Schultz, K., Baird, C. E., and Sutherland, E. W., 1973b, *Proc. Natl. Acad. Sci. U.S.A.* **70**:3889–3893.
Schultz, J., 1975, *J. Neurochem.* **24**:495–502.
Schumm, D. E., Morris, H. P., and Webb, T. E., 1974, *Eur. J. Cancer* **10**:107–113.
Seifert, W. E., and Rudland, P. S., 1974, *Nature (London)* **248**:138–140.
Sharma, S. K., Klee, W. A., and Nirenberg, M., 1975, *Proc. Natl. Acad. Sci. U.S.A.* **72**:3092–3096.
Sharp, G. W. G., Hynie, S., Lipson, L. C., and Parkinson, D. K., 1971, *Trans. Assoc. Am. Physicians* **84**:200–211.
Sheppard, H., 1970, *Nature (London)* **228**:567–568.
Sheppard, J. R., 1971, *Proc. Natl. Acad. Sci. U.S.A.* **68**:1316–1320.
Singer, A. L., Sherwin, R. P., Dunn, A. S., and Appleman, M. M., 1976, *Cancer Res.* **36**:60–66.
Smith, C. G., 1974, *Adv. Enzyme Regul.* **12**:187–204.
Smith, J. W., Steiner, A. L., Newberry, W. M., Jr., and Parker, C. W., 1971, *J. Clin. Invest.* **50**:432–441.
Smith, R. S., Sherman, N. A., and Coffey, R. G., 1974, *Int. Arch. Allergy* **47**:586–597.
Sobel, B. E., Henry, P. D., Robison, A., Bloor, C., and Ross, J., Jr., 1969, *Circ. Res.* **24**:507–512.
Solomon, S. S., Brush, J. S., and Kitabachi, A. E., 1970, *Science* **169**:387–389.
Solomons, C. C., and Millar, E. A., 1972, *Drug. Ther.* **2**(3):13–15.
Steiner, A. L., Kipnis, D. M., Utiger, R., and Parker, C. W., 1969, *Proc. Natl. Acad. Sci. U.S.A.* **64**:367–373.
Steiner, A. L., Wehmann, R. E., Parker, C. W., and Kipnis, D. M., 1972, *Adv. Cyclic Nucleotide Res.* **2**:51–61.
Stoner, J., Manganiello, V. C., and Vaughan, M., 1974, *Mol. Pharmacol.* **10**:155–161.
Strom, T. B., Carpenter, C. B., Garovoy, M. R., Austen, K. F., Merrill, J. P., and Kaliner, M., 1973, *J. Exp. Med.* **138**:381–393.
Sutherland, E. W., 1970, *J. Am. Med. Assoc.* **214**:1281–1288.
Sutherland, E. W., and Robison, G. A., 1969, *Diabetes* **18**:797–819.
Swislocki, N. I., 1970, *Anal. Biochem.* **38**:260–269.
Szego, C. M., and Davis, J. S., 1969, *Life Sci.* **8**:1109–1116.
Taylor, A. L., Davis, B. B., Pawlson, L. G., Josimovich, J. B., and Mintz, D. H., 1970, *J. Clin. Endocrinol. Metab.* **30**:316–324.
Taylor, W. A., and Sheldon, D., 1974, *Int. Arch. Allergy* **47**:696–707.
Thomas, E. W., Murad, F., Looney, W. B., and Morris, H. P., 1973, *Biochim. Biophys. Acta* **297**:564–567.
Thompson, W. J., Johnson, D. G., Lavis, V. R., and Williams, R. H., 1974, *Endocrinology* **94**:276–278.
Tucci, J. R., Lin, T., and Kopp, L., 1973, *J. Clin. Endocrinol. Metab.* **37**:832–835.
Voorhees, J. J., Stawiski, M., Duell, E. A., Haddox, M. K., and Goldberg, N. D., 1973, *Life Sci.* **13**:639–653.

Walsh, D. A., and Ashby, C. D., 1973, *Recent Prog. Horm. Res.* **29**:329–359.
Watson, J., 1975, *J. Exp. Med.* **141**:97–111.
Weber, T. H., and Goldberg, M. L., 1976, *Exp. Cell Res.* **97**:432–435.
Wedner, H. J., Dankner, R., and Parker, C. W., 1975, *J. Immunol.* **115**:1682–1687.
Weiss, B. (ed.), 1975, *Cyclic Nucleotides in Disease,* 410 pp., University Park Press, Baltimore, Maryland.
Weiss, H. J., 1975, *N. Engl. J. Med.* **293**:531–540, 580–588.
Weissman, G., Goldstein, I., Hoffstein, S., Chauvet, G., and Robineaux, R., 1975, *Ann. N. Y. Acad. Sci.* **256**:222–231.
White, J. G., Goldberg, N. D., Estensen, R. D., Haddox, M. K., and Rao, G. H. R., 1973, *J. Clin. Invest.* **52**:89a.
Whitfield, J. F., MacManus, J. P., Boynton, A. L., Gillan, D. J., and Isaacs, R. J., 1974, *J. Cell. Physiol.* **84**:445–458.
Wright, T. C., and Price, R., 1975, *Anal. Biochem.* **67**:342–346.
Yamamoto, I., and Webb, D. R., 1975, *Proc. Natl. Acad. Sci. U.S.A.* **72**:2320–2324.

Index

Acetylcholine
  in asthma, 216
  augmented cell lysis and, 50
  cGMP and, 7-8, 15, 204
  carbachol, 16
ACh, *see* Acetylcholine
Acidic proteins, phosphorylated, 15-16
Acne conglobata, 297
ACTH, corticosteroids and, 215
Activated macrophages, characteristics of, 88-89
Active site chemotactic factors, 129
Adenosine triphosphate, *see* ATP
Adenylate cyclase
  in asthma therapy, 217
  ATP and, 48
  in cAMP formation, 204
  GTP level and, 211
  isoproterenol and, 48
  in platelets, 76
  in S49 mutants, potential value of, 336-337
Adjuvant arthritis, 153
α-adrenergic antagonists, in asthma treatment, 212
α-adrenergic receptors, 6-7, 80, 209
β-adrenergic blockade theory, 209-212
β-adrenergic catecholamines, 7, 331
β-adrenergic receptors, 48, 80
AFP(α-fetoprotein), 270-271
Alkylating agents, as immunodepressants, 257
Allergy
  cyclic nucleotides in, 203-221
  immediate-hypersensitivity type, 203-204
Alloimmunity regulation, cyclic nucleotides in, 47-57
Amines
  cell binding to, 348-350
  insoluble configurations of, 345-348
  vasoactive, 75
p-aminobenzoic acid, 316
Aminopeptidase-M, 118
Aminophylline, 48, 54
AMP (adenosine monophosphate) production, lymphocyte receptors and, 332
Anaphylaxis, eosinophil chemotactic factor of, *see* Eosinophil chemotactic factor of anaphylaxis; *see also* Slow-reacting substance of anaphylaxis
Antiallergic drugs, 203-221
Antianaphylatoxin antibody, 273
Antiarthritic agents, 232-233
Antibody affinity, assessment of, 320-321
Antibody-coated target cells, K-cell mediated lysis of, 52
Antibody-forming cells, 353
  precursors of, 29
Antibody production, antibody influence in, 273
Antibody specificity, assessment of, 319-320
Antibody synthesis
  control of, 42-43
  cyclic nucleotides as intracellular mediators in induction of, 29-41
  induction and paralysis of, 30-31
Antibody titer, assessment of, 321
Antibody (-ies)
  antidrug, 316-321
  detection of, 317-319
  digoxin-specific, 328-329
  in immunoassays, 321-326
  lipopolysaccharides and, 289
  T-cell function and, 273
Antidrug antibodies, 316-321
Antigen(s)
  artificial conjugated, 315
  thymus-dependent, 30
  thymus-independent, 30
  in tolerance induction models, 272
Antigen-antibody aggregates, Hageman factor and, 127
Antigen-antibody reactions, 272-274
Antihistamines
  is asthma therapy, 216
  histamine release and, 103
Antiinflammatory agents or drugs, 68, 151-152
  defined, 228
  immune response and, 227-241

Antiinflammatory agents or drugs (*cont'd*)
lymphocytes and, 228-230
macrophage secretory activity and, 239-240
nonsteroid, 231-232
topically active, 151
Antilymphocyte globulin, 89, 260
Antineoplastic agents, 266
Antirheumatic agents, 228
Arachidonic acid
lecithin and, 14
synthesis and metabolism of oxidation products of, 146
hydroperoxide, 217
Arylsulfatase A, SRS-A and, 122
Arylsulfatase B, 121
Aspirin
as antiinflammatory drug, 228, 231
PG biosynthesis and, 67
Asthma
β-adrenergic blockade theory in, 209-212
antihistamines in, 216
ATPase activity in, 220
atropine and, 215-216
chemical mediators, 208-209
chlorphenesin and, 218-219
corticosteroids in, 213-215
cromolyn in, 218
defined, 207-208
drugs used in treatment, 212-219
hetrazan and, 218
pathology, 207-212
phosphodiesterase inhibitors in, 213
prostaglandins in, 216-218
receptor imbalance in, 219
sympathomimetic amines and antagonists in, 212-213
Ataxia telangectasia, 297, 304
ATP (adenosine triphosphate), 2
adenylate cyclase and, 48
cAMP formation from, 204
ATPase
agents acting on, 6-7
in asthma therapy, 220
Atropine, in asthma therapy, 215-216
Autonomic nervous system, 81
Azathioprine, as immunodepressant, 236, 254-259

Bacillus anthracis, 87
Bacillus Calmette-Guérin, 280-281
action of, 283
in cancer therapy, 284-285
mycobacterial fractions of, 281-282
therapeutic uses of, 283-285
Bacterial lipopolysaccharide, as probe of T helper cell function, 34-35, *see also* Endotoxin, Lipopolysaccharides
Basophils
desensitization of, 108
histamine formation within, 115
in immune response, 227
kallikrein of anaphylaxis, 109, 208
B cells
inactivation of by cAMP, 33-34
paralytic pathway in, 30-31
T-cell-independent antigens in, 31
B-cell expression, intracellular mediators of, 31-32
BCG, *see* Bacillus Calmette-Guerin
Besnoitia jellisoni, 88
Biological control, dualism concept in, 61, 68
BK-A, *see* Basophil kallikrein of anaphylaxis
B lymphocytes, *see also* B cells
cAMP as differentiation signal in, 40-41
in immune response, 227
insulin receptors on, 362-367
mitogen-induced, 34-37
Bone marrow, promonocytes and monocytes in, 234-237
Bronchoconstrictors, in asthma therapy, 217-281
Brucella abortus, 87
Brucella infections, 295
Brucella suis, 87
Burkitt's lymphoma, 363, 366-367

Caffeine, on platelet phosphodiesterase activity, 76
Calcitonin, radioreceptor assay for, 381
Calcitonin receptors, on lymphoid cells, 375
Calcium
cGMP and, 18-20, 207
in histamine release, 105
in mitogenic action, 12-13
in proliferative processes, 39
cAMP (cyclic 3′, 5′-adenosine monophosphate), *see also* Cyclic nucleotides
action of in lymphocytes, 2, 4
adenylate cyclase in formation of, 204
β-adrenergic responses and, 209-210
agents that increase production of, 4-6
anomalous increases in, 22
in antigen-induced release process, 102
antiinflammatory effects of, 68
antiproliferative role of, 5
in asthma therapy, 219
ATP and, 204
in B cell antigenic signals, 31
calcium level and, 40

cAMP (*cont'd*)
cancer and, 406-407
catecholamines and, 65
cell function control by, 64
cell functions and, 206
cholera enterotoxin and, 49, 104
Concanavalin A (Con A) and, 10-11
dibutyryl, 32-34, 48, 53, 64, 72, 76, 334-335, 351, 400
as differentiation signal in B lymphocytes, 40-41
in DNA synthesis, 39
exogenous and endogenous, 173, 176
formation of, 204
in histamine release, 107-108
inactivation of B cells by, 33-34
insulin and, 371-372
intracellular actions of in platelets, 76
as intracellular mediator of expression of B-cell pathways, 41-42
as intracellular mediator of platelet function inhibition, 76-77
levels in lymphocytes, 2, 4
lipophilicity of, 76
measurement of, 393-394
in mediator release, 101
MIF and, 73, 176-177, 181-182, 186-187
mitogen stimulation by, 39
mitogenesis and, 334
monobutyryl, 33
mutants and, 335
PGEs and, 156-158
$PGF_{2\alpha}$ and, 148
PHA and, 10-11
phagocytosis and, 72
phosphorylation and, 3
platelet release and, 77
prostaglandins and, 23, 48, 55, 70, 80, 103, 145
receptor function and, 334-339
as "second messenger system," 1, 48
serine esterase and, 114
stimulating effects of, 32-33, 39
in target cell destruction, 54-55
in target cell lysis, 48
THF and, 23
cAMP synthesis, prostaglandins and, 145
cAMP phosphodiesterase, 5, 70, 82, 207
inhibition of, 23, 213
theophylline and, 102, 213
cAMP receptors, cell regulation and, 337-338
Cancer therapy
BCG in, 284-285
Corynebacteria in, 287
Cancer therapy (*cont'd*)
cyclic nucleotides and, 406-407
levamisole in, 298
lipopolysaccharides in, 290-291
Candidiasis, mucocutaneous, 300
Carbamylcholine, 189
in cytotoxicity, 55
Carbodiimide, water-soluble, 316
Carrageenan paw edema, 151-152
Catecholamines
β-adrenergic, 331
in asthma therapy, 209, 212
cAMP and, 65, 73, 204
Cell binding, to amine conjugates, 348-350
Cell chromatography, effect of, 350
Cell separation
cell receptors and, 341-345
physiologic function and, 339-341
Cellular immunity, macrophage proliferation and, 90-91; *see also* Immunity
cGMP (cyclic 3′, 5′-guanosine monophosphate), *see also* Cyclic nucleotides
acetylcholine and, 7-8
agents that increase production of, 7-9, 204-207
in bioregulation of cellular processes, 61-83
biosynthesis of, 68, 204-207
calcium and, 12-13, 18-20, 207
cell function control by, 64
collagen and, 77-78
Concanavalin A and, 11-12
corticosteroids and, 215
cytotoxicity and, 52
dibutyryl, 39
in DNA synthesis, 38
in histamine release, 105
as intracellular mediator in B cells, 31, 41-42
and intracellular mitogen signal, 18-20
in leukocytes, 2, 4
in lymphoid cells, 33
lysosomal enzyme release and, 65
MIF and, 177
platelet release and, 77
as proliferation signal, 37-40
in RNA polymerase activity, 17-18
as second messenger, 1, 48, 206
SRS-A generation and, 115
stimulatory effects of, 32-33, 51
Sutherland's criteria for, 400
in target cell destruction, 54-55
in Yin-Yang hypothesis of biological control, 61-62
cGMP dependent protein kinase, 4, 207
cGMP phosphodiesterase, 3, 70, 82

Chalones, lymphocytic, 268-269
Chemical immunopotentiators, 292-299
Chemical mediators
  characteristics of, 115
  generation and release of, 114-115
Chemotactic product, 154
Chemotaxis
  in anaphylaxis, 116-119
  prostaglandins in, 153-154
Chlorambucil, 258
Chloroquine, 240
Chlorphenesin, 73
  in asthma therapy, 218
Chlorpheniramine, 103
Chlorpromazine, 103
Cholera enterotoxin, *see* Cholera toxin
Cholera toxin
  cAMP and, 49, 52
  enterotoxin
    antigen-induced immunosuppression and, 351
    histamine release and, 104
  immunoglobulins and, 349
Cholinergic receptors, 50
Chromosomes, "marker," 362
Chronic mucocutaneous candidiasis, 300
Colchicine
  microtubule disruption and, 106-107
  in MIF action, 185
Collagen, cGMP and, 77-78
Colony-stimulating factor, 94-95, 283
Complement, 133-138
Complement effector sequence, 134, 136-137
  activation of, 137-138
  biologically active products of, 135
  activation, amplification, and function of, 132
Complement
  inhibition of, 321
  modulation of, 137-138
  physiochemical characteristics of, 134
Complete Freund's adjuvant, 280
Con A (concanavalin A), 10-11
  cGMP and, 11-12, 37
  guanylate cyclase stimulation by, 39
  interferon (IF) induction in lymphocytes by, 193, 334
  and lymphocytes, 15
  thymopoietin and, 22-23
Conjugates, characteristics of, 317
Convertase formation, 133-136
Corticosteroids, *see also* Glucocorticoids; Steroids
  in asthma therapy, 213-215
  cell-mediated immunity and, 230
  in immune response, 228-231
  lymphoid tissues and, 229
  macrophages and, 238
Corynebacteria, 285-287
Corynebacterium granulosum, 93, 285, 287
Corynebacterium parvum, 285
  human immune parameters and, 287
  and immune system of animals, 286-287
CP, *see Corynebacterium parvum, Corynebacterium granulosum*
Cromolyn, in asthma therapy, 218
Cryptococcus neoformans, 88, 238
CSF (colony-stimulating factor), 94-95, 283
Cultured B lymphoid cells, 364-365
Cultured T lymphocytes, insulin receptors on, 367-369
Cy, *see* Cyclophosphamide
Cyclic 3′,5′-adenosine monophosphate, *see* cAMP
Cyclic 3′,5′-guanosine monophosphate, *see* cGMP
Cyclic nucleotides, *see also* cAMP, cGMP
  abnormalities, diseases with, 401-405
  agents that alter levels of, 205
  allergy and, 203-221
  in alloimmunity regulation, 47-57
  in antibody synthesis induction, 32-34
  assays for, 389-407
  biochemistry of, 2-4, 204-207
  bioregulatory mechanisms in, 82
  biosynthesis and degradation of, 82, 204-207
  in B lymphocyte proliferation and differentiation, 32-42
  cancer and, 406-407
  in cell regulation, 1, 61-83
  extraction of, 390
  in graft-vs.-host proliferation, 52-53
  in histone acetylation, 17
  intracellular levels of, 206-207
  as intracellular mediators in antibody synthesis, 29-43
  as intracellular messengers, 2
  lymphocyte nuclear activation and, 15-18
  manipulation of, 42
  measurement of, 392-393
  metabolism of, 204-207
  production of, 2, 4
  proliferative stimuli and, 9, 396-397
  purification of, 390-392, 399
  in regulation of immune system, 405-406
  in thymocyte differentiation, 22-24
  in T lymphocyte proliferation and differentiation, 1-43
  variation of with leukocyte concentration, 395
Cyclizine, 103
Cyclophosphamide
  as immunodepressant, 258-264
  lymphocyte subpopulations and, 261
Cytochalasin B, 62-64, 70

Cytotoxic cells, precursors to, 353
Cytotoxic-T-lymphocytes, target cell lysis and, 50, 54-55

Delayed hypersensitivity
macrophage activation and, 89
steroids and, 252
Deoxycorticosterone, 237
Deoxycytidine kinase, 266
Desensitization, of basophils, 108
Dexamethasone, 150, 237, 239
Digoxin-specific antibodies, biological properties of, 327-328
Dinitrochlorobenzene, 283
Diphenhydramine, 103
DNA synthesis
cAMP and, 39
cGMP and, 38
IF production and, 194
immunodepression and, 265
lymphoid inhibitor and, 269
DNCB (dinitrochlorobenzene), 283
Double stranded complementary RNA homopolymers
immune response to, 292-294
therapeutic applications of, 294-295
T lymphocytes and, 293
Drug immunoassay methods, applications of, 324-326
Drugs
antibody properties of, 326-328
antiinflammatory, *see* Antiinflammatory agents or drugs
immunoassay of, 315-328
radiolabeling of, 318
dsRNA, *see* Double stranded complementary RNA homopolymers
DTIC (dimethyl-1-triazenoimidocarbazole), 257, 261-262

EACA (ε-aminocaproic acid), 138
ECF-A (eosinophil chemotactic factor of anaphylaxis), 109, 208
generation of, 114
Eicosatetranoic acid, 154
Endocrine system, PMNs and, 81
Endotoxin, in macrophage activation, 97
Eosinophil arylsulfatase B, 121
Eosinophil chemotactic factor of anaphylaxis, 109, 117-118
Eosinophils, in immune response, 227
Epinephrine, 76
asthma and, 209
β-receptors and, 80
in mitosis, 24
E-rosette formation, 303

Erythrocytes, insulin receptors on, 360-361
Escherichia coli, 153, 238
Eukaryotic organisms, 16

Factor XII, *see* Hageman factor
α-Fetoprotein, 270-271
Fibroblast growth factor, 38
Flufenamic acid, 217
Fluorescent hormone conjugates, 352-353
5-Fluoruracil, 262
Freund's adjuvant, 280

Glucagon, 47
Glucocorticoids, 228
as antiinflammatory agents, 68
as immunodepressants, 250-253
lymphocyte activation products and, 237-238
prostaglandins and, 150
Gluconeogenesis, 3
Glycogenolysis, glucagon and, 47-48
Gold and gold salts, in rheumatoid arthritis, 233, 240
Graft-vs.-host reaction, 20, 47, 52-53, 286
Gram-negative bacteria, endotoxins of, 287-288, *see also* Endotoxin, Lipopolysaccharides
Granulocytes, insulin receptors on, 361
Granulomatous disease, 297
Guanylate cyclase, 2, 204
adenylate cyclase activation and, 211
calcium activation of, 68, 206
cGMP formation and, 204
stimulation of, 79
Guinea pig MIF
antigen requirement and antigen-binding property of, 171
characteristics of, 168-170
GVH, *see* Graft-vs.-host reaction

Hageman factor (Factor XII)
activation of, 126
amplification of, 131
defined, 125
feedback activation of by plasma kallikrein, 129
proenzyme substrates of, 128-131
Hageman-factor-dependent system, 125-132
inhibition of, 131
interaction with other mediator systems, 138
pharmacological modulation of, 138
Hageman factor fragments, 126-128
Hapten, conjugation of, 316-317
Hapten-protein conjugates, formation of, 316-317
Heparin, in mast cell mediator release, 118
HETE (eicosatetranoic acid), 154
Hetrazan, in asthma therapy, 218-219

HGG (thyroid-dependent antigen human IgG), 36-37
hGH, *see* Human growth hormone
Histamine
antihistamines and, 331
antigen and, 107-108
bronchopulmonary actions of, 117
cGMP in control of, 105
eosinophilotactic activity of, 117
formation of, 115
inhibition of histamine release by, 103
pathobiological effects of, 115-116
separation of cells with receptors for, 353-354
Histamine methyl transferase, 121
Histamine release
calcium and, 105
general properties of, 101-102
Histamine-RSA conjugates, 341-347
Histones, acetylation of, 15, 17
Hormone receptors, *see also* Receptors
donor regulation of, 382-383
polypeptide, 381
Hormones
in cAMP and cGMP formation, 204
low-molecular-weight, receptors for, 331-354
polypeptide, *see* Polypeptide hormones
Human growth hormone
insulin-receptor concentration and, 383
on lymphoid cells, 373-375
radioreceptor assay for, 380-381
Hydrocortisone, 81, 181, 237, 239
Hypersensitivity, immediate, *see* Immediate hypersensitivity

Ibuprofen, 127
Interferons (IF), 193-195, 267-268, 301
Imidazole, 38, 70
LMC and, 51, 55
PHA and, 8
in target cell lysis, 51
Imipramine, 103
Immediate hypersensitivity
allergy of, 203-204
chemical mediators of, 116-117
mast cell mediators and, 113-121
modulation of mediators by, 120-122
Immune response
antiinflammatory drugs in, 227-241
BCG and, 283-284
dsRNA and, 292-293
levamisole in, 296
prostaglandins in, 155
T and B lymphocytes in, 227-228
Immunity, passive transfer of, 89-90
Immunization, hapten-protein conjugates in, 317
Immunoadjuvants, 279
antigenicity and, 283
Immunoassays
antibodies in, 321-325
applications of, 324-326
limitations and problems in, 323-324
Immunodeficiency, levamisole in, 297
Immunodepression, *see also* Immunosuppression
evaluation of in humans, 248-249
selective, 266
therapeutic, 266
Immunodepressive agents, 245-274
antibody production and, 247
defined, 246
mechanism of, 266
nonspecific biological, 267
Immunologic control, perspectives for, 272-274
Immunopharmacology, goal of, 279
Immunopotentiation
interferons and, 301
mechanism of, 279-305
synthetic, 298
thymic hormones in, 302-304
Immunopotentiator, defined, 279
Immunoregulatory α-globulin, 269-270
Immunosuppression, *see also* Immunodepression
"histamine receptors" in, 350-352
interferon in, 268
Immunosuppressive agents, *see* Immunodepressive agents
Immunotolerance, histamine receptors and, 350-352
Indomethacin, 217, 228, 231
as antiinflammatory agent, 152
lysosomal enzyme levels and, 239
PG biosynthesis and, 67
THF and, 23
Infections, levamisole in, 297
Inflammatory diseases, models for, 151-153
Inflammatory response, prostaglandins in, 155; *see also* Antiinflammatory agents
Inhibitor, low-molecular weight lymphoid, 269
Inosiplex, immunoenhancing and, 299
Insulin, 6-7
binding interactions of, 383
cAMP and, 371-372
cGMP and, 7, 55-56
cytotoxic T lymphocytes and, 56
LMC and, 55
radioreceptor assay for, 377-380
in target-cell lysis, 50
Insulin receptors
in circulating cells, 360
in cultured B lymphocytes, 362-367
in cultured T lymphocytes, 367-368

Insulin receptors (*cont'd*)
on erythrocytes, 360-361
on granulocytes, 361
on lymphoid cells, 361-373
on mononuclear leukocytes, 57
Interferons, 193-195, 267-268
in immunopotentiation, 301
Ionophores, divalent cation, 66
IRA (immunoregulatory α-globulin), 269-270
Isoproterenol, 4-5, 23, 48, 70, 217
cAMP and, 55

Job's syndrome, 297

Kallikrein, basophil, *see* Basophil kallikrein of anaphylaxis
K-cell mediated lysis, cGMP and, 52
Kinin-generating sequence, 129-130
Kinin-forming pathway, inhibition of, 132
Kininogen, 129
Komuro-Boyse induction assay system, 22-23

Latex, in phagocytosis, 72
Lecithin, arachidonic acid and, 14
Lentinan, 291
Leukocyte receptors, cAMP action and, 334-338
Leukocytes
cAMP and cGMP in relation to, 2, 4
peripheral blood mononuclear, *see* Peripheral blood mononuclear leukocytes
pharmacological control of mediator release from, 101-110
Leukotaxis, prostaglandins and, 153
Levamisole, 38, 233, 295-298
action of, 296-297
cAMP and, 70, 296-297
in cancer therapy, 298
cGMP and, 70
in immune response, 296
therapeutic uses of, 297-298
Lipopolysaccharides, 31, 287-291
action of on cells of immune system, 290
antibody production and, 289
antigen and, 289
bacterial, 34-35
B lymphocyte and, 288
in cancer therapy, 290-291
cGMP levels and, 37, 41
HGG and, 36-37
inductive pathway and, 36
mitogenic activity of, 36-37
paralytic pathway and, 36-37
radioactive, 35
synergy with antigen, 35
Listeria monocytogenes, 88, 253, 296
peritoneal macrophages infected with, 90
LKs, *see* Lymphokines
LMC, *see* Lymphocyte-mediated cytotoxicity
LPS, *see* Lipopolysaccharides
LTs, *see* Lymphotoxins
Lymphocyte(s), *see also* B lymphocytes; T lymphocytes
biology of, 5
cAMP action in, 4
Con A and, 10-11
in immune response, 227
insulin and, 6
macrophage and, 91-93
PHA binding to, 9
postthymic, 303
Lymphocyte-mediated cytotoxicity, 47
cGMP and, 55
cholera toxin effects in, 49
cholinergic enhancement of, 55
imidazole and, 51, 55
Lymphocyte mitogens, 34
Lymphocyte nuclear activation, cyclic nucleotides and, 15-18
Lymphocyte proliferation
cyclic nucleotides and, 1-43
hormonal and pharmacological modulation in, 4
nonsteroidal antiinflammatory drugs in, 231-232
Lymphocyte receptors
in inflammatory and immunologic processes, 332-334
"physiologic" importance of, 332-334
probing of, 338-339
Lymphocyte response, histamine level and, 104
Lymphocytic chalones, 268-269
Lymphoid cell receptors, 369-376
radioreceptor assay of polypeptide hormones using, 376-377
Lymphoid cells
calcitonin receptors on, 375-376
hGH receptors on, 373-375
insulin receptors on, 361-369, 373
polypeptide hormone receptors on, 357-384
Lymphoid tissues, corticosteroids and, 229
Lymphokines, 163-197; *see also* Migration-inhibitory factor
chemotactic, 188-190
defined, 163-164
functional classification of, 196
in immunity and nonimmunologic processes, 195-197
immunopotentiation and, 300-301
in vivo realities of, 195-197

Lymphokines (*cont'd*)
  physiologic control and pharmacological modulation of, 187-188
Lymphotoxins, 190-193
  in immune reaction, 273
  pharmacological modulation of, 192
Lysosomal enzyme(s)
  in macrophage activation, 95-97
  bioregulation of secretion, 62, 69
  cAMP and, 66, 72
  platelets and, 75

Macrophage(s), *see also* Mononuclear phagocytes
  activated, *see* Activated macrophages
  antiinflammatory drugs and, 239-240
  in cell-mediated immunity, 87
  corticosteroids and, 238-249
  cytotoxic activity of, 269
  in immune response, 234
  interaction with lymphocyte, 91-93
  regulation of, 71-74
Macrophage activation, *see also* Activated macrophages
  delayed hypersensitivity and, 89
  in vitro, 91
  in vivo, 87-88
  lymphokines and, 92
  lysosomal enzyme induction in, 95-97
  MIF and, 178-179
  molecular aspects of, 87-98
  other mechanisms of, 97
Macrophage arming factor, 237
Macrophage chemotactic factor, 283
Macrophage division
  cellular immunity and, 90-91
  mitogenic factor and, 93
  in vitro, 93-94
Macrophage function
  pharmacological modulation of, 72-73
  regulation of, 61-83
  theoretical considerations and future directions in, 74
Macrophage mitogenic factor, 93
  macrophage activation and, 94
  mechanism of, 95
Macrophage motility, mechanism of, 172-173
"Marker" chromosomes, 362
Mast cell
  generation, function, and disposition of chemical mediators of, 113-123
  reactions, IgE-dependent, 122
Meclofenamic acid, 217
Mediators
  modulation of, 121
  pharmacological control of release, 101-110
  types of, 108-109
Melphalan, 256, 261-262
6-Mercaptopurine, 236, 257
  as immunodepressant, 254-258
Metabolic disorders, receptor alterations in, 381-382
Methotrexate, as immunodepressant, 262-267
Microtubules, reactions with, 106-107
MIF (migration inhibitory factor), 73-74, 92, 301
  action of, 174-178
  administration of to animals, 179-181
  antisera and, 183
  azathioprine and, 256
  cAMP and, 73, 181, 186-187
  cellular origin of, 165-166
  cGMP and, 177
  characterization and isolation of, 167-168
  colchicine and vinblastine in, 185
  detection of *in vivo,* 181
  electrophoretic motility and, 175
  enzymatic properties of, 175
  exogenous cAMP and, 176
  of guinea pig, 168-172
  interference with, 185-187
  in vivo, 179, 181
  lymphocytes and, 332
  lymphokines and, 164-165
  macrophage activation and, 178-179
  macrophage motility and, 172-173
  macrophage proliferation and, 74
  mechanism of action of, 172
  neutralization of, 184-185
  partial purification of, 167
  PGE formation and, 154
  pharmacological modulation of, 182-187
  physiologic control of, 181-182
  production of, 166-167, 182-184
  promotion of, 185
  receptor for, 173-174
  RNA and, 183
  skin reactive factor and, 180
  steroids and, 252
  T-cell stimulation and, 283
Mitogen action, *see also* PHA
  calcium in early events of, 12-13
  cyclic nucleotides and, 9
  lymphocyte, 34
  other components of, 13-15
  responsiveness, 20
Mixed lymphocyte cultures
  allogeneic T lymphocytes and, 47
  modification of by cyclic nucleotides, 53-54
  responsiveness in, 20
MLC, *see* Mixed lymphocyte cultures
MMF, *see* Macrophage mitogenic factor
Monocytes, in bone marrow, 234-237

Mononuclear phagocytes, 234
glucocorticoids and, 237-238
insulin receptors in, 57
in vitro cell model systems of, 71-72
isolation and purification of, 72
physiologic functions of, 71
regulation of, 71-74
MTX-L-asparaginase, 262
mRNA synthesis, 20
Muscarinic agonists, 66
Mutant cells, selection of, 335-336
Mycobacteria, 91
Mycobacterial fractions, 281-283
Mycobacterium tuberculosis, 87-88

NCF-A (Neutrophil chemotactic factor of anaphylaxis), 118-119
Neutrophil
bioregulation and pharmacological modulation of, 64-67
chemotaxis, 63
Niridazole, 183
Nonsuppressible insulinlike activity, 377-379
Norepinephrine, 76
asthma and, 209
NSILA, *see* Nonsuppressible insulinlike activity

Organophosphorus esterase inhibitors, 193

PAF (platelet activating factor), 119-120, 208
Paralytic pathway
in B cells, 29-31
LPS and, 36-37
Parathyroid hormone, 377
Pasteurella pestis, 87-88
PDE, *see* Phosphodiesterase
Penicillamine, 232
Peripheral blood mononuclear leukocytes, 361-362
PGs, *see* Prostaglandins
PHA (phytohemagglutinin), 3, 5; *see also* Mitogen action
binding of to lymphocytes, 9
calcium uptake and, 39
cAMP and, 10-11
Corynebacteria and, 286
cGMP and, 8, 37
immunodepressive activity of, 271-272
intracellular events and, 18-20
lymphocytes and, 334
as mitogenic agent, 95
Phagocytes, mononuclear, *see* Mononuclear phagocytes
Phagocytosis
cAMP and, 72
inhibition of, 66
by mononuclear phagocytes, 71
Pharmacological augmentation, of target-cell lysis, 50-51
Phentolamine, 76, 211
Phenylbutazone, 217, 228, 231
Phorbol myristate acetate, 38, 70, 151
Phosphodiesterase, 207
aminophylline and, 48
inhibition of, 32
protein kinase and, 336
Phosphodiesterase inhibitors, in asthma therapy, 213
Phospholipid metabolism, changes observed in, 14
Phosphoribosyl pyrophosphate synthetase, 3-4
Phosphorylation
of acidic proteins, 15-16
cAMP and, 3
cGMP and, 15-16
Physiologic function, cell separation on basis of, 339-341
Phytohemagglutinin, *see* PHA
Phytomitogens, 5-6, 271-272, *also see* PHA, Con A, Mitogen action,
Pinocytosis, 89
Plasma factors, 125-138
modulation of, 131-132
Plasma plasminogen proactivator, 125, 130-131
Plasma thromboplastin antecedent, 128
Plasminogen proactivator, 125, 130-131
Platelet(s)
in vitro cell model systems and, 75-76
physiologic functions of, 74-75
regulation of, 74-83
Platelet activating factor, (PAF), 119, 208
Platelet aggregation, dibutyryl cAMP and, 76
Platelet function
bioregulation and pharmacological modulation of, 76-78
in vitro vs. *in vivo* findings in, 79-80
regulation of, 61-83
Platelet plasma membrane, properties of, 81
Platelet release, cGMP and, 77
Pleiotypic response, in B-cell expression, 31
PMA, *see* Phorbol myristate acetate
PMNs, *see* Polymorphonuclear leukocytes, Neutrophil
Pokeweed mitogen, 267, 286
Poly A:U
antibody response and, 293
in macrophage activation, 97
Polymorphonuclear leukocytes
autonomic nervous system and, 81
cAMP inhibition and, 83
cGMP stimulation and, 83
lysing of antibody-coated tumor cells by, 56
in vitro cell model systems and, 62-64, 67-68
motility of, 67

Polymorphonuclear leukocytes (*cont'd*)
physiological functions of, 62
regulation of, 61-83
SRS-A activity and, 109
Polynucleotides, 292
Polypeptide hormone receptors, 358-359
on lymphoid cells, 381
negative cooperativity of, 383
Polypeptide hormones
cell-surface receptors and, 358-359
radioreceptor assay of, 357-384
tissue responses to, 357-358
Polysaccharides, in immunology, 291-292
Prednisolone, 239
Prekallikrein, 125
feedback activation of Hageman factor by, 129-130
Procarbazine, as immunosuppressive agent, 157
Procarbazine hydrochloride, in skin graft survival, 54
Progesterone, 237
Proinsulinlike component, 378
Promethazine, 103
Promonocytes, in bone marrow, 234-237
Properdin pathway, 136
Propranolol, 331
Prostaglandin(s) (PG)
antiinflammatory agents and, 152
$F_{2\alpha}$, 148-149
in asthma therapy, 216-218
cAMP and, 23, 48, 55, 70, 80, 103
biological function of, 147-149
in chemotaxis, 153-154
Ia-alloantigen and, 40
in immune and inflammatory responses, 145-158
immunosuppressive role of, 51, 156-157
intercellular messenger role of, 154-156
leukotaxis and, 153-154
pathophysiologic role of, 67
in platelet function regulation, 78
primary, 146
suppressive action of, 52, 156-157
type A (PGA), 149
type E (PGE), 48, 145, 147-148
adjuvant arthritis and, 153
in asthma therapy, 217
cAMP and, 157-158
heat, pain, and erythema associated with, 158
type F(PGF), 148-149
MIF stimulation in formation of, 154
urate crystal edema and, 152
type F (PGF), 148-149
Prostaglandin–glucocorticoid interrelationships, 149-150, 214
Prostaglandin synthetase inhibitors, 158, 217
Protein kinase
cAMP- and cGMP-dependent, 16
cyclic nucleotides and, 16, 206
functions of, 336
Prothymocyte, differentiation of, 24, 40
PRPP, *see* Phosphoribosyl pyrophosphate synthetase
PWM, *see* Pokeweed mitogen
Pyrazalones, 217

Radiolabeled drug
separation of unbound from antibody-bound, 323
specific binding of, 319-320
Radioreceptor assay
for calcitonin, 381
for human growth hormone, 380-381
for insulin and insulin-related peptides, 377-380
of polypeptide hormones, 376-377
Receptors
cell regulation of, 337-338
in cell separation, 341-344
histamine, 350-352
insulin, *see* Insulin receptors
polypeptide hormone, 357-384
probing of, 338-339
Recognition sites, hormone interaction with, 357
Rheumatoid arthritis
gold salts and, 240
penicillamine and, 232
Rickettsia infections, 295
RNA polymerase stimulation, cGMP and, 18
RNA synthesis, 3
cAMP and, 17
cGMP and, 15
initiation of, 16
modification of, 17
RSA (rabbit serum albumin), 341-345

Saccharomyces cerevisiae, 291
Salmonella typhimurium, 238
Serotonin, 76
Sheep red blood cells
antibody suppression and, 156
cyclophosphamide and, 258-260
immune responses to, 32
Skin, erythema of, 151
Skin allograft rejection, steroids and, 252
Skin grafts, procarbazine hydrochloride in, 54
Skin reactive factor, MIF and, 180
Slow-reacting substance of anaphylaxis
asthma and, 208
degradation of, 121

Slow-reacting substance of anaphylaxis (*cont'd*)
formation of, 114
inflammatory process and, 332
in mast cell mediator release, 119
PMNs and, 109
release of from lung tissue, 108
Sodium aurothiomalate, 233
SRBC, *see* Sheep red blood cells
SRS-A, *see* Slow-reacting substance of anaphylaxis
Staphylococcus aureus, 88, 238
Steroids, *see also* Corticosteroids; Glucocorticoids
hydroxyl group of, 316
as immunodepressants, 250-254
in vivo effects of, 250
lymphocyte activation process and, 250
monocyte-macrophage system and, 253
in organ transplantation, 252
Streptococcus vaccine, 290
Sutherland's criteria, for cGMP, 400-401
Sympathomimetic amines, in asthma treatment, 212

TAME (*p*-toluene sulphonyl-L-arginine methyl ester), 109
Target-cell lysis, *see also* LMC
cholinomimetic augmentation of, 50
insulin stimulation of, 50
pharmacological abrogation of, 48-49
pharmacological augmentation of, 50-52
T-cell independent antigens, *see* Thymus-independent antigens
T-cell precursors, factors influencing, 21
Testosterone, 24
TF, *see* Transfer factor
T helper cell function, bacterial LPS and, 34-35
Theophylline, 5, 48, 73, 213
antiinflammatory effects of, 68
in cAMP production, 102
poly A:U and, 32
THF (thymic humoral factor), 22-23
Thiopurines, as immunodepressants, 256
Thrombin, 76
Thymic factors
cellular immunity and, 302-303
therapeutic applications of, 303-304
Thymic hormones, in immunopotentiation, 302-304
Thymic humoral factor, 22-23
Thymocyte differentiation, *see also* Prothymocyte
cyclic nucleotides and, 22-24
hormone induction and, 20-22
Thymopoietin, 20-22, 303
Thymosin, 303
Thymus-dependent antigens, 30
Thymus-derived lymphocytes, *see* T-lymphocytes; *see also* T-cells
Thymus-differentiation antigen markers, 20
Thymus gland, in cell-mediated immunity, 20
Thymus-independent antigens, 30
T lymphocytes
in immune response, 227
prothymocyte and, 24
Toxoplasma gondii, 88
Toxoplasma immunity, 92
Toxoplasma-sensitive spleen cells, 91
Transcortin, 228
Transfer factor, 299
cGMP and, 300
in Wiskott-Aldrich syndrome, 300
Trichinella spiralis, 88
Triethylene melanine, 258
Tritium, in drug labeling, 318
T-suppressor cells, 251

Ubiquitin, 23
Ultraviolet light, erythema and, 151
Urate crystal edema, 152-153

Vinblastine, on MIF action, 185

Wiskott-Aldrich syndrome, 297, 300, 304
WSA (water-soluble analog), 283

Yin-Yang hypothesis, of biological control, 61, 68

Zymosan, 70, 72
glucan derived from, 291-292

MIX
Papier aus verantwortungsvollen Quellen
Paper from responsible sources
FSC® C105338

If you have any concerns about our products,
you can contact us on
ProductSafety@springernature.com

In case Publisher is established outside the EU,
the EU authorized representative is:
Springer Nature Customer Service Center GmbH
Europaplatz 3, 69115 Heidelberg, Germany

Printed by Libri Plureos GmbH
in Hamburg, Germany